Drugs and Behavior

An Introduction to Behavioral Pharmacology

Third Edition

William A. McKim
Memorial University of Newfoundland

PRENTICE HALL, Upper Saddle River, New Jersey 07458

Library of Congress Cataloging-in-Publication Data

McKim, William A.
    Drugs and behavior : an introduction to behavioral pharmacology /
William A. McKim. — 3rd ed.
      p. cm.
    Includes bibliographical references and index.
    ISBN 0–13–377128–8
    1. Psychopharmacology. 2. Psychotropic drugs. I. Title.
    [DNLM: 1. Behavior—drug effects. 2. Psychotropic Drugs—
therapeutic use. 3. Psychopharmacology. QV 77 M158d 1996]
    RM315.M36 1996
    615′.78—dc20
    DNLM/DLC   96–33685
    for Library of Congress   CIP

Acquisitions editor: Nicole Signoretti
Editorial director: Charlyce Jones Owen
Editorial/production supervision
  and interior design: Darrin Kiessling
Copy editor: Peter Reinhart
Cover designer: Bruce Kenselaar
Buyer: Tricia Kenny
Marketing manager: Michael Alread

This book was set in 10/12 Times Roman by Pine Tree
Composition, Inc. and was printed and bound by R R
Donnelley & Sons Company. The cover was
printed by Phoenix Color Corporation.

 ©1997, 1991, 1987 by Prentice-Hall, Inc.
Simon & Schuster/A Viacom Company
Upper Saddle River, New Jersey 07458

Cover image from Dunhill, 1954, p. 4.

Printed in the United States of America
10 9 8 7 6 5 4 3 2 1

ISBN 0-13-377128-8

Prentice-Hall International (UK) Limited, *London*
Prentice-Hall of Australia Pty. Limited, *Sydney*
Prentice-Hall Canada Inc., *Toronto*
Prentice-Hall Hispanoamericana, S.A., *Mexico*
Prentice-Hall of India Private Limited, *New Delhi*
Prentice-Hall of Japan, Inc., *Tokyo*
Simon & Schuster Asia Pte. Ltd., *Singapore*
Editora Prentice-Hall do Brasil, Ltda., *Rio de Janeiro*

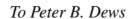

To Peter B. Dews

Contents

Chapter 7
THE BARBITURATES AND BENZODIAZEPINES   141

Chapter 8
TOBACCO   166

Chapter 9
CAFFEINE AND THE METHYLXANTHINES   191

Chapter 10
PSYCHOMOTOR STIMULANTS   212

Preface

Behavioral pharmacology is developing quickly. You sometimes do not see this rapid development when you stand too close and pay attention to one or two restricted areas within the field. But when you stand back and go through the exercise of trying to update a comprehensive review such as an introductory text, the pace of development—the progress that has been made even in the space of five years—appears overwhelming.

In the third edition of *Drugs and Behavior,* I have tried to capture some of the recent developments in behavioral pharmacology, but at the same time not lose sight of where the field has been. In the limited space available in a text of this nature, achieving this balance has become quite a challenge. Necessarily I have not been able to include everything I wanted. Hard decisions had to be made.

Since the second edition was published, there have been a number of new developments in several areas. These include new families of drugs such as the SSRIs and atypical antipsychotics, a receptor and an endogenous ligand for THC, new insights into the neurochemistry of psychosis and depression and new drugs to treat these diseases, a renewed political and scientific interest in nicotine and smoking, and increased interest in caffeine as an addicting drug. These are some of the areas that have received increased attention in the third edition.

Barbiturates are now infrequently used in medical practice, their use in research has dwindled, and they appear infrequently on the street scene. Nevertheless, many landmark studies were done with barbiturates, and no text would be complete without an extensive discussion of them. In the first edition, I included barbiturates and benzodiazepines in one chapter. In the second edition I gave each a chapter of its own. In this edition I have put them back together again.

Great strides have been made in research on drug self-administration using laboratory animal models of human abuse of drugs, and interesting new laboratory techniques have been developed to study the reinforcing effects of drugs in humans. One of the more interesting developments has been the application of economic theory to understanding drug consumption. Economic theory holds great promise for many reasons. Not only does it explain how and why drug use increases, but it suggests methods, such as providing alternative sources of reinforcement, by which drug use can also be decreased. The third edition discusses some of these issues.

In a book of this nature, aimed at students who do not have a technical background, there is a limit to the amount of neurophysiology that can be presented. It is a challenge to strike a balance between keeping it simple and making the field make sense. Understanding behavioral pharmacology requires a grasp of certain neural mechanisms. Students need to know about synapses, transmitters, receptor sites, action potentials, and so on; otherwise, much of what behavioral pharmacologists do does not make sense. In this edition I have extended the neurophysiology a bit further by introducing students to ion channels. Previous editions did not elaborate on the mechanisms by which receptors were able to create EPSPs and IPSPs. In my teaching I found this was a serious omission that hampered the students' grasp of what was actually going on at synapses. When I introduced students to ion channels, even though this approach was a bit more technical, it actually made neurotransmission easier to understand. I have discussed this move with several teachers of neurophysiology who have had similar experiences and who agree that such concepts are well within the grasp of second-year college students, even those who claim to be uninterested or even intimidated by things technical.

This book would not have been possible without the assistance of many people, including those mentioned in the earlier editions upon which the third edition is based. In this edition I would like to acknowledge the help of my family, who not only assisted with many technical matters but also tolerated my absence of body and mind while the book was being written; my colleagues, both at Memorial University of Newfoundland and many other institutions around the world, who read many drafts, pointed out many errors, and made many suggestions; my students who suffered through many teaching experiments and nearly unreadable drafts of the manuscript; and the technical and office staff in the psychology department at Memorial University. These people include, but are not limited to, Michael Aman, Kim Butler, Geoff Carre, Marilyn Carroll, Carolyn Harley, Gene Heyman, Gerard Martin, Andrew McKim, Edna McKim, Heather McKim, Kathleen McKim, Richard Neuman, Brenda Noftle, Krista Pirez, John Podd, Sam Revusky, John Scott, and Bernice St. Croix.

I would also like to acknowledge the helpful comments of the following people who served as reviewers for the publisher: W. Jeffrey Wilson, Indiana University-Purdue University, Fort Wayne; and John P. Broida, University of Southern Maine.

Apart from taking credit where such credit is due, none of these people can be held in any way responsible for any errors or problems in the book because I did not always follow the advice I was given.

W.A.M.

CHAPTER

1

Drugs: Some Basic Pharmacology

NAMES OF DRUGS

One of the more confusing things about studying drugs is their names. Most drugs have at least three names, and it may not always be apparent which name is being used at any given time.

Chemical Name

All drugs have a *chemical name*. This is in formal chemical jargon, and a chemist can usually tell by looking at the name what the molecule of the drug looks like. Here is the chemical name of a drug: 7-chloro-1,3-dihydro-1-methyl-5-phenyl-2H-1,4-benzodiazepin-2-one. As you can see, it is full of chemical terminology, letters, and numbers. The numbers refer to places where different parts of the drug molecule are joined. Just to make things more complicated, there are different conventions for numbering these parts of molecules. As a result, the same drug will have different names if different conventions are used.

Generic Name

Once a drug becomes established, its chemical name is too clumsy to be useful, so a new, shorter name is made up for it, the *generic name* or *nonproprietary name*. The generic name for the drug whose chemical name we just struggled through is *diazepam*. You can see that the generic names bears some resemblance to the chemical name. There are conventions for making up generic names that are handy to know because they are clues to the nature of the drug. For example, most barbiturate drugs end in *al*, like *secobarbital*, and most local anesthetics end in *caine*, as in *procaine*.

For the most part, textbooks (including this book) and scientific discussions of drugs use the generic name.

Trade Name

When a drug company spends many millions of dollars to invent and develop a new drug, it can patent the drug for a number of years so that no other company can sell it. The drug company does not sell the drug under its generic name. Instead, it makes up a new name called the *trade name* or *proprietary name*. The trade name for the drug we have been discussing is *Valium*. After the patent expires, other companies can sell the drug, or they can make it under license from the owner of the patent, but they frequently sell it under different trade names. Therefore, there can be many different trade names for the same drug.

Because drug companies sell their products under trade names, people in the medical profession are most familiar with these names and are most likely to use them. So if you are given a prescription for a drug by a physician and you are told the name of the drug, you may not be able to find it listed in this or any other text that uses generic names. Trade names can be distinguished from generic names because the first letter is capitalized.

DESCRIBING DOSAGES

All of modern science uses the metric system, and drug doses are nearly always given in *milligrams (mg)*. A milligram is 1/1,000 of a gram (there are a little over 28 grams in an ounce).

It is generally true that the effect of a drug is related to its concentration in the body rather than the absolute amount of drug administered. If the same amount of a drug is given to individuals of different sizes, the drug will reach a different concentration in the body of each individual. To ensure that the drug is present in the same concentration in the brains of all subjects or patients, different doses are given according to body weight. For this reason, in research papers, doses are usually reported in terms of milligrams per *kilogram (kg)* of body weight, for example, 6.5 mg/kg. (A kilogram is equal to 2.2 pounds.)

Reporting doses in this manner also helps when comparing research on different species. If you account for such other factors as metabolic rate and body composition, a dose of 1 mg/kg in a monkey will be roughly comparable to a dose of 1 mg/kg in a human.

Dose Response Curves

To get a true picture of the effect of a drug, it is usually necessary to give a range of doses of the drug. The range should cover a dose so low that there is no detectable effect and doses so high that increases in dose have no further effect. It is usual to plot the effect of this range of doses on a graph with the dose indicated on the horizontal axis and the effect on the vertical axis. This type of figure is called a *dose response curve (DRC)*. Figure 1–1 shows a typical DRC. It shows the effect of caffeine on the mouse's rate of responding on an FI schedule. (Schedules will be explained in Chapter 2.)

Note that the scale on the horizontal axis is graduated logarithmically. It is generally found that a small change in low doses can have a big effect, but an equally small change in a large dose has no effect. Plotting doses on a log scale allows a wide range of doses to be reported and permits greater precision at the low end of the dosage range. Log scales became common when it was found that many physiological effects of a drug showed up as a straight line when plotted on a log scale.

In the example just used, the drug effect was a measure of response rate, but there are other types of DRCs where the effect is a discrete binary variable rather than a continuous one. For example, we could not use this type of curve if we wanted to report a DRC for effectiveness of a drug as an anesthetic. Subjects are either anesthetized or they are not. If the vertical axis simply read "yes" or "no," we would not have any sort of a curve. When a binary variable is used, DRCs are constructed differently.

This sort of problem is handled by working with groups of subjects. Each group is given a different dose of the drug, and the percentage of subjects in each group that show the effect is then plotted. An example of this sort of DRC is

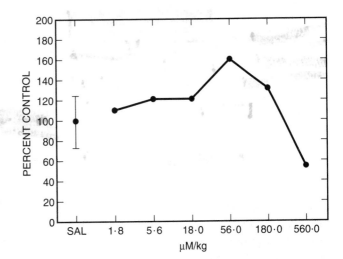

Figure 1–1 The dose response curve for the effect of caffeine on rate of responding by a mouse being reinforced on an FI schedule with food. (Adapted from McKim, 1980.)

given in Figure 1–2. This hypothetical experiment is designed to establish the DRC for loss of consciousness and the lethal effects of a fictitious new drug, "endital." In this experiment there are 12 groups of rats. Each group is given a different dose of endital, from 0 mg/kg, a placebo, to 110 mg/kg. The vertical axis of the graph shows the percentage of rats in each group that showed the effect. The one curve shows how many rats lost consciousness, and the other curve shows the percentage of rats in each group that died.

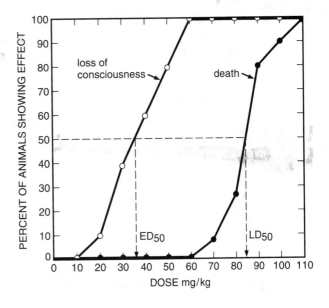

Figure 1–2 Results of a hypothetical experiment in which 12 groups of rats were each given a different dose ranging from 0.0 (a placebo) to 110 mg/kg. One curve shows the percent of animals in each group that lost consciousness and the other shows the percent that died at each dose. The ED_{50} and the LD_{50} are also indicated.

ED$_{50}$ and LD$_{50}$. A common way of describing these curves and comparing the effectiveness of different drugs is by the ED$_{50}$. The ED$_{50}$ is the *median effective dose*, that is, the dose that is effective in 50 percent of the individuals tested. The ED$_{50}$ for losing consciousness for endital in Figure 1–2 is 35 mg/kg. By checking the next curve, you can see that the dose of endital that killed 50 percent of the rats was 84 mg/kg. This is known as the *median lethal dose*, or the LD$_{50}$.

It is also common to use this method to refer to other effective and lethal doses. Whereas the LD$_{50}$ is the dose at which 50 percent of animals die, the LD$_1$ is the dose that kills 1 percent of subjects, and the ED$_{99}$ is a dose that is effective in 99 percent of cases.

Drug Safety

When new drugs are being developed and tested, it is common to establish the LD$_{50}$ and the ED$_{50}$ to give an idea of the safety of a drug. Obviously, the farther the lethal dose is from the effective dose, the safer the drug. The *therapeutic index (TI)* is sometimes used to describe the safety of a drug. This is the ratio of the LD$_{50}$ to the ED$_{50}$; TI = LD$_{50}$/ED$_{50}$. The higher the index, the safer the drug. The TI of endital calculated from Figure 1–2 would be 84/35 = 2.4.

Drug safety may also be described as a ratio of the ED$_{99}$ and the LD$_1$.

POTENCY AND EFFECTIVENESS

Potency and *effectiveness* (or *efficacy*) are terms that are sometimes used to describe the extent of a drug's effect. They do not mean the same thing. When you are comparing two drugs that have the same effect, *potency* refers to differences in the ED$_{50}$ of the two drugs. The drug with the lower ED$_{50}$ is the more potent. For example, if you compared LSD and a drug called lysergic acid amide, a related hallucinogen found in morning glory seeds, you would find that lysergic acid amide is 10 times less potent than LSD in producing a hallucinatory experience. In other words, the nature and extent of the effect of lysergic acid amide would be the same as LSD if you increased the dose of lysergic acid amide by a factor of 10.

Effectiveness refers to differences in the maximum effect that drugs will produce at any dose. Both aspirin and morphine are analgesics or painkillers. When dealing with severe pain, aspirin at its most effective dose is not as effective as morphine. To compare these two drugs in terms of potency would not be appropriate. They both might produce analgesia at the same dose and thus be equally potent, but the extent of the analgesia would be vastly different.

MAIN EFFECTS AND SIDE EFFECTS

It is generally accepted that no drug has only one effect. In most cases, however, only one effect of a drug is wanted, and other effects are not wanted. It is often common to call the effect for which a drug is taken the *main effect* and any other effect a *side effect*. If a drug is taken to treat a disease symptom, that is its main effect, and anything else it might do, harmful or otherwise, is a side effect.

Very often the distinction between the two is arbitrary. Aspirin, for example, has several physiological effects; it brings down fever, it reduces swelling and inflammation, and it slows the blood's ability to clot. If you take aspirin because you have a high temperature, the temperature-reducing effect is the main effect, and the other two are side effects. The inhibition of blood clotting is a potentially harmful effect because it can cause bleeding into the stomach, which can have serious consequences for some people. Recently it has been shown that this anticlotting effect can be useful. Strokes are caused by a clot of blood getting caught in the brain. Many physicians believe that taking one aspirin a day can reduce the chances of stroke in people at high risk for stroke. In this case, the anticlotting effect would be the main effect, and any other effects that the aspirin might be having would be the side effects.

It is often the aim of research with drugs to try to find a drug that has a very specific main effect that is therapeutically useful and has minimal side effects. When dealing with behaviorally active drugs, the ability of a drug to be abused or create an addiction is considered a dangerous side effect. To a drug user, however, the psychological effect of the drug is vitally important, and any other effects the drug may have on the body are considered unimportant or undesirable.

DRUG INTERACTIONS

When two drugs are mixed together, their effects can interact in several ways. If one drug diminishes the effect of another, this interaction is called *antagonism*. Drug antagonism is established by plotting two DRCs, one for the drug alone and a second one for the drug in the presence of the other drug. If the DRC is shifted to the right by adding the new drug, this result indicates antagonism between the drugs.

If adding the new drug shifts the DRC to the left, this result indicates that the drugs have an additive effect. If drugs have an effect together that is greater than you might expect simply by adding their effects, this is called a *superadditive effect*, or *potentiation*. It is not always obvious whether a drug interaction is additive or superadditive, but there is one situation where the distinction is clear. If one drug has no effect alone but increases the effect of a second drug, potentiation is clearly occurring.

Careful determination of how drugs interact can tell us a great deal about the mechanism of drug action. For example, if we give a drug that is known to block a certain type of receptor and find that it antagonizes a specific effect of another drug, we can guess that the second drug probably interacts with that type of receptor to produce that effect (see Chapter 4).

TOLERANCE

In the year 63 B.C., Mithradates VI, king of Pontus, tried to commit suicide by poisoning himself. Mithradates was a great leader and a great warrior; he had defeated the Roman legions and spread his influence over Asia Minor, but in 63 B.C. he had been defeated by the Roman general, Pompey, and his son had just led a successful revolt against him. To end it all, the king took a large dose of poison, but it had no effect on him. He was finally forced to have one of his Gallic mercenaries do the job. What was the source of the king's resistance to poison? Well, it appears that Mithradates was also a good pharmacologist. Throughout his life he lived in great fear of being poisoned, so to protect himself, he repeatedly took increasing doses of poison until he could tolerate large amounts without ill effects. This effect has been called *mithradatism* (Lankester, 1889) after the king, or *tolerance*, as we know it today. Mithradatism was also practiced by a number of historical figures including Vespasia, the mother of the Roman emperor Nero, and by the infamous Lucretia Borgia.

Drug tolerance is defined either as the decreased effectiveness of a drug that results from the continued presence of the drug in the body or as the necessity of increasing the dose of a drug in order to maintain its effectiveness after repeated administrations. The term *tolerance* is frequently used in a way that suggests that all the effects of a drug diminish at the same rate, but this is usually not the case; some effects of a drug may develop tolerance very quickly, some other effects may only show tolerance slowly, and some effects may never show tolerance no matter how often the drug is given. One of the effects of morphine, for example, is nausea and vomiting. This effect shows rapid tolerance, but the ability of morphine to constrict the pupils of the eyes shows no tolerance at all, no matter how long the drug is taken. Because tolerance develops at different rates to different effects of a drug, it is apparent that there must be many mechanisms responsible for tolerance.

Once tolerance develops, it does not last indefinitely. Tolerance tends to disappear with the passage of time after the use of a drug has been discontinued. As with the development of tolerance, its disappearance may take place at different rates for different drug effects.

Tolerance to one drug may well diminish the effect of another drug. This phenomenon is called *cross-tolerance*. Cross-tolerance is usually seen between members of the same class of drugs. All opiate drugs, for example, will show cross-tolerance. Cross-tolerance is sometimes taken as evidence that the drugs may be producing their effect by common mechanisms.

It is usually assumed that a drug must be given repeatedly many times before tolerance can occur, but some effects of some drugs may show tolerance after only one or two administrations. This type of tolerance is known as *tachyphylaxis*. It is also possible to demonstrate that tolerance may develop during the course of a single administration of a drug. As we shall see later in this chapter, after a drug is taken into the body, the level of the drug in the blood rises and then falls. With some drug effects it has been shown that the effect of the drug is greater at a specific blood level soon after administration when the levels is rising than at that same point later when the level of the drug is falling. This finding indicates that tolerance developed during a single administration. This is called *acute tolerance*. A good example of acute tolerance is given in Chapter 6.

Very rarely it is noted that the effects of a drug increase with repeated administration. Such an effect has been reported with amphetamines. This is known as *reverse tolerance* or *sensitization*.

Metabolic Tolerance

As discussed later in this chapter, *metabolic tolerance* arises from an increase in the rate at which the body is able to metabolize and get rid of a drug. For the most part this is a result of enzyme induction, an increase in the level of the enzyme the body uses to destroy the drug. When a drug is given repeatedly, it may induce or increase the action of the enzyme the body uses to destroy it. With increases in the rate of metabolism, a given amount of a drug will not reach the same peak levels and will not last as long, so that more and more of the drug will be needed to produce the same effect.

Physiological Tolerance

Physiological tolerance is also known as *cellular* or *pharmacodynamic* tolerance. These terms generally describe a type of tolerance that arises from adjustments made by the body to compensate for an effect of the continued presence of a drug. These adjustments may involve entire physiological systems, or they may take place at the level of the synapse. For example, if a drug blocks a receptor at a synapse, the body might attempt to compensate for the blockage by creating more receptors so that the transmitter at the synapse can be restored to normal functioning. It might also cause more transmitter to be released from the presynaptic neuron to help overcome the blockage. (See Chapter 4.)

Behavioral Tolerance

It has often been demonstrated that tolerance can be influenced by learning and conditioning processes. In other words, through experience with a drug, an organism can learn to decrease the effect that drug is having. This learning can use both instrumental and respondent conditioning processes. Before an extensive discussion of these effects, it will be necessary to have a good grasp of the principles of conditioning and learning. These topics will be covered more extensively in Chapter 2, and behavioral tolerance is described more fully in Chapter 3.

DEPENDENCE AND WITHDRAWAL SYMPTOMS

Probably no word in the field of drug research causes more misunderstanding or has been abused more than the term *dependence*. It is generally used in two ways: (1) to describe a state where discontinuation of a drug causes *withdrawal symptoms*, and (2) to describe a state where a person compulsively takes a drug.

At one point it was believed that the two states were exactly the same. It was assumed that the reason why people compulsively took a drug was that they were afraid of withdrawal. It is now known that this assumption is not correct, but the word "dependence" is still often used this way. (To make matters worse, sometimes a distinction is made between "physical dependence" and "psychological dependence," but this will be discussed in more detail in Chapter 5.) As a result of this early assumption, the word "dependence" took on a life of its own and may now be used by some to indicate compulsive use without presuming that the mechanism is fear of withdrawal. In any case, much confusion arises because the word is used as an explanation rather than a description of a state of affairs. Too often we hear people say such things as "Sally is dependent on that drug," as though this were an explanation of Sally's drug taking—it is not. At best, it only describes the way Sally uses the drug.

Withdrawal symptoms are physiological symptoms that occur when the use of a drug is stopped or decreased. Different drugs produce different sorts of withdrawal symptoms, but drugs of the same family generally produce similar withdrawal. Withdrawal can be stopped almost instantly by giving the drug that has been discontinued. Usually, if the discontinued drug is not available, another drug of the same family will also stop withdrawal. This phenomenon is known as *cross-dependence*. Withdrawal usually begins some hours after the use of a drug has been stopped, but it can also be produced by giving an antagonist drug. Naloxone is a powerful antagonist to morphine and rapidly blocks all morphine effects soon after it is given. When naloxone is given to morphine-dependent humans and nonhumans, severe withdrawal can be seen in minutes.

Tolerance and dependence are closely related. Tolerance to a drug may occur without dependence, but withdrawal symptoms are never seen in the absence of tolerance. Withdrawal symptoms are usually thought of as the expression of the adjustment that the body has made to the drug. With repeated administration of a drug, the body changes its functioning and adjusts to the physical changes the drug produces. Later, when the drug is stopped and its effects disappear, it takes some time for the body to readjust to its absence. This readjustment is withdrawal. For this reason, the physiological changes seen in withdrawal are usually opposite to the effects of the drug. For example, constipation is one of the more marked effects of heroin use, and one of the major symptoms of withdrawal from heroin is diarrhea.

Withdrawal symptoms may vary in intensity from one drug to another. In some cases withdrawal symptoms may be so slight that they can only be detected with sensitive instruments, and the individual might not notice them. In other cases withdrawal can be so severe as to cause death. The extent of withdrawal may also depend on the dose and administration schedule of the drug. Generally, high doses produce more severe withdrawal. And usually, withdrawal is worse if the drug is administered continuously rather than occasionally.

PHARMACOKINETICS

Drugs do not have an effect on all body tissues. As a matter of fact, most drugs only influence the operation of the body at specific and limited places called *sites of action*. A drug may get into the body, but unless it gets to its site of action, it will have no effect. It is therefore important to have an understanding of how drugs get from their place of administration to the place where they act. Some foods and medications may contain large amounts of valuable nourishment and medicine, but simply swallowing them or otherwise putting them in your body is no guarantee that they will have the desired effect. It is also true that the way a substance is administered not only can determine whether it gets to its site of action but also affects how fast it gets there and how much of it gets there.

ROUTES OF ADMINISTRATION

Route of administration refers to the method used to get a drug from outside the body to some place under the skin. This purpose can be accomplished by taking advantage of the body's natural mechanisms for taking substances inside itself, such as digestion and breathing, or the drug can be artificially placed under the skin by means of injection. Of course, some substances can be directly absorbed through the skin, but this is not a common route of administration for recreational or medical purposes.

Parenteral Routes of Administration

Parenteral refers to routes of administration involving injection through the skin, although the literal meaning of the term suggests all routes that do not involve the digestive system. The term was appropriate when first used, but since then, inhalation has become another common medical route of administration that, technically, is parenteral. In practice, the term refers only to injection into various parts of the body. Parenteral routes are further subdivided, depending on the specific point in the body where the drug is to be left by the needle.

Vehicle. Before a drug can be injected, it must be in a form that can pass through a syringe and needle; that is, it must be liquid. Since most drugs are in a dry powder or crystalline form (the word *drug* is derived from the French *drogue,* meaning "dry powder"), it is necessary to dissolve a drug in some liquid before it can be injected. This liquid is called a *vehicle.* The choice of a vehicle can be important for a number of reasons. To begin with, the vehicle should be inert or totally inactive both with respect to the drug that is to be dissolved in it and with respect to the physiology of the organisms into which it is to be injected. These considerations do not normally present a problem for most behaviorally active drugs, since they tend to dissolve well in water and remain stable for long periods of time in water solution. Pure water is not totally inert with respect to the physiology of the body, and so a weak salt solution is used instead. Body fluids contain dissolved salts, and the most common vehicle is *normal* or *physiological saline,* a solution of 0.9 percent sodium chloride (ordinary table salt), which matches body fluids in concentration and does not irritate the tissues it is injected into. Normal saline, therefore, meets the requirements of a good vehicle for most of the drugs used in behavioral pharmacology; it dissolves drugs and does not interact with either the drug or the organism.

In some cases the drug to be injected does not dissolve in water. The active ingredient in marijuana, tetrahydrocannabinol (THC), is an example of such a drug, and it requires a special vehicle. One solution to this problem is to use alcohol as a vehicle, since alcohol will not only dissolve the THC but will also keep it from deteriorating in solution. Dissolving a drug in alcohol presents other problems for the behavioral researcher because alcohol is not physiologically inert. It also may cause behavioral changes that are sometimes difficult to separate from the effects of the drug dissolved in it.

Once the drug is in liquid form and the syringe is filled, the needle can be inserted into various places in the body and the drug and vehicle injected to form a small bubble, or *bolus.* There are four common parenteral routes, depending on the site where the drug is to be placed.

Subcutaneous. The term *subcutaneous* in published material is frequently abbreviated *s.c.* and in jargon is called "sub-q." As the name suggests, in this route of administration the drug is injected to form a bolus just under the skin or cutaneous tissue. In most laboratory animals, the injection is usually made into the loose skin on the back between the shoulders. For medical purposes in humans, s.c. injections are usually done under the skin of the arm or thigh, but the hand or wrist is sometimes used to self-administer heroin—a procedure sometimes referred to as *skin popping*.

Intramuscular. In the *intramuscular (i.m.)* route, the needle is inserted into a muscle, and a bolus is left there. In humans, the most common muscle used for this purpose is the *deltoid* muscle of the upper arm or the *gluteus maximus* muscle of the buttock. To receive such an injection, the muscle must be fairly large, so i.m. injections are seldom given to rats and mice. They are more frequently given to monkeys. This route of administration is common also in pigeons, where the injection is given into the large breast muscle.

Intraperitoneal. The abbreviation for the *intraperitoneal* route is *i.p.*, and as the name suggests, the needle is inserted directly into the peritoneal cavity. The peritoneum is the sack containing the visceral organs such as the intestines, liver, and spleen. The aim of an i.p. injection is to insert the needle through the stomach muscle and inject the drug into the cavity that surrounds the viscera. It is not desirable to inject the drug directly into the stomach or any of the other organs, since doing so could be harmful and could cause hemorrhaging and death. At the very least, injection into an organ is likely to alter the animal's reaction to the drug.

Intraperitoneal injections are commonly used with rats and mice because they are easy and safe and cause the animal very little discomfort. They are much less convenient in larger animals and are almost never given to humans. At one time rabies vaccine was commonly given to humans via this route, but this is no longer the case.

Intravenous. In an *intravenous (i.v.)* injection, the end of the needle is inserted into a vein, and the drug is injected directly into the bloodstream. This procedure is more popularly known as *mainlining*. Before an i.v. injection can be given, it is necessary to find a vein that comes close enough to the surface of the skin that it can be pierced with a needle. In humans, this is usually the vein on the inside of the elbow. The most common procedure is to wrap a tourniquet around the upper arm between the injection site and the heart. Since veins carry blood toward the heart, the tourniquet will dilate or enlarge the vein and make injection into the vein easier.

When the end of the needle is inserted into the vein, the tourniquet is removed, and the drug is injected when normal blood flow is resumed. This is essentially the same procedure used when blood is removed for a blood test. One difficulty with i.v. injections, however, is that a vein cannot be used too frequently or it will collapse and simply stop carrying blood. When veins have collapsed in the arms, other veins in the wrists, hands, and feet may be used, but these are more difficult to strike accurately with a needle.

In laboratory animals, i.v. injections are not commonly used by behavioral pharmacologists because veins close to the surface of the skin are unusual in rats, mice, and pigeons, and the procedure is not easy in unrestrained animals. Fur and feathers also make the location of such veins difficult. When i.v. injections are necessary, they are usually accomplished by means of a permanently implanted *catheter*. A catheter is a tube that is surgically implanted into the body. One end of the tube is at a site inside the body, while the other end is outside. In rodents and monkeys, venous (in a vein) catheters are usually inserted in the jugular vein with the free end of the tube emerging from the animal's back. When an intravenous injection is required, the syringe is attached to the end of the catheter outside the body, and the drug is injected. Researchers frequently use this type of preparation to study self-administration of drugs by animals, since the catheter may be attached to a motor-driven pump that the animal can control by pressing a lever (see Chapter 5). These catheters are fairly permanent and may last for months before they have to be replaced.

ABSORPTION FROM PARENTERAL SITES

With intravenous injections, the drug is put directly into the blood, but when other sites are used, the drug must be absorbed into the circulatory system. The rate at which a drug gets into the blood from an injection site is determined by a number of factors associated with blood flow to the area. Generally, volume of blood flow is greater to the peritoneal cavity than to the muscles and greater to muscles than under the skin. As a result, absorption is fastest from an i.p. injection and slowest from an s.c. injection.

Heat and exercise can speed absorption from i.m. and s.c. sites because they increase blood flow to muscles and skin. Thus an i.m. injection will be absorbed faster if the muscle is exercised after the injection, and the drug from a subcutaneous site will get into the blood faster if heat is applied to the area and more slowly if the area is chilled.

To be absorbed, a drug must pass through the walls of the *capillaries*. A capillary is a tiny tube through which blood flows. Through the walls of capillaries, nutrients and oxygen pass out of the blood into body tissues, and waste products and carbon dioxide pass into the blood and are removed. Blood leaves the heart and is distributed around the body in arteries. The arteries divide into smaller and smaller branches until they become capillaries so small in diameter that blood cells can just pass through. The blood in capillaries is eventually collected in veins, which carry the blood back to the heart.

The walls of the capillaries are made up of a single layer of cells. Between the outer membranes or coverings of these cells are small openings, or *pores*, through which the nutrients, waste products, and drugs may pass freely. The only substances in the blood that cannot move in and out of the capillaries through these pores are red blood cells and large protein molecules, which are trapped inside because they are larger than the pores.

Injected drugs pass into capillaries and the bloodstream by simple *diffusion*. Diffusion is the process by which a substance tends to move from an area of high concentration to an area of low concentration until the concentrations are equal in both areas. If a drop of food coloring is placed in the corner of a tub of still water, it will remain as a highly colored drop for a short period of time. The forces of diffusion will soon distribute the coloring evenly throughout the tub of water. The same principle determines that a drug injected into a muscle or under the skin will move from the area of high concentration (the bolus at the site of the injection) into the blood, an area of low concentration, until the concentrations in the two places are equal. The drug from an injection site will move through the pores into the blood in the capillaries surrounding the injection site. Since this blood is constantly circulating and being replaced by new blood with a low concentration of drug, more will be absorbed as the blood circulates through the area.

Areas that are serviced by many capillaries will absorb drugs faster than areas that have few capillaries. Since muscles use more oxygen, they have a richer capillary supply than the skin; it is for this reason that absorption into the blood is faster from i.m. injections than from s.c. injections. Drugs injected into the peritoneum have access to an even greater number of capillaries, and consequently i.p. injections are absorbed even more rapidly.

Absorption through capillary walls is not a factor in intravenous injections, since the drug is placed directly into the blood. Blood in the veins is transported to the heart and then redistributed around the body after a short detour through the lungs. Since the body has about 6 liters of blood and the heart pumps these 6 liters once a minute, the drug in most i.v. injections is distributed around the body about a minute after injection.

Depot Injections

Some drugs need to be taken continuously or chronically to prevent the symptoms of a disease or disorder from appearing. The antipsychotic drugs (see Chapter 12) are examples of drugs that sometimes need to be taken continuously for many years. Often people do not like to take these drugs and do not continue to use them after release from hospital, with the result that they are readmitted regularly with recurring psychotic symptoms. In such cases it is possible to give *depot injections*. With depot injections, the drug is dissolved in a high concentration in a viscous oil (often sesame oil), which is then injected into a muscle, usually in the buttock. The drug then slowly diffuses from the oil into the body fluids over a long period of time. A single depot injection of an antipsychotic drug can be effective as long as four weeks. This technique usually only works with drugs that are highly lipid-soluble (to be discussed shortly) and prefer to remain dissolved in the oil; otherwise they would be released too quickly. Fortunately, antipsychotic drugs have this property (Lemberger et al., 1987).

INHALATION OF GASES

Since every cell in the body requires oxygen and gives off carbon dioxide as a waste product, the body has developed a very efficient system for absorbing gases from the air and distributing them quickly and completely throughout the body: the lungs. When drugs in the form of gases or vapor are breathed into the lungs, they take advantage of this system and consequently get into the blood very rapidly.

The lungs are an extremely efficient gas exchange system. Their inside surface is convoluted and contains many pockets of air so that the total surface area exposed to the air is very large. This entire area is richly supplied with blood by capillaries, which are close to the surface. When gas is inhaled, it dissolves in the moist surface of the lungs and by diffusion passes through capillary walls and enters the circulating blood. Figure 1–3 shows the circulation to and from the lungs. As can be seen in this figure, after blood returns to the heart through the veins, it is pumped directly to the lungs. Here the carbon dioxide is released into the air, and oxygen in the lungs is absorbed into the blood. The blood then returns directly to the heart and is pumped around the body. One of the main arteries from the heart goes directly to the brain. Consequently, drugs dissolved in the blood in the lungs are delivered very quickly to the brain.

The principle that governs the movement of gases from inhaled air into the blood and from the blood into the air within the lungs is diffusion. Gases move from areas of high concentration to areas of low concentration. If the concentration of drug in the inhaled air is higher than in the blood, the drug will move from the air into the blood, but if the reverse is true, the drug passes out of the blood into the air and is ex-

Figure 1–3 The circulatory system, showing how the heart circulates blood through the lungs before sending it around the rest of the body and the brain.

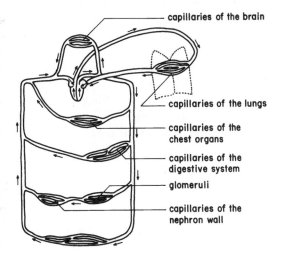

- capillaries of the brain
- capillaries of the lungs
- capillaries of the chest organs
- capillaries of the digestive system
- glomeruli
- capillaries of the nephron wall

haled. Thus the inhalation of gases provides a means of controlling drug levels in the blood with considerable precision. This ability is one reason volatile gases are used widely as general anesthetics and inhalation is the favored route of administration for anesthesia.

INHALATION OF SMOKE AND SOLIDS

Volatile gases and solvent vapors are not the only substances administered through the lungs. Drugs that occur naturally in some plants may be administered by burning the dried plant material and inhaling the smoke. Tobacco, opium, and marijuana are traditionally ingested in this manner. When the dried plant material is burned, the active ingredient remains in the smoke, either as a vapor or in tiny particles of ash that are inhaled into the lungs. When contact is made with the moist surface of the lungs, the drug dissolves and diffuses into the blood. The major difference between smoke and volatile gases is that the drug in the smoke particles will not revaporize after it is dissolved in the blood and consequently cannot be exhaled. These drugs must stay in the body until they are excreted by other means.

Powdered drugs such as cocaine, heroin, and tobacco snuff are sometimes sniffed into the nostrils. This practice is known as intranasal administration. What happens to the drug when given in this manner is unclear. It appears that most of the drug sniffed in the nose is dissolved in the moist *mucous membranes* of the nasal cavities and is absorbed into the blood from there. Some drug enters the lungs, while more runs down the throat into the stomach and digestive system and may be absorbed there. Although the nasal cavity is not as richly supplied with blood as the lungs and the area is not designed to transport substances into the blood, it is a reasonably efficient system for getting drugs into the blood.

The problem with administration of solids and smoke by inhalation is the susceptibility to damage of all the tissues in the respiratory system. Smoke from burning marijuana and tobacco contains many substances in addition to the active drug; there are tars, hydrocarbons, and other chemicals created by the burning process. In time, these substances may cause respiratory diseases such as emphysema, asthma, and lung cancer and may decrease the ability of the lungs to absorb oxygen and eliminate carbon dioxide from the blood. In addition, when most substances burn in air, carbon monoxide gas is given off. Carbon monoxide is a very toxic gas because it blocks the ability of the blood to carry oxygen.

In the experimental laboratory, drugs are seldom administered by inhalation. The major difficulty is that to make an animal inhale a gas or smoke, it is usually necessary to confine it in a closed environment filled with gas or smoke. Laboratory animals will generally not inhale gases voluntarily, and even if they do, the total amount of drug consumed is difficult to determine. The uncertainty about total dose and the technical problems of administration make this a cumbersome and unpopular route of administration in behavioral pharmacology.

ORAL ADMINISTRATION

Figure 1–4 shows the digestive system. Drugs absorbed into the body through the digestive system are taken into the mouth and swallowed, hence the term *peroral (p.o.)*. Sometimes substances can get into the digestive system by other means. As just explained, snuff from the nostrils can sometimes get down the throat and be swallowed.

A drug may be taken into the mouth and not swallowed, as with chewing tobacco. Although this is technically an oral administration, the absorption into the body is through the *buccal membranes*, or mucous membranes of the mouth, not the digestive system.

The digestive system may also be entered via its other end. Suppositories placed in the rectum

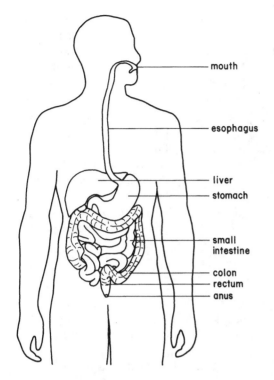

Figure 1–4 The digestive system, showing the location of the liver.

mouth

esophagus

liver
stomach

small intestine

colon
rectum
anus

also cause the drug to be absorbed into the blood. Such absorption is not as reliable as oral administration, but it can be used to advantage to give medication when it is impossible to give it orally (for example, when a patient or animal is unconscious or vomiting).

THE DIGESTIVE SYSTEM

After a drug is swallowed, it goes directly to the stomach. The stomach churns and secretes strong acids to break down food pieces and turn them into a liquid, which is then released slowly into the intestines, where nutrients are absorbed. Drugs may be absorbed from the stomach, but it is in the intestines where absorption is most efficient. The rate at which a swallowed drug will be absorbed may be determined by the speed with which it gets through the stomach to the intestine. Since solid food tends to be held in the stomach, taking a drug with a meal generally slows its absorption. When a drug is taken on an empty stomach, it passes quickly into the intestine and is absorbed rapidly.

The walls of the intestines are lined with capillaries to absorb nutrients from food, and these capillaries also absorb drugs. To get to the capillaries, however, the drug must pass through the membrane of the intestinal wall. All body tissue is made of cells, and all cells are surrounded by a membrane. Figure 1–5 shows the cross section of a typical membrane in the body. Most membranes are primarily made up of what is called a *lipid bilayer*. *Lipid* is another name for fat, and the membrane consists of two layers of fat molecules held tightly together. Each lipid molecule has a clump of atoms at one end and two chains of atoms at the other. The lipid molecules in a membrane are organized so that the clumps point to the outside and the tails point inward. Large molecules of protein are embedded in the lipid bilayer, and these have rather specific functions that will be described in Chapter 4.

For a drug molecule to pass through a wall of cells such as those in the lining of the intestine, there must be pores or holes large enough to allow it to diffuse through, or it must be able to dissolve in lipids. Since there are no pores in the lining of the intestines and stomach, a drug must be lipid-soluble to be absorbed from the digestive system.

All drug molecules vary in their degree of lipid solubility in their normal state, but when a molecule of a drug carries an electric charge, its lipid solubility is greatly diminished. Such a charged molecule is called an *ion*. Ions are not lipid-soluble and consequently pass through membranes very poorly. When a drug is dissolved in a fluid, some or all of its molecules become ionized. The percentage of ionized molecules in a solution is determined by (1) whether the drug is a weak acid or a weak base, (2) whether it is dissolved in

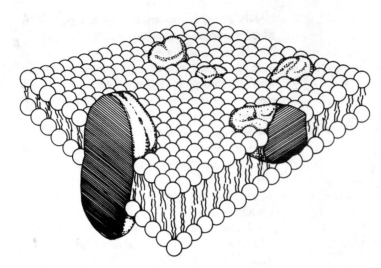

Figure 1–5 A cross section of a typical membrane, showing that it is made up of two layers of lipid molecules with their long chains pointing inward. Embedded in this lipid bilayer are large molecules of protein that serve special functions (see the text). (From "The Fluid Model of the Structure of Cell Membranes," J. J. Singer and G. L. Nicholson, *Science*, Vol. 175, pp. 720–731, February, 1972.)

an acid or a base, and (3) its *pKa*. The pKa of a drug is the pH at which half of its molecules are ionized.

The easiest way to understand pKa is to imagine the following experiment with a fictional drug called "damital." A fixed amount of damital is dissolved in each of 15 bottles; each bottle contains a liquid with a different pH ranging from 0 to 14. A solution's pH is a number that describes the degree to which it is either an acid or a base. On this scale, 7 is completely neutral, numbers less than 7 indicate increasing acidity, and numbers greater than 7 indicate increasing alkalinity.

After we dissolve the damital in each bottle, we then determine the percentage of damital molecules that are ionized and plot the results in Figure 1–6. As you can see from this figure, the pH at which half of the damital molecules are ionized is 5.

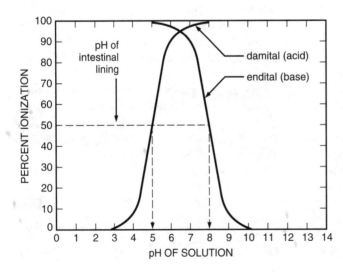

Figure 1–6 The percentage of ionized molecules in two fictional drugs dissolved in solutions with different pHs. Damital, a weak acid, becomes more highly ionized as the pH becomes more basic (higher numbers). Endital is a weak base, and it becomes more highly ionized at acid pHs. By drawing a horizontal line at the 50 percent ionization level we can determine the pKa of each drug: damital, 5.0, and endital, 8.0. Caffeine is a weak base with a pKa of 0.5. Try to figure out what its curve would look like.

Most drugs are either weak acids or weak bases. Damital is a weak acid. If we do this experiment again with a drug that is a weak base, we see something different. One line in Figure 1–6 is a plot for an imaginary base, "endital." As you can see, the curve for the acid damital starts with 0 percent ionization at the acid end of the scale, and ionization increases as it moves toward the base end. Just the opposite is true for endital, the base. It starts with 100 percent ionization in the acids, but its percentage of ionization decreases as the solution gets more basic. The pKa for endital is calculated in the same way as for damital. In this case, the pKa for endital is 8. As you can see, it is possible by knowing whether a drug is an acid or a base and by knowing its pKa to predict the degree to which it is likely to be ionized in a solution of known pH. The pH at the lining of the intestine is 3.5. In Figure 1–6, we can see that damital is about 5 percent ionized at this pH and endital is completely ionized. Since ionized molecules are not lipid-soluble and do not pass through membranes, we can conclude that endital will not be very effective when taken orally, whereas damital will be readily absorbed.

Morphine is a base, with a pKa of about 8. Since bases are highly ionized at low (acid) pHs and the curve drops at increasing pHs, we can predict that morphine will be poorly absorbed from the digestive system, and it is.

In general, most bases like morphine are poorly absorbed when taken orally, but their absorption depends on their pKa. For example, caffeine is a base, but it has a pKa of 0.5. Its ionization curve drops off very quickly at low pHs, and consequently it is almost entirely nonionized at pHs encountered in the digestive system. Caffeine, therefore, is readily absorbed when taken orally.

It should be pointed out that significant absorption will take place even if only a small percentage of molecules are not ionized. For example, if 97 percent of a drug is ionized at digestive-system pHs, only 3 percent will be lipid-soluble, but as soon as that percentage diffuses through the membrane and is removed by the blood, 3 percent of the remaining drug loses its charge, so the 97 percent ionization figure will stay constant for the drug remaining in the digestive system. The newly nonionized 3 percent now diffuses into the blood, and 3 percent more can lose its ionization. This process will continue until equilibrium is reached; that is, the concentration of nonionized molecules is the same on either side of the membrane. For this reason it is not appropriate to think that the percentage of nonionized drug is all that is absorbed. Rather, the percentage of nonionized molecules determines the number of molecules available for absorption at any period of time and therefore determines the rate of absorption.

ION TRAPPING

Until now we have been assuming that pH is the same on either side of a membrane, but this is not the case in the digestive system. The pH of the digestive system is usually acidic and can range from 1.5 to 7, but the pH of the blood on the other side of the membrane is slightly basic, about 7.5. As a result, the percentage of nonionized molecules of a given drug will differ on either side of the membrane.

As an example of how this process works, we shall examine aspirin (acetylsalicylic acid, sometimes called ASA). As the name suggests, this is an acid. It has a pKa of about 3.5. Thus, at the pH of the stomach, it is about 50 percent ionized, and half of its molecules will be lipid-soluble and free to diffuse across membranes and enter the blood. Diffusion will keep the nonionized molecules moving into the blood until the concentration of nonionized molecules is the same on both sides. But the pH of the blood is about 7.5, and aspirin is more than 99.99 percent ionized at this pH. Therefore, nearly all of the drug molecules that cross the membrane into the blood become ionized and are trapped there. As nonionized molecules diffuse into the blood, more and more ionized molecules in the digestive system lose their charge in order to maintain the 50 percent ionization level, and these can then diffuse across the membrane to be trapped there when they ionize.

You can get some idea of the extent to which ion trapping can concentrate a drug by remembering that nonionized molecules diffuse until they reach equal concentration on either side of a membrane. With a drug like aspirin, for example, one molecule in two in the digestive system will not be ionized, but in the blood one molecule in 10,000 will not be ionized. If the nonionized molecules are in equal concentration, then for every molecule in the digestive system there is only one other that is ionized, but in the blood, for every nonionized molecule there are more than 10,000 that are ionized. Thus there will be more than 5,000 times more aspirin molecules in the blood than in the digestive system.

Because of ion trapping, drugs that are acids tend to concentrate on the side of a membrane with the higher pH, and bases tend to concentrate on the side with the lower pH. The greater the difference in pH between the sides of a membrane, the greater this tendency.

The pH of the contents of the intestines tends to become less and less acidic further from the stomach, so bases are more and more easily absorbed as they pass through the digestive system. Furthermore, consumption of substances that change the digestive pH, such as antacids, can alter the absorption of many drugs.

DISTRIBUTION OF DRUGS

Even though most drugs get spread widely around the body, they tend to be concentrated in particular places and segregated from others. This process is called the *distribution* of a drug.

Lipid Solubility

Nonionized molecules of different drugs have different degrees of lipid solubility, which are usually expressed in terms of the *olive oil partition coefficients*. To test lipid solubility, equal amounts of olive oil and water are placed in a beaker, and a fixed amount of drug is mixed in. Later the oil and water are separated, and the amount of drug dissolved in each is measured. Drugs that are highly lipid soluble are more highly concentrated in the oil. Poorly lipid soluble drugs mostly end up in the water. This test, while not perfectly accurate, predicts reasonably well the degree to which a drug will dissolve in fat tissue in the body.

It has been stressed that lipid-soluble substances can get through membranes easily, but this capacity also means that highly lipid soluble drugs tend to stay in lipids wherever they encounter them. Consequently, highly lipid soluble drugs tend to concentrate in body fat outside the central nervous system. Since few drugs have any effect in body fat, all of a drug dissolved in fat is, in effect, inactive. Very often, the body fat acts like a sponge, absorbing a drug and taking it away from its site of action and diminishing its effect. Later the drug is slowly released back into the blood from the fat over a long period of time.

Distribution to the Central Nervous System

Many years ago it was discovered that when certain types of dyes were injected into the blood, they would be distributed to all extracellular fluids except those in the brain and the spinal cord. It was hypothesized then that there was a special barrier between blood and brain that protected the central nervous system from free diffusion of materials out of the blood. This became known as the *blood-brain barrier*. It has now been established that the blood-brain barrier is a result of special cells in the central nervous system that wrap themselves around the capillaries and block the pores through which substances normally diffuse. These provide a solid lipid barrier so that non-lipid-soluble substances have great difficulty getting into the brain.

Active and Passive Transport across Membranes

It is frequently important for the body to get non-lipid-soluble substances across membranes, so special transport mechanisms exist. These may be either passive or active.

In the passive transport mechanism, it appears that the non-lipid-soluble molecule attaches itself to a carrier or specialized molecule that diffuses across the membrane, releasing the normally non-lipid-soluble substance on the other side. In this way a substance can move from areas of high to low concentration on either side of a membrane as though it were lipid-soluble.

An active transport mechanism is similar to a passive mechanism except that it can work against normal diffusion by concentrating a substance on one side of a membrane. This is an active process that requires the expenditure of energy and takes place only in living membranes. Mechanisms such as *ion pumps*, which maintain electrical potentials of nerve cells (see Chapter 4), are examples of active transport systems. The blood-brain barrier has a number of such systems, many of which actively remove undesirable substances from the brain and some of which selectively concentrate substances in the brain.

Protein Binding

The blood contains a number of large protein molecules that cannot diffuse out of the pores in the capillaries because of their size. Some drugs attach themselves, or *bind*, to these protein molecules so strongly that they remain attached until metabolized and consequently never get to their site of action.

The Placental Barrier

The blood supply of the fetus and the mother is not continuous, and nutrients are transferred to (and waste products from) the blood to the unborn child through a membrane similar to the blood-brain barrier. This transfer takes place in the placenta, the organ connected to the fetus that attached to the wall of the uterus. Most behaviorally active drugs can be transferred from the mother's blood through the placenta to the fetus. Highly lipid soluble substances cross more easily than drugs with low lipid solubility. Drug concentration in the blood of the fetus usually reaches 75 to 100 percent of that of the mother within five minutes of administration. Thus there appears to be very little protection for the fetus from any drug the mother takes.

EXCRETION AND METABOLISM

There are some substances, such as heavy metals like lead and mercury, that the body is not very good at getting rid of. Levels of these substances can build up over time and accumulate to high and toxic concentrations. In most cases, however, the body has fairly efficient systems to rid itself of unwanted substances. It has already been described how volatile gases can be eliminated in exhaled breath. Small amounts of many drugs are eliminated in sweat, saliva, and feces, but the major job of elimination is done by the kidneys and the liver, the "dynamic duo" of excretion.

The Kidneys

The kidneys are two organs about the size of a fist located on either side of the spine in the back. Their primary function is to maintain the correct balance between water and salt in body fluids. Along with the excretion of excess water in the form of urine, the kidneys can also excrete molecules of unwanted substances (H. W. Smith, 1961). They function as a complex filtering system that physically removes certain substances from the blood. Figure 1–7 shows the *nephron*, the functional unit of the kidney. Each kidney has millions of nephrons, which all work in more or less the same way.

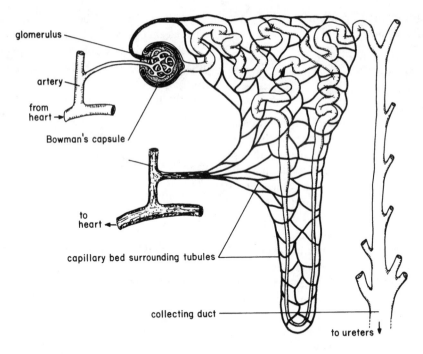

Figure 1–7 A drawing of a nephron showing the capillaries of the glomerulus that filter fluid out of the blood into the nephron, and the capillary bed that reabsorbs water, nutrients, and lipid-soluble drugs into the blood. All material that is not reabsorbed is excreted in the urine.

The nephron is essentially a long tube. At one end of the tube is a cuplike structure called *Bowman's capsule,* and inside Bowman's capsule is a clump of capillaries called the *glomerulus.* The other end of the nephron empties into collecting tubes, which in turn empty into the *urinary bladder.* The capillaries in the glomerulus have pores in their membranes, and most of the fluid in the blood that flows through these capillaries passes into Bowman's capsule and down the nephron. The remaining blood, which contains red and white cells and large protein molecules that are too large to pass out of the pores, continues out of the glomerulus and then moves through another bed to capillaries that surround the nephron along most of its length. At this point most of the fluid and other substances are absorbed through the nephron wall back into the blood, and whatever is not reabsorbed passes through the length of the nephron and is excreted from the body in the urine.

The kidney works not by filtering impurities out of the blood but by filtering everything out of the blood and then selectively reabsorbing what is required. Reabsorption in the nephron is accomplished by the mechanisms just described: diffusion, lipid solubility, and active and passive transport. All lipid-soluble substances diffuse through the nephron wall back into the blood unless there is a selective transport mechanism working against this diffusion. Desirable substances that are not lipid-soluble, such as glucose (blood sugar), have a transport mechanism that successfully reclaims them into the blood. Unless they have special transport systems, ionized or non-lipid-soluble substances tend to be excreted because they are not reabsorbed.

As with the digestive system, pH influences the degree of ionization and as a consequence can influence reabsorption. Urine tends to be acidic and blood is basic, so, similar to the digestive system, acids tend to concentrate on the blood side of the nephron wall and bases tend to be retained in the urine and are excreted more easily. The pH of the urine can be manipulated and made either more acidic or basic, which means that the excretion of drugs can also be manipulated. A similar process can also be used to facilitate the excretion of certain drugs in overdose cases. For example, one of the drug families involved frequently in overdoses is barbiturates, which are weak acids. Making the urine basic tends to ionize the barbiturate molecules, thus preventing their reabsorption. The kidneys can be assisted in the excretion of barbiturates by making the urine basic.

The Liver

The liver is a large organ located high in the abdomen under the diaphragm (see Figure 1–4). Its function may best be compared to that of a chemical factory where molecules are modified and rearranged to form new substances useful to the body and to change substances that are toxic to the body. These molecular changes are achieved by molecules called *enzymes*. An enzyme is a *catalyst*, or a substance that controls a certain chemical reaction. The enzyme takes part in the reaction, but when the reaction is finished, the enzyme is released unchanged and is free to participate in another reaction in the same way. Without the presence of the enzyme, the reaction would proceed very slowly or would not take place at all. The body controls chemical reactions by controlling the amount of enzyme available to act as a catalyst.

A good example of an enzyme is *alcohol dehydrogenase*. Someone with a background in chemistry can usually tell what the enzyme does by its name. To begin with, most enzymes end in *ase*. In the case of alcohol dehydrogenase, the enzyme removes hydrogen from a molecule of alcohol and makes it into *acetaldehyde*.

The process of restructuring molecules is referred to as *metabolism*, and the products of metabolism are called *metabolites*. In general, metabolites are either more useful to the body or less toxic than the original substance, and where drugs are concerned, the process is sometimes called *detoxification*. Although this term is appropriate some of the time, metabolites are not always less active or less toxic than the original drug. Chloral hydrate, psilocybin, and THC, the active ingredient of marijuana, are good examples of substances whose metabolites can be more active than the original drugs from which they are formed.

Another general rule is that metabolites are usually more likely to ionize. This is very important for the functioning of the kidneys as described earlier, since ionized molecules cannot be reabsorbed into the blood through the nephron wall and consequently can be excreted more easily. In this way the liver and kidneys work together to rid the body of unwanted substances; the liver changes the molecules into more ionized forms to be filtered out by the kidneys.

Rate of Excretion

The kidneys operate most efficiently when the concentration of a drug in the blood is high. As concentration falls off, the kidneys cannot filter out the drug at the same rate, and as a result, the curve that plots the level of a drug in the blood over time is not a straight line, but tends to level off to an asymptote as in Figure 1–8. Because of this trailing off, the rate of excretion for most drugs can be described in terms of a *half-life*.

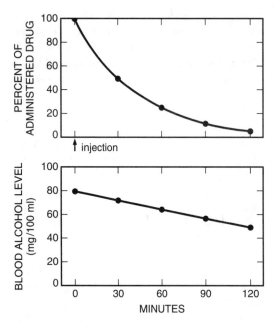

Figure 1–8 The top panel shows a typical excretion curve for a drug like nicotine that has a half-life of about 30 minutes. The bottom panel shows the excretion function for alcohol, which is excreted at a constant rate (about 15 mg/100 ml of blood per hour). Because the excretion function for alcohol is a straight line, the concept of half-life does not apply.

This is the time taken for the body to eliminate half of a given blood level of a drug. In the example given in Figure 1–8, half the original blood level is eliminated in 30 minutes. Thirty minutes later the level has fallen to 25 percent of the original level, and 30 minutes after that it is down to 12.5 percent. Every 30 minutes the body gets rid of half the drug circulating in the blood, so the half-life of the drug is 30 minutes.

The excretion of most drugs can be described in terms of half-life, but there is one important exception: alcohol. If the blood level of alcohol is above a low minimum level, the excretion curve for alcohol is a straight line, as in Figure 1–8. The half-life does not apply to alcohol.

FACTORS THAT ALTER DRUG METABOLISM

A number of factors can influence the rate of metabolism of drugs in the liver and, consequently, the intensity and duration of a drug effect. A great many individual differences in response to drugs can be explained in terms of variations in drug metabolism and enzyme systems that change according to such factors as age, species, and past experience with drugs.

Stimulation of Enzyme Systems

Levels of a given enzyme can be increased by previous exposure to a specific drug that uses that enzyme or some other enzyme system. This process is known as *enzyme induction* and is responsible for the development of *metabolic tolerance* discussed earlier in this chapter. A good example of such a process is an increase in levels of alcohol dehydrogenase in the livers of heavy drinkers. Those who drink a great deal are able to metabolize alcohol faster than nondrinkers and are therefore more resistant to its effects.

The effects of alcohol are not limited to inducing alcohol dehydrogenase. It can also stimulate the enzymes that metabolize barbiturates; this fact partly explains why heavy drinkers are much less sensitive than nondrinkers to the effects of barbiturates.

Depression of Enzyme Systems

When two drugs that use the same enzyme are introduced into the body at the same time, the metabolism of each will be depressed because both will be competing for the enzyme. Again we turn to the metabolism of alcohol as an example. Alcohol dehydrogenase converts alcohol to acetaldehyde, which is in turn converted into something called *acetyl coenzyme A* by another enzyme, *aldehyde dehydrogenase*. Disulfiram (Antabuse) is a drug that competes with acetaldehyde for this enzyme, causing acetaldehyde levels to increase in the body because the enzyme is not readily available to metabolize it (see Figure 1–9). Acetaldehyde is toxic and causes sickness and discomfort, so people who take disulfiram and then drink alcohol will get sick because of the buildup of high acetaldehyde levels. Disulfiram is sometimes used in the treatment of alcoholics to discourage drinking; alcoholics will feel well and stay that way if they refrain from ingesting alcohol, but as soon as they take a drink, they will feel ill.

Age

Enzyme systems are not fully functional at birth and may take time to develop properly. For this reason, immature members of a species may metabolize drugs differently from adults or may not metabolize them at all. For example, the liver of a newborn human first converts theophylline to caffeine and then metabolizes caffeine very slowly. In adults theophylline is metabolized directly without this intermediate stage. Theo-phylline is similar to caffeine and is found in tea but is sometimes given to newborn babies to stimulate breathing. In infants the effects of theophylline are greatly enhanced because of the intermediate stage of metabolism involving caffeine. For this reason, doses must be small and closely monitored to avoid overdose. A similar problem is encountered when drugs are given to a woman immediately before she gives birth. Drugs given at this time cross the placental barrier and circulate in the blood of the fetus. As long as the child's circulatory system is connected to the mother, the mother's liver can handle the drug, but if the baby is born and the umbilical cord is cut before all the drug is metabolized, the drug remains in the infant's body and is dependent solely on the baby's immature liver for metabolism, which may take many days.

There can also be impairments in metabolism at the other end of the life span. Liver functioning is less efficient in elderly people, so physicians prescribing for elderly patients should reduce doses considerably.

Figure 1–9 Steps in the metabolism of alcohol. Note that disulfiram (Antabuse) stops this reaction at a point that causes a buildup of acetaldehyde.

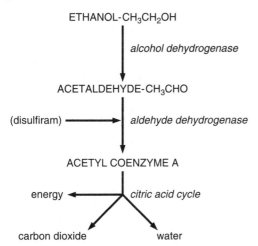

Species

The vast majority of research in behavioral pharmacology uses species other than human beings. Studies are usually done on rats, mice, pigeons, or primates. It is important to understand how differences in drug metabolism can alter the intensity and duration of a similar dose in different species. As an example, the levels of alcohol dehydrogenase are quite different in different species. The liver of a rat or mouse contains about 60 percent of the alcohol dehydrogenase per gram in a human liver, but the liver of a guinea pig contains 160 percent of the level in a human liver. The liver of a rhesus monkey has a concentration of alcohol dehydrogenase similar to that of a human liver. As you can see, the same experiments on the guinea pig, rat, or human might reach quite different conclusions.

COMBINING ABSORPTION
AND EXCRETION FUNCTIONS

The effects of a drug change over time to reflect increasing and decreasing drug levels after administration. When these effects over time are plotted on a graph, the result is usually called a *time course*. The drug effect is usually represented on the vertical axis and time on the horizontal axis. Figure 1–10 is a time course for the concentration of drug in the blood after administration. In this graph there are three curves. One shows the time course of absorption of a drug from the site of administration. This curve is hypothetical because it assumes that while the drug is being absorbed, the liver and kidneys are not working and no excretion is going on. The second curve is a hypothetical excretion curve; it shows the rate of excretion of a drug but assumes instantaneous absorption. In reality, neither of these curves would exist. What is usually seen is a combination of both. This is shown in the third curve, which has both an ascending and a descending phase indicating both absorption and excretion. The absorption rate of any given drug and thus the shape of this curve will vary, depending on the route of administration.

Figure 1–11 shows typical curves for various routes of administration. When drugs are given intravenously, the absorption phase is very steep, the drug achieves high levels, and it is metabo-lized and excreted quickly. When given orally, the absorption is slow and blood levels do not reach the same high concentrations seen after i.v. administration, but the drug lasts much longer in the body. Intramuscular and subcutaneous routes are intermediate between i.v. and oral routes. The route of administration can determine whether a drug reaches high levels for a short period or lasts a long time at low levels. If the function of a drug depends on maintaining constant blood levels, as with antibiotics, oral administration is preferred. If it is necessary to achieve very high levels for brief periods, the drug is best given intravenously.

One major difficulty with slower routes of administration is the delay in feedback or knowledge of effect. This can be an important feature in the recreational self-administration of drugs. When a drug is taken orally, there is a considerable delay between its consumption and the onset of peak effect. During this delay, the user may consume more drug before fully knowing what effect the first dose is having; the result may be that too much drug is ingested. When a drug is given by a faster route, feedback is more immediate, and the dosage can be monitored more closely. A good example of this problem is phencyclidine, or PCP, which is discussed in Chapter 15. This substance was introduced to drug users in the 1960s but never achieved much popularity. In the 1970s, however, it became more widely

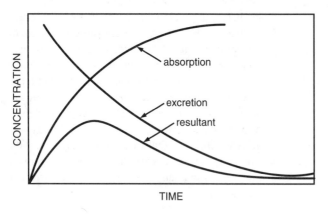

Figure 1–10 This figure shows a theoretical absorption curve that we might see if there were no excretion going on at all. Also shown is a theoretical excretion curve, one that we might see if absorption and distribution were instantaneous. The third line shows the resultant of these two theoretical processes. This curve is typical of the time course for blood level of most drugs.

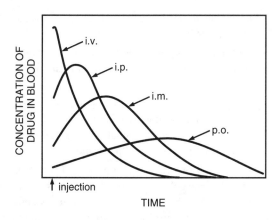

Figure 1–11 The time courses for blood levels of a drug given by different routes of administration.

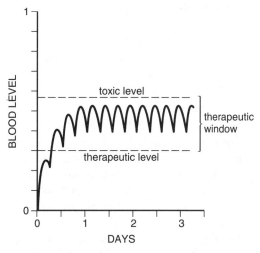

Figure 1–12 The therapeutic window is the range of blood concentrations of a therapeutic drug between a level so low that it is ineffective (therapeutic level) and a level so high that it has toxic side effects (toxic level). When drugs are taken chronically, it is important that the drug be given in the right dose and at the right frequency so that blood levels remain in the therapeutic window as shown here.

used. Many theories attempt to explain this increase in use, but the most convincing points out that in the 1960s the drug was taken orally like LSD and people frequently took too much, resulting in unpleasant consequences. In the 1970s users switched to either smoking or sniffing the drug. This faster absorption gave better control of blood levels, and use of the drug became more popular.

The Therapeutic Window

When drugs are administered for therapeutic purposes, it is important that just the right level of the drug be maintained in the blood. If the drug reaches too high a level, there will be an increase in unwanted side effects and no increase in the therapeutic effect. If the drug falls below a certain level, it will not have a therapeutic effect at all. The drug must be given in such a way that the concentration in the blood stays between a level that is too high and one that is too low. This range is called the *therapeutic window*. Figure 1–12 illustrates this therapeutic window.

For drugs that are absorbed slowly and excreted slowly, it is usually not difficult to achieve a dosing regime that keeps the blood level within

this window, but this is more complicated for drugs that are absorbed rapidly and excreted rapidly. One such drug is lithium carbonate, which is given to people with bipolar disorder (see Chapter 13). Lithium has a rather narrow therapeutic window (the effective dose and a dose that causes side effects are very close). Lithium is also absorbed and excreted rapidly, so it must be given in small doses as many as four times a day. To help solve this problem, pills have been developed in which the lithium is embedded in a material that dissolves slowly to delay its absorption and hence its peak blood level. Using this sort of medication makes it easier to keep the blood level within the therapeutic window and reduce the number of doses to two a day.

CHAPTER SUMMARY

- Drugs have three different kinds of names. The *chemical name*, the *generic name,* and at least one *trade name*.

- *Dose response curves (DRCs)* are curves that show changes in the effect of a drug that are produced by changes in the dose.

- The ED_{50} (*median effective dose*) is the dose of a drug that will have a particular effect in 50 percent of the subjects to whom it is given. The LD_{50} (*median lethal dose*) is the dose of a drug that will be lethal to 50 percent of the subjects.

- The safety of a drug can be described by the TI (*therapeutic index*), which is the LD_{50} divided by the ED_{50}.

- When comparing two drugs that have the same effect, the drug with the lower ED_{50} is the more *potent*. The drug with the greater maximum effect is the more *effective*.

- All drugs have a number of effects. The one of primary interest is the *main effect*, and all others are *side effects*.

- If one drug shifts the DRC of a second drug to the right, the drugs are said to be *antagonistic*. If the DRC is shifted to the left, the effects are *additive*. *Potentiation* or *superadditive* effects are seen if the effects of a drug mixture are greater than what might be expected if the effects were simply added together.

- If a drug is taken repeatedly, it will become less and less effective, and hence more drug will be needed to achieve a consistent effect. This change is known as *tolerance* and may occur at different rates for different drug effects.

- The term *dependence* is sometimes used as an explanation of excessive drug use, but it should only be used to describe a state where *withdrawal symptoms* will occur if the drug is stopped or the dose is decreased.

- Parenteral administration may be *subcutaneous, intramuscular, intraperitoneal,* or *intravenous*.

- Drugs in the form of gases, vapors, and smoke may be inhaled into the lungs and enter the blood. Drugs that are inhaled reach the brain more quickly than any other route.

- Molecules of drugs that are *ionized* (have an electric charge) are not *lipid-soluble* and cannot be absorbed from the digestive system. The rate of absorption of a drug can be altered by changing the pH of the digestive system.

- Drugs that are not lipid-soluble have difficulty passing through membranes and get into the brain slowly because of the *blood-brain barrier*. Highly lipid-soluble drugs are sometimes absorbed rapidly into body fat and released slowly.

- In the kidney, most of the fluid in the blood is released into one end of the *nephron*, and as it passes through, water and nutrients are reabsorbed. Ionized drugs and many drug metabolites are not reabsorbed, pass through the length of the nephron, and are *excreted* in the urine.

- Drugs are eliminated from the body by the *liver*, which changes the drug molecules by the process of *metabolism*, and by the *kidneys*, which filter out both the drug and the *metabolites* produced by the liver. The liver controls metabolism by *enzymes*, which are *catalysts* that speed up certain chemical reactions.

- The *half-life* is the time taken for the body to get rid of half of the circulating drug.

- The *therapeutic window* refers to the range of blood levels of a drug between the lowest effective dose and a dose so high that there are undesirable side effects.

2

Research Design and the Behavioral Analysis of Drug Effects

RESEARCH DESIGN

All scientific experimentation can be thought of as a search for a relationship between events. In behavioral pharmacology the researcher is usually trying to find the relationship between the presence of a drug in an organism and changes that occur in the behavior of that organism. In most true experiments, one of these events is created or manipulated by the experimenter, and the other event is measured. The manipulated event is called the *independent variable*, and the observed event is called the *dependent variable*. The independent variable in behavioral pharmacology is usually the amount of drug put into the organism; that is what the researcher manipulates. The dependent variable is usually some change in the behavior of that organism, and this is what the researcher measures. Later in this chapter we will discuss some of the more commonly used measures of behavior or dependent variables.

Experimental Research Design

Experimental Control. It is not enough to give a drug and observe its effect. For an experiment to be meaningful, the experimenter must be able to compare what happened when the drug was given with what would have happened if the drug had not been given. In other words, the experiment needs a *control*. A controlled experiment is one in which it is possible to say with some degree of certainty what would have happened if the drug had not been given. This permits comparisons to be made between drug and nondrug states. For example, a researcher could give several subjects each a pill containing THC, the active ingredient in marijuana, and observe that everyone tended to laugh a great deal afterward. These observations would not be worth much unless the research could demonstrate that the increased laughter was a result of the drug and not a result of the subjects' expectations or of nervousness about being observed or some factor other than the presence of the drug in the body. As with most behavioral experiments, many factors could influence the results, so it is essential to be sure that the drug, and not something else in the procedure, caused the laughter.

The only truly reliable way to do this experiment and eliminate all possible causes of the laughter apart from the drug would be to have a time machine and, after the experiment, go back and, under exactly the same circumstances, give the same subjects identical pills *not* containing any drug. Comparisons could then be made between the amount of laughter with and without the drug, since all other factors (the subjects, the situation, the time of day, and so on) would be the same. Only then could we be sure the laughter was caused by the drug and nothing else.

Since there is no such thing as a time machine, the behavioral pharmacologist must compare the behavior of a drugged subject with either (1) the drug-free behavior of that subject under similar conditions or (2) the behavior of other drug-free subjects under similar conditions.

Within-Subject Designs.   The first alternative is called a *within-subject* design. In this strategy, careful observations are made of a subject's behavior under specific conditions, and when the behavior appears to be stable and predictable, it is then possible to give the drug and make comparisons between drugged and nondrugged behavior. In other words, subjects serve as their own controls.

Let us say, for example, that we are interested in the effect of amphetamine on the feeding behavior of rats. In a within-subject design, the researcher carefully measures the daily food consumption of several rats until the measures are constant for each animal. The researcher then injects a dose of amphetamine into each rat and measures food consumption for that day. Meaningful comparisons can now be made between food consumption on drug and nondrug days, since the researcher has a pretty good idea of how much each animal would have eaten if it had not been given the drug.

Between-Subject Design.   The same experiment could also be done using a *between-subject* design. In this strategy, a number of rats are randomly assigned to two groups. One group, the experimental group, would get the amphetamine, and the other, the control group, would not get any drug. The food consumption of both groups could then be compared.

Comparisons of Between- and Within-Subject Designs.   The type of design used by the behavioral pharmacologist is usually determined by the type of dependent variable being measured in the experiment. If the measure is stable from day to day, like eating, within-subject designs can be used, but if the dependent variable is subject to systematic change, the researcher is forced to use a between-subject design. Exploratory behavior is a good example of such a measure; on the first exposure to a new cage, a rat will usually spend considerable time moving around and exploring, but on the second day it may be habituated to the surroundings and may just sit and lick its whiskers. A within-subject design could not be used to study exploratory behavior because the behavior changes from day to day. We would not know whether the change was due to the drug or to habituation. A between-subject design would be appropriate because both the experimental and control groups could be compared on the first exposure to the new cage, and habituation would not be a factor.

The difficulty with the between-subject design is that responses of individuals may vary a great deal. By chance we may get very curious rats in one group and very lazy rats in another. The differences in groups would then be due to differences in rats and not to the effects of the drug. We could get around this difficulty by having large groups, which would decrease the likelihood that all the curious or lazy rats would end up in one group. This procedure would require much more work and have the additional disadvantage that the final results would be in terms of group averages, which sometimes hide important information that is more apparent in work with individual subjects.

The advantage of the within-subject design is that more perfect control conditions can be achieved because each subject is its own control. The disadvantage is that it can only be used with behavioral measures that are not likely to change when repeated. Within-subject experiments usually take more time, but they do not require as many subjects.

Statistical Testing

In some within-subject and most between-subject designs, some sort of statistical tests are needed to determine the probability of differences observed between drug and nondrug measures. Such tests are necessary because differences could be due to chance variations from day to day and from subject to subject. When a researcher finds a difference in the means of the groups, a statistical test can tell how often such a difference would be likely to occur by chance if there were no drug effect. Box 2–1 gives a numerical example of how statistical tests are used.

Placebo Controls

To be completely useful, a control condition must be as similar as possible to the experimental condition except for one variable: the presence or absence of the drug. In our example in which the effect of amphetamine on rats' eating was determined, the control procedure could have been improved. As you recall, we had two groups: one was injected with amphetamine, and the other was not injected at all. It is quite possible that the anxiety of being stuck by a needle suppressed eating by itself and the amphetamine had nothing

to do with the results. For this reason, behavioral pharmacologists always use a control condition that involves the injection of the vehicle alone (see Chapter 1). On control days in within-subject designs and for control subjects in between-subject designs, an injection of normal saline would be given. Subjects in the experimental group or on drug days would be treated identically, except they would have the drug dissolved in the saline.

Such careful controls are especially important with human subjects because of a phenomenon known as the *placebo effect*. A *placebo* is a totally inert substance that causes no physiological change but is administered as though it were a drug. If people believe they are getting a drug that will have a specific effect, they will frequently show that effect even though the drug does not cause it. This placebo effect makes careful control an absolute necessity when evaluating the clinical effectiveness of newly developed medicines because patients will frequently show an effect they expect the drug to produce. For example, let us suppose that we are testing a new pain reliever. We go to a hospital and give the drug to a group of patients who are in postoperative pain and tell them that this new drug should relieve their distress. The next day we find that 68 percent of the patients report that their pain was relieved. By itself, this is not a useful experiment because we do not know how many patients would have reported the same thing without the drug. To do this experiment the proper way, it would be necessary to have two groups of patients. Both groups would be told they were getting a pain reliever, but only one group would get the new drug; the other would be given an identical pill containing only sugar. The next day, pain ratings would be taken from all the patients, and comparisons could be made.

Further precautions must be taken in an experiment of this nature. It has been known for some time that an experimenter can influence the outcome of research without knowing it. For example, if the researcher knows which patients have

BOX 2–1   An Example of the Use of a Statistical Test

A mythical experiment was done to determine the effect of amphetamine on food consumption in rats. The experiment was a between-subject design with 10 rats in each group. Both groups were treated identically except that the rats in one group were given amphetamine before eating and the rats in the other group were given a placebo injection of the vehicle, normal saline. The amount eaten by each rat is given in the following table:

CONTROL GROUP		EXPERIMENTAL GROUP	
Rat Number	Food Eaten (grams)	Rat Number	Food Eaten (grams)
1	18	11	17
2	22	12	14
3	23	13	12
4	17	14	25
5	28	15	15
6	20	16	16
7	16	17	20
8	22	18	21
9	21	19	13
10	18	20	11
Mean	20.5		16.4

The researcher found that the amphetamine group ate a mean of 16.4 g of food and that the control rats ate a mean of 20.5 g of food. On the basis of this difference, could the experi-

been given a placebo, the researcher might unconsciously change the manner in which the patients are interviewed or even make systematic mistakes in recording data. To eliminate this possibility, it is usually necessary to conduct the experiment so that neither the doctors and nurses giving the drug nor the researchers interviewing the patients for the pain ratings know which patient is in which group. This procedure is called a *double blind,* and it is essential because it eliminates the possibility of any experimenter bias effects.

When a new drug is being tested for use in the treatment of a disease, the standard design is what is known as a *three-groups design.* One group is given the experimental drug to be tested, a second group is given a placebo, and a third group is given an established drug with known therapeutic effect. These three groups permit the researchers to answer a number of important questions. Comparisons between the drug and the placebo group show whether the drug caused any improvement; comparisons between the placebo control and the established drug group indicate whether the research measures were sensitive enough to detect an improvement; and comparisons between the experimental and established drug groups tell whether the new drug has any

menter conclude that amphetamine reduced food intake? To answer this question, a statistical test is needed.

The most appropriate statistical test for this type of experiment is what is known as a *t* test. This test takes into account the variability in each group, and on the basis of certain assumptions, it can tell the experimenter how many times the experiment would have to be repeated to get this big a difference between the means just by chance.

In this case the *t* test tells the experimenter that if the drug had no effect and the experiment was done 100 times, a difference this big could occur as often as 10 times just by chance. This result is normally not good enough. Most behavioral researchers insist that their results be explained by chance no more than five times in 100, or as they say, with a probability of less than 5 percent ($p < .05$). If the probability level is greater than .05, the result is generally considered to be negative. If you read original research reports, you will see the results of statistical tests reported something like this: ($t = 2.09$, $df = 18$, $p < .1$). The first two numbers are values associated with the statistical test, and the final number is the probability level (in this case it is less than 10 percent).

There are many types of statistical tests for many different research designs. However, they all end up telling you the same thing: How often you would expect to get the results by chance if there were no drug effect (Ferguson, 1966).

When using a within-subject strategy, a statistical test is sometimes not necessary. Most research using operant techniques examines the behavior of three or four experimental subjects in great detail and under carefully controlled experimental conditions. Nondrugged performance is very reliable, so when the drug is given, it is readily apparent whether there are any drug-produced changes in behavior, and statistical analyses are not necessary.

advantage over established treatment (Overall, 1987).

NONEXPERIMENTAL RESEARCH

A good deal of what we know about drugs is a result of research that does not involve experiments. As explained earlier, experiments attempt to find relationships between two events, a manipulated event and a measured event. Nonexperimental research looks for a relationship between two measured events. A good example is the discovery of a relationship between smoking during pregnancy and infant mortality. It was shown some time ago that there was a higher rate of infant death among babies born to women who smoked during pregnancy than among babies born to nonsmoking mothers (see Chapter 8). In this research nothing was manipulated; there was no independent variable. The two events, smoking and infant mortality, were measured and found to be related.

One major difficulty with this sort of finding is that we cannot assume a causal relationship between the two related events. We know that children born to smoking mothers are more likely to die, but we cannot conclude that smoking *causes* the infants' deaths. The relationship might be due to some third factor that causes both events. For example, it may be that women smoke because they have a biochemical imbalance that causes their bodies to need the nicotine in cigarettes. This imbalance might also be responsible for the higher infant mortality rates. The only way we could be sure that the smoking caused the infant mortality would be to do a true experiment by finding two groups of pregnant women and forcing one group to smoke. If there were a difference in infant mortality between the two groups, we would be in a good position to propose a causal relationship. Of course, such an experiment is out of the question on ethical grounds and could never be done with humans. For this reason, we are going to have to be satisfied with relational rather than causal data on many issues of drug effects in humans.

THE STUDY OF BEHAVIOR

Behaviorism

Contemporary psychology should not really be called "psychology" at all. The name is derived from the Greek word *psyche*, meaning "mind," and it literally means "the study of mind," which it is not. Modern psychology has its roots in both physiology and philosophy. It is from philosophy that it derives its name, but its methods and subject matter are closer to physiology.

Early psychologists attempted to study the mind scientifically but met with very little success because they used a method of gathering data called *introspection*. Introspection is the internal observation of what is going on in one's own mind. Introspection failed to make it as a scientific method because it violated one of the principal requirements of science: that its subject matter be public. This means that the data must be available for everyone to observe. Introspection, by its very nature, could not be a source of scientific information.

In the early part of the twentieth century, an American psychologist, John B. Watson, founded a school of psychology known as *behaviorism*, which has become the basis of contemporary Western psychology. Watson rebelled against the study of the mind and any other concept that could not be defined in terms of observable and measurable phenomena, claiming that the real subject matter for psychologists should be behavior. Behavior was public, measurable, and reproducible and consequently was amenable to the scientific method. As a result of Watson's influence, most experimental psychologists today are behaviorists, although the old terms *psychology* and *psychologist* are still used as widely as ever.

Psychologists and pharmacologists who study the effects of drugs on behavior sometimes refer to their field as *psychopharmacology*, which is simply a combination of the words *psychology* and *pharmacology*. Purists prefer to use the term *behavioral pharmacology*. Today the term *psychopharmacology* is most often used to describe the field that studies the effects of drugs on psychiatric symptoms—a merging of the concerns of both psychiatry and pharmacology.

Introspection

Unstructured Introspection. Introspection, or the study of internal mental processes as used by early psychologists, did not succeed as a scientific method and is not particularly helpful as a tool in behavioral pharmacology. This is not to say that unstructured verbal descriptions of drug-produced internal states are not useful to the researcher. On the contrary, they guide and inspire more systematic study, but the accounts themselves are not adequate data for the scientists unless they are collected in a systematic or structured fashion.

Many chapters in this book provide accounts of the experiences of people who have taken various drugs. These can give us some indication of how the drug affected the writer at that time and can be fascinating, but by themselves they can only give readers some indication of how they might feel if they took a similar dose of the drug. These accounts alone cannot provide data that can be used to predict or understand the action of the drug in terms that scientists can find useful.

Systematic Introspection. Introspection by itself is of no value to the behaviorist, but the acts of introspecting and the subsequent verbalization are behavior that can be studied. If a psychologist sticks a pin into a subject's finger, the pain will be quite real to the subject but is available only to the subject and not the experimenter for study. However, if the psychologist asks, "Does it hurt?" and the subject answers, "Yes," the answer is public and scientifically useful. Similarly, when a drug is given to an experimental subject who hallucinates, the visions seen are the subject's own and cannot be studied, but the subject's responses to the visions can be recorded, analyzed, measured, and subjected to any kind of behavioral test. The scientific usefulness of such responses will, to a large extent, depend on the care with which they are collected and the skill with which they are analyzed.

Systematic self-reporting is also useful in human research when studying the effects of drugs on internal states such as moods. Rather than just asking subjects how they feel, the researcher can use scales that measure a particular aspect of how the drug makes a person feel. One example of such a scale is the *Profile of Mood States (POMS)*, a paper-and-pencil test that asks subjects to describe on a five-point scale how each of 72 adjectives applies to them at a particular moment. These 72 items give a score on eight independent subscales: anxiety, depression, anger, vigor, fatigue, confusion, friendliness, and elation. Scales such as these give a reliable and quantifiable measure of a subject's internal state. See Chapter 10 for an example.

The *Addiction Research Center Inventory (ARCI)* is a similar test developed specifically to assess the abuse potential of drugs. The complete questionnaire consists of 550 true/false items covering a broad range of physical and subjective effects. This scale can then be given to a person after taking a new drug, and its subjective effect can be compared with any of these other drug classes (Haertzen & Hickey, 1987). The assumption is that drugs with similar subjective effects, particularly euphoric effects, will be similarly abused.

LEVEL OF AROUSAL

The concept of arousal level has been around for a long time and is the basis for a number of important psychological theories. In the course of a day, we all experience changes in arousal that normally range from deep sleep to mild excitement. Arousal level is thought of as one continuous variable so that the arousal level at a specific time can be characterized as being at a point on that scale and moving in either direction. Figure 2–1 shows the scale of arousal level and indicates the normal range of arousal encountered by us all in the course of a day.

The scale of arousal can continue beyond the normal ranges in both directions into pathological or abnormal states. At the low end it goes beyond deep sleep to coma and death, and at the

Figure 2–1 The range of arousal levels. Normal arousal varies between deep sleep and excitement, but drugs and disease may cause arousal to move out of the normal range.

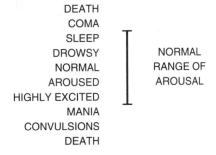

high end excitement ranges into mania, convulsions, and death.

EEG

One device used to measure the level of arousal is the *electroencephalograph*, or *EEG*. The EEG consists of a number of electrodes that are attached to the scalp and detect differences in electrical potential between points on the scalp and a neutral part of the body. These potential differences are amplified and recorded by pens on a sheet of paper that moves at a constant rate. The changes in the potential detected by these electrodes show up as wavy lines on the paper, and these tracings indicate electrical activity in the brain.

When an individual is attached to an EEG, the recording pen will always be moving in response to electrical activity in the brain, and the pattern of movement can be read as an indication of the level of arousal. In an alert individual, the EEG will usually show *beta waves*, which are small and have a frequency greater than 12 hertz (Hz; waves per second). A relaxed individual with closed eyes will show smooth, regular waves. These are *alpha waves* and have a frequency of between 8 and 12 Hz. As a person becomes more relaxed, the waves get larger and the cycles get longer.

Sleep

During sleep, these waves may slow to 1 to 2 Hz and are called *delta waves* or *sleep spindles*. As a person goes to sleep, there are five distinct stages that can be recognized with the EEG. These stages are characterized by slower and slower frequency, except the last stage, known as *paradoxical* or *REM sleep*.

Over the course of a night, the EEG reading shows the brain cycling through these five stages. Every 90 minutes or so the brain appears to wake up; it shows a normal waking EEG including beta waves, even though the individual is still sound asleep. Recordings from muscles show that they are even more relaxed than normal, yet the subject has a wide-awake EEG; thus the term *paradoxical sleep*. This is also known as rapid-eye movement (REM) sleep because careful observation shows that during these periods, the eyeballs are moving rapidly under closed lids. Figure 2–2 shows the typical progression through the stages of sleep during the course of a night.

The physiological and psychological significance of REM sleep has only recently been studied, but it is known that dreaming is associated with REM, and people deprived of REM sleep suffer from changes in intellectual ability, motivation, and personality. REM sleep is altered by many drugs.

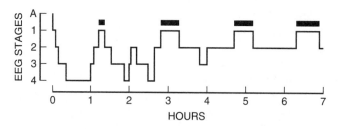

Figure 2–2 Typical cycles of sleep during a night. Sleep stage is indicated on the vertical axis from A (awake) through four stages of sleep. Solid bars show periods of REM sleep. These tend to be more frequent and of longer duration in the latter part of the night. (Dement & Kleitman, 1957.)

Arousal, Mood, and Activity

Arousal level is also associated with moods. It is usually assumed that depression in the nervous system is accompanied by a placid, tranquil mood that deepens to a groggy disorientation and finally sleep. At the other end of the scale, the stimulated nervous system produces speeded activity and feelings of pleasure and excitement until a state of *mania* results and the individual is confused, delirious, and highly agitated. The colloquial classification of drugs as "uppers" and "downers" is based on this presumed relationship between mood and state of arousal, but it cannot always be assumed that arousal has anything to do with mood. For example, the stimulation and jitters caused by many stimulant drugs such as caffeine are considered unpleasant, as is the depressed, sedated state caused by the antipsychotic drugs. By contrast, opiates, which cause a depressed, dreamy state, and cocaine, which causes high arousal, produce euphoria.

It should also be pointed out that *arousal and activity are not the same thing*. High arousal does not necessarily mean more activity, and low arousal does not mean less activity. This statement is especially true with regard to drug-altered arousal. The so-called stimulants may be stimulants so far as mood is concerned because they make people feel happy or aroused or "stimulated," but it is a mistake to think that they inevitably make organisms more active. The effect that any drug has on behavior depends far more on the behavior being measured and on the organism than on the nature of the drug. This is also true of the drugs classed as depressants. They are called depressants because they make people feel less activated, but it does not follow that they make the user less active.

MEASURING PERFORMANCE IN HUMANS

Some tasks, such as driving a car, are of great interest to the behavioral pharmacologist and are studied through elaborate tests and simulations of real-life conditions. Although findings from these tests are directly applicable to the task studied, it is generally better to study the basic intellectual and behavioral processes used in these more complex skills and apply the findings more generally to a greater variety of tasks that use the same basic skills. Most tests of human performance can be categorized according to whether they measure perceptual, intellectual, or motor abilities.

Perceptual Performance

Thresholds. A number of tests and techniques have been developed to measure the acuity of the senses, particularly sight and hearing. Sensitivity changes are reported as changes in *thresholds*. The term *absolute threshold* refers to the lowest value of a stimulus that can be detected by a sense organ. It is a measure of the absolute sensitivity of the sense organ. *Difference thresholds* are measures of the ability of a sense organ to detect a change in level or locus of stimulation. If a threshold increases, it means that the intensity of the stimulus must be increased in order for it to be detected. In other words, the sense has become less keen. A lowering in threshold means that a sense has become more sensitive.

One common measure of visual acuity, the ability of the eye to detect detail, is *critical frequency at fusion (CFF)*. If the speed with which a light flickers is increased, eventually a point will be reached where the light no longer flickers and appears to be steady. This is the critical frequency at fusion, and it is sensitive to many drugs. The ability to detect flicker is a reliable measure of how well the visual system is functioning. To measure the functioning of hearing, an auditory flicker fusion test has also been developed.

Another sense that seems to be influenced by drugs is judgment of the passage of time. This can be measured in several ways; most commonly, a subject is presented with a standard time interval and then asked to create a similar interval or to judge which of a number of intervals is similar to the standard.

Cognitive Performance

Vigilance. Vigilance tasks do not test the ability of an observer to detect the presence or absence of a stimulus at threshold but rather to detect a specific signal in a group of signals. This type of task measures the ability of the brain to identify specific information; it is a task of cognitive functioning rather than perception.

An example of a vigilance task would be to go over a page of text and count the words that contain the letter *o*. The task is basically easy, but if you have only 10 seconds to do it, it presents quite a challenge. Other varieties of vigilance tests require the subject to monitor several dials at once and report when one shows a reading different from the others. After an hour or two, this task can be quite challenging.

Other tests of intellectual functioning include the ability to perform addition and subtraction mentally, to learn lists of words, to sort cards, and to name colors.

Memory and Learning. Numerous tests have been developed over the years to evaluate learning, memory, and recall. These tests involve presenting material, either verbal, such as a list of words, or visual, like a series of pictures, and then at a later time testing the subject to see if the material has been learned or can be recalled. Such testing can be done either by asking the subject to reproduce the material—for example, to recall the words or pictures—or by asking the person to recognize the material. The entire process of learning and testing may take place while the subject is under the influence of the drug, or the effect of the drug on different stages of the process can be determined by giving the drug during either the learning phase or the recall phase.

Motor Performance

Reaction Time. One of the simplest measures of motor performance is reaction time. The reaction time apparatus is basically a telegraph key connected to a timer. The experimental subject is instructed to press the key as fast as possible at a given signal. The timer starts at the beginning of the signal and stops when the key is depressed. This is the reaction time. Usually the signal is either a sound, such as a tone or a buzzer, or a light. Reaction time is normally faster to a sound than to a visual stimulus.

In a choice reaction time test, there are a number of stimuli and a number of different response keys. The subject is instructed to press a different key for each stimulus. When the task is made more difficult in this way, reaction time slows considerably.

Tapping Rate. Another measure of motor performance is tapping rate. In this task the subject taps with a stylus on a metal plate, and the number of taps in a fixed period of time is counted.

Hand Steadiness. Hand steadiness also is measured with a very simple apparatus. The experimental subject is instructed to hold a stylus in a hole drilled in a metal plate. The stylus and the metal plate are both connected to a low-amperage electrical source, and every time the stylus touches the metal plate, it operates a counter. If the hand is held steady, the stylus will not touch the metal often, but with an unsteady hand, the edges of the hole will be touched frequently.

Pursuit Rotor. A common machine for measuring not only motor behavior but also the ability to coordinate the hand and the eye is the pursuit rotor. With this device, the subject is instructed to hold the end of the stylus on a point on a rotating disk. The total time the subject is able to hold the stylus on the moving spot is a measure of hand-eye coordination.

Driving. Because driving is such a necessary and common activity, it is important to know the effect many drugs have on the ability of a person to operate an automobile. Determining the effect of a drug on driving ability, however, is not as easy as it might seem. To begin with, driving is a complex activity requiring many skills of perception, motor control, and judgment. There is much more involved than simply moving a car from one place to another. Researchers have tried to assess driving skill by using many different strategies. Some simply have their subjects drive a car through city traffic and have professional driving instructors rate their performance on a number of factors. One difficulty with this approach is that the demands of the task will be different for each person tested because traffic conditions are constantly changing, but the main problem is that it is unethical to permit subjects to drive in real traffic and endanger their lives and the lives of others if there is any danger that their skills might be impaired by drugs.

To get around these problems, researchers sometimes have their subjects operate a vehicle around a closed course where various demands are made on the skill of the driver. This approach is more artificial but safer, and because the task is the same for each subject, comparisons are more easily made between and within subjects.

One difficulty with using a real car is that it is sometimes difficult to measure a subject's performance accurately. You can tell if the subject knocks over a pylon, but you will not be able to determine whether the error resulted because the object was not seen, the subject could not estimate the speed of the car, or the reaction time was too slow. To answer such questions, many researchers do not use cars at all; they use computerized driving simulators that are capable of measuring a subject's reaction time, steering ability, and ability to react to specific crises. It is even possible to measure the subject's eye movements while driving.

MEASURING BEHAVIOR IN NONHUMANS

Unconditioned Behavior

The simplest measure of behavior in nonhumans is how much of it there is. Such measures are usually referred to as *spontaneous motor activity (SMA)*. SMA may be measured in a number of ways, but usually the animal is placed in an *open field*, a large open box, and its movements are measured. This is sometimes done by drawing a grid on the floor of the open field and counting the number of times the animal crosses a line. Sometimes the measure of activity is recorded automatically; light beams are shone across the floor, and photocells count the number of times these beams are broken by the moving animal.

Much can also be learned simply by observing the behavior of animals after they have been given drugs. Some classes of drugs cause the animal to exhibit stereotyped behavior, which is the continuous repetition of a simple act such as rearing or head bobbing. Other drugs may cause sleep or convulsions.

Conditioned Behavior

Learned behavior is frequently classified by whether it is a result of *respondent* or *operant* conditioning. This distinction does not represent two types of learning; rather, it arises from attempts to condition two different types of behavior, reflexive or voluntary. Respondent conditioning is also known as *classical* or *Pavlovian conditioning,* since it was the first type of learning to be studied systematically and was first investigated by Ivan Pavlov, the great Russian physiologist.

Respondent behavior is reflexive in the sense that it is under the control of well-defined stimuli in the environment. When a dog salivates at the sight of food, the salivation is respondent behavior under the control of the stimulus of food.

Pavlov found that if he paired the sight of food with a neutral stimulus such as a ringing bell, the bell alone would come to elicit the salivation. Although Pavlov's studies of drug effects on respondent conditioning were some of the very first studies in behavioral pharmacology, such studies are rare in behavioral pharmacology today.

Operant behavior is behavior that appears to be voluntary and is not elicited by any apparent stimulus in the environment. Operant behavior may be conditioned if it is followed by a reinforcing stimulus such as food. A dog that learns to beg for food at the table is demonstrating operant conditioning. The begging is the operant, and it is maintained by the occasional delivery of food that the begging provides. If begging no longer results in the delivery of food, the begging stops.

The principles of operant conditioning are thought to apply to nearly all behavior of all animals. Operant behavior is usually studied in the laboratory using a *Skinner box*. A Skinner box is a small cage attached to an apparatus that will deliver small quantities of food or water. It also contains a *manipulandum*, something that the animal can manipulate or move (a bar, lever, or knob, for example). Figure 2–3 shows a Skinner box for a rat. In this box there is a food delivery system that delivers one small pellet of rat food at a time. The manipulandum is a lever on the wall near the food dish.

To study operant conditioning, it is usual to use an animal that has been deprived of food or water so that these can act as rewards for performing the desired operant (in this case, pressing the lever). Each lever press is detected electronically and causes food to be delivered. In this way the rat is rewarded, or *reinforced*, each time it makes the desired response. Once the rat has learned this response, it makes it frequently and reliably. However, the first time it is placed in the box, it may not depress the lever on its own, so a procedure called *shaping* is used. In shaping, the researcher first reinforces the rat for going near the lever. Then, when the rat is approaching the lever reliably, the researcher waits until the rat touches the lever before delivering food. Eventually the behavior of the rat is shaped by rewarding closer and closer approximations of the desired behavior until it is pressing the lever and being rewarded electronically.

Schedules of Reinforcement

To maintain this behavior, it is not usually necessary to reward the rat with food every time it presses the lever. Animals will usually respond many times for one reinforcement, and in most operant research this approach is required. Sometimes reinforcement is given after a specific number of responses, and sometimes reinforcements are given on the basis of time. The term *schedule of reinforcement* refers to the pattern

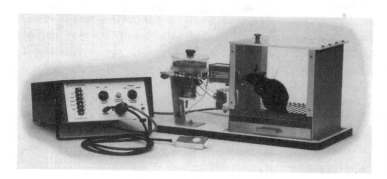

Figure 2–3 A Skinner box for a rat. (Courtesy of Gerbrands Corporation, Arlington, Massachusetts 02174.)

that determines when reinforcements are to be given.

Each schedule of reinforcement engenders a characteristic pattern of responding that will be seen no matter what the species or organism or the type of reinforcer. These patterns are reliable and predictable, and they are sensitive to the effects of many drugs. Behavioral pharmacologists have found them a useful means of analyzing the behavioral effects of drugs because specific schedules are more sensitive to some drugs than others, and similar drugs affect schedule-controlled behavior in a similar manner.

Not only do schedules provide a powerful method for analyzing and classifying drugs, but the study of the effects of drugs on operant behavior is useful in other respects. It is believed that most human behavior, while very complex, is ultimately controlled by reinforcements just as the behavior of the animal in a Skinner box is. It is believed that by carefully studying the effects of a drug on operant behavior, we can provide valuable information that will help us understand the effects of the drug on the behavior of humans.

Ratio Schedules

When reinforcement is based on the number of responses an animal makes, the schedule is known as a *ratio schedule*. On a *fixed ratio (FR)* schedule, the animal is required to make a fixed number of responses in order to be reinforced. For example, on an FR 30 schedule, every 30th response produces a reinforcement. If only 29 responses are made, the reinforcement is never given. A *variable ratio (VR)* schedule is similar except that the number of required responses varies randomly so that at any given time the occurrence of a reinforced response cannot be predicted. A VR 30 schedule will produce a reinforcement every 30 responses on the average. FR schedules usually engender a pattern of responding where there is a pause after each reinforcement followed by responding at a high rate until

the next reinforcement occurs. VRs usually cause a steady rate of responding with few pauses.

Interval Schedules

On an interval schedule, an animal's responding is reinforced only if a period of time has elapsed since some event such as a previous reinforcement. Responses that the animal makes during that time are recorded on the cumulative record but do not influence the delivery of reinforcement. On a *fixed interval (FI)* schedule, a response is reinforced only after a fixed time has elapsed. A typical example might be an FI 3 schedule where the animal must wait three minutes after the delivery of a reinforcement for a response to be reinforced again. Responding on an FI is characterized by a pause after reinforcement followed by an ever-increasing response rate until a high rate of responding is reached, which remains constant until the next reinforcement is given. On a *variable interval (VI)* schedule, the interval is randomly determined, and the animal shows fast, consistent rate of responding with no pauses. When a value is specified for a VI, such as VI 2, this indicates that the interval is an average of two minutes long.

Avoidance Schedules

Not only will animals learn to press a lever to obtain appetitive rewards like food, but they will also learn to avoid unpleasant stimuli such as electric shocks. Avoidance schedules are of two basic types, signaled or unsignaled.

On a *signaled avoidance* schedule, the animal is given a stimulus such as a buzzer or a light as a warning that a shock is coming. The warning comes several seconds before the shock, and if the animal makes a response during that time, the warning stimulus is turned off and the shock never comes. If the animal does not respond, the shock comes on, and the animal can then *escape* from the shock by responding.

This type of avoidance task has proved to be a valuable tool in analyzing the effects of drugs. It has been found that drugs useful in treating anxiety in humans interfere with an animal's ability to avoid shock. These drugs block avoidance behavior during the signal but do not have any effect on the animal's ability to turn off or escape from the shock when it does come. This finding shows that the drug has not interfered with the ability of the animal to respond but has selectively blocked the motivation to avoid the shock.

In *unsignaled avoidance* (also known as *Sidman avoidance)*, shock is programmed at regular intervals. Every time a response is made, the shock is postponed for a period of time. If the animal responds at a steady rate, it can avoid getting the shock, but if it pauses longer than the scheduled shock interval, it will receive a shock. As the name suggests, the shock is not signaled, and the only cue as to when it is coming is the passage of time.

Punishment.   Responding that is maintained by appetitive rewards may be suppressed if it is also punished with electric shocks. This behavior is usually measured by having the animal respond on a VI schedule that produces a steady rate of responding. At various times during a session a stimulus is turned on lasting for a minute or two. During this stimulus each response is followed by a shock. Responding during this stimulus will be suppressed. The frequency and intensity of the shock can be manipulated to produce a specific amount of suppression. Some varieties of drugs, such as barbiturates, increase the frequency of behavior that has been suppressed by punishment. Other drugs, such as amphetamine, lack this ability.

Stimulus Properties of Drugs

Another method of analyzing the effects of drugs is by their stimulus properties, that is, their ability to act as a discriminative stimulus in a discrimination learning task. In this type of task, a hungry animal, usually a rat, is given a choice of two levers to press. In some sessions lever A will be reinforced, and in other sessions lever B will be reinforced. The reinforcement is on an FR 20 schedule so that without a cue to guide it, the rat will not know which lever will produce the food until it has made at least 20 responses. In this situation the only cue is the presence of a drug. On days when lever A is reinforced, the rat is injected with a drug, but on days when lever B is reinforced, it is injected with saline. After a short period of training, the rat will learn to discriminate between the drug and saline, and on drug days it starts off responding on lever A and on saline days it starts off on lever B. Thus the first 20 responses on any given day will show whether the rat thinks it has been injected with the drug or saline.

Animals are capable of discriminating even low doses of most drugs, but this is not the most interesting aspect of the type of drug state discrimination. We can do several things in this experiment that will tell us a great deal about the drug. One often-used test is to give the rat a different drug and see how it causes the rat to behave. If the rat makes the response usually made to the training drug, it is said to *generalize* to that drug, and this result tells us that the two drugs are perceived as similar by the rat. Usually rats will generalize to drugs that are members of the same class. These responses can be helpful in screening new drugs.

Drug state discrimination studies are also useful in determining the biochemical mechanisms by which a drug produces its subjective effects. This is done primarily through the use of antagonist drugs. For example, it can be demonstrated that the stimulus properties of amphetamine can be blocked by the drug AMPT. AMPT blocks the enzyme that creates the catecholamine neurotransmitters (see Chapter 4). This finding tells us that the subjective effects of amphetamine depend on catecholamines in the brain.

Similar techniques have been used in human research where subjects are given two capsules and asked to guess which one contained a drug similar to a previously administered test drug. In addition, standardized tests of subjective effects such as the ARCI have been used to assess the similarity of the subjective effects of two drugs.

DEVELOPMENT AND TESTING OF PSYCHOTHERAPEUTIC DRUGS

Before any new drug can be put on the market it must undergo rigorous development and testing to prove that it is effective and safe. Only then will it be approved by governmental agencies for sale as a medicine. In the United States approval is granted by the Food and Drug Administration (FDA).

Because we do not really understand the biochemical basis of mental illness, we cannot specifically design drugs in the laboratory with any certainty that they will have a desired effect on psychiatric symptoms. Instead, the laboratories of pharmaceutical companies synthesize many new chemicals they think might be effective. These drugs are then screened using nonhumans to determine first if they are toxic and then whether they have effects similar to known therapeutically useful drugs. It is known, for example, that drugs that are useful in treating anxiety will block avoidance responding in doses that have no effect on escape responding. Drugs that are useful in treating depressive illness will block the depression in behaviors caused by reserpine. In fact, many of the procedures described earlier in this chapter are used in the initial screening process of behaviorally active drugs.

When a new drug appears to be reasonably safe and shows interesting behavioral properties in nonhumans, it goes to phase 1 of human testing, which assesses the toxicity and side effects of the drug on healthy human volunteers. In phase 2 the drug is tested on patients under very carefully supervised conditions. If phases 1 and 2 show that the drug has minimal toxic effects and also has a potential therapeutic effect, it then goes to phase 3, expanded clinical trials, which are usually carried out in university teaching hospitals and other institutions and often use the three-groups design discussed earlier. This research is usually carried out by a number of independent investigators under contract to the pharmaceutical companies. If phase 3 investigations are successful, the drug is licensed and marketed. The research, however, does not stop here. Phase 4 involves the accumulation of data on the success of the drug as used in the clinic and attempts to identify adverse effects that were not apparent in the short-term testing of the early stages. In phase 4 improved dosing schedules may be developed, and individuals who are at risk of having adverse reactions to the drug can be identified (Baldessarini, 1985, p. 5).

As you can imagine, the entire process can be very expensive. It is usually paid for by a pharmaceutical company. In exchange for all this expense, the company is granted a patent giving it the exclusive right to sell the drug for a period of time so that it can recover its investment and make a profit.

CHAPTER SUMMARY

- Scientific experiments consist of an *independent variable* that is manipulated by a researcher and a *dependent variable* that is measured. In most experimental research in behavioral pharmacology, the independent variable is the presence of drug in the body and the dependent variable is some aspect of behavior.

- Treatment of control subjects in an experiment should be as similar as possible to treatment of experimental subjects. For this reason, control subjects are usually given a *placebo*, an inactive substance administered in exactly the same way as the drug. This procedure controls for differences that result from the act of drug administration.

- To determine whether the differences between experiment and control conditions mean anything, a statistical test is often used. Statistical tests tell the researcher how frequently there would be differences as large as in the experiment if the drug had no effect at all and all differences were due to chance alone.

- In *nonexperimental* drug research, when relationships between two measured variables are found, one cannot assume the existence of any causal relationships between variables.

- Although the name *psychology* literally means "the study of the mind," modern psychology is the study of behavior.

- *Level of arousal* ranges from deep sleep to mild excitement but may extend into pathological states of mania and convulsions at the upper end and coma and death at the low end. Arousal level is only partly related to both mood and general activity.

- In one stage of sleep, *REM sleep*, there is an activated EEG and eyeballs move under closed lids. REM sleep occurs in cycles about every 90 minutes throughout the night.

- The performance of the senses is determined by measuring their *threshold*. *Vigilance* tests measure the ability to detect a certain signal in a group of signals. Motor performance may be measured by simple or choice reaction time, tapping rate, hand steadiness, or pursuit rotor tests.

- Conditioned behavior may be of two types, *respondent* or *operant*. In respondent conditioning, involuntary reflexive behavior is brought under the control of a previously neutral stimulus. This is also known as *classical* or *Pavlovian conditioning*. In operant conditioning, voluntary behavior is brought under control by delivery of contingent reinforcements or rewards.

- When reinforcement is not given for every response but is given according to some pattern, the pattern is called a *schedule of reinforcement*.

- Animals can also be trained to *avoid* and *escape* a noxious stimulus such as an electric shock.

- Animals can be trained to make one response after being given a drug and different response after being given saline or a different drug. The responses of an animal trained to discriminate a drug can be a useful tool in testing the biochemical mechanisms of a drug.

3

Drug State Conditioning, Behavioral Tolerance, and Dissociation

In Chapter 2 we looked at conditioned behaviors as dependent variables in drug research; that is, we asked how drugs affect conditioned behavior. In this chapter we will look at some ways in which conditioning can alter the effects of drugs and can explain phenomena such as tolerance and withdrawal. We will also discuss dissociation, a demonstration of how drugs can alter memory and learned behavior.

CLASSICAL CONDITIONING OF DRUG EFFECTS

At the end of the nineteenth century, Ivan Pavlov and his colleagues in St. Petersburg, Russia, first discovered and demonstrated the principles of respondent conditioning (also known as classical conditioning) that were outlined in Chapter 2. Researchers in Pavlov's laboratory were also the

first to show that the effects of a drug could be conditioned to neutral stimuli present at the time the drug was having its effect. One of these experiments was conducted in the following manner:

A dog was given a small dose of apomorphine subcutaneously and after one to two minutes a note of definite pitch was sounded during a considerable time. While the note was still sounding the drug began to take effect upon the dog: the animal grew restless, began to moisten its lips with its tongue, secreted saliva and showed some disposition to vomit. After the experimenter had reinforced the tone with apomorphine several times it was found that the sound of the note alone sufficed to produce all the active symptoms of the drug, only in a less degree [experiments by Podkopaev]. (Pavlov, 1927, p. 35)

Later they were able to show that after a number of injections, the preliminaries to the injection and the administration procedure itself were sufficient to produce the salivation and other effects of the drug even though no drug was given. In Pavlov's terminology, the drug was the unconditioned stimulus (UCS); the effects of the drug, the salivation and vomiting, were the unconditioned response (UCR); the stimuli preceding the drug were the conditioned stimuli (CS); and the salivation and nausea produced by these stimuli alone were the conditioned response (CR).

Since these classical experiments, conditioned drug effects have been demonstrated many times in many different laboratories. It has also been demonstrated that withdrawal responses can be conditioned in a similar manner by presenting a neutral stimulus during withdrawal symptoms (Goldberg & Schuster, 1970). The conditioning of drug effects to neutral stimuli has been used to explain a number of drug-related phenomena. For example, heroin addicts will sometimes inject themselves with water and other ineffective substances when they are unable to get the drug they require. Such procedures ease withdrawal symptoms most likely because they cause a conditioned drug effect. In addition, former heroin addicts who have gone through withdrawal will frequently experience withdrawal symptoms when they return to places where they have experienced withdrawal before. As the following example illustrates, there can be little doubt that these conditioned withdrawal symptoms play an important part in the relapse to drug use in post-dependent addicts (O'Brien, 1976).

The patient was a 28-year-old man with a ten-year history of narcotic addiction. He was married and the father of two children. He reported that, while he was addicted, he was arrested and incarcerated for six months. He reported experiencing severe withdrawal during the first four or five days in custody, but later he began to feel well. He gained weight, felt like a new man, and decided that he was finished with drugs. He thought about his children and looked forward to returning to his former job. On the way home after his release from prison, he began thinking of drugs and feeling nauseated. As the subway approached his stop, he began sweating, tearing from his eyes, and gagging. This was an area where he had frequently experienced narcotic withdrawal symptoms while trying to acquire drugs. As he got off the subway he vomited onto the tracks. He soon bought drugs and was relieved. The following day he again experienced craving and withdrawal symptoms in his neighborhood, and he again relieved the symptoms by injecting heroin. The cycle repeated itself over the next few days and soon he became readdicted. (O'Brien, 1976, p. 533)

The conditioning of drug effects and withdrawal symptoms is more complicated than it would appear at first because the unconditioned response to the drug and the conditioned response are not always the same. In the example from Pavlov's lab, the effect of the apomorphine was to cause salivation, and the effect of the tone, or CS, after it had been paired with the apomorphine also was salivation. Atropine is a drug that blocks the secretion of saliva and causes a dry mouth. You might expect that, after conditioning, a stimulus associated with atropine would also cause a dry mouth. In fact, it has the opposite effect; if injections of atropine are paired with a stimulus, that stimulus will cause *excessive* salivation, not a dry mouth.

A number of experiments have demonstrated these "paradoxical" effects, and some researchers have suggested that the majority of conditioned drug effects are in the direction opposite to the unconditioned effect of a drug (S. Siegel, 1983). As we shall see shortly, this phenomenon has an important role in the development of tolerance.

The reason why some drug effects condition one way and other effects condition in the opposite direction is not well understood, but in 1982 a compelling theoretical explanation was put forward by Rolff Eikelboom and Jane Stewart of Concordia University in Montreal. Figure 3–1 outlines how their theory works. The theory makes two assumptions. The first is that bodily functions are controlled by self-adjusting feedback mechanisms similar to the one in this figure, a model of the system that controls the amount of saliva in the mouth. If saliva levels are too low or too high, the sensory input from the mouth sends messages to the central control center, which in turn causes the salivary glands either to work harder or to slow down to keep the levels just right.

The theory also proposes that what actually gets conditioned to the CS is the activity in the central nervous system (CNS) at the time the CS is presented. If the effect of the drug is to stimulate the salivation center in the CNS, then a CS paired with the drug will produce salivation as well. Such an effect is produced by apomorphine, as can be seen in Figure 3–1. If a neutral stimulus is presented at the same time as apomorphine, that stimulus will come to produce salivation.

The picture is somewhat more complex if the effect of the drug is in the peripheral nervous system (PNS). Eikelboom and Stewart maintain that events in the PNS are not conditioned, but if the CNS tries to compensate for the effect, the compensation is what gets conditioned. For example, atropine causes a dry mouth because it blocks the synapses that control the salivary glands, and these stop operating. This is an effect in the PNS

and cannot be conditioned to a CS. Next, the sensors in the mouth detect the lack of saliva and send messages to the central control center in the CNS that the mouth needs more saliva. This center becomes activated and commands the salivary glands to secrete, which they are unable to do because of the drug. In other words, because of the dry mouth, the CNS salivation center is activated. If a stimulus is paired with atropine administration it will also be paired with an activation of the central system even though the mouth is dry. Later, when the CS is presented without the atropine, the conditioned response will be an activation of the central control center, and this will cause an excess of saliva.

Since most functions in the body work on this type of feedback control system, most conditioned drug effects can be thought of in the same way. Most drug effects that are a result of activity in the CNS will have the UCR the same as the CR, but if the drug effect is on the PNS, the CR will be the opposite of the UCR.

BEHAVIORAL TOLERANCE

In Chapter 1 we discussed several types of tolerance, but discussion of behavioral tolerance was deferred to this chapter because it depended on a knowledge of conditioning, both operant and respondent. There are two types of *behavioral tolerance*: One is based on operant conditioning and the other on classical or respondent conditioning. The operant type of behavior tolerance takes place when the organism learns through operant conditioning to change behavior to compensate for the effect the drug is having.

One of the first experiments in this area was done by Judith Campbell and Lewis Seiden at the University of Chicago (Campbell & Seiden, 1973). They trained rats to respond for food reinforcement on a DRL schedule. On this schedule the animal is reinforced only if it waits for a fixed period of time between responses. In other words, it is reinforced for responding at a low

Figure 3–1 This model proposed by Eikelboom and Stewart (1982) explains the opposite conditioning effects of apomorphine and atropine on salivation. See the text for further explanation.

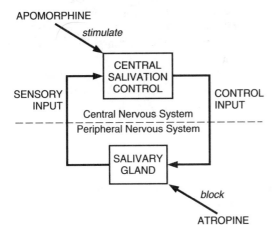

rate. When amphetamine is given it stimulates responding, and the rat loses reinforcements because it cannot wait long enough between responses. For 28 sessions, Campbell and Seiden gave amphetamine to one group of rats immediately before placing them in a Skinner box where they were reinforced on a DRL schedule. Another group of rats was given the same number of injections and the same number of sessions on the DRL schedule, but the amphetamine was given after the DRL trials. Over the period of the experiment, the amphetamine-pretreated rats developed tolerance and were able to obtain more and more reinforcements, but when the other rats were tested on the DRL with amphetamine, they performed as though they had never received the drug; they had no tolerance. If the tolerance shown by the first group was the result of metabolic and physiological changes, if should have shown up in both groups. The only explanation for the difference is that the rats learned to alter their behavior to compensate for the change that the amphetamine caused.

The same effect can occur in humans with alcohol. At exactly the same blood alcohol levels, the behavior of heavy drinkers is frequently less severely affected by alcohol than the behavior of nondrinkers. The reason could be that the drinkers have had a chance to practice behaving normally while intoxicated, and the abstainers have not.

Many tolerance effects can also be explained by classical conditioning. This type of research was pioneered by Shepard Siegel of McMaster University in Hamilton, Ontario. Siegel investigated the development of tolerance to the analgesic effect of morphine. To test analgesia, he placed rats on a metal plate that was heated to 54 degrees Celsius. After a few seconds on this plate, rats normally lift a forepaw to their mouth as if they were licking it. This test is known as the *paw lick test*, and the measure of analgesia is the latency or the length of time the rat waits before licking. After an injection of morphine, the paw lick latency increases, indicating that the

morphine has reduced the animal's sensitivity to pain. With repeated trials, the latency tends to get shorter and shorter as tolerance to the morphine develops (S. Siegel, 1975).

In Siegel's experiment, he was able to demonstrate that rats would show tolerance to the analgesic effects of morphine only if they were given the paw lick test in the same room where repeated morphine injections had been experienced earlier. Animals given morphine in the colony room where they were normally housed and tested in a different room had long latencies similar to those of animals that had never been given morphine at all. The tolerance to morphine was dependent on the environment in which the drug had been experienced.

To explain this effect, Siegel proposed that the special environment that is always associated with the drug acts like a CS and becomes conditioned to the drug effect, but the CRs that it elicits are compensatory. The environment associated with the administration of the drug elicits physiological responses opposite to the effect of the drug. These changes help prepare the rat for the drug and diminish its effect; that is, they cause tolerance.

In support of his theory, Siegel was also able to show that if he injected a rat with saline and gave it the paw lick test in an environment that had previously been associated with repeated injections of morphine, the animal would show hyperalgesia, an increased sensitivity to pain. This hyperalgesia is the compensatory response that had been produced by the morphine environment through conditioning.

Box 3–1 gives another example of how this type of tolerance can protect humans and nonhumans from a heroin overdose.

Behavioral Tolerance and Withdrawal

Just as learning processes can explain some tolerance, learning may also be responsible for withdrawal. Earlier we saw how compensatory responses may be conditioned to a particular en-

BOX 3–1   The Mystery of Heroin Overdose

One of the greatest risks of being a heroin addict is death from heroin overdose. Each year about 1 percent of all heroin addicts in the United States die from an overdose of heroin despite having developed a fantastic tolerance to the effects of the drug. In a nontolerant person the estimated lethal dose of heroin may range from 200 to 500 mg, but addicts have tolerated doses as high as 1,800 mg without even being sick (Brecher and the editors of Consumer Reports, 1972). No doubt, some overdoses are a result of mixing heroin with other drugs, but many appear to result from a sudden loss of tolerance. Addicts have been killed one day by a dose that was readily tolerated the day before. An explanation for this sudden loss of tolerance has been suggested by Shepard Siegel of McMaster University and his associates Rily Hinson, Marvin Krank, and Jane McCully.

Siegel reasoned that the tolerance to heroin was partly conditioned to the environment where the drug was normally administered. If the drug is consumed in a new setting, much of the conditioned tolerance will disappear, and the addict will be more likely to overdose. To test this theory, Siegel and associates ran the following experiment (S. Siegel et al., 1982):

Rats were given daily intravenous injections for 30 days. The injections, either a dextrose placebo or heroin, were given in either the animal colony room or a different room where there was constant white noise. The drug and the placebo were given on alternate days, and the drug condition always corresponded with a particular environment so that for some rats the heroin was always administered in the white noise room and the placebo was always given in the colony. For other rats the heroin was always given in the colony and the placebo was always given in the white noise room. Another group of rats served as a control: These were injected in different rooms on alternate days but were injected only with the dextrose and had no experience with heroin at all.

All rats were then injected with a large dose of heroin: 15 mg/kg. The rats in one group, labeled the ST group, were given the heroin in the same room where they had previously been given heroin. The other rats, the DT group, were given the heroin in the room where they had previously been given the placebo.

Siegel found that 96 percent of the control group died, showing the lethal effect of the heroin in nontolerant animals. Rats in the DT group who received heroin were partly tolerant, and only 64 percent died. Only 32 percent of the ST rats died, showing that the tolerance was even greater when the overdose test was done in the same environment where the drug had previously been administered.

Siegel suggested that one reason that addicts suddenly lose their tolerance could be that they take the drug in a different or unusual environment like the rats in the DT group. Surveys of heroin addicts admitted to hospitals suffering from heroin overdose tend to support this conclusion. Many addicts report that they had taken the near-fatal dose in an unusual circumstance or that their normal pattern was different on that day (S. Siegel et al., 1982).

vironment where the drug is repeatedly given. Later, if the animal is placed in that environment without the drug, it will show the conditioned compensatory responses. Since compensatory responses are physiological changes opposite to the drug's effect, they are just like withdrawal responses; therefore, some aspects of withdrawal are learned and may be associated with specific stimuli and situations (S. Siegel, 1983). In the example of conditioned withdrawal symptoms given earlier, where the addict's eyes tear and he begins sweating when he comes into the subway station where he had previously acquired drugs, it is possible that what he felt was his body preparing itself for an injection of heroin that it had become conditioned to expect in that environment.

DISSOCIATION

Learning while under the influence of a drug may not be easily recalled after the effects of the drug have worn off, and, conversely, information learned while drug-free is not easily recalled when intoxicated. This phenomenon, known as *dissociation*, has been recognized for many years but has been systematically investigated only since 1945.

The first account of dissociation appeared in 1830 in a British medical text. It was related by George Coombe, who stated that "before memory can exist, the organs require to be affected in the same manner, or be in a state analogous to that in which they were, when the impression was first received" (quoted in S. Siegel, 1982, pp. 257–258). As an example of this phenomenon, Coombe cited the case of an Irish porter who had lost track of a valuable parcel while drunk. Later, while sober, he was unable to remember anything about it. The next time he was intoxicated, however, he remembered exactly where he had put it.

The same effect was also used in the plot of a famous British detective novel, *The Moonstone*

by Wilkie Collins, published in 1868. In this novel the detective finds a valuable diamond that was hidden for protection by a young man while he was under the influence of *laudanum*. Laudanum was a patent medicine that contained opium and was widely used by many writers in the nineteenth century (see Chapter 11). The jewel was found when the young man took laudanum again and remembered where he had hidden it (S. Siegel, 1982).

Dissociation research often uses the following design: Experimental subjects are assigned to four groups, and they all learn a task on day 1 and are tested for recall on day 2. Group 1 gets a drug on both training and testing days, group 2 gets the drug during training but not during testing, group 3 get no drug on training days and drug during testing, and group 4 does not get the drug on either day. The design and results of this type of experiment are shown in Table 3–1. Typically, subjects in groups 1 and 4 on day 2 are able to recall the training they received on day 1, but the subjects in both groups 2 and 3 have difficulty remembering what they learned on day 1 because of the change in drug state between these two days.

Dissociation has been demonstrated in a number of species, with many drugs and using a variety of memory tests (Overton, 1972), and it may actually be a cause of much day-to-day forgetting. It has been shown that many drugs we consume regularly every day in moderate doses such as coffee, tobacco, and alcohol, especially when consumed together, can cause dissociation in a memory task that involved learning a route through a simple map (Lowe, 1988).

Dissociation also may have an important influence on drug self-administration because it means that much of what we learn about drug taking while we are not under the influence of the drug may not be easily remembered after we take the drug. An alcoholic, for example, may experience the adverse and punishing consequences of drinking while sober and therefore may not remember these consequences while drunk. Drug

TABLE 3–1   The Design of a Typical Dissociation Experiment. On the training day, subjects are taught a task, and on the testing day, they are tested for recall of that task. For groups 1 and 4 the state does not change, but subjects in groups 2 and 3 are tested under drug states different from training. If the drug causes dissociation, subjects in both groups 2 and 3 have difficulty remembering.

Group	Training Day	Testing Day	Result
1	Drug	Drug	Memory
2	Drug	Saline	No memory
3	Saline	Drug	No memory
4	Saline	Saline	Memory

education programs are always aimed at people while they are sober. Information acquired in this state may have little influence on a person after he or she takes a drug.

CHAPTER SUMMARY

- Pavlov was the first to demonstrate that stimuli paired with the administration of a drug a sufficient number of times will eventually come to elicit some of the effects of the drug through *classical conditioning* processes. Later research has shown that quite often the effect that becomes conditioned is a physiological response opposite to the unconditioned effect of the drug, or a *compensatory response*.

- According to one theory, drug effects caused by a drug's direct action on the CNS will be conditioned directly. That is, the *conditioned effect* will be similar to the drug effect. But if the drug effect arises from the action of the drug outside the CNS, what will be conditioned is the opposite or compensatory response, which represents an attempt of the CNS to compensate for the anticipated effect of the drug.

- It has been demonstrated that if a drug interferes with the ability of an organism to obtain reinforcement, tolerance will develop quickly, but drug effects that do not interfere with reinforced behavior develop little, if any, behavioral tolerance.

- *Conditioned tolerance* is dependent on the stimuli associated with drug administration. Stimuli that are always present when a drug is given will come to elicit conditioned compensatory responses that diminish the effect of the drug. This tolerance does not occur when the drug is given in the absence of these stimuli.

- *Dissociation* occurs when learning that takes place during intoxication is not recalled well in the sober state, and vice versa.

4

Neurophysiology, Neurotransmitters, and the Nervous System

Virtually all behavior is under the control of the nervous system, and the effect of most behaviorally active drugs can ultimately be traced to a direct or an indirect action on some aspect of the functioning of the nervous system. It is therefore necessary to have at least a rudimentary grasp of the normal functioning of the nervous system to understand the behavioral effect of drugs.

THE NEURON

Like all other tissues in the body, the nervous system is made up of cells. Some of these cells, called *glial* cells, are not excitable, and provide structural and metabolic functions in the nervous system. The other cells, called *neurons,* are excitable and function to transmit and analyze information. They are responsible for receiving sensory information from the outside, for integrating informa-

tion, for storing information, and for controlling the action of the muscles and glands—everything that we see and understand as behavior.

Nerve cells come in many shapes and sizes, but they all have a number of identifiable parts. A typical nerve cell is shown in Figure 4–1. Like all other cells in the body, it has a *nucleus* that contains genetic information and controls the metabolism of the cell. The cell is covered by a *membrane* and is filled with a fluid called *cytoplasm.* All nerve cells have a *cell body,* which is the largest part of the cell and contains the nucleus. Arising from the cell body are several structures. At one end are projections called *dendrites.* These divide into smaller and smaller fibers. The *axon* is a long process attached to the cell body at the *axon hillock* which is located at the opposite end of the cell body from the dendrites. The axon is usually covered by a layer of fatty material called the *myelin sheath.* The

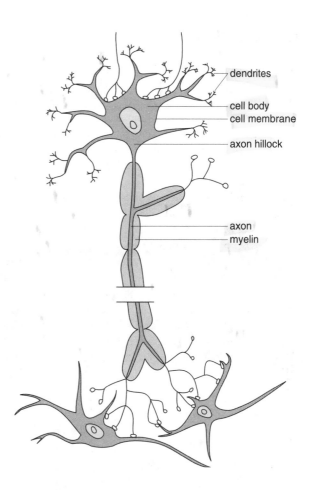

dendrites

cell body
cell membrane

axon hillock

axon
myelin

Figure 4–1 A typical nerve cell. Note that in this case the neuron receives input from synapses from several other nerve cells at its dendrites and cell body and that it also has synapses on other nerve cells.

myelin sheath is an extension of a special type of glial cell that wraps itself around the axon.

As we have seen in Chapter 1, cell membranes are made up of two layers of lipid molecules (see Figure 1–5) with large protein molecules embedded. In nerve cells these large protein molecules have special functions that make the cells excitable and capable of conveying, storing, and integrating information. These actions are accomplished by controlling the flow of ions through the membrane.

Resting Potential

If we take two very fine wires and insert one inside a neuron and place the other just outside the membrane, and then attach the wires to a voltmeter, we will see that there is a difference in electrical charge; the inside is slightly negatively charged with respect to the outside. A voltmeter is a device that measures differences in electrical potential between two places, the same sort of instrument used to test batteries. This potential difference across the membrane is called the *resting potential*. The resting potential varies from cell to cell but is usually about –70 millivolts. (One millivolt is 1/1,000 volt. A standard flashlight battery has a charge of 1.5 volts.) The reason for this potential difference is that there is an uneven distribution of ions between the inside and the outside of the cell. Ions are particles that possess an electrical charge. The ions described in Chapter 1 were usually large drug molecules; the ions that are responsible for the resting potential of a cell are ionized molecules of the elements potassium (K^+), sodium (Na^+), and chlorine (Cl^-), although some larger molecules of amino acids are also involved. The resting potential exists because there are more positively charged ions than negatively charged ions outside the cell, and the opposite is true inside the cell.

Three processes are responsible for this uneven distribution of ions. The most important of these is an active transport mechanism known as an *ion pump*. Ion pumps are specialized molecules that selectively move ions from one side of a membrane to another. In the case of nerve cells, an ion pump, known as the Na^+/K^+ pump, moves Na^+ ions to the outside and K^+ ions to the inside, but it moves 3 Na^+ ions out for every 2 K^+ ions it moves in, thereby creating an excess of positive ions outside the membrane (see Figure 4–2).

Two other processes are also at work. One is simple diffusion, the tendency for a substance to move from an area of high concentration to an area of lower concentration. The other is electrostatic charge, the tendency for similar electrical charges to repel each other and opposite electrical charges to attract each other; that is, positive ions are repelled by the net positive charge outside the membrane and attracted to the negative charge inside. The reverse is true for negative ions.

If the membrane were completely permeable to ions, diffusion and electrostatic charge would drive ions unevenly distributed by the ion pumps back across the membrane as fast as the pumps could move them, but membranes are not permeable to ions. The only way that ions can move across the membrane is through specialized holes, or channels in the membrane. These are called *ionophores* or *ion channels*. Like ion pumps, ion channels are also large molecules embedded in the cell membrane. They are special-

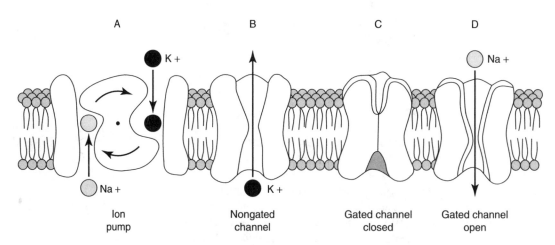

Figure 4–2   *A* shows a representation of an ion pump moving potassium ions (K^+) into a cell through a membrane and sodium ions (Na^+) out of a cell. *B* shows a nongated ion channel that is always open and allows particular ions (in this case, K^+) to move back out of the cell. *C* and *D* show a gated Na^+ ion channel. In panel *C* it is closed, but panel *D* shows it in its open configuration allowing Na^+ back into the cell.

ized so that they will only allow certain ions to pass through and only let them through at a particular rate. There are ion channels for K^+, Na^+, and Cl^-. (There are also channels for calcium Ca^{++} ions, but these are not involved in the resting potential and have a special function described later.) There are two types of ion channels, ones that are always open, and ones that are gated. *Gated ion channels* open and close in response to specific circumstances (see Figure 4–2).

Normally, the nongated channels do not permit ions to flow through the membrane fast enough to neutralize the ion pumps, so that there remains a net positive charge outside. This fact explains the resting potential. However, it should be clear that anything that speeds or slows the passage of ions through the membrane can increase or decrease the resting potential.

Action Potential

The resting potential of a neuron can be increased or decreased. An increase in the resting potential is called *hyperpolarization*, and a decrease is called *depolarization*. We can hyperpolarize a cell by inserting a fine electrode (a fine wire similar to the one described to measure the resting potential) into a neuron and applying electricity that makes the inside even more negative than the outside. The more current we apply, the greater the hyperpolarization. When the current is turned off, the cell returns to its normal resting potential. We can depolarize the cell by reversing the polarity of our electrode and make the inside of the cell less negative with respect to the outside, but depolarizing a neuron can lead to some startling changes. Small amounts of depolarization simply cause the resting potential to decrease, and when the electricity is turned off, the normal resting potential returns, but if the neuron is depolarized past a certain point called the *threshold*, the entire resting potential and the process that maintains it break down.

This breakdown occurs because of special gated ion channels that are sensitive to the voltage difference between the inside and outside of the cell. These *voltage gated ion channels* open when the potential difference is reduced beyond the *threshold*. When they open, they allow the free flow of ions across the membrane. First, sodium channels open and Na^+ ions rush into the cell driven by their concentration gradient (there are many more outside than inside) and their electrostatic charge (they are positively charged, and the outside has a net positive charge). As a result the resting potential of the membrane is neutralized. In fact, the polarity is actually reversed slightly. When this condition occurs, the sodium ion channels close and potassium channels open. Potassium (K^+) ions rush out of the neuron, driven by their concentration gradient and the transient positive charge created by all the Na^+ ions that just entered. Along with the ion pumps this process restores the resting potential.

This breakdown and restoration of the resting potential is known as an *action potential,* and it occurs very quickly. Some cells are capable of producing and recovering from many hundreds of action potentials each second. The term "firing" is often used to indicate an action potential. It is by means of action potentials that the cells in the nervous system integrate and convey information.

The All-or-None Law

Action potentials are always the same no matter how strong a stimulus produces them. As long as a stimulus is strong enough to depolarize a cell to the threshold, it will cause an action potential. Increases in the depolarizing stimulus beyond this point will not change the action potential in any way; regardless of the strength of the stimulus, the action potential will always be the same. This principle is known as the *all-or-none law*.

If all action potentials are the same, how then does a neuron convey information about the strength of the stimulus that is depolarizing it? This information is reflected in the rate at which action potentials are generated. If a depolarizing stimulus is applied continuously to a cell, it will cause the cell to produce repeated action potentials. Weak stimuli that produce low levels of depolarization will permit the membrane a bit of time to recover between action potentials, but more intense depolarization caused by stronger stimuli permits less recovery time between action potentials. As a result, the stronger the depolarizing stimulus, the faster the membrane will fire.

Conduction of Action Potentials

When an action potential is generated at a point on the membrane of an axon, it does not stay there. The Na^+ ions that move into the cell through the ion channels also move sideways along the inside surface of the membrane because of diffusion and electric charge, and this movement reduces the resting potential of the surrounding membrane; that is, it depolarizes it. This depolarization causes the voltage gated ion channels to open and causes another action potential immediately beside the first. In its turn, this new action potential will depolarize the membrane next to it, and so the action potential will sweep across the surface of the membrane away from the stimulus that produced it. In the nervous system, action potentials are generated on the membranes of cell bodies at the axon hillock and move along axons in this way.

Depending on the type of axon, an action potential can move as fast as 100 meters a second. The presence of the myelin coating on the axon greatly speeds the conduction of action potentials along the axon. Myelinated axons can conduct much faster than unmyelinated ones.

Action Potentials from Sensory Neurons

We have seen how action potentials are created when a section of a neuron's membrane is depolarized past its threshold and how the action potential moves along an axon, but the action potentials we have discussed have been artificially created with a stimulating electrode inserted into the cell. Where do natural action potentials come from? Action potentials arise in neurons from several sources. One of these is the outside world. Sensory neurons are specialized nerve cells that are depolarized or hyperpolarized by events in the environment. In the skin are neurons whose cell bodies are depolarized by touch, sending action potentials along their axons into the brain and causing us to experience the sensation of feeling. The stronger the stimulation is, the greater the depolarization is and the faster the sensory neurons generate action. The skin also has nerve cells that are specialized to detect heat, cold, and pain. Cells in the ear are depolarized by vibration, and cells in the muscles are depolarized by movement. In fact, all that we know about the outside world comes to our brains in the form of action potentials generated by these specialized receptor neurons.

THE SYNAPSE

We still have not come to the most interesting part: How neurons communicate with one another. A nerve cell is like any other cell in the body—it is completely surrounded by a membrane. For the information received from the outside world to get from the sensory receptor neuron to other neurons in the brain, there must be a mechanism for one cell to communicate with another. Electron microscopes show that although the membranes of adjacent neurons come extremely close to each other, their membranes never touch, and there is no way that an action potential on one cell can directly depolarize the membrane of another cell. The way in which neurons communicate across this gap is of vital interest to the behavioral pharmacologist because it is this process that is altered in one way or another by many drugs that affect behavior.

Information is transferred between neurons at *synapses*. Synapses occur at the end of the axon of one cell where it terminates close to the dendrites and cell body of another cell. The end of the axon of the first cell may divide into many branches, and these small branches are intertwined with the dendrites of the second cell. Where the axons and dendrites come close to each other, synapses may be found. Figure 4–3 is a schematic drawing of a typical synapse. It is characterized by a swelling called the *terminal bouton* at the termination of the branch of the axon of the presynaptic cell (the cell sending the information) and a thickening on the membrane of the cell body or dendrite of the postsynaptic cell (the cell receiving the information) immediately beneath the bouton. Between the terminal bouton and the postsynaptic cell is a gap call the *synaptic cleft*. Another feature of the synapse is a number of spherical structures in the terminal bouton called *synaptic vesicles.*

Action at a Synapse

When an action potential arrives at the terminal bouton, calcium (Ca^{++}) channels open, and the flow of calcium ions into the cell causes a chemical called a *neurotransmitter* to be released from the synaptic vesicles into the synaptic cleft. The neurotransmitter is stored in the vesicles, and when the action potential arrives, the vesicles move to the membrane at the synaptic cleft and release the neurotransmitter through the cell wall into the cleft. The neurotransmitter diffuses across the cleft, where it comes in contact with the membrane of the postsynaptic cell.

Embedded in the membrane of the postsynaptic cell are specialized molecules called *receptor*

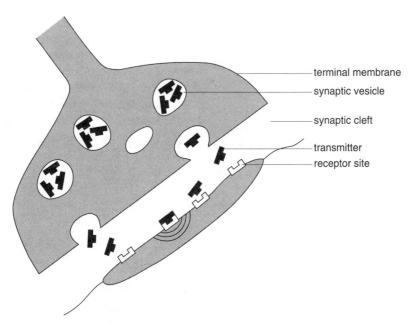

terminal membrane

synaptic vesicle

synaptic cleft

transmitter

receptor site

Figure 4–3 This schematic drawing of a synapse shows the molecules of transmitter normally stored in vesicles being released into the cleft in response to the arrival of an action potential. The transmitter molecules diffuse across the cleft and occupy receptor sites on the membrane of the postsynaptic cell. These events cause changes in the excitability of the postsynaptic cell membrane, either making it easier (excitation) or more difficult (inhibition) to fire.

sites or *recognition sites*. Receptor sites are designed so that molecules of the neurotransmitter will briefly join with them much like a key fitting into a keyhole. When a neurotransmitter with the right configuration (the key) attaches to a receptor site (the keyhole), it causes certain changes to occur in the postsynaptic cell, changes that often result in shifts in its resting potential or a change in its biochemistry. Such changes can be brought about in a number of direct and indirect ways.

Fast-Acting Transmission

In some synapses, receptor sites are connected to a gated ion channel and cause it to open or close. This process is illustrated in Figure 4–4. Depending on the ion channel, this could either increase or decrease the resting potential of the membrane.

Excitation. If the presynaptic cell is producing action potentials at a high rate and it has many synapses on the cell body and dendrites of the postsynaptic cell, a great deal of neurotransmitter will be released and the resting potential of the postsynaptic cell will be strongly affected.

When the transmitter causes the receptor sites to open gated ion channels that permit positively charged ions into the cell, the resting potential will drop closer to the action potential threshold. In other words, the membrane will be depolarized. Depolarization of the postsynaptic membrane has a special name: *excitatory postsynaptic potential (EPSP)*. The faster a presynaptic cell fires, the more neurotransmitter it will release at its synapses and the greater the EPSP it will cause. If enough EPSPs are being produced at the same time, the postsynaptic cell may be depolarized past its threshold, and it will create action potentials in its axon. As described in the section on the all-or-none law, the more the postsynaptic cell is depolarized past its threshold, the faster the cell will fire.

Inhibition. There are also synapses where the neurotransmitter will inhibit the firing of the postsynaptic cell. At these synapses the neurotransmitter causes the receptor site to open ion channels that permit negatively charged ions into the cell. The resting potential increases; that is, the postsynaptic membrane becomes hyperpolarized. As a result, it is harder for the cell to produce action potentials. This condition is called an *inhibitory postsynaptic potential (IPSP)*.

Summation of Excitation and Inhibition. Any neuron in the nervous system may have both inhibitory and excitatory synapses controlling its polarization. The rate at which it fires is determined by the sum of EPSPs and IPSPs occurring at its cell body and dendrites at any given time. Thus it is possible for transmission of information from one cell to another to be modified by activity at inhibitory synapses from a third cell.

The degree to which one cell can influence the firing rate of another depends largely on the number of synapses it has on the cell. If it has many, its influence will be extensive, but if it has only a few, its effect will not be great. A single nerve cell may have a number of synapses on any number of other cells, and so its activity can influence many other cells at once. In addition, a single cell can have synapses on it from many other cells. The firing rate of a cell is determined

Figure 4–4 *A,* a receptor-gated ion channel in the closed configuration. *B,* a transmitter molecule occupying the receptor site and the channel in the open configuration.

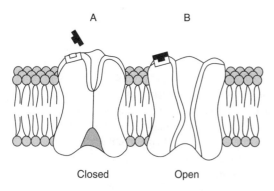

A   B

Closed   Open

by the sum total of all the depolarization and hyperpolarization caused by all the activity at all the synapses on its cell body and dendrites at any particular moment.

In general, the summation of excitatory and inhibitory activity takes place on the cell body and dendrites of a cell. The membrane of the dendrites and cell body is not able to produce action potentials. These are generated at the axon hillock where the axon is attached to the cell body. The net effect of IPSPs and EPSPs generated on the cell body and dendrites is reflected in the degree of depolarization at the axon hillock where action potentials are generated.

Slow, Long-Acting Transmission

Some receptor sites are not connected directly to a gated ion channel; their influence on ion channels is indirect and consequently somewhat slower. In this case, when the transmitter interacts with the receptor site, a special molecule is released inside the postsynaptic cell. This molecule is called a *second messenger,* and it can do a number of things inside the postsynaptic cell. Often, a second messenger interacts with gated ion channels from the inside with effects similar to the directly gated ion channels, as shown in Figure 4–5, or the second messenger can alter the operation of nongated ion channels in a way that has the effect of changing the resting potential or its sensitivity to other stimuli.

Neuromodulation and Long-Term Changes in Synaptic Functioning

Second messengers can also trigger a host of biochemical changes that can alter the entire functioning of the cell; such effects can be quite long-lasting, even permanent. Because some of these effects are designed to alter the responsiveness of the postsynaptic cell to the actions of other neurotransmitters—for example, to increase the number or sensitivity of receptor sites—they are called *neuromodulators* rather than neurotransmitters. While a neurotransmitter

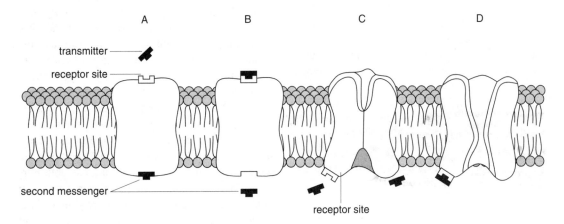

Figure 4–5   This figure shows how second messengers work. Panels *A* and *B* show that when a receptor outside the cell membrane is occupied by a transmitter molecule, it causes the release inside the cell of a molecule of a second messenger. Panels *C* and *D* show that the second messenger then interacts with a receptor on the inside of a gated ion channel, in this case causing it to open. Second messengers may do a great many other things in the postsynaptic cell as well.

causes an immediate short-acting effect on the membrane potential (EPSP or IPSP), a neuromodulator causes a slow, long-acting effect on the reactivity of the postsynaptic cell, modifying its responsiveness to other neurotransmitters. It may either increase or decrease the action of the neurotransmitter, or it may shorten or prolong its activity. Many of the substances that act as neurotransmitters in one synapse may also be neuromodulators at other synapses.

It has been shown that second messengers can have effects that permanently alter the functioning of a cell such as changing the way genetic information is expressed in the cell's biochemistry. Such long-lasting or permanent changes are thought to be the mechanism used by the nervous system to store long-term memories.

Terminating Synaptic Action

The arrival of action potentials at the terminal bouton causes the release of a transmitter into the synaptic cleft that causes changes in the membrane of the postsynaptic cell, but it is important to have some mechanism to get rid of the transmitter when the presynaptic terminal bouton stops receiving action potentials. Otherwise, the transmitter would stay in the cleft and continue to influence the postsynaptic cell. Every synapse has some system to accomplish this purpose. It is usually accomplished in one of two ways. Either the synapse contains an enzyme that destroys the transmitter if it stays in the cleft for any length of time, or the presynaptic cell has a means of reabsorbing the transmitter and then recycling it. The latter process is called *reuptake*.

NEUROTRANSMITTERS

A number of substances are known to be neurotransmitters, and many more are believed to serve that function. In fact, in recent years as many as 50 different substances have been identified as neurotransmitters, and it is likely that

there are many others. One of the earliest discovered and best understood is *acetylcholine (ACh)*. There also is a family of neurotransmitters called *biogenic amines* or *monoamines* that is composed of the *catecholamines (CA)*, which include *epinephrine (E), norepinephrine (NE), dopamine (DA)*, and one *indoleamine, serotonin*, which is sometimes known as *5-hydroxytryptamine (5-HT)*. *Histamine* also acts as a neurotransmitter. While it is chemically classed as a biogenic amine, histamine is chemically quite different from the other amines.

Some transmitters are amino acids. Three of the most common are *gamma-aminobutyric acid (GABA)*, *glycine*, and *glutamate*. Many of these amino acids are found normally in all cells in the body, where they serve metabolic and other biochemical functions, but in some neurons they can be transmitters as well.

Peptides are a number of amino acids linked together in a long chain. Peptides that act as neurotransmitters include *somatostatin, vasopressin, oxytocin, prolactin, growth hormone, substance P*, and *insulin*. There are also a number of substances known as *enkephalins* or *endorphins*. You may recognize many of these names because they have been known for years as hormones. A hormone is a chemical messenger released by a gland in the body. It circulates throughout the body and has an effect on some biological process distant from the place it is released. Many of these peptides were first identified as hormones and given appropriate names, such as growth hormone. It is now clear that the body uses many of these substances as both hormones and neurotransmitters. In fact, when you think about it, the two functions are similar; hormones carry messages over long distances, and neurotransmitters are messengers over very short distances. The distinction between a hormone and a neurotransmitter may not always be clear. Table 4–1 lists some of the substances believed to be neurotransmitters.

It was established many years ago that a neuron always produces the same neurotransmitter at

TABLE 4–1 Neurotransmitters in the Central Nervous System

Acetylcholine (ACh)
Biogenic amines (monoamines)
  Catecholamines
    Norepinephrine (NE)
    Dopamine (DA)
    Epinephrine (E)
  Indoleamine
    Serotonin (5-hydroxytryptamine, 5-HT)
  Others
    Histamine
Amino acids
  Gamma-aminobutyric acid (GABA)
  Glycine
  Glutamate
  Proline
Peptides
  Substance P
  Morphine-like substances
    Enkephalins
    Endorphins
  Thyrotropin-releasing factors
  Somatostatin
  Vasopressin
  Growth hormone
  Prolactin
  Insulin

every one of its synapses. This principle is known as *Dale's law*, named after Sir Henry Dale, its proposer. This law is still believed to be true, although it is now known that some neurons may release more than one transmitter from their synapses. Even in these cases, however, all synapses of a particular cell release the same transmitter or transmitters. Neurons are classified according to the neurotransmitters they use. Those that use acetylcholine are called *cholinergic* neurons. Since another name for epinephrine is *adrenaline* (used primarily in Europe), synapses that use epinephrine and norepinephrine are called *adrenergic* and *noradrenergic.* Those that use *dopamine* are *dopaminergic,* those that use *serotonin* are *serotonergic,* and so on.

Even though each neuron always releases the same transmitter, its effect can be quite different on different cells. The effect of a transmitter depends on the receptor site, not the transmitter, and any transmitter may have a number of different receptor sites. These receptor sites may cause IPSPs or EPSPs; they may be directly connected to an ion channel or they might use a second messenger. Thus a substance released from the vesicles into the cleft can be either an excitatory or inhibitory neurotransmitter, or a neuromodulator.

Drugs and Neurotransmission

As you can see, the transmission between nerves is a chemical process, and it is primarily at synapses that drugs have the opportunity to interfere with the process. Substances administered from outside the body can find their way to synapses and alter these processes in many different ways. Externally administered drugs can mimic neurotransmitters by occupying some or all of the receptor sites that cause the drug's effect (*agonism*). Drugs sometimes occupy receptor sites and have no effect. This action blocks the transmitter from having its normal effect (*antagonism*), as illustrated in Figure 4–6. Other ways that drugs can alter synaptic transmission include decreasing the activity of enzymes that

Figure 4–6 Drug transmitter molecules compete for the transmitter's receptor sites. A receptor site may be occupied by the drug molecule, keeping the transmitter molecule out, but the drug is not the correct shape to activate the receptor in the same way the transmitter would. Therefore, the drug blocks the receptor, and the effectiveness of the transmitter is reduced.

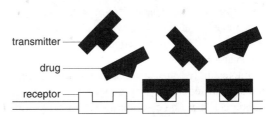

either create or destroy a transmitter, altering the reuptake of a transmitter, altering the activity of a second messenger, and interfering with the operation of ion channels.

Acetylcholine

Acetylcholine (ACh) is synthesized in cholinergic cells and stored in the synaptic vesicles. When an action potential arrives at the terminal bouton, the vesicle releases the ACh into the synaptic cleft, where it interacts with receptor sites on the surface of the postsynaptic cell. The synaptic cleft also contains an enzyme called *acetylcholinesterase (AChE)* that breaks down the ACh whenever it comes in contact with it. Thus the ACh does not remain in the synaptic cleft for very long. As explained earlier, every neuron must have a mechanism for deactivating the neurotransmitter or removing it from the cleft so the postsynaptic cell has a way of knowing when the action potentials stopped arriving at the terminal bouton. Because of the AChE, the neurotransmitter is removed from the cleft as soon as the presynaptic cell stops releasing ACh. Several drugs interfere with the activity of the AChE and consequently interfere with transmission across cholinergic synapses. This is the mechanism of action of many commonly used insecticides and even some older nerve gases such as *sarin*.

Some drugs alter the functioning of cholinergic synapses by acting at the ACh receptor sites. Although all ACh receptor sites are stimulated by ACh, they can be classified according to other substances that can affect them. *Nicotinic* cholinergic receptors are stimulated by nicotine and blocked by a drug called *curare*, a poison used by South American Indians on the point of their spears and arrows. *Muscarinic* cholinergic receptors are stimulated by *muscarine* and blocked by drugs like *atropine* and *scopolamine* (see Chapters 8 and 15).

Interestingly, muscarinic and nicotinic receptor sites differ in the way they alter the postsynaptic cell. Nicotinic receptors are directly connected to a gated ion channel, but muscarinic receptors use a second messenger.

Biogenic Amines (Monoamines)

The catecholamines E, NE, and DA and the indoleamine 5-HT all work in a similar way, so we will consider them together. The catecholamine neurotransmitters are made by the body from *tyrosine,* a substance found in food. Figure 4–7 shows the metabolic steps of this process. The tyrosine is converted into L-dopa, which is then converted to DA and used by dopaminergic neurons. Some DA is converted into NE, and E is created from the NE by another step. Each step in the conversion of tyrosine to E is controlled by a special enzyme. 5-HT is converted from *tryptophan,* another substance found in food, in two steps using two enzymes.

The biogenic amines E, NE, DA, and 5-HT are stored in vesicles in the terminal bouton, where they are protected from two enzymes that destroy them: *monoamine oxidase (MAO)* and *catechol-*

Figure 4–7 Metabolic pathway for the manufacture of catecholamine neurotransmitters showing the enzyme responsible for each step.

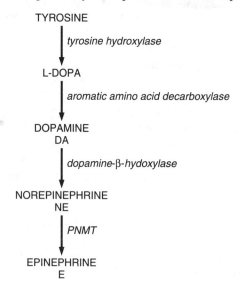

O-methyltransferase (COMT). Like ACh, these neurotransmitters are released into the cleft when an action potential arrives, but they are deactivated by a slightly more complex mechanism. After these neurotransmitters diffuse across the synapse and interact with receptor sites, they are reabsorbed into the terminal bouton, where they are again stored in the vesicles and recycled. Any transmitter not protected in this way is destroyed by MAO and COMT.

Other drugs, such as the amphetamines, stimulate these synapses by causing a leakage of the neurotransmitter into the cleft and increasing the amount of neurotransmitter released when an action potential arrives. Drugs such as cocaine and some antidepressants block reuptake so that the transmitter stays in the cleft longer. Activity at synapses that use monoamines as neurotransmitters are also stimulated by drugs that block the activity of MAO (see Chapter 12).

Each biogenic amine can have a number of different receptor sites. Epinephrine and norepinephrine work at two types of receptors, *alpha* (α) and *beta* (β) adrenergic receptors, and each of these has two subtypes, α_1 and α_2, and β_1 and β_2. Dopamine has at least six receptor types, but there are two main ones, D_1 and D_2. These are found in different dopaminergic brain systems. Drugs used to treat psychotic disorders selectively block D_2 receptors, but some of the newer antipsychotic drugs also have effects on other dopamine receptors (see Chapter 12).

Serotonin has four main types of receptors: 5-HT_1, 5-HT_2, 5-HT_3, and 5-HT_4. In addition, there are four subtypes of the 5-HT_1 receptor. The 5-HT_3 receptors are connected to a gated ion channel, but the rest use a second messenger system.

Gamma-Aminobutyric Acid (GABA)

Most of the neurotransmitters mentioned so far are either excitatory or inhibitory depending on the nature of the receptor site; GABA, however, is believed to be a universal inhibitory neurotransmitter in all parts of the brain. It produces its inhibitory effect directly by opening a Cl^- ion channel, permitting negatively charged chloride ions to flow inward along their concentration gradient. This action hyperpolarizes the membrane and makes it more difficult to create an action potential. Like the other amino acid transmitters, GABA is removed from the cleft by a reuptake mechanism.

Depressant drugs like the barbiturates and the benzodiazepines (e.g. Valium, see Chapter 7) enhance these inhibitory properties of GABA by increasing its ability to open the chloride ionophore. Convulsant drugs like bicuculline block GABA by occupying its receptor.

Glutamate

Glutamate is the major excitatory transmitter in the brain. It has a number of receptor sites that work in a complex fashion and are dependent on the presence of several other substances. One of its receptors operates through a second messenger system, but mostly, glutamate causes excitation by directly opening ion channels that allow positively charged ions to cross the membrane. One of these channels can be blocked by the hallucinogenic drug phencyclidine (PCP or angel dust; see Chapter 15).

Peptides

Peptides are long chains of amino acid molecules attached in a specific order. Unlike other neurotransmitters that can be synthesized directly in the terminal bouton, these transmitters are formed in the cell body and transported to the synapse before they are stored in vesicles.

Peptides can be classified into several groups. One such group is the opioid-type peptides. These are generally formed from a chain of amino acids manufactured elsewhere in the body. Some chains, varying in length from 16 to 30 amino acids, are known as *endorphins,* and shorter chains of five animo acids are called *enkephalins.* There are known receptor sites for these peptides in the brain and other places in the body. Opiates such as morphine and heroin activate these same receptors. Opioid peptides have several types of receptors: the *mu*, the *kappa,* and the *sigma* receptors. Most of the analgesic and reinforcing effects of morphine are mediated by the mu receptor.

We do not understand the action of peptides as well as we do the biogenic amines and simple amino acids, but it is clear that some act as neuromodulators as well as neurotransmitters (see Chapter 11).

THE NERVOUS SYSTEM

The nervous system can be divided into various parts, but the most basic distinction is between the *central nervous system (CNS)* and the *peripheral nervous system (PNS).* The CNS is made up of the brain and spinal cord, and the PNS is everything outside the brain and spinal cord. In both the CNS and PNS, neurons are organized in a similar manner; cell bodies tend to be located together, and the axons from these cells also tend to stay together and run as a bundle of axons between clusters of cell bodies. We therefore find that the nervous system is made up of groups of cell bodies and bundles of axons running between these groups of cell bodies. In the PNS these groups of cell bodies are called *ganglia* (the singular is *ganglion),* and the bundles of axons are called *nerves.* In the CNS the cell body groups are called *nuclei* (singular, *nucleus)* or *centers*, and the bundles of axons are called *tracts.* Because axons are generally covered with myelin, which is white, the nerves and tracts usually appear white and are called *white matter.* The unmyelinated cell bodies are called *gray matter.*

The Peripheral Nervous System

Somatic Nervous System. The PNS may be divided into two functional units, the *somatic nervous system* and the *autonomic nervous system.* The somatic system is made up of all the sensory nerves from most of our conscious senses, such as the nerves running from the sensory receptors in the eyes, ears, and skin to the CNS. The somatic nervous system also contains the motor nerves, which have their cell bodies in the spinal cord and send axons directly to the striated muscles (muscles over which we normally have voluntary control). The motor nerves control these muscles at *neuromuscular junctions,* which are very much like synapses. Acetylcholine (ACh) is the transmitter at most neuromuscular junctions, and the receptor sites are of the nicotinic cholinergic type.

Autonomic Nervous System. Whereas the somatic system usually carries information into the CNS from our conscious senses, the autonomic nervous system (ANS) is concerned with sensory systems that we are not usually aware of, such as information about blood pressure and blood gases, the functioning of the intestines, and levels of hormones. The somatic system controls the muscles over which we have voluntary control; the ANS controls the muscles of the heart and intestines, secretions of glands, and other regulatory systems over which we normally have no conscious control.

The autonomic nervous system really has two divisions. The one that is dominant most of the time and generally keeps the internal functioning of the body operating smoothly is called the *parasympathetic nervous system.* The other autonomic system, called the *sympathetic nervous system,* is connected to the same internal organs as the parasympathetic system, but it comes into operation at times of stress and danger and takes over from the parasympathetic system. Its function is to prepare the body for sudden expenditure of energy such as is required for fighting or running. Blood is directed away from the digestive system to the arms and legs, the pupils dilate, and heart rate and breathing rate increase. This series of changes is called the *fight-or-flight response.*

The parasympathetic and sympathetic nervous systems are anatomically, functionally, and neurochemically distinct, and both systems are influenced by a number of drugs. The parasympathetic system uses acetylcholine as a transmitter to control glands and muscles. Consequently, drugs that alter transmission at cholinergic synapses interfere with parasympathetic functioning. Perhaps the best example of such drugs is atropine, which is a cholinergic muscarinic blocker or *anticholinergic*. Atropine has been used by optometrists to dilate the pupils in the eye so that the retina of the eye can be examined. When atropine is placed in the eye, it blocks the receptor sites at the parasympathetic neuromuscular junctions. Since the parasympathetic system can no longer control the size of the pupils, they dilate. The muscles that control the lens are also under parasympathetic control, so the atropine makes vision blurry as well. Some drugs, such as tricyclic antidepressants and antipsychotics (see Chapters 12 and 13), have anticholinergic side effects that include blurred vision and a dry mouth.

The primary transmitter in the sympathetic system is epinephrine (adrenaline). In times of stress, the adrenal gland secretes epinephrine into the blood, directly stimulating receptors in the sympathetic system and causing the fight-or-flight response. Drugs such as amphetamine and cocaine that stimulate adrenergic synapses will also cause sympathetic arousal.

The Central Nervous System

Spinal Cord. The CNS has two basic parts, the brain and the spinal cord. While some integration of information and reflex activity goes on within the cord, it functions primarily as a relay station transmitting information from the sensory nerves into the brain and carrying motor commands from the brain to the muscles. The central part of the cord is composed of gray matter and shaped in cross section somewhat like a butterfly, as seen in Figure 4–8. It is made up of cell bodies and synapses. Axons from sensory nerves enter the gray matter of the cord from the side nearest the back (dorsal side), and motor axons leaving

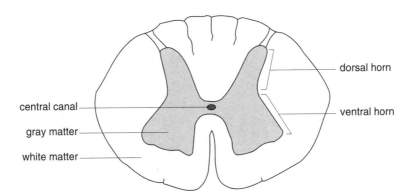

Figure 4–8 A cross section of the spinal cord showing the white and gray matter. Axons of sensory nerves come in through the dorsal (toward the back) horn and form synapses in the gray matter. Cell bodies in the ventral (toward the front) horn send axons to the muscles out the ventral side of the cord. The white matter consists of bundles or tracts of myelinated axons running between the brain and different parts of the body.

the cord do so from the side nearest the front (ventral side), as illustrated in Figure 4–8. The ventral horn of the gray matter of the cord contains the cell bodies of the *motoneurons,* the neurons that directly control the action of muscles. This area also mediates many reflexes. The dorsal horn contains cells that convey sensory information. Surrounding the gray matter are a number of tracts of axons running both up and down the cord from the brain to various parts of the body.

Brain. It has been estimated that the brain contains 10^{11} neurons (that is, 100,000,000,000). On average, each neuron has synapses on 1,000 other neurons and receives an average of 10,000 synapses (Costa, 1985). Obviously, the brain is a complicated structure made up of numerous nuclei and complex fiber tracts that connect them in many ways. For this reason, the brain has been called a "great raveled knot." In recent years neuroscientists have made great strides in unraveling this knot, but it still contains many mysteries and is the subject of intensive study. The brain is too

complex a structure to be explained in a simple fashion, but we will attempt to introduce some of the features that appear to be important in an understanding of many drug effects. Figure 4–9 is a drawing of the brain with some of the structures noted.

Medulla. The area at the base of the brain where the spinal cord arises is called the *medulla.* For the most part it is made up of fiber tracts running to and from the spinal cord to higher centers in the brain. A number of nerves of the autonomic nervous system enter and leave the brain at the medulla, and many of them have control centers located there. The proper functioning of these centers depends on the general level of arousal in this area of the brain. One of these centers is very sensitive to many drugs: the respiratory center, which controls breathing. Many drugs, such as the barbiturates, opiates, and alcohol, depress this center and consequently depress breathing. Death from an overdose of most drugs is usually a result of suffocation because the respiratory center is depressed to the point where

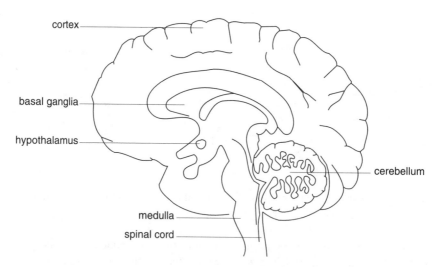

Figure 4–9   A cross section of a human brain showing the location of some of the structures mentioned in the text.

breathing stops. Quite often, people who survive drug overdoses have brain damage because of low oxygen levels in the blood resulting from extended depression of the respiratory center. If you should ever be in a position to help someone who has taken an overdose of such a drug, it is important to stimulate or maintain breathing, either by keeping the person aroused and awake or by artificial respiration.

Another center located in this part of the brain that is sensitive to drugs in the vomiting center. This center is able to monitor the blood and can cause vomiting, presumably to rid the digestive system of a poison that has just been ingested. Some drugs, such as the opiates and nicotine, stimulate this center and cause nausea and vomiting even though the drug was inhaled or injected.

Reticular Activating System and Raphé System. There are two diffuse projection systems that originate in the medulla and run forward into the higher parts of the brain. They are the *reticular activating system (RAS)* and the *Raphé system*.

The RAS in a complicated interconnection of diffuse centers and branching fiber tracts connected in such a way that when one part is excited, the entire system becomes activated. The RAS receives input from axons of sensory nerves that run past the RAS on their way from a sense organ to the sensory areas of the cortex. Thus the RAS is activated by incoming stimulation. The RAS projects a diffuse net of axons forward into the entire cortex and higher parts of the brain so that when it becomes active, so does the entire brain. One function of the RAS is to maintain levels of activation in the cortex and thereby control the level of arousal. Because GABA is an inhibitory neurotransmitter, drugs such as barbiturates, which enhance GABA activity, decrease the ability of neurons in the RAS to fire repeatedly and consequently decrease arousal. If the RAS of an animal is damaged, it will fall into a coma.

Unlike the RAS, which causes arousal, parts of the Raphé system cause sleep. The Raphé system is also made up of a number of nuclei, but they are not interconnected in the same way as the RAS. Artificial stimulation of some Raphé nuclei causes sleep, and damage to them produces an animal that seldom sleeps. This finding shows that sleep is not just a lack of stimulation in the RAS but an active process as well. The Raphé nuclei use serotonin as a neurotransmitter, and drugs like PCPA that alter serotonin activity also seem to interfere with sleep.

A number of centers in the Raphé system send axons forward to the limbic system and the forebrain through the medial forebrain bundle. These projections are thought to be part of an MA system that governs mood and may be the site of action for a class of antidepressants called specific serotonin reuptake inhibitors (SSRIs) of which fluoxetine (Prozac) is the best known example.

Locus Coeruleus. The *locus coeruleus* is a nucleus in the lower brain that sends axons to the limbic system and cortex through the medial forebrain bundle. Its synapses use NE as the transmitter. It is believed that the locus coeruleus contains about 50 to 70 percent of the noradrenergic neurons in the brain. This system, along with several other similar systems (such as the serotonergic forebrain projections of the Raphé system), projects to the higher brain centers through the medial forebrain bundle and is known to be involved in the control of mood. Depression is believed to be a result of abnormal functioning of these systems.

The activity of the locus coeruleus is controlled by a large inhibitory input of synapses that release GABA. In addition to mood, activity in the locus coeruleus is believed to be associated with fear, panic, and anger. *Positron emission tomography (PET)* shows that the locus coeruleus and the places in the brain where it sends its axons become highly active when people are having panic attacks. Drugs like the benzodiazepines (e.g., Valium) that increase the inhibitory effect of GABA are known to relieve anxiety, and drugs like amphetamine and cocaine that stimulate adrenergic synapses can cause anxiety.

Rebound overactivity in the locus coeruleus is also known to be a cause of withdrawal effects from opiates. Drugs that block certain adrenergic receptors can also alleviate much of the distress of opiate withdrawal and withdrawal from other drugs as well (Gold & Miller, 1995a).

Cerebellum. Just inside the skull, above the medulla, is a structure known as the *cerebellum*. The cerebellum functions as part of the motor system. Voluntary actions are initiated and controlled by an area of the cortex (discussed later) higher up in the brain known as the motor cortex. Cell bodies in the motor cortex send axons directly to the spinal cord through fiber bundles that travel through the brain stem. There is, however, much more to the motor system than this. Signals to the muscles from the cortex are refined and modified by two other centers in the brain, the basal ganglia and the cerebellum. The cerebellum receives direct input both from the motor cortex and from the muscles themselves via the spinal cord. It compares these two signals and modifies the output of the cortex both by direct actions on its signals as they pass through the brain stem and by fibers connected back to the cortex. These feedback loops make possible smooth and accurate muscle movements. Another function of the cerebellum is controlling the movement of the eye from one fixation point to another, and it also seems to be involved in learning.

People with damage to the cerebellum are slow and clumsy and often appear to be intoxicated with alcohol. It is quite likely that many of the motor effects of alcohol are due to a specific effect on the cerebellum.

Basal Ganglia. The *basal ganglia* are located just under the cortex. They include two nuclei known as the *caudate nucleus* and the *putamen*. They are part of an area of the brain known as the *striate cortex* or *striatum*. Like the cerebellum, these nuclei are important in the smooth regulation of voluntary bodily movement. The basal ganglia receive signals from all areas of the cortex and send fibers back to the motor cortex, and other parts of the cortex responsible for motor planning and thinking. Parkinson's disease is a result of a malfunction of the basal ganglia. People suffering from Parkinson's disease have tremors, rigidity in the limbs, and difficulty initiating movement. The disease is usually progressive over many years and leads eventually to death. It has been demonstrated that Parkinson's is due to a depletion of DA in the synapses of axons that terminate in the basal ganglia. In many cases the symptoms of Parkinson's disease can be alleviated if the patient is given L-dopa, the metabolic precursor of DA. The L-dopa is absorbed into the brain and transformed into DA, which then increases activity at these synapses in the basal ganglia. We also know that drugs like the antipsychotics, which block DA, have side effects that resemble Parkinson's disease (see Chapter 12).

The system that directly connects the motor cortex to the muscles is called the *pyramidal motor system,* and consequently the system involving the basal ganglia is sometimes called the *extrapyramidal motor system.*

In addition to motor control, the basal ganglia have other functions that include control of eye movement, memory for locations in space, and some thought processes.

Periaqueductal Gray. Another system that runs through the central part of the brain is the *periaqueductal gray* or *central gray*. It has two functions of interest. The first is involved in the perception of pain. The periaqueductal gray serves as one of several relays for axons that carry pain signals from the dorsal horn of the spinal cord to the cortex. This area is rich in receptor sites for opiate drugs such as morphine and their endogenous counterparts, endorphins and enkephalins. These neurons send axons to the spinal cord where they inhibit the neurons that convey pain signals from the body to higher levels of the brain. They do so both by direct inhibition and by stimulating other neurons that release endogenous opiates in the spinal cord. Thus opiate drugs can block pain by stimulating cells in the periaqueductal gray and the spinal cord.

Also located in the periaqueductal gray is a system that has been described as a "punishment" system. These are sites where electrical stimulation appears to have a punishing effect on experimental animals. Animals will learn to perform a task in order to avoid stimulation in this area. It has not been determined whether the pain perception and the punishment functions of these systems are related, but it is certainly tempting to speculate that they are.

Limbic System. Just under the cortex is a series of interconnected nuclei known as the *limbic system*. Structures in the limbic system are related to the control of motivations and emotions and seem to be the site of action of many drugs. One of the more complex structures in the limbic system is the *hypothalamus*. Lesions in specific parts of the hypothalamus can either induce excessive eating or drinking, or can abolish eating or drinking in experimental animals.

It is also in the hypothalamus that some *reinforcement* or *pleasure centers* are located. Humans and nonhumans will learn to press levers or engage in activities that are followed by electrical stimulation in these areas of the brain. It is thought that the reinforcement centers are stimulated when a hungry organism eats or a thirsty organism drinks or any other motivation is fulfilled. The function of such systems is to ensure that the organism will repeat actions that led to the satisfaction of the drive. They have been called pleasure centers because humans sometimes report experiencing pleasure when these areas of the brain are stimulated electrically.

Many reinforcement centers of the brain are associated with the fiber tract called the *medial forebrain bundle*, which carries axons that run in both directions between lower centers in the brain and the hypothalamus and other limbic system structures.

One important reinforcement system called the *mesolimbic system* has been identified as a fiber tract whose cell bodies are located in the *ventral tegmental area (VTA)* in the midbrain. The axons of these neurons run through the medial forebrain bundle and terminate in synapses in the limbic system, forebrain, and other structures. In the limbic system, many fibers from the VTA have synapses in the *nucleus accumbens (ACC)*. Because these fibers use DA as a neurotransmitter, and some are known to have receptor sites for morphinelike transmitters on their cell bodies in the VTA, drugs like amphetamine, cocaine, and morphine can stimulate them. This stimulation is probably the source of the *rushes,* or intense feelings of pleasure that these drugs cause, as well as the powerful tendency to repeat actions that lead to the administration of the drug (see Chapter 5). Malfunctions of the mesolimbic system also appear to be an important cause of schizophrenia (see Chapter 12).

Other limbic system structures include the *amygdala* and the *septum*. Among other connections, these centers receive serotonergic input from the Raphé nuclei. Lesions in the amygdala cause normally aggressive experimental animals to become calm and placid, but when the amygdala is stimulated, animals become aggressive and attack other animals. Lesions in the septum also cause emotional changes. Although it is not known how drugs affect neurotransmitters in the limbic system, it appears that there are many benzodiazepine receptors located in this region. The benzodiazepines enhance the inhibitory effects of GABA, and this increased inhibition in the limbic system may be one mechanism by which the benzodiazepines, such as chlordiazepoxide (Librium) and diazepam (Valium), reduce aggression in nonhumans and produce a calming effect (see Chapter 7).

Cortex. The *cortex* makes up the uppermost surface of the brain and virtually covers the rest of the brain. It is convoluted and gives the brain the appearance of a walnut. Because of its convolutions, most of the cortex cannot be seen. If it were flattened out it would cover an area of 2.5 square feet.

The cortex is undoubtedly the most complex and advanced part of the brain, and its neurochemistry is not well understood, but glutamate and GABA are known to be prominent excitatory and inhibitory transmitters here. Dissociative anesthetics like PCP and ketamine are known to act at these receptors for glutamate, and these drugs probably have their effects directly on the cortex.

One of the functions of the cortex is to handle the integration of sensory information. Information from each sense is projected to a different part of the cortex, where it is analyzed. The cortex also has areas that are responsible for voluntary motor control. These areas send axons directly to the interneurons in the spinal cord that control the motoneurons and consequently the muscles (pyramidal motor system). Other axons from this area go to the basal ganglia and the cerebellum, which modify the direct output of the motor cortex and coordinate bodily movement (extrapyramidal motor system).

The cortex also has language areas that permit us to recognize speech and written language and enable us to speak and write. Most importantly, the cortex is responsible for the higher mental processes of thought and cognition. Understanding of the anatomy and neurochemistry of these complex processes is still elusive.

DEVELOPMENT OF THE NERVOUS SYSTEM

In the early 1960s a drug called thalidomide was prescribed to many pregnant women to treat the nausea of morning sickness. Unfortunately, the drug interfered with the developing fetus, and many of these mothers gave birth to babies with missing or severely malformed limbs. Since the time of thalidomide, it has become widely recognized that drugs consumed by a mother during pregnancy can alter the development of the fetus. Drugs that cause such malformations are called *teratogens* (literally, "monster makers").

The developing nervous system is particularly vulnerable to disruption by drugs, and there is reason to believe that behaviorally active drugs are especially potent teratogens for two reasons. First, in order to be behaviorally active, drugs must readily penetrate the brain, and this property also gives these drugs easy access across the placenta to the body of the developing fetus. Second, drugs that act to alter the functioning of neurotransmitters are particularly dangerous to the developing nervous system because of the way the nervous system develops.

The growth of the nervous system is a complex and delicate process involving the formation, migration, and interconnection of billions of nerve cells. All these cells form during the first 12 weeks of life. During this time, therefore, brain cells are forming at a rate of 150,000 cells a minute. These cells do not develop in the part of the adult brain they are destined to occupy. Many neurons have to migrate from one place in the brain to another. This journey must take place only at particular times in the development of the brain and in the appropriate order, or else the brain will develop incorrectly. Once these cells reach their target area, their growth is still not completed. They must send out their axons along prescribed paths to make contact with other cells in the developing brain. In addition, they must then form synapses with these other cells.

It is now believed that the formation, differentiation, and migration of cells, the projection of axons, and the formation of synapses are under chemical control. Chemicals are released by different parts of the developing brain, and the migrating cells and axons move either toward or away from these sources of chemicals. It is now believed that these control chemicals are the same substances used as neurotransmitters in the adult brain. Consequently, if a mother consumes a psychoactive drug at crucial times during the development of the fetal brain, it could interfere with the delicate chemical signaling taking place in the developing brain of the fetus. If these chemical control signals are altered, masked, or inhibited, the development of the fetal brain may be disrupted (Abel, 1989).

Such disruptions may cause severe brain malformation of the sort seen in the fetal alcohol syndrome described in Chapter 6, or they may be much less apparent disruptions in the functioning of the brain that can be detected after careful systematic study of the organism's behavior. This kind of damage is called *functional teratology* or *behavioral teratology*. Functional teratology is an exciting and comparatively new field of research. Most functional teratology research has been done on laboratory animals, and the exact significance for humans is still not clear. What is clear is that exposure to low levels of behaviorally active drugs during certain stages of fetal development can cause alterations in the functioning of the nervous system, which can be apparent at many stages throughout the organism's life span (Boer et al., 1988).

CHAPTER SUMMARY

- Nervous tissue is made up of nerve cells called *neurons,* which are excitable. Their excitability depends on the breakdown of the *resting potential,* the difference in electrical charge between the inside and the outside of each cell. The resting potential is a result of an uneven distribution of ions inside and outside of the cell.

- The flow of ions across the cell membrane is controlled by ion channels that can be either passive or gated—that is, opened and closed either by the presence of a chemical or by a change in the resting potential.

- When the cell is stimulated (depolarized) to a certain point, ion channels open and the resting potential is destroyed. This condition is called an *action potential.* The resting potential then quickly restores itself.

- Action potentials move along the axon away from the *cell body* along the cell's *axon* to *synapses* very near the cell body and *dendrites* of another neuron. They stimulate the second neuron by releasing a chemical called a *neurotransmitter* into the tiny gap between the cells.

- The transmitter interacts with *receptor sites* on the cell, thus either increasing the excitability of the postsynaptic cell (depolarizing it) or inhibiting it (hyperpolarizing it), depending on the nature of the receptor.

- Whether a cell produces action potentials in its axon depends on the sum of the excitation and inhibition at all the synapses on its dendrites and cell body at any given time.

- *Acetylcholine, epinephrine, norepinephrine, dopamine, serotonin, GABA,* and some *peptides* are all neurotransmitters.

- The nervous system has two major divisions. The *central nervous system (CNS)* is made up of all the neurons in the brain and spinal cord; all other neurons make up the *peripheral nervous system (PNS),* which is further divided into the *somatic* and the *autonomic nervous systems.* The autonomic nervous system also has two parts: the *parasympathetic* system, which controls the vegetative involuntary functions of the body on an ongoing basis, and the *sympathetic* nervous system, which prepares the body for the sudden expenditure of energy, the *fight-or-flight response.*

- The central part of the spinal cord is gray matter (cell bodies) surrounded by white matter (myelinated axons), which is made up of fiber bundles of axons running to and from the brain.

- The *medulla* at the base of the brain controls breathing and other autonomic functions. The *cerebellum* controls the smooth movement of muscles. The *reticular activating system* controls arousal. The *Raphé system,* conversely, is important in causing sleep.

- The *locus coeruleus* is a center in the lower brain that sends NE projections to the limbic system and the cortex. It is associated with anxiety and panic and seems to be responsible for withdrawal from opiates. The *central gray* is important in mediating responses to pain. It contains opiate receptors and is one site of action for the analgesic effects of the opiates.

- The *limbic system* controls emotions and motivation. It is made up of a number of centers including the *hypothalamus* which controls eating and drinking and contains *reinforcement centers.*

- The *cortex* makes up the uppermost surface of the brain and receives direct input from many senses. It also has direct control over voluntary movement. The cortex contains centers that permit us to recognize speech and written language and enable us to speak and write.

- The development of the brain is a complex process that involves the formation, migration, and connection of billions of neurons. Because migration and synapse formation are controlled by substances that also function as neurotransmitters, drugs that interfere with neurotransmitters can be *teratogens,* meaning that they can severely disrupt the development of the nervous system.

SUGGESTED READINGS

Abel, E. (1989). *Behavioral teratogenesis and behavioral mutagenesis.* New York: Plenum.

Boer, G. J., Feenstra, M. G. P., Mirmiran, M., Swaab, D. F., & Van Haaren, F. (1988). *The biochemical basis of functional teratology: Progress in brain research,* Vol. 73. Amsterdam: Elsevier.

Kandel, E. R., Schwartz, J. H., & Jessell, T. M. (1991). *Principles of neural science.* Norwalk, CT: Appleton & Lange.

5

Dependence, Addiction, and Self-Administration

EXPLAINING DRUG SELF-ADMINISTRATION

It often happens that people understand the least the things they do most frequently. It may seem obvious why people take drugs, at least to themselves, but can we depend on these "obvious" insights to formulate a scientific theory of drug taking? When we drink a beer, smoke a cigarette, or drink a cup of coffee, we are taking a drug, and if we are asked why, most of us can come up with an answer that sounds reasonable: "Because I like it," "It wakes me up," or "I need to unwind after a long, hard day." Likewise, there may be equally obvious reasons for the drug use of others: "Losing his wife drove him to drink" or "She turned to LSD in order to understand herself." These are reasonable statements, but even though they may satisfy us and those around us, the history of research into drug use shows that self-analysis and "obvious" explanations have led researchers down many

dead-end paths and should be approached with caution.

In this chapter we will be discussing three models of drug abuse or addiction: two fairly old ones, the disease model and the physical dependence model, and one more recent one, the positive reinforcement model. These are not so much theories of drug abuse as they are sets of assumptions about the nature of drug abuse, and so we will use the term *model* rather than *theory*. These models are not mutually exclusive; that is, if one is correct, the others are not necessarily all wrong. However, some of the assumptions made by one model may directly conflict with the assumptions of another. Some of these models have been around for such a long time that they have had a powerful influence on the way we think about drug abuse, and their influence has been so great that they have even influenced the language we use to talk about drug abuse.

From the time when people first started to try to understand the nature of drug abuse, they noticed a number of "obvious" characteristics of drug abuse that they felt ought to be explained. First, it appeared that the behavior of drug addicts was distinctly different from normal behavior, and second, there were considerable individual differences in the development of drug abuse. As we proceed through this chapter, you will see that these "obvious" characteristics of drug abuse are not necessarily correct, but they did have a strong influence on the development of our ideas about addiction.

THE "ABNORMALITY" OF DRUG ABUSE

It appears that the behavior of addicts toward their drug does not follow "normal" rules of behavior. The characteristics of addictive behavior that set it apart from normal, ordinary behavior is that it is compulsive (it seems to be beyond the voluntary control of the individual) and it can be extraordinarily self-destructive. Intuitively, we expect people to do things that cause them pleasure and avoid pain, but addicts seem to behave differently. They spend virtually all their time, to the exclusion of nearly everything else, obtaining and administering their drug. Very often they do so at the expense of their jobs, their families, and most certainly their comfort. This kind of behavior makes it easy to suppose that there is no point in looking for an explanation of addiction among the rules that govern "normal" behavior and suggests that there is something "abnormal," possibly a disease state, that is responsible for these "irrational" actions.

Drugs appear to have very different effects on different people. For example, two people may have an equal exposure to alcohol, but one may become an alcoholic and the other may not. Because different people have the same opportunities to use a drug and only some end up under its control, it seems that the mechanisms responsible

for the addiction must be in the person rather than in the drug.

DEVELOPMENT OF THE DISEASE MODEL

Before the middle of the nineteenth century, people who had problems with drugs were considered to be deficient in character, moral fiber, willpower, or self-control; in other words, they were sinners or criminals. Consequently, addiction to drugs was a problem for priests and clerics to understand, and for the legal system to deal with. These ideas were challenged on two fronts.

On the one hand, a powerful social reform movement was under way in England and North America that advocated reform of a variety of social problems of the time such as child labor, slavery, poverty, and the treatment of criminals—including "inebriates" (alcoholics). One organization inspired by this movement was the American Association for the Cure of Inebriates which was established in 1870 and became the forerunner of the temperance movement. Its first principle was "Inebriety is a disease." Its seventh principle went on to declare:

Facts and experience indicate clearly that it is the duty of the civil authorities to recognize inebriety as a disease, and to provide means in hospitals and asylums for its scientific treatment, in place of the penal methods by fine and imprisonment hitherto in use, with all [their] attendant evil. (Jaffe, 1992, p. 17)

In addition to the social reform movement, other changes came about largely because the other widely abused drugs of the period were morphine and opium. Opium is the raw extract of the opium poppy and was usually consumed in the form of laudanum, a mixture of opium and alcohol. Morphine is the principal active ingredient in opium and was usually injected. Laudanum was sold as a patent medicine, and morphine was widely used by physicians to treat a number of ailments (see Chapter 11). It was logical, then, to think of abuse of these drugs a problem that physicians should solve (Berridge & Edwards, 1981).

This change in perception of drug abuse from sin to disease led to the adoption of a new terminology. Toward the end of the nineteenth century the temperance and antiopium social movements started using the term *addiction* to refer exclusively to the excessive use of drugs, and it replaced terms like *intemperance* and *inebriety* (Alexander & Schweighofer, 1988). The medical profession also adopted the term *addiction* and started using it as a diagnosis and an explanation of excessive drug use, thereby giving it the implication of a disease. This use is still common.

Even though the concern about drug use moved from the cleric to the physician, earlier notions about morality and sin were slow to change. Instead of being a lack of willpower, addictions became a "disorder of the will," immorality became a "moral disorder," and treatments were very often based on the teaching of self-control and self-discipline with liberal doses of prayer and worship. Physicians were no better equipped to handle addiction as a disease than were priests to handle it as a sin.

The disease model of alcoholism seemed to fade until the middle of the twentieth century when the Alcoholics Anonymous movement gained prominence and influence. One of its most influential theorists, E. M. Jellinek, focused attention on the issue and eventually wrote a book called *The Disease Concept of Alcoholism* (Jellinek, 1960).

The idea that addiction is a disease became formalized first with alcoholism, which was declared a disease by the World Health Organization in 1951 and the American Medical Association in 1953 (Room, 1983). The concept soon found its way into the popular press and even the courts where, because it was a disease, alcoholism became an excuse for diminished respon-

sibility for one's actions (Heyman, in press). By implication, then, all forms of drug addiction became a "disease."

Some of the appeal of the disease model is that it accommodates well the observations that drug abuse is not "normal," that it is a special type of behavior that does not seem to follow normal rules. Because it is a disease state, the usual rules that govern behavior do not apply to the behavior of addicts, at least as far as their use of drugs is concerned. The disease model also fits well with the observation that some people become addicted and others do not in the same way that a disease may strike only some.

As we have seen, thinking about drug abuse as a disease also has profound implications for therapy. At the heart of the issue is whether the addict really has any control over drug taking. If the abuse of drugs can be considered a sickness rather than an immoral or criminal activity, it is therefore beyond the control of the abuser, who then requires treatment rather than punishment. This view also justifies spending money on research on drug abuse in the same way that money is spent by government agencies on other diseases.

Disease or Disorder?

Currently drug dependence is formally classified as a "disorder" by the DSM-IV, the *Diagnostic and Statistical Manual of Mental Disorders,* fourth edition, of the American Psychiatric Association, published in 1994. The DSM-IV lists conditions considered to be mental disorders and presents standardized criteria by which these disorders may be recognized and diagnosed. These criteria are strictly descriptive and are not meant to give an indication of the nature of an underlying disease process. The DSM-IV does not use the term *disease,* but it defines *disorder* as

a clinically significant behavioral or psychological syndrome or pattern that occurs in an individual and is associated with present distress (e.g., a painful symptom) or disability (i.e., impairment in one or more important areas of functioning) or with a significantly increased risk of suffering death, pain, disability or an important loss of freedom. (American Psychiatric Association, 1994, p. xxi)

This definition specifically excludes deviance or criminal behavior. While the DSM-IV does not use the term *disease,* it is clear that *disorder* is, in fact, a synonym for *disease.*

The DSM-IV distinguishes between the terms *substance dependence* and *substance abuse.* (See Box 5–1) Being recognized in the DSM-IV is important for a number of reasons. Even though it does not use the word, inclusion in the DSM-IV means that dependence and substance abuse can be considered a "disease" under the law, at least insofar as physicians in the United States are able to charge for treating the condition.

The ICD-10 is a similar catalog of diseases issued by the World Health Organization (WHO, 1993). The ICD-10 distinguishes between *harmful use* and *dependence syndrome* with criteria similar to substance dependence and abuse in the DSM-IV.

Problems with the Disease Model. There are some problems with the disease model, the main one being that the nature of the "disease" has never been identified. What sort of disease is it, and how can a disease make people take drugs? There have been a number of attempts to explain the abuse of specific drugs in terms of a disease process; for example, it has been suggested that alcoholism is a result of a type of food allergy to the grain from which alcohol is manufactured, but such attempts have been limited to a specific drug and have never been particularly convincing.

There has never been a comprehensive disease theory that suggests a mechanism that can account for all types of addictions as a single disease. Perhaps this is not necessary, but considering the similarity of different addictions, it would be scientifically pleasing—and much more useful—if one theory could explain many different addictions. The continued absence of any disease mechanism that can account for the compulsive use of specific drugs or addictive behavior in general makes it increasingly difficult to accept the belief that addiction is a pathological condition.

There are those who argue that the fact that we do not understand the origins or the mechanism of the disease does not mean it is not a disease (Maltzman, 1994). In fact, we recognized many conditions such as diabetes and polio long before science could explain them in terms of biochemical deficiencies or viruses. Nevertheless, one might expect after all this time that some sort of disease process would have been discovered that would explain the compulsive use of at least one drug.

In spite of the declarations of the American Association for the Cure of Inebriates, there were no "facts and experience" to indicate that alcoholism was a disease, and there was no "scientific treatment." The issue was whether the alcoholic could control his or her drinking. Social reformers believed on the basis of their experience that an alcoholic had lost control over drinking and therefore could not be held responsible for his or her actions. The only possible explanation for this was that the person was "sick." In other words, the disease was presumed to exist because this was the only rational explanation at the time for the loss of control. It turns out that it is not the only explanation. As we shall see later in this chapter, rejecting the "disease" model of addictions does not mean that we must accept that drug consumption is always under voluntary control and return to older "moralistic" explanations of drug use and treatment.

The physical dependence model described in the next section attempts to provide a "physiological" mechanism that can explain compulsive drug use. It has been widely accepted, but physiological dependence is not a "disease," and, as we shall see, as a mechanism it cannot by itself account for the use of drugs.

BOX 5–1 DSM-IV Definitions of Psychoactive Substance Dependence and Abuse. (American Psychiatric Association, 1994, pp. 181–183)

Criteria for Substance Dependence

A maladaptive pattern of substance use, leading to clinically significant impairment or distress, as manifested by three (or more) of the following, occurring at any time in the same 12 month period:

(1) tolerance, as defined by either of the following:
   (a) a need for markedly increased amounts of the substance to achieve intoxication or desired effect
   (b) markedly diminished effect with continued use of the same amount of the substance
(2) withdrawal, as manifested by either of the following:
   (a) the characteristic withdrawal syndrome of the substance
   (b) the same (or a closely related) substance is taken to relieve or avoid withdrawal symptoms
(3) substance is often taken in larger amounts or over a longer period than was intended
(4) there is a persistent desire or unsuccessful efforts to cut down or control substance use
(5) a great deal of time is spent in activities necessary to obtain the substance (e.g., visiting multiple doctors or driving long distances), use of the substance (e.g., chain smoking), or recovering from its effects
(6) important social, occupational or recreational activities are given up or reduced because of substance use
(7) the substance use is continued despite knowledge of having a persistent or recurrent physical or psychological problem that is likely to have been caused or exacerbated by the substance (e.g., current cocaine use despite recognition of cocaine induced depression, or continued drinking despite recognition that an ulcer was made worse by alcohol consumption)

Specify if:
With Physiological Dependence: evidence of tolerance or withdrawal (i.e., either item 1 or 2 is present)

Without Physiological Dependence: no evidence of tolerance or withdrawal (e.g., neither item 1 or 2 is present)

Criteria for Substance Abuse
A. A maladaptive pattern of substance use leading to clinically significant impairment or distress, as manifested by one (or more) of the following, occurring within a 12 month period:
   (1) recurrent substance use resulting in failure to fulfill major role obligations at work, school or home (e.g., repeated absences or poor work performance related to substance use; substance-related absences, suspensions or expulsions from school; neglect of children or household)
   (2) recurrent substance use in situations in which it is physically hazardous (e.g., driving an automobile or operating a machine when impaired by substance use)
   (3) recurrent substance-related legal problems (e.g., arrests for substance-related disorderly conduct)
   (4) continued substance use despite having persistent or recurrent social or interpersonal problems caused or exacerbated by the effects of the substance (e.g., arguments with spouse about consequences of intoxication, physical fights)
B. The symptoms have never met the criteria for Substance Dependence for this class of substance

DEVELOPMENT OF THE PHYSICAL DEPENDENCE MODEL

Early biochemical explanations of addiction drew attention to the sickness that develops when a user of opium or morphine tries to stop. These explanations proposed a hypothetical substance called an *autotoxin*, a metabolite of opium that stayed in the body after the drug was gone. This autotoxin had effects opposite to opium and when left in the body made the person very sick. Only opium or a related drug could antagonize the extremely unpleasant effects of the autotoxin and relieve the sickness. It was believed that the sickness was so unpleasant that the relief provided by opium was responsible for the continuous craving for more opium (Tatum & Seevers, 1931).

Later the existence of the autotoxin was disproved. The sickness that remained after the drug was gone was called a *withdrawal symptom* or *abstinence syndrome,* and more accurate explanations were developed to account for it (see Chapter 1), but avoidance of withdrawal was still regarded as the explanation for opium use and the compulsive craving for the drug. The term *physical dependence* or *physiological dependence* was used to describe the state where the discontinuation or reduction of a drug would cause withdrawal symptoms.

Because alcohol was the other major addicting drug at the time and because alcohol also causes severe withdrawal symptoms, it was logical for scientists to consider avoidance of withdrawal as a general explanation for the excessive use of all drugs. The ability of a drug to cause physical dependence (and consequently withdrawal), became accepted as the universal indication of an addicting drug, and the presence of physical dependence became the defining feature of an addict and an addiction.

This assumption became crystallized in the language developed to talk about drug use. The term *dependence* came to describe two separate effects that were synonymous in the minds of scientists at the time. Dependence meant both (1) the state where a drug produces "physical dependence"—that is, withdrawal symptoms occur when the drug is stopped—and (2) the compulsive self-administration of a drug. In addition, because the development of tolerance seems to be a necessary condition for physical dependence (see Chapter 4), many laboratories studied tolerance presuming that they were in fact, studying dependence. As a result, *tolerance* was used by some as a synonym for *dependence*. This term is seldom used in this way today.

This model of drug abuse, which we shall call the physical dependence model, is still widely accepted. It seems to account rather well for the apparent "abnormality" of drug addiction. If you accept that withdrawal sickness is exceptionally unpleasant, this model explains why addicts work so compulsively to get their drug. Similarly, fear of severe withdrawal can also explain why drug abuse is so self-destructive. Drug-seeking behavior is different from normal behavior because the motivation for drugs is so extreme. According to this view, physically dependent individuals are willing to sacrifice almost anything to avoid having to go through withdrawal. This view of the addict is still commonly presented in movies and on television.

By itself, the physical dependence model does not explain individual differences as well as the disease model does, but the two models are not incompatible, and often they are combined. For example, there could be a disease that alters the rapidity with which a person develops physical dependence, or there might be a disease that changes a person's sensitivity to drugs or drug withdrawal. Such a disease would make a person more vulnerable to developing a physical dependence.

One of the strengths of the physical dependence model is that it is more general than the disease model and can apply to any drug that causes dependence. It seems to work well for abuse of the opiates, alcohol, and barbiturates, but it does not offer an explanation for the use of many other drugs like cocaine and cannabis that do not cause obvious withdrawal sickness at abused doses.

There was also a widespread belief that only "depressants" (opiates, alcohol, etc.) would create physical dependence, and only these drugs would cause "true dependence" (Tatum & Seevers, 1931). "Stimulant" drugs like cocaine, by definition, were not addicting.

Habituation. One way of handling addictions to non-dependence-producing drugs was to suggest that a different mechanism was responsible for the use of these drugs. In 1931, Tatum and Seevers suggested that the term *drug habituation* (meaning habit forming) be used for drugs that do not create physical dependence. "Habituation is a condition in which the habitué desires a drug, but suffers no ill effects on its discontinuance" (Tatum & Seevers, 1931, p. 108). Addiction referred to behavior that was harmful to the individual, but habituation was much less serious and caused little harm (Winger, Hoffmann, & Woods, 1992, p. 17). The term was later used by the World Health Organization into the 1950s, but it is not widely used anymore.

Psychological Dependence. In addition to coining the word *habituation,* in 1931 Tatum and Seevers suggested the adoption of "some non-committal term such as psychic addiction" (p. 119). This concept later was developed into the concept of *psychological dependence.*

The fact that physical dependence did not explain the compulsive and destructive use of cocaine and other drugs became increasingly troublesome to theorists. Following the lead of Tatum and Seevers, the term "psychological dependence" became widely used. It expanded the dependence model by assuming that drugs such as cocaine caused unobservable psychological withdrawal symptoms, that is, "psychological" or "psychic" dependence. In short, "psychological dependence" presumed that there was some sort of "psychological" as opposed to "physical" withdrawal that caused a craving for a drug. This "psychological" withdrawal was not observ-

able—it took place in the brain and did not have any outward manifestations apart from the fact that the user became highly motivated to take the drug. It was assumed that the brain could not function normally without the drug and this inability manifested itself subjectively to the user as a "craving." Behaviorally, psychological dependence created an "impaired control of psychoactive substance use" (American Psychiatric Association, 1987, p. 166).

The term *psychological dependence* presents a serious conceptual problem, however. The difficulty is that it cannot be used as an explanation because it involves circular reasoning. For example, if we say that we know that John is "psychologically dependent" because he uses a drug excessively, we cannot say that John uses a drug excessively because he is "psychologically dependent." The term may be used as a description of a state of affairs, but it cannot be used as an explanation. This problem does not arise with physical dependence because there is independent evidence that physical dependence exists: withdrawal symptoms. Apart from the excessive drug use itself, there is no independent evidence that psychological withdrawal and consequently psychological dependence exist.

Because of its past association with explanations that involve fear of withdrawal and the circularity of logic that it suggests, the term *psychological dependence* will not be used in this text; however, many writers do use the term in a somewhat different manner. It is commonly used in a generic sense to refer to any excessive use of drugs that cannot be explained by physical dependence and fear of physical withdrawal. When the term is used in this way, it may include drug use motivated by a desire to experience the "pleasurable" effects of drugs, and it may include behavioral mechanisms we will be discussing in the next section on the positive reinforcement model (Grilly, 1989; Ray & Ksir, 1993).

Problems with the Physical Dependence Model. There are two problems with the physical dependence model and any disease mechanism that uses its assumptions. To begin with, we now know that powerful compulsive drug abuse can develop to substances like cocaine and marijuana that cause only mild (if any) withdrawal, and second, recent research has shown that even with drugs like heroin that can cause physical dependence, many people (and laboratory animals) can become addicts without developing physical dependence. In fact, the definition of substance dependence in the DSM-IV recognizes that it is possible to be dependent without being physically dependent, although it suggests that the presence or absence of physical dependence should be noted in the diagnosis.

DEVELOPMENT OF THE POSITIVE REINFORCEMENT MODEL

One assumption that was widely made up until the mid-1950s and held back the development of new ideas and properly controlled scientific research was that addictive behavior was uniquely human. Attempts to create "addictions" in other species had generally been unsuccessful. As early as the 1920s it was shown that laboratory animals could be made physically dependent if they were forced to consume a drug like morphine or alcohol, but it could never be shown that they would make themselves physically dependent (then believed to be the defining feature of addiction) if a drug were freely made available to them. Even animals made physically dependent by forced consumption seldom continued to consume a drug when alternatives were made available. The sociologist A. R. Lindesmith, for example, wrote the following in 1937: "Certainly from the point of view of social science it would be ridiculous to include animals and humans together in the concept of addiction" (quoted in Laties, 1986, p. 33).

The reluctance of laboratory animals to show the compulsive and self-destructive drug taking that humans so often exhibit also led people to

believe addiction must be caused by something that makes humans different from nonhuman animals. This line of reasoning supported an older, moralistic view that since humans had "free will" and nonhumans did not, humans could "sin" by choosing to take drugs, and this "sin" was punished by the misery of addiction.

Another more scientific explanation originated in the physical dependence model. It was that nonhuman animals could never become addicted to a drug because they were not capable of learning the association between an injection and relief from withdrawal sickness, which occurred 15 or 20 minutes later (Goldberg, 1976). Whatever the explanation, it was widely accepted that there was no point in using laboratory animals to study addictive behavior of humans.

In the absence of laboratory techniques that could test it, the physical dependence model seemed to account nicely for addiction and was virtually unchallenged until a few simple technological breakthroughs were made in the 1950s. At that time a number of researchers began to show that laboratory animals would learn to perform behavior that resulted in drug injection. This line of research expanded quickly when the technology was developed that allowed drug infusions to be delivered intravenously to freely moving animals by means of a permanently implanted catheter (see Figure 5–1). With this one development, our whole view of drug self-administration changed.

Because of the pervasive influence of the physical dependence model, in these early studies it was assumed that physical dependence was essential for drug self-administration. Thus rats and monkeys were first made physically dependent on morphine by repeated injections. Then they were placed in an operant chamber and were given the opportunity to press a lever that caused a delivery of morphine through a catheter. The animals quickly learned to respond. It became obvious that the drug infusion was acting like a more traditional positive reinforcer such as food or water (Thompson & Schuster, 1964).

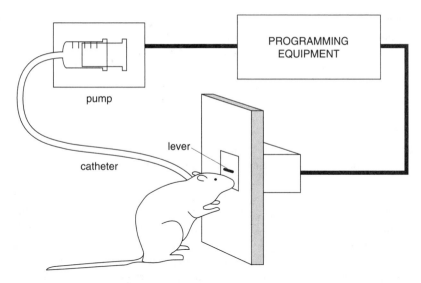

Figure 5–1   A schematic drawing of the drug self-administration preparation for the rat. The rat presses the lever which causes the activation of the pump by the programming equipment. The pump injects a specific amount of a drug solution through a catheter that has been implanted into the jugular vein near the rat's heart.

The role of physical dependence was further explored by Charles Schuster and his colleagues who showed that animals that were not physically dependent would self-administer doses of morphine so low that no physical dependence ever developed (Schuster, 1970). It was also demonstrated that rats would press a lever to give themselves infusions of cocaine and other stimulants that do not cause marked withdrawal symptoms (Pickens & Thompson, 1968).

These and many other studies have clearly demonstrated that many of the assumptions of both the disease model and the physical dependence model are not correct. They have shown that while physical dependence can be an important factor controlling the intake of some drugs, it is not necessary for drug self-administration and cannot serve as the sole explanation for drug taking. These studies also showed that drug self-administration behavior obeys the same laws that govern the "normal" behavior of all animals in similar situations. There is no advantage to considering drug abuse as a disease; it can be understood in terms of operant conditioning theory.

The model of drug taking that has developed as a result of these studies we shall call the positive reinforcement model. This model assumes that drugs are self-administered because they act as positive reinforcers and that the principles that govern behavior controlled by other positive reinforcers apply to drug self-administration. The remainder of this chapter will be devoted to a discussion of the positive reinforcement model and the insights it has provided into drug self-administration in both human and nonhuman animals.

Often people use the term *positive reinforcement* interchangeably with pleasure, euphoria, or some sort of positive affect. It is true that stimuli that act as positive reinforcers are often reported to give pleasure that is frequently assumed to be a cause of behavior (e.g., "I do it because it makes me feel good"), but there are plenty of examples of stimuli that can act as positive reinforcers that do not cause pleasure. In fact, there are circumstances where an electric shock can be a positive reinforcer (Kelleher & Morse, 1968). Traditionally, a positive reinforcer has been defined only in terms of its effect on behavior; that is, it is any stimulus that increases the frequency of behavior it is contingent on (see Chapter 2). Over the years many have speculated on the nature of positive reinforcement, suggesting, for example, that it is a result of such things as drive reduction, drive induction, and consummatory behavior (Domjan, 1993). Later in this chapter we will present information linking positive reinforcement to the activity in certain parts of the brain. This is clearly a complex area that is not well understood; however, it is clear that it is a mistake simply to equate positive reinforcement with the experience of pleasure.

Self-Administration via Other Routes. Over the years it has been demonstrated that laboratory animals will administer drugs to themselves through a variety of routes, including intragastric (i.g.) (direct injection through a cannula into the stomach), intracranial (direct injection of tiny amounts of drug through a cannula into specific parts of the brain), intracerebroventricular (injection through a cannula into the ventricles in the brain), and inhalation (pulmonary administration). Laboratory animals will also consume drugs orally (Meisch & Lemaire, 1993).

Before the development of the technology of i.v. self-injection, virtually all attempts to get nonhuman animals to take drugs had been by making the drug available for oral consumption. It turns out that this is a perfectly acceptable route, but earlier researchers were not aware of some particular problems that must be overcome using this route. To begin with, most drugs have an aversive and unpleasant taste, and most animals require special training to overcome this natural aversion. In addition, all animals have a protective mechanism called *flavor toxicosis*

learning. If the animal experiences almost any kind of altered state or sickness after it experiences a novel taste, it will assiduously avoid that taste in the future. In addition to these aversive protective mechanisms, there is a delay between the consumption and the reinforcing effect because absorption from the digestive system is comparatively slow. This delay diminishes the reinforcing capacity of the drug (Meisch & Lemaire, 1993).

Another reason why earlier researchers who used the oral route were discouraged about using laboratory animals is that even if they could get their animals to consume the drug, the animals voluntarily administered amounts that were never so extensive that the animals became physically dependent. Physical dependence was considered to be the only legitimate indicator of addiction at the time, so the experiments were considered failures. In more recent times, techniques have been developed to overcome the natural protective mechanisms, and the defining characteristics of drug use and abuse are better understood. Much of what we know today about drug use, especially alcohol, has come from experiments with laboratory animals using oral administration.

DRUGS AS POSITIVE AND NEGATIVE REINFORCERS

To demonstrate that any event can be a positive reinforcing stimulus, you must be able to show that it will increase the rate of behavior of a response that it is contingent on. That is, if you wish to demonstrate that an infusion of a drug is acting as a positive reinforcer for lever pressing, it is necessary to show that the frequency of lever pressing will increase if it is reliably followed by an infusion of drug, and will decrease when it is no longer followed by the drug.

To illustrate this point we will look at a classic experiment performed by Pickens and Thompson and published in 1968. In this experiment, rats were implanted with catheters so that they could receive infusions of cocaine into the jugular vein. The rats were placed in a small chamber that was equipped with two levers and a stimulus light. The rats lived in these chambers permanently and were provided with food and water. From 9 A.M. to 11 P.M. an infusion of 0.5 mg/kg cocaine HCl was administered to each rat in response to a depression of one of the levers on a continuous reinforcement (CRF) schedule. Responding on the other lever had no effect. Within a few days each rat was responding at a steady rate of about 8 to 12 infusions per hour on the lever that produced the infusions. There were virtually no responses on the other lever.

Pickens and Thompson were aware that there could be other explanations for the increase in the rate of lever pressing. For example, the increases could be due to a general stimulating effect of cocaine on the behavior of the rats. In other words, the rats might just hit the lever accidentally, and the resulting infusion of the stimulant cocaine would cause the animal to be more active. This increased activity in turn might cause more accidental lever presses and, consequently, more activation caused by more of the drug.

To demonstrate that this was not the case, Pickens and Thompson included some control conditions in their experiment that demonstrated conclusively that the reason for the lever pressing was the reinforcing effect of the cocaine rather than any activation effect of the drug. As shown in line *A* of Figure 5–2, responding occurred only when the drug infusions were contingent on the lever presses. The second half of line *A* shows that the rat stopped pressing when cocaine was delivered at the same rate by the experimenter independently of rat's behavior.

Line *B* in Figure 5–2 shows that extinction of responding occurred if saline placebo infusions were substituted for the cocaine infusions after each lever press. As you can see, when the cocaine infusions were stopped, there was a short

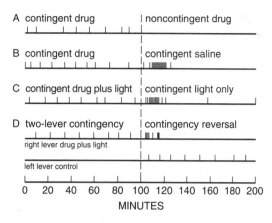

Figure 5–2   Data from the experiment by Pickens and Thompson (1968). Vertical lines indicate the occurrence of lever presses throughout the 200 minutes of each session in various stages of the experiment. See the text for experimental details.

burst of lever pressing before the rat stopped responding. This pattern is typically observed at the beginning of extinction.

In this experiment each infusion was accompanied by a light. Line *C* shows that the light by itself was not responsible for lever pressing. The two lines at *D* show what happened when the contingency was switched from one lever to the other. This result shows clearly that the rat's choice of levers also switched. Its behavior was being controlled by the contingency between the lever press and the drug infusion rather than any other property of the drug or the situation.

Pickens and Thompson showed that rats would also respond on fixed ratio (FR) schedules for cocaine reinforcement and that the pattern of lever pressing generated by the schedule was similar to the pattern FR schedules generate with other positive reinforcers.

Since these early studies, it has been demonstrated that laboratory animals will self-administer many different drugs. Table 5–1 lists some of these drugs and the species that have been used.

Some Drugs That Have Been Found to Be Self-Administered, Not Self-[Administered] and Avoided by Nonhuman Species

	Self-Administered	Not Self-Administered	Avoided
	Baboon, rat, rhesus monkey		
Amphetamine	Baboon, rat, dog, rhesus monkey		
Aspirin		Rhesus monkey	
Caffeine	Rat, rhesus monkey	Rhesus monkey	
Cathinone	Rhesus monkey		
Chloropromazine		Rat, rhesus monkey, squirrel monkey	Rhesus monkey
Cocaine	Baboon, cat, pig, rat, rhesus monkey, squirrel monkey		
Diazepam	Rhesus monkey	Baboon	
Ethanol	Rat, rhesus monkey		
Haloperidol	Rat	Rhesus monkey	
Heroin	Rat, rhesus monkey		
Imipramine		Rhesus monkey	Rhesus monkey
LSD		Rhesus monkey	
MDA	Baboon		
Mescaline		Rhesus monkey	
Methadone	Rat, rhesus monkey		
Midazolam			
Morphine	Dog, mouse, rat, rhesus monkey		
Naloxone		Rat	
Nicotine	Baboon, dog, rat, rhesus monkey		
PCP	Baboon, dog, rat, rhesus monkey		
Procaine	Rat, rhesus monkey		
Scopolamine		Rat, rhesus monkey	
THC	Rat, rhesus monkey	Rhesus monkey	

Sources: Yokel (1987), pp. 4–9; Hoffmeister and Wuttke (1975).

Drugs as Aversive Stimuli

Before proceeding with a more detailed analysis of drug self-administration, we should note that some drugs do not act as positive reinforcers and some even have aversive properties; that is, laboratory animals will work to shut off infusions of some drugs or learn to perform tasks to avoid receiving such infusions. In the avoidance training task described in Chapter 2, laboratory animals are taught to make a response to turn off a stimulus that always precedes an electric shock. To demonstrate that some drugs have aversive properties, a similar procedure is used except that a drug infusion replaces the shock. Table 5–1 lists some drugs that have been demonstrated to

have aversive properties. They include LSD, antipsychotic drugs such as chlorpromazine, and the antidepressant imipramine.

The Positive Reinforcement Paradox

While it is clear that drugs act as positive reinforcers, it is not intuitively obvious how this model can account for some aspects of addictive behavior. As described earlier, the consequences of using some drugs can, indeed, be painful and unhealthy and ought to be punishing enough to make an organism stop using them. For example, when cocaine and amphetamine are made freely available to a monkey for a period of time, very often it will refuse to eat or sleep for extended periods, the drug will cause it to mutilate parts of its body, and ultimately the monkey will die of an overdose or bleed to death from its own self-inflicted wounds, not unlike the economically and physically destructive human behavior motivated by cocaine in some humans. It may seem paradoxical that behavior motivated by positive reinforcement should persist in the face of such punishing consequences. Addicts themselves often acknowledge that continued drug use creates an aversive state they generally would like to avoid or terminate. For this reason drug users often seek treatment for their addiction. How can an event like the administration of a drug be both positively reinforcing enough to make people continue to use it, and at the same time be aversive enough to motivate people to stop. As Gene Heyman of Harvard University asks, "If addictive drug use is on balance positively reinforcing, then why would a user ever want to stop?" (Heyman, in press, p. 16).

Such a paradox is not unique to drugs. There are many examples where consumption of more traditional reinforcers such as food is destructive and causes pain. People often overeat, become obese, and experience physical discomfort, health risks, and social censure. Sexual activity also acts as a reinforcing stimulus. It has positive reinforcing effects but can also have the potential to cause unpleasant and undesirable consequences such as sexually transmitted diseases and unwanted pregnancy. In fact, most positive reinforcers, including drugs, can have negative destructive effects that can motivate people to seek treatment to help them stop.

One of the reasons that positive reinforcing effects continue to control behavior is that they are immediately experienced after behavior, whereas the punishing and painful effects are often delayed. One well-understood principle of operant conditioning is that if a consequence is delayed, its ability to control behavior is diminished. Thus if a drink of alcohol causes pleasure within minutes and a hangover a number of hours later, it is the pleasure rather than the hangover that will be more likely to determine whether the person will drink again. When punishing consequences occur infrequently and after a considerable delay, no matter how severe they might be, they are less likely to exert as much control over behavior as immediate gratification.

There are other things we know about operant behavior that can help us understand this paradox. They will be discussed in the section on choice later in this chapter.

SELF-ADMINISTRATION IN HUMANS AND NONHUMANS

Many hundreds of studies have explored the drug-taking behavior of laboratory animals. In fact, we now probably know more about nonhuman drug taking than we do about human drug taking. The successes achieved by studying laboratory animals using operant techniques has prompted some scientists to adopt these research strategies to study human behavior. These techniques were pioneered by Nancy Mello and Jack Mendelson at the McLean Hospital in Belmont, Massachusetts. In this research, paid volunteers live in a research ward in a hospital so that they may be kept under constant medical supervision and their health and behavior may be carefully monitored. They are given the opportunity to perform some operant task such as pushing a button or riding an exercise bicycle to earn tokens or points that they are able to exchange for injections of a drug. This type of situation is analogous to the operant task with laboratory animals and can probably tell us a great deal more about drug self-administration than simply observing the behavior of addicts in their natural environment. For example, researchers are able to test the effect of different doses of drugs, compare different types of drugs, and contrast drugs with placebos. They can also manipulate other variables such as availability, route of administration, and work required, and they can even check the effects of other drugs administered at the same time. They can also carefully measure and observe changes in other sorts of behavior that might be caused by the test drug. Although the situation may be artificial, it permits researchers to exercise considerable precision and control, which is not possible in any other circumstance (Mello & Mendelson, 1987).

One disadvantage of this method is that it can present an ethical dilemma when it comes to using naive or inexperienced subjects. It would be unethical to use inexperienced or nonaddicted subjects in research of this type if it involved unrestricted exposure to drugs like heroin that are known to be habit forming. Such a procedure would introduce subjects to the reinforcing effects of a drug, an experience they might not otherwise have. Only people who have a history of drug use or previous exposure to a specific drug are generally permitted to participate in these experiments.

Operant techniques have been further refined to allow some testing of humans outside the laboratory or research ward. In this sort of research, normal human volunteers are asked to report to the laboratory every morning and asked to swallow a capsule of a particular color. On alternate days they take a capsule of a different color. Usually one color is a drug and the other is a placebo. When they have been exposed to both, they then are asked to choose which one they want to take. If the drug is a reinforcer, it will be chosen more often than the placebo. While this procedure has the advantage of not being carried out in an artificial laboratory environment, a considerable amount of precision is lost. There are also some ethical restrictions on the type and dose of drug that can be given.

Similarities and Differences between Human and Nonhuman Animals

Type of Drug. Comparisons of human and nonhuman behavior in controlled studies like these have made it quite clear that there is not a great deal of difference between species (Griffiths, Bigelow, & Henningfield, 1980). Table 5–1

lists some of the drugs that have been demonstrated to be positive reinforcers in laboratory animals. As you can see, laboratory animals will take most of the drugs that humans use, with some interesting exceptions. Nonhumans do not seem to find drugs we classify as hallucinogens to be reinforcing, and nonhumans do not readily self-administer THC (the active ingredient in cannabis). We do not understand the nature of these species differences. They could represent differences in biochemistry, but it is also possible that some aspect of the testing situation (dose or route of administration) might be inappropriate for nonhuman species.

Patterns of Self-Administration. Not only do nonhumans appear to self-administer similar drugs, but the patterns of self-administration are also similar. Figure 5–3 shows the record of a rhesus monkey self-administering alcohol (ethanol) and of a human volunteer in a research ward of a hospital who could earn drinks of alcohol by pressing a button. The records are very similar. Both subjects worked for the alcohol in an erratic pattern, and both subjects voluntarily experienced periods of withdrawal, a pattern quite similar to alcohol consumption patterns of alcoholics in more natural settings. As we proceed through this book and examine the self-administration patterns of humans and nonhumans, many more similarities will become apparent.

OPERANT ANALYSIS OF DRUG SELF-ADMINISTRATION

Abuse Potential

A number of interesting operant techniques have been used to provide us with a wealth of information about the factors that can influence the self-administration of drugs. For example, operant techniques have been used to assess the *abuse potential* or *abuse liability* of different drugs. It has become important to be able to assess abuse potential of new drugs as they are developed, and

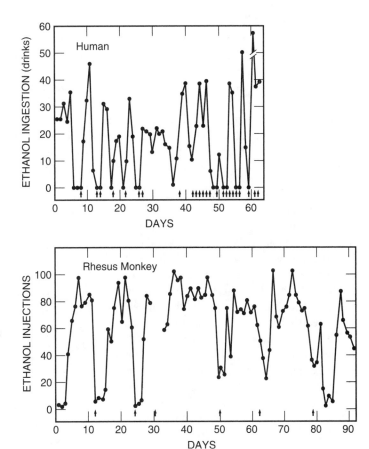

Figure 5–3 The similarity between the patterns of self-administration of ethanol in a human and a rhesus monkey under continuous drug availability. The arrows indicate the occurrence of withdrawal symptoms. Top: data from an experiment where a volunteer earned tokens by pressing a button. The tokens could be exchanged for drinks. Bottom: intake of ethanol by a rhesus monkey pressing a lever for intravenous infusions. (Adapted from Griffiths, Bigelow, and Henningfield, 1980, p. 19.)

abuse potential is becoming an important consideration in the legal classification of drugs. In operant terms, abuse potential can be thought of simply as reinforcing ability.

Rate of Responding. With traditional reinforcers we know that the greater the reinforcement, the faster an organism will respond. For example, rats will respond faster for three food pellets than they will for one pellet. We might expect then that animals will respond faster for drugs that are more reinforcing, but rate of responding has some problems. One is that drugs have different durations of action, and a long-acting drug might well be self-administered at a slower rate than a short-acting drug merely be-

cause the effect of each dose lasts longer. In addition, rate of responding depends on the animal's ability to make a response. Many drugs have effects that interfere with their own self-administration. For example, monkeys will give themselves infusions of anesthetic doses of pentobarbital, which immediately cause the animal to go to sleep. Such a drug may be highly reinforcing, but it could not be self-administered at a high rate. Conversely, many drugs such as cocaine could stimulate their own self-administration.

Progressive Ratio. These problems can be avoided by using a *progressive ratio* schedule. In this schedule, the subject is required to work for a drug infusion on an FR schedule that consistently gets longer. The schedule may start at FR 50, and after the first reinforcement is received it might change to FR 100, then to FR 200, and so on. At some point, known as the *breaking point,* the demand of the schedule will be too high, and the organism will stop responding. Presumably, highly reinforcing drugs will motivate the animal to work harder than drugs that are not so reinforcing, and will consequently have a higher breaking point.

Choice. The choice procedure is fairly simple. With laboratory animals, two levers are presented. There is a period when one lever will cause an infusion of drug A and the other lever has no consequences. This is followed by a period when the second lever will cause an infusion of drug B and the first lever has no consequences. This procedure ensures that the animal has an equal exposure to both drugs A and B. Following this phase of the experiment, both levers will dispense their drugs, and the animal is given the opportunity to respond on either lever. Presumably, the animal will respond more on the lever that delivers the more reinforcing drug.

These techniques have shown that psychomotor stimulants in general and cocaine in particular are the most robust reinforcers yet encountered. Cocaine is extensively used to train laboratory animals to self-administer drugs, and it has become a standard against which other drugs are often compared (Yanagita, 1975).

Dose of Drug. These techniques have also demonstrated that larger doses of any drug are generally more reinforcing than smaller doses, although some studies suggest that there may not be much difference between very large doses. In fact, reinforcing ability may decline when very large doses are used (Brady et al., 1987; Depoortere et al., 1993).

Genetic Differences

Even though the positive reinforcement model of drug self-administration emphasizes that environmental and schedule variables are of primary importance in controlling drug self-administration, the model does not preclude the possibility that biochemical and genetic differences between individuals may be responsible for variations in drug use. In fact, operant drug self-administration techniques can be used to test the reinforcing properties of drugs in different strains of laboratory animals and to test the possibility that certain aspects of an animal's biochemistry could alter drug-taking behavior (George, Ritz, & Elmer, 1991).

It has been known for some time that different strains of laboratory rats and mice differ in alcohol consumption. In fact, both alcohol-preferring and alcohol-avoiding strains of rats have been selectively bred in the laboratory. In addition, there is now evidence that there is a significant genetic contribution to the risk of becoming alcoholic (Schuckit, 1985, 1992): Men with a family history of alcoholism are at greater risk of becoming alcoholic themselves.

It seems that this genetic predisposition is not unique to alcohol. Frank George of the University of New Mexico and Stephen Goldberg at the National Institute on Drug Abuse in Baltimore have shown that different strains of rats and mice have different preferences for cocaine. Similar genetic differences have also been shown in the consumption of opiates (George & Goldberg, 1989).

Relief of Unpleasant Symptoms

It would be reasonable to assume that drugs that have therapeutic effects—ones that relieve an unpleasant symptom—might be self-administered for that reason. In fact, it has often been suggested that alcohol is used by some people to relieve the symptoms of stress or depression. Similarly, the motivation for abuse of diazepam (Valium) might be to protect against the distress of anxiety. Thus people experiencing high stress and anxiety might be particularly susceptible to the overuse of alcohol or diazepam.

A team of researchers at the University of Chicago, which includes Harriet de Wit and Chris Johanson, has successfully tested some of these assumptions using a variation on the choice procedure with human subjects. In this procedure, volunteers report to the lab every morning for a number of days. Each day they are given a capsule to consume at that time. On days 1 and 3 they get a capsule of one color, and on days 2 and 4 they get a capsule of a different color. On the next five days they are given their choice of color. By definition, the more reinforcing pill will be chosen more frequently. Using this technique with normal volunteers as subjects, de Wit and Johanson (1987) found that there is generally no preference for diazepam over a placebo. This result is somewhat surprising because diazepam is an extensively prescribed drug suspected of being overused.

The researchers reasoned that diazepam might be preferred and excessively used only by very anxious people, so they selected their subjects using a diagnostic test for anxiety. Surprisingly, they did not find that highly anxious people consistently chose diazepam over the placebo even though the anxious subjects reported that the drug reduced their anxiety and rated it more highly than the placebo.

In addition to testing diazepam in various populations, these researchers also found that amphetamine, which improves mood and decreases appetite (see Chapter 10), was not preferentially chosen by people who were depressed or overweight (de Wit & Johanson, 1987, p. 568; de Wit, Uhlenhuth, & Johanson, 1987).

Understanding drug use as a form of self-medication to relieve unpleasant psychological states has considerable intuitive appeal, but as yet there are few laboratory data to support the idea.

Task Demands

It seems clear from human experience that people often choose to use a drug or not depending on the demands of the situation they expect to be in. For example, they may not choose to drink alcohol if they know that they will be driving, or they may take a stimulant if they know that they will be driving long distances at night. Until recently, task demand has not been systematically examined, but recent experiments by Kenneth Silverman and his colleagues at Johns Hopkins Medical School have shown that this variable can affect drug choice in human subjects.

Silverman had volunteers ingest color-coded capsules containing either triazolam, a short acting benzodiazepine tranquilizer (see Chapter 7), d-amphetamine (a stimulant, see Chapter 10), or a placebo. Then they were required to engage in either of two activities. They participated in either a vigilance task where they stared at a computer screen for 50 minutes and were required to respond when a star appeared, or a relaxation task where they were required to lie on a bed for 50 minutes without moving. Seven of eight subjects reliably chose the amphetamine capsules when they knew that the vigilance task was to follow and all eight always chose the triazolam when they knew that would be in the relaxation situation (Silverman, Kirby, & Griffiths, 1994).

In a later experiment (Silverman, Mumford, & Griffiths, 1994) it was shown that subjects reliably chose a capsule containing 100 mg of caffeine rather than a placebo before the vigilance activity. Thus it appears that task demand can either enhance or diminish the reinforcing value of a particular drug.

Other Deprivations and Motivations

Hungry animals will drink more alcohol than satiated animals. It was always assumed that they did so because alcohol has calories that can supply the hungry animal with energy. It turns out, however, that hunger also stimulates the self-administration of many other drugs that have no calories, including cocaine and phencyclidine (PCP, a dissociative anesthetic, see Chapter 15), and thirst seems to have the same effect as hunger (Carroll & Meisch, 1984). As yet, there have been no studies of deprivation effects on drug self-administration in humans.

Previous Experience with Other Drugs

In general, most research shows that slower-acting drugs in the benzodiazepine family, such as diazepam (Valium), are not self-administered. As you can see from Table 5–1, diazepam is listed in the "not self-administered" column, but this is not always the case. Diazepam is also listed in the "self-administered" column. It turns out that an important determinant of whether diazepam is self-administered is past experience with sedative hypnotic or depressant drugs such as barbiturates. In a study with baboons, Bergman and Johanson (1985) found that animals did not self-administer diazepam when they were switched to it from cocaine, but did self-administer diazepam to some degree when switched to it from pentobarbital.

This difference does not appear to be unique to baboons. Other research using the choice procedure has consistently found no preference for diazepam over a placebo in normal population of volunteers, but similar experiments conducted with moderate alcohol users, people who consume an average of one drink a day, find a marked preference for the diazepam. In a different experiment, subjects living on a hospital research ward did work for the a benzodiazepine when given the opportunity, but they were all former sedative abusers (de Wit & Johanson, 1987).

Previous Experience with the Same Drug

In naive laboratory animals, caffeine does not appear to be a robust reinforcer. In one experiment, only 2 out of 6 monkeys self-administered caffeine spontaneously. The 4 monkeys that did not give themselves caffeine were then given automatic infusions of caffeine for a period of time. It was then shown that caffeine would act as a reinforcer in 3 of these 4 monkeys (Deneau, Yanagita, & Seevers, 1969). It has been demon-strated repeatedly that a history of either self-administration or passive exposure to a drug can enhance the drug's reinforcing ability (Goldberg, 1976, pp. 304–305; Samson, 1987).

Physical Dependence

It has already been demonstrated that physical dependence is not necessary for drug self-administration, but does it play any role in drug taking? Extensive research has not been attempted, but it appears that withdrawal can influence the strength of the reinforcing effect of many drugs. For example, early research on the self-administration of morphine showed that the rate of self-administration will increase if the animal is denied the opportunity to self-administer for a period of time and starts experiencing withdrawal symptoms (Thompson & Schuster, 1964).

In another study, Tomoji Yanagita (1987) compared the breaking points on a progressive ratio for animals that were physically dependent with animals that were not. Physical dependence was established in some animals by giving them pretreatments with a drug, and control animals were pretreated with a placebo. The breaking points on a progressive ratio schedule for the drug were determined for both groups of animals. Yanagita used this procedure with morphine and codeine and showed that animals that were physically dependent on both drugs had higher breaking points than controls. He also showed that physical dependence on ethanol caused only a slight increase in ethanol's breaking point, but the same effect was not seen with diazepam (Valium).

CHOOSING TO USE DRUGS

We have already looked at choice behavior in this chapter when experimental subjects are given the opportunity to chose between two different drugs or different doses of a drug. In this section, we look at situations where a choice is made between a drug and some other nondrug alternative, and we examine the factors that can influence the choice.

Even though it is useful to consider drug use in terms of positive reinforcement, it is clear that a single positive reinforcer does not act on behavior in isolation. Nevertheless, the effects of positive reinforcement are often studied in isolation; the organism is in an insolated chamber with only one reinforcing stimulus available, and only one response such as pressing a lever is recorded. This, of course, is a highly contrived, artificial situation. It is useful when we desire to reduce or eliminate the effects of uncontrolled variables on behavior, but it can only help us understand the basic building blocks of behavior. In reality, the world we live in and the effects of positive reinforcers are much more complex.

A rat in a Skinner box may press a lever at a high rate, a low rate, or not at all, but when it is not pressing the lever it does not stop behaving. It may be sniffing, scratching, exploring, sleeping, or engaging in a myriad of other activities, all controlled by reinforcers not immediately apparent to us. Thus the rate at which a rat presses a lever is influenced not only by the reinforcer we have programmed to follow a lever press, but by all the other reinforcers available to the rat at that instant. In other words, at any given moment, the rat distributes its activity among a number of possible responses, all controlled by a number of positive or negative reinforcers. How an organism chooses to distribute its behavior among all these alternatives presents a number of interesting and important questions that have been the focus of recent research in behavioral pharmacology laboratories.

The slogan "Just say no to drugs" suggests that the alternative to using a drug is doing nothing. In fact, it is better to think of the decision to take a drug, not as a choice between drug taking and not drug taking, but as a choice between taking a drug and doing something else. Thinking this way, it becomes apparent that the decision to use a drug may have as much to do with the avail-ability and value of the alternatives as with the availability and reinforcing value of the drug. To understand drug taking, then, we need to know more than the schedule, availability, and reinforcing value or abuse liability of the drug; we need to know what other activities and reinforcers are available to the organism in its environment. It will also help to understand how people and other animals make choices between alternatives.

Making Choices

Some time ago, psychologists started studying concurrent schedules of reinforcement. On these schedules, animals are presented with two levers and are free to press either one. Reinforcers are made available on both levers. These levers may vary in amount of reinforcer delivered and schedule of reinforcement, and the dependent variable is how the experimental subject distributes its responses between the levers.

For example, a pigeon in a Skinner box may be presented with two response keys, a red one provides a grain reinforcement on a VI 5-min. schedule. A green key presents the same amount of grain on a VI 10-min. schedule; that is, in the same time period pecking the red key has the potential to produce twice as many reinforcements as the green key. How does the pigeon handle this situation? It could just peck the red key and ignore the green key. If it chose this course, however, it would not receive all the reinforcers available to it. On a VI schedule, the longer the pigeon waits after receiving a reinforcement, the more likely it is to be reinforced, thus the more time it spends pecking the red key, the more likely it will be missing reinforcements from the green key, and vice versa. What happens in this situation is that the pigeon distributes its responses to each key in proportion to the reinforcements that key produces.

The Matching Law. Richard Herrnstein of Harvard University first described the kind of behavior mentioned in the preceding paragraph and proposed the *matching law* to describe it. The matching law simply states that *the relative rate of responding on an alternative will match the relative rate of reinforcement on that alternative* (Domjan, 1993, p. 178). Thus our pigeon would respond twice as often on the red key as the green key. As you can see, according to the matching law, the experimenter could easily change responding on the red key, not by altering the schedule on that key, but by changing the schedule on the green key. If the schedule on the green key changed from a VI 10-minute to a VI 2.5-minute schedule, then according to the matching law, the pigeon would now spend twice as much time on the green key as it would on the red key.

In this key-pecking situation the matching law makes it easy to predict mathematically how the pigeon will distribute its pecks between two alternatives. Real life is much more complicated. Not only do different stimuli vary in their capacity to function as reinforcers, as we have seen already with drugs, but the reinforcing value of a stimulus can also be modified by numerous factors including amount, delay, and the current physiological state of the organism. Nevertheless, the same principle applies; an organism will distribute its behavior among different alternatives in proportion to the relative reinforcement each alternative provides.

Thus, in real life the proportion of a person's behavior that is reinforced by the administration of a drug may have as much to do with the presence and scheduling of other nondrug reinforcers as it does with the reinforcing capacity of a drug. In human terms, this idea suggests that if drugs are available, environmental factors such as boredom, poverty, unemployment, and a lack of economic opportunity or social interaction will contribute to the development of the strength of drug use habits. It is little wonder then that drug and alcohol abuse are common in places like economically depressed inner cities, prisons, and battle zones. This association between economic and social deprivation has been noted many times, and it has usually been attributed to "stress." Rather than stress, however, it may be that the crucial variable contributing to drug use in these situations is the lack of opportunity to obtain reinforcement from any other source.

For example, studies of U.S. servicemen in Vietnam showed that many were using high-grade heroin on a regular basis while in Vietnam. On their return to the United States, the vast majority stopped using the drug (Robbins, Davis, & Goodwin, 1974) even though many were physically dependent and it was still readily available. It is likely that in Vietnam there were few sources of reinforcement available apart from drugs, but after the servicemen had returned to the United States, more incompatible activities such as employment and family activities were available to them to compete with drug use. It is easier to say no to drugs if you are busy doing something else.

In an interesting experiment, Bruce Alexander and his colleagues at Simon Fraser University in British Columbia contrived an analogous situation in the laboratory with rats. They showed that rats in a social environment where they have an opportunity to engage in other activities such as social interaction, mating, fighting, and nest building do not consume as much morphine as rats who are isolated in cages in the traditional manner of laboratory research (Alexander et al., 1981).

Looking at drug use in terms of competing activities can also help us understand some of the factors that can lead to initial use of drugs, how to improve drug therapies, and how to prevent relapse to drug use after therapy (Carroll, 1995). In an environment where the influence of alternative positive reinforcers is minimized because they are difficult to achieve or unavailable, the impact of introducing a new reinforcer such as a drug might be considerable, and it could easily come to dominate most behavior, especially if it is readily available and not expensive. Once this dominance is established, the effect might be difficult to reverse.

Sudden decreases in the opportunity to obtain competing nondrug reinforcement could also contribute to relapse in former drug users. It has been shown, for example, that former alcoholics are more likely to return to using alcohol at times when there are disruptions in work and family life (Vuchinich & Tucker, 1988, p. 188), and conversely, good therapeutic outcomes are much more likely in individuals with a stable work and family history (Vaillant, 1992).

Individual Differences. Although a given drug may be equally reinforcing to two individuals and be available to both individuals on the same schedule, factors such as the availability of other reinforcers and the relative demand other reinforcers make on behavior could modify the control exerted by that drug on each individual. This type of analysis could well explain why the same drug could control vastly different amounts of behavior in different individuals and different amounts of behavior in the same individual in different environments.

Rational Economic Theory

The alternative to the matching law, one traditionally favored by economists, is based on the assumption that behavior is rational. It assumes that organisms strive to maximize total reinforcement, that is, will distribute responses in such a way as to receive the most reinforcement in the long run. In other words, organisms respond in a pattern or strategy that will make sure that they get the most possible benefit from any situation *over an extended period of time*. Such theories are called *molar* theories, and they assume that evolution has led to the development of behavioral processes that maximize reinforcement (Domjan, 1993, p. 184).

In some cases, like the pigeon choosing between two VI schedules, the matching law and rational economics both predict the same sort of behavior, but there are circumstances where they make quite different predictions.

The following example illustrates the difference between matching and rational economic theory. Say you have a choice of fishing from a small pond where there are lots of fish and they are easy to catch, and the ocean where there are lots of fish too, but they are harder to catch. In the small pond, every fish you remove means that there will be fewer fish left to breed, so that if you take fish out too fast, the numbers will decrease over time. In the ocean, however, there are so many fish that you cannot remove them fast enough to affect the rate of reproduction. Where are you going to fish? The matching law would predict that you would fish more in the small pond because that is where there is the highest rate of reinforcement. You would continue to fish there until the probability of catching a fish falls below that of catching a fish in the ocean. Then you would switch. On the other hand, economic theory would say that it is to your benefit to catch fish in the pond no faster than they can reproduce, and you would spend more time fishing in the ocean because, in the long run, you will catch more fish in total from both sources.

It may come as no surprise to anyone who watches television advertising ("Buy now and make no payments till next year"), that studies show that most human and nonhuman animals seem to be using matching when it comes to most choice situations. In other words, most organisms appear to use rather shortsighted bookkeeping to determine relative reinforcing values of various alternatives and not look at "the big picture."

Apart from traditional laboratory species like rats and pigeons, matching has been shown in cows, college students, and free-ranging animals in natural settings, and the reinforcements have been food, money, shock avoidance, verbal praise, or getting the right answer (Heyman, in press).

Positive Reinforcement Paradox Again. This shortsightedness, at least in part, offers a means of understanding the positive reinforcement paradox discussed earlier. Why is it that a behavior supposedly maintained by positive reinforcement continues in the face of adverse consequences that are often sufficient to make the addict "want" to stop using the drug? Such a question is only a paradox if we assume that people use a molar or rational strategy in the choice to use drugs.

Gene Heyman of Harvard University (Heyman, in press) has formulated an explanation that involves two main assumptions. The first is that the choice behavior is controlled by the matching law rather than rational economics, that is, that organisms only use a short-term bookkeeping scheme and choose a particular alternative on the basis of which one is more likely to produce reinforcement. They do not look at the long term and decide which behavior will ultimately be the most beneficial. Heyman's second assumption is that when you use a drug, it diminishes the value of other conventional reinforcers that control competing activity. The use of alcohol, for example, can disrupt relationships with one's spouse or interfere with work and thereby diminish reinforcement normally available from the family or the workplace. This diminished availability of competing reinforcement could in turn lead to more drinking.

If matching mechanisms control choice to use drugs and if drugs are able to diminish the value of competing activities, you can see how it is possible for drug use to spiral out of control, eventually reaching a state where the drug controls an addict's life and causes pain, deprivation, and anguish even though it is a positive reinforcer.

BEHAVIORAL ECONOMICS: PRICE AND DEMAND

The study of the factors that contribute to how people will spend their time and money has not been of interest only to psychologists. As we have seen in the previous section, economists have been thinking about similar problems for years. They have been studying how a consumer distributes money among a variety of consumer goods and what happens to the demand for these goods when the price increases and decreases. These lines of inquiry are basically similar, and research in both areas has yielded surprisingly consistent results. The application of economic principles to understanding operant behavior is called *behavioral economics*.

One of the most basic questions that can be asked in behavioral economics is about the effect of increasing the price of a commodity on the demand for that commodity. If the price of a commodity increases, a drug for example, does the demand for the drug go down, or do consumers of that drug continue to use it the same way in spite of the increased cost?

Economists identify two possibilities here. If consumers continue to spend the same amount for the drug as before even though they are not able to purchase as much, demand is said to be *inelastic*. But if people start spending less for the drug in response to a price increase, demand is said to be *elastic*. Goods considered necessities like food, water, and shelter usually show inelastic demand, but luxury items like entertainment and travel often show elastic demand.

An experiment conducted by Marilyn E. Carroll (1993) of the University of Minnesota illustrates how this research is done and how the results are often presented. She used rhesus monkeys who were trained to press a lever on a FR schedule to receive access to a drinking tube that delivered water containing phencyclidine (PCP). She tested the monkeys at a number of different FR values, 4, 8, 16, 32, 64, and 128. The results are shown in Figure 5–4. On these graphs, the horizontal axis gives the cost of the drug in terms of the number of responses that must be made to receive each milligram of drug. The vertical axis on the left panel presents the demand for the drug, that is, the total amount of drug consumed. Both the axes are on logarithmic scales—the standard manner of presenting such data. As you can see from the left panel (for now,

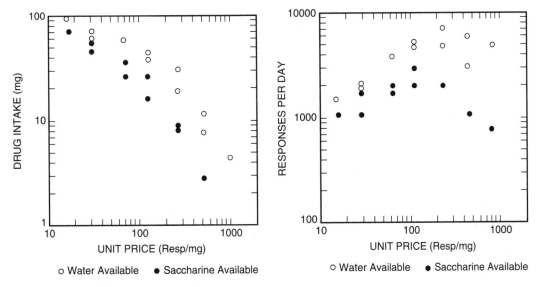

Figure 5–4 Demand curves for monkeys responding on FR schedules of 4, 8, 16, 32, 64, and 128 to receive access to a drinking tube that delivered water containing phencyclidine (PCP). For both graphs the horizontal axis gives the cost of the drug in terms of the number of responses that must be made to receive each milligram of drug. *Left:* The vertical axis presents the demand for the drug, that is, the total amount of drug consumed per day. *Right:* The horizontal axis is also unit price in responses per milligram of drug, but the vertical axis is total responses, that is, total expenditure per day. Both the axes are on logarithmic scales, which have become the standard manner of presenting such data. The open circles indicate responding when water was present, and the closed circles show responding when a sweet-tasting saccharin solution was present. (Carroll, 1993.)

just pay attention to the open circles), as the cost of each delivery of PCP increases, the demand for PCP drops. The slope of the curve can tell us whether the demand is elastic or inelastic. If the slope is between 0 and −1.0, it shows that the demand does not decline as fast as the price increases (the consumer is spending just as much or more on the commodity); that is, demand is inelastic. Negative slopes with an absolute value greater than −1.0 show that the consumer is spending less and less on the drug as price goes

up and that the decrease is proportionally greater than the price increase; that is, demand is elastic.

The bottom graph also presents interesting information. In this graph, the horizontal axis is also unit price in responses per milligram of drug, but the vertical axis is total responses—that is, total expenditure. As cost increased up to 415 responses per milligram of drug, responding also increased. At higher costs, however, responding declined. These results show that at lower costs (up to 415 responses/mg), demand is inelastic (total spending for the drug increased or remained the same), but a point was reached where demand became elastic (spending declined). This sort of pattern seems to be typical of many drugs. This situation is analogous to the progressive ratio schedule discussed earlier where the schedule requirements for a reinforcer are increased to a point where the organism stops responding for it. A review by Bickel and his coworkers (Bickel et al., 1990) showed a similar function in ten different experiments using a variety of drugs including cocaine, barbiturates, d-amphetamine, and ketamine in rhesus monkeys, squirrel monkeys, and rats.

Substitution

One factor that economic studies have shown to influence elasticity is the availability of other related consumer goods. Apart from being completely *independent*, two products may be *substitutes*; for example, when the price of beef goes up, consumers may buy more chicken. Also, two commodities may be *complements* to each other; that is, when the price of one product goes up, the use of both products may decline. For example, if people always put butter on their bread and the price of bread increases, consumption of both bread and butter may decline.

There has been some interesting research on how the availability of substitutes can influence the demand functions described previously—for example, what sort of reinforcers can substitute for drugs, and what effect the availability of a substitute will have on elasticity of demand for a drug. The answers to these questions have important implications for treatment strategies and for public drug control policy.

Drug Substitutes. In one experiment (DeGrandpre et al., 1993), subjects in a laboratory were given the opportunity to use a limited amount of money to purchase either their own preferred brand of cigarettes, which were expensive, or another less preferred brand that was rel-
atively cheap. When they were given a large amount of money, they chose their preferred brand, but when the amount of money they were given to spend decreased, they tended to choose the less preferred, cheaper brand. In total, however, no matter which brand they consumed, their daily intake of nicotine did not change. The cheaper brand was able to substitute for the preferred brand, but only when income was reduced.

Nondrug Substitutes. It might not be too surprising to find that one drug can substitute for itself or that one drug can substitute for a similar drug, but it appears that the availability of nondrug reinforcers can also substitute for a drug. An interesting experiment demonstrated that if rats were allowed to have access to a sweet sugar solution, their oral consumption of a morphine solution dramatically decreased. When the sweet solution was removed, morphine consumption returned to original levels. Sweet solutions have been shown to reduce amphetamine and ethanol self-administration as well (Kanarek & Marks-Kaufman, 1988; Carroll, 1993). It also seems that access to a simple running wheel has the same effect on drug intake as the sweet solution (Kanarek & Marks-Kaufman, 1989).

In the research by Carroll (1993) described previously, the unit price of PCP was increased, and there was a reduction in the use of the drug by rhesus monkeys. The research went on to show that if the monkeys were provided with a nondrug substitute for the PCP, in this case access to a sweet-tasting saccharin solution, the monkeys did not work as hard for PCP, and that the demand for PCP dropped much faster when the saccharin was present. The graphs of Figure 5–4 show what happened when the substitute was available (solid circles) compared with a control condition when water was available (open circles). When the saccharin was available, the demand for the drug significantly decreased. In the right graph you can see that without saccharin, the monkeys increased their responding for PCP up to a cost of 415 responses per milligram, (open circles), but when the saccharin was available, responding peaked at 160 responses per milligram (solid circles) and then declined. The fact that saccharin was substituting for the PCP was indicated by an increase in saccharin consumption as the PCP consumption declined. What this research shows is that the effect of a price increase on demand for a commodity depends on the availability of competing commodities.

It is worth noting that this effect of the saccharin substitute was much greater when there was a very high work requirement for the PCP. At the lower FR values (FR 4), PCP intake was only reduced by about 21 percent by making the saccharin available, but the availability of saccharin reduced PCP intake by more than 87 percent at the higher FR values (FR 128).

You will recognize the similarity between this discussion and the discussion of choice. The analysis of behavior in terms of economics—that is, price and demand—essentially boils down to a study of factors that govern how we choose between alternatives. Both lines of research clearly show that drug use will increase or decrease depending on the cost (availability) of alternatives (substitutes).

THE NEUROANATOMY OF REINFORCEMENT

In the 1950s, James Olds and Peter Milner (1954) at McGill University discovered that electrical stimulation of certain areas of the brain would act as reinforcement; that is, rats would learn to perform a task in order to cause the stimulation. It is now clear that these circuits are the location of the mechanisms of positive reinforcement. They are systems in the brain that are activated when an organism performs a task that contributes to the survival of the organism or the species, and their function is to ensure that such behavior will be repeated. Thus, if a hungry animal finds food after turning over a rock and eats it, the reinforcement mechanisms will be activated. As a result, the animal will be more likely to turn rocks over the next time it gets hungry. In other words, it will have learned where to find food. These systems appear to be an intricate development of evolution that has permitted organisms to be maximally flexible in adapting their behavior to an ever-changing environment (J. H. Campbell, 1971). Drugs act as positive reinforcers because they activate these reinforcement systems directly and artificially "reinforce" their own administration.

We have no way of knowing what any organism experiences when the brain's reinforcement system is activated, but we do know that in humans, when these systems are stimulated electrically, a feeling of pleasure is reported. It is certainly tempting to speculate that it is this pleasure that "rewards" the behavior that caused it and motivates the organism to repeat such actions, but the situation is probably much more complicated. We have already seen that events can be reinforcing without being pleasurable. In fact, T. E. Robinson and K. C. Burridge (1993) have speculated that there are two separate systems in the brain, one that is responsible for "liking" and another that controls "wanting." They say that drugs primarily activate the "wanting" system, and it is for this reason that drugs can cause such intense cravings, sometimes in the absence of the experience of intense pleasure.

Since the 1960s, considerable work has been done on reinforcement systems, and we now have a good understanding of their location and their neurochemistry. We also know that the activation of at least one of these systems is responsible for the reinforcing properties of two major classes of self-administered drugs, opiates like morphine and heroin and psychomotor stimulants like cocaine and amphetamine (Bozarth, 1983).

Although other theories propose more complex reinforcing pathways of drugs in the brain (Dworkin & Smith, 1987), Figure 5–5 presents

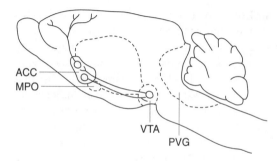

Figure 5–5 The major centers in the rat brain stimulated by opiates. Axons from the nucleus accumbens (ACC) synapse in the ventral tegmental area (VTA). This is part of a system that mediates reinforcement. Also shown is the medial preoptic area (MPO), which controls the effect of opiates on body temperature, and the periventricular gray (PVG), which mediates the analgesic effect of opiates. The PVG also is responsible for sedation and physical dependence. (Bozarth, 1983, pp. 352, 355.)

the simplest and most widely accepted theory, known as the dopamine hypothesis, advanced by Bozarth and Wise (Bozarth, 1983). It shows the location of the reinforcing system in the brain of a rat that mediates reinforcing effects of opiates, cocaine, and amphetamine. The cell bodies are located in a part of the brain known as the *ventral tegmental area (VTA)*, and they send their axons forward to an area known as the *nucleus accumbens (ACC)*, via the *medial forebrain bundle* where they synapse on other cells, which send axons into the forebrain and many other places. It is thought that the ACC sends axons back to the VTA where their synapses release an endogenous opiate, thus creating a loop (Vaccarino, Schiff, & Glickman, 1989).

It is known that rats will work to have morphine and other opiates injected directly into the area of the VTA where the cell bodies of this system are located. In addition, the transmitter released by these cells in the ACC is dopamine, and

amphetamine and cocaine injected directly into this area are also reinforcing. The intravenous self-administration of both opiates and psychomotor stimulants stops when the VTA-ACC system is damaged. Furthermore, drugs such as the antipsychotics, which block the effects of dopamine, also block the reinforcing properties of both the opiates and the psychomotor stimulants.

The system shown in Figure 5–5 looks fairly simple and involves only two brain centers. It is quite likely, however, that many other parts of the brain are also involved. Do other self-administered drugs also activate this system? It appears that they do either directly or indirectly (Gold & Miller, 1995b; Wise, 1995).

Research that involves direct injection of opiates into the brain has uncovered another interesting fact about the relationship between opiates and physical dependence. Figure 5–5 also shows different areas of the brain where opiates have a direct effect. You can see that an area known as the *medical preoptic area (MPO)* controls the effect of opiates on the animal's body temperature. Another area, the *periventricular gray area (PVG),* seems to be responsible for several other effects of opiates including analgesia, sedation, and the development of physical dependence. This means that opiates injected directly into the VTA that cause reinforcement do not also cause physical dependence. Since nondependent rats will work to inject opiates into the VTA and not into the PVG, this is compelling evidence that the motivation for self-administration of opiates is positive reinforcement rather than fear of withdrawal (Bozarth & Wise, 1984).

Earlier it was shown that sweet tasting solutions were effective in acting as substitutes for a variety of drugs. A number of studies have demonstrated that sweet tastes seem to cause the release of endogenous opiates and catecholamines in the brain and result in an activation of reinforcement centers. This may be the neurological mechanism by which such stimuli are able to substitute for reinforcing drugs (Hoebel, et al. 1989; Carroll, 1995).

CHAPTER SUMMARY

- Historically, the abuse of drugs was viewed as an abnormal type of behavior which could not be explained by the same rules that govern normal behavior. This belief was held because drug abuse appeared to be particularly compulsive and self-destructive.

- Originally people who abused drugs were thought to be deficient in willpower or morality, and drug abuse was thought to be a problem for the clergy and the church to handle. Later the medical profession became involved in attempts to treat people who were abusing opium and morphine because these substances were widely used as medicines. At about this time the term *addiction* became exclusively applied to excessive drug use and took on the connotation of disease.

- Despite explanations involving biochemical deficiency and allergies, the disease of addiction has never been identified, and excessive drug use has never been successfully explained as a disease.

- The physical dependence model suggests that excessive drug use is motivated by a fear of withdrawal symptoms that occur when a person stops using a drug. Proponents of the dependence model explain the abuse of drugs that do not cause physical dependence by suggesting that these drugs cause *psychological dependence*.

- Prior to the 1950s, when it became known that nonhumans would give themselves drugs in the same manner as humans, it was easily demonstrated that some assumptions of the disease model and the physical dependence model were not correct.

- Experiments with nonhumans showed that physical dependence was not necessary for self-administration.

- Researchers came to realize that drug administrations could control the behavior of organisms in the same way as more traditional positive reinforcers like food and water.

- The rate at which an organism self-administers a drug is not a good indication of the reinforcing ability of that drug, because many drugs have effects that interfere with their own self-administration.

- *Progressive ratio schedules* demonstrate how hard an organism will work for a single administration of a drug. Choice between drug and nondrug alternatives has also been used as measures of drug reinforcement.

- Deprivation from other reinforcers (for example, hunger) and previous experience with a drug will increase drug self-administration, while the presence of withdrawal symptoms seems to have little effect.

- One environmental influence that can diminish drug self-administration is the availability of other reinforcers. If other reinforced behaviors are available, an organism will reduce drug intake.

- Organisms will distribute their behavior among a number of tasks in accordance with the rate of reinforcement on each task. This is known as the *matching law*. Humans and nonhumans tend to assess reinforcement frequency in a rather short time frame, so that serious negative consequences that occur at a distance in time after a choice is being made often do not have a great influence on that choice. *Rational economic theory* predicts a *molar* strategy in which an organism maximizes total reinforcement over an extended period of time.

- Sometimes drugs can come to control behavior because the use of those drugs diminishes the availability of other reinforcers that could compete with the drug.

- The application of economic principles to understanding operant behavior is called *behavioral economics*. Drug use can be understood in terms of behavioral economics. If people spend less on a commodity when the price increases, the demand is said to be *elastic*. If they do not decrease spending on the drug (or increase spending), the demand is said to be *inelastic*. For many drugs, demand is inelastic up to a point where it becomes elastic.

- Demand can be influenced by other commodities. Commodities are *substitutes* when the drop in demand for one is accompanied by an increase in demand for the other. They are *complements* when a decrease in demand for one is accompanied by a decrease in demand for the other.

- Both drug and nondrug reinforcers can serve as substitutes for drugs.

- It has been demonstrated that there are places in the brain, the *ventral tegmental area* and the *nucleus accumbens*, that mediate reinforcement, and drugs like cocaine and the opiates appear to stimulate these areas directly. A completely different area seems to be responsible for the development of physical dependence.

6

Alcohol

SOURCE OF ALCOHOL

Alcohol is a chemical term that covers a class of substances only a few of which are ever consumed. Some members of this class are *isopropyl alcohol*, used as rubbing alcohol; *methanol (methyl alcohol)*, or *wood alcohol*; and *ethanol (ethyl alcohol)*, the stuff we drink. These other alcohols can be consumed and have behavioral effects similar to ethanol, but they are rather toxic and are normally only consumed by accident. In this book, as in most others, the term *alcohol* will be used to refer to ethanol. Where other alcohols are intended they will be mentioned by name.

Fermentation

The alcohol we drink is made largely by *fermentation*. When sugar is dissolved in water and left exposed to the air, the mixture is invaded by tiny microorganisms called *yeasts*. Yeasts thrive in this environment by eating the sugar, and they multiply rapidly. The metabolic processes of the yeasts convert the sugar into ethanol and *carbon dioxide (CO$_2$)*. The CO$_2$ rises to the top in bubbles, and the alcohol remains. More and more yeasts produce more and more alcohol until all the sugar is used up or the yeasts are unable to continue.

The type of beverage you get from fermentation is determined by the source of the sugar. Almost any vegetable material containing sugar may be used, but the most common are grape juice, which is fermented to make wine, and grains, which are fermented to make beer. Modern fermentation is done with special yeasts rather than the wild variety. Yeasts are living organisms and have been bred and selected over the centuries for particular types of fermentation. Because yeasts can tolerate only low levels of alcohol, fermented beverages do not have alcohol levels much above 10 to 15 percent.

Distillation

There is some debate about the discovery of *distillation*. Alcoholic spirits may first have been distilled in Arabia. The process of distillation, known only to alchemists, was a jealously guarded secret, and little was committed to writing until the Dominican scholar Albertus Magnus described the process in detail in the thirteenth century (Austin, 1985, p. 92). The process of distillation is quite simple. It starts with ordinary fermentation of a sugary substance. When fermentation is completed, the mixture is heated. Since alcohol has a lower boiling point than water, the vapor or steam given off will have a higher content of vaporized alcohol than the original product. When this vapor is condensed by cooling, the resulting fluid will also contain a higher percentage of alcohol. Of course there is no reason why the condensed spirits cannot be redistilled again and again until the resulting fluid has the desired level of alcohol. The traditional method among moonshiners for determining whether they have distilled their product sufficiently is to take a teaspoon of the stuff and set it on fire. When the fire has burned off all the alcohol, the spoon is tipped, and if more than a drop of water remains, the liquid is distilled again.

Brandy is the result of distilling wine, and whiskey is distilled from fermented grains. Brandy and whiskey were the first popular spirits. Today we have rum, distilled from fermented molasses, and schnapps, which traditionally is distilled from fermented potatoes. Gin and vodka are made from a mixture of water, flavoring, and pure alcohol distilled from any source. Distilled spirits, or *hard liquor,* usually have an alcoholic content of about 40 to 50 percent by volume. In addition to these hard liquors are the *liqueurs,* which are sweetened and flavored. Some well-known liqueurs are crème de menthe, which is flavored with mint; Cointreau, which has an added flavor of oranges; and the famous Greek drink ouzo, which has an anise flavor.

Midway between the distilled and fermented beverages are the *fortified wines,* such as sherry, port, madeira, and muscatel, which were developed during the Middle Ages. These are blends of wine with extra alcohol added to boost the alcohol content to about 20 percent. Vermouth is a flavored fortified wine developed in Turin in the eighteenth century.

MEASUREMENT OF ALCOHOL CONTENT

The description of alcohol content has always been confusing. Percentage figures may be given either by volume, as in the United States, or by weight, as in Britain. Alcohol has a specific gravity of about 0.79 (this means that a quantity of alcohol will weigh 79 percent as much as the same volume of water), and therefore a ratio based on volumes will have less alcohol than the same ratio based on weight. In other words, a drink that is 50 percent alcohol by volume will be about 40 percent alcohol by weight. In Britain, alcoholic content has customarily been described in terms of *proof.* The term has its origin in the British navy, which traditionally issued all its sailors a ration of rum every day. The navy had to buy vast quantities of rum, and its purchasers developed a rather ingenious way of testing the alcohol content. They would mix the rum with gunpowder and try to light it. If it burned, this was "proof" that it was at least 50 percent alcohol by weight. Thus *proof spirits* means a liquor with 50 percent alcohol. The term *overproof* refers to spirits with a content greater than 50 percent. It later became customary to assign a proof number to liquor. Liquor that is 50 percent alcohol is 100 proof, so the proof number is twice the percentage of alcohol by weight. The British stuck to the custom of calculating the percentage by weight, whereas in the United States alcohol content is described by volume. Therefore, British proof spirits have a higher alcoholic content than American spirits with the same proof number. Fortunately, it is becoming more common to have the percent alcohol content of a beverage printed clearly on the label of bottles in unambiguous terms.

ORIGIN AND HISTORY

Alcohol has been used from before recorded history, and its use is so widespread that few cultures in the world do not use alcohol regularly. Historically, it appears as though native North American cultures and cultures in the Pacific Islands are among the few peoples that did not discover fermentation on their own (Falk & Feingold, 1987, p. 1507). One of the reasons for the widespread use of alcohol is that it is very easy to make. The first alcohol that humans consumed was probably in the form of fermented honey or fruit.

Deliberate fermentation probably began with the development of agriculture when Neolithic people learned to cultivate grains and the grapevine. These developments probably took place around 6000 B.C. in a region south of the Black Sea that is now Armenia. An abundance of uncultivated grapes grow in this area (Austin, 1985).

The earliest written set of laws, the Code of Hammurabi, written in the year 2225 B.C. in Assyria, sets forth some rules for the keeping of beer and wine shops and taverns. The ancient Egyptians were also known for their drinking. The Egyptian Book of the Dead from about 3000 B.C. mentions the manufacture of a drink called *hek*, which was a form of beer made from grain (Bickerdyke, 1971). Herodotus, the Greek historian, tells the story that at a rich man's feast in ancient Egypt it was the custom to have a man carry around the image of a corpse in a coffin and show it to all the guests saying, "Drink and make merry, but look on this for such thou shalt be when thou are dead" (R. G. McCarthy, 1959, p. 66). The ancient Egyptians as well as the Assyrians and the Babylonians drank beer primarily because their climate was more suitable for the growing of grains than grapes, but they also drank a great deal of wine. It was probably the Egyptians who taught the Israelites to make wine and beer before the Exodus to the Promised Land (Firebaugh, 1972).

There is much evidence that the Greeks, who were supposed to be "temperate in all things," may not always have been so temperate where wine was concerned. Plato had much to say about the effects of alcohol. In *The Law*, Plato said:

When a man drinks wine he begins to be better pleased with himself and the more he drinks the more he is filled full of brave hopes, and conceit of his powers, and at least the string of his tongue is loosened, and fancying himself wise, he is brimming over with lawlessness and has no more fear or respect and is ready to do or say anything. (Laws I, 649a–b, translation Jowett, 1931, p. 28)

Though the early Romans had little trouble with wine, there was a great deal of insobriety and debauchery in the later days of the Roman Empire, for which the later Roman emperors such as Nero, Claudius, and Caligula became notorious. The fall of the Roman Empire has been blamed on the consumption of wine—not so much as a result of the alcohol but because wine at the time was fermented and stored in vessels made of lead, and an additive was put in the wine to enhance the flavor and stop fermentation. This additive had a very high lead content, and it is believed that most of the Roman nobility who drank wine suffered from lead poisoning, of which mental *inability* is a symptom (Nriagu, 1983).

Before the Romans brought grapes, and subsequently wine, to the British Isles, the main alcoholic beverages were beer made from barley, mead from fermented wild honey, and cider from fermented applies. The Romans introduced grapes to Britain, but the vine never thrived in the British climate, and wine, as today, was primarily imported. After the Romans left Britain, so did the grape, but the Saxons carried on the tradition of heavy drinking with mead, ale, and cider. Taverns and alehouses were established in about the eighth century and quickly acquired such a bad reputation that priests were not allowed to enter (French, 1884).

After the Norman Conquest in 1066, drinking became more moderate and wine was reintroduced, but the English were still heavy drinkers. "You know that the constant habit of drinking has made the English famous among all foreign nations," wrote Peter of Blois (French, 1884, p. 68).

Though distillation had been known for some time, it did not make its presence felt in England until the sixteenth century, when a number of Irish settlers started manufacturing and distributing *usquebaugh*, which became, in English, *whiskey*. Imported brandy from France was also becoming popular. After the restoration of the monarchy in 1660, distilleries were licensed, and the popularity of gin spread like an epidemic. (Gin is raw alcohol flavored with the juniper berry, which in Dutch is *genever*. Through misunderstanding, the drink became known as *Geneva dose* and later as *gin*.) The appalling conditions brought on by this "gin epidemic" are amplified in Figure 6–1, "Gin Lane," an illustration by William Hogarth depicting the streets of London in the early 1700s.

Between 1684 and 1727 the consumption of distilled spirits increased from about half a million gallons to over 3.5 million (French, 1884, p. 271). These figures do not include the large quantities of rum and brandy smuggled into the country to escape high duties and tariffs. This epidemic raised such concern that the government passed a desperate series of laws aimed at curtailing the use of liquor, but nothing had much effect. Finally, in 1742 when consumption reached 19 million gallons, Parliament finally found something that worked: it banned the distillation of grain altogether for a number of years and then closely regulated the manufacture of spirits. By 1782 consumption had dropped to 4 million gallons. But these laws were to expire and their enforcement was to relax over the next 50 years. By the early part of the nineteenth century, things were almost as bad as before.

The English propensity for strong drink was transported across the Atlantic to the colonies. Colonial Americans were also hearty drinkers, and alcohol played a large part in their lives.

So highly did the colonies prize booze that their statutes regulating its sale spoke of it as "one of the good creatures of God, to be received with thanksgiving." . . . Harvard University operated its own brewery, and commencements grew so riotous that rigid rules had to be imposed to reduce "the Excesses, Immoralities and Disorders." . . . Workmen received part of their pay in rum and their employees would set aside certain days of the year to total inebriety. (Benjamin Rush, quoted in Kobler, 1973, pp. 25–26)

Before the American Revolution, there had been some success in regulating taverns and drinking, but this control weakened after independence.

Americans perceive liberty from the crown as somehow related to the freedom to down a few glasses of rum. Did not both freedoms give a man the right to choose for himself? . . . As a consequence drinking houses emerged from the war with increased vitality and independence and the legal regulation of licensed premises waned. (Rorabaugh, 1979, p. 35)

Consumption continued to increase to prodigious levels, followed by a precipitous decline between 1830 and 1860. This decline can be attributed to the efforts of one agency alone: the temperance movement.

In both England and the United States, there had always been people who openly condemned the use of alcohol, and there were organized movements against drinking and alcohol consumption. In the late 1700s in the United States, the champion of temperance was Dr. Benjamin Rush, a physician who wrote widely about the dangerous physical, social, and moral effects of alcohol. In 1785, Rush published one of the first influential temperance documents, "An Inquiry into the Effects of Ardent Spirits."

Although Rush's writings were not heeded at the time, they inspired the American temperance movement of the early nineteenth century, which

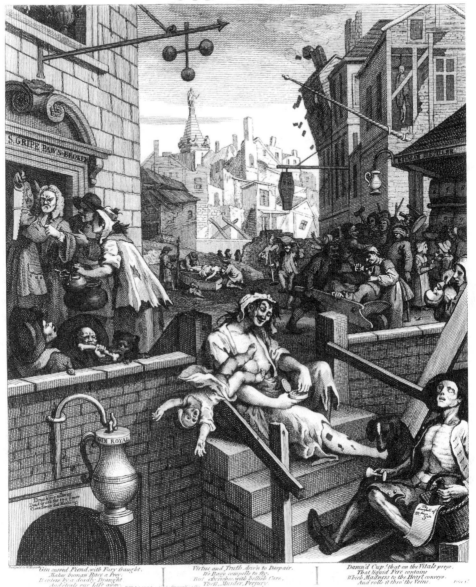

Figure 6–1 "Gin Lane," an engraving by Hogarth characterizing the social state of affairs in England during the "gin epidemic" in the mid-eighteenth century. Note that the only businesses prospering belong to the pawnbroker and the coffin maker. (Courtesy of the Print Collection, Lewis Walpole Library, Yale University.)

was more successful than any similar movement before or since. The temperance movement at that time was successful because it was philosophically in tune with the moral tenor and ideals of the new republic, and socially it filled exactly the same function as drinking. "Some men sought camaraderie at the tavern, others in their local temperance organization" (Rorabaugh, 1979, p. 189). In addition, a religious revival was sweeping the United States at the time. Total abstinence provided a symbolic way to express conversion and faith, and booze provided a target for righteous zeal.

The temperance movement was not content to rely on the force of moral persuasion to dry up the country. During this period the movement attracted enough power to have alcohol prohibition laws enacted in 11 states and two territories. Soon a national Prohibition party was founded, and the temperance reformers set their sights on the federal government. Their vigorous campaign culminated in 1917 with the ratification of the Eighteenth Amendment to the U.S. Constitution. This was the "noble experiment," Prohibition. It was passed for the most part without referendum at a time when most legislatures were paying attention to World War I, and there was little opposition.

Because it did not have widespread public support, the law was virtually unenforceable and provided a vehicle for the rapid development and funding of mobsters and organized crime. Alcohol that was not manufactured in the United States was smuggled in from Canada and elsewhere in vast quantities.

It finally became apparent to both Herbert Hoover and Franklin Roosevelt, candidates in the 1932 presidential election, that Prohibition did not have popular support. One month after Roosevelt's victory, a Twenty-First Amendment to the Constitution was drafted that would void the Eighteenth. Within two months it was passed by

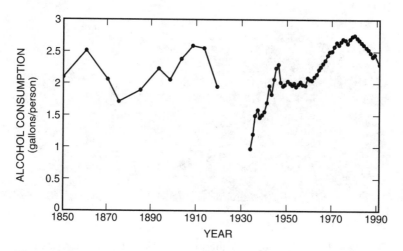

Figure 6–2 Yearly alcohol consumption in gallons per person of raw alcohol from 1850 to 1990 in the United States. Note that there are three peaks in consumption about sixty years apart. The gap in the early part of the twentieth century is due to Prohibition. Note the short-lived increase in consumption in the years following World War II. (Williams, Clem & Dufour, 1993.)

both the House and the Senate, and on December 5, 1933, the 36th state, Utah, ratified it, and it was signed into law. Prohibition had lasted almost 14 years.

After Prohibition ended, alcohol consumption rates increased steadily until they peaked in about 1979 (White, 1993). Spurred by movements such as MADD (Mothers against Drunk Driving), consumption has begun to decline in response to an increasing concern with health and a decreasing public tolerance of drugs in general and the harm that they do. There are those such as David Musto, a medical historian at Yale University, who predict that history is likely to repeat itself and that this decline will continue into the early twenty-first century and be followed by another drinking backlash (Kolata, 1991).

Figure 6–2 shows that American consumption of alcohol appears to go through cycles with consumption peaks about 60 to 70 years apart. These peaks have been followed by a decline in use. Historians have pointed out that these periods of decline were accompanied by a preoccupation with health and morality and a public concern over the harm that alcohol was doing, and both were followed by a fairly sharp increase in consumption. It appears as though the United States has begun a phase of decreasing alcohol use.

MEASURING ALCOHOL LEVELS IN THE BODY

Alcohol levels are usually measured in terms of the concentration of alcohol in whole blood. This is known as the blood alcohol level or BAL. The BAL may be measured directly by taking a blood sample, but more often a breath sample is taken and analyzed using a device known as a Breathalyzer. It has been well established that alcohol concentration in the breath reliably reflects the concentration in the blood, and so the results of a Breathalyzer are reported as "blood alcohol level" rather than "breath alcohol level."

Metric Measurements and Percent

It is usual for BAL to be expressed in terms of milligrams (mg) of alcohol per 100 milliliters (ml) of whole blood. (A milligram is 1/1,000 gram; a milliliter which is 1/1,000 liter; 100 ml is equal to a deciliter, or dl.) Blood alcohol level may also be described as a percent of alcohol in the blood. Conversion between these measures is not difficult and only involves moving the decimal point three places to the left or right. For example, a BAL of 80 mg per 100 ml (or 80 mg/dl) is the same as 0.08 percent.

SI Units

There has been a recent trend to start reporting drug concentrations in SI units (Système International d'Unités), and many journals report alcohol concentrations this way. The SI unit for drugs, including alcohol, is millimoles per liter (mmol/l). To convert the metric measures to SI units you must first convert milligrams of alcohol to millimoles and then convert deciliters of blood to liters. The first step is accomplished by dividing the milligrams by the molecular weight of alcohol, 46.07. Thus, 80 milligrams becomes (80/46.07 = 1.74) 1.74 millimoles. A liter is 10 deciliters; thus 80 mg/dl is equivalent to 17.4 mmol/l. By combining these steps, you can convert milligrams per 100 ml to mmol/l, simply by dividing by 4.607.

ROUTE OF ADMINISTRATION AND PHARMACOKINETICS

Figure 6–3 shows the theoretical time course for the level of alcohol in the blood after taking a single drink. This curve can be considered as being made up of several phases. The part of the curve labeled *A* is the absorption phase, where absorption is taking place much more rapidly than excretion. The next phase, labeled *B* and *C,* is the plateau phase, where absorption tapers off and excretion starts to lower alcohol levels. During this phase blood levels peak. If absorption

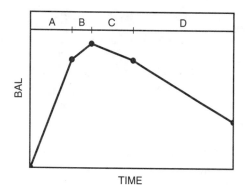

Figure 6–3 Theoretical time course for BAL after taking a single drink. Part *A* is the absorption phase, where absorption is taking place much more rapidly than excretion. Phase *B* and *C* is the plateau phase, where absorption tapers off and excretion starts to lower alcohol levels. During this phase blood levels peak. If absorption has been rapid, there may also be a brief period immediately following the peak when the decline in blood levels is rapid. This rapid decline is caused by the distribution of alcohol out of the blood to other parts of the body. During the excretion phase, *D,* absorption is complete and alcohol is eliminated from the body at a constant rate.

has been rapid, there may also be a brief period immediately following the peak when the decline in blood levels is rapid as a result of the distribution of alcohol out of the blood to other parts of the body. After the plateau phase comes the excretion phase, *D,* during which alcohol is eliminated from the body at a constant rate.

ABSORPTION

Alcohol is normally administered orally, and absorption takes place in the digestive tract. Since the molecules of alcohol cannot be ionized, the pH of neither the digestive system nor the blood has an effect on absorption.

Alcohol readily dissolves in water, and it may pass into the blood from the stomach, intestines, or colon, but it is absorbed most rapidly from the small intestine. In addition, as long as the alcohol stays in the stomach it is subjected to fairly high levels of alcohol dehydrogenase, the main enzyme that destroys alcohol. This destruction of alcohol in the stomach is called *first pass metabolism.* After solid food has been eaten, the digestion process usually keeps the food in the stomach for a period of time before it is released in small quantities into the intestines. Thus the longer alcohol stays in the stomach, the more slowly it will be absorbed into the blood and the less of it there will be to be absorbed because of first pass metabolism. In general, absorption of alcohol is faster on an empty stomach, and more will get into the body. Even though peak blood levels are higher when there is no food in the stomach, the peak will occur at about the same time, and it will take about the same time for blood levels to return to zero (Watkins & Adler, 1993).

It has also been shown that some medicines such as *cimetidine* (Zantac) and *ranitidine* (Tagamet), which are commonly used to reduce stomach acidity in people who have ulcers, can increase blood alcohol levels created by a given amount of alcohol. These drugs, known as H_2-receptor antagonists, are widely prescribed. It has been found that some H_2-receptor antagonists reduce stomach levels of alcohol dehydrogenase, and this action protects alcohol from first pass metabolism. One study showed that the amount of alcohol that entered the blood was increased by 17 percent after ranitidine treatment for one week. The effect was even greater with cimetidine. The effects of cimetidine and ranitidine are greatest when alcohol is taken on a full stomach. On an empty stomach (or in the case of alcoholics) there is little first pass metabolism in the digestive system in any case (DiPadova et al., 1987, 1992).

There also appear to be gender differences in first pass metabolism. Women appear to have lower levels of alcohol dehydrogenase in their stomachs than men, and consequently more of the alcohol a woman drinks gets into the blood, resulting in higher BALs in a woman than the same amount of alcohol would produce in a man of similar size (Whitfield & Martin, 1994; Frezza et al., 1990). It has been speculated that this difference could be one reason why women are more vulnerable than men to the acute and chronic complications of alcoholism including alcoholic liver disease.

Interestingly, abstainers reach lower peak BALs than moderate drinkers. The reason for this difference is not clear, but it may also have to do with different degrees of first pass metabolism in people who never drink (Whitfield & Martin, 1994).

The time to reach the maximum blood levels after drinking is highly variable between individuals and situations, but the time to reach the beginning of the plateau (*B* in Figure 6–3) is usually about an hour with the peak about 15 minutes later. After a few drinks, however, absorption rates seem to increase, and the peak and plateau will be reached 20 to 25 minutes sooner (Ditmar & Dorian, 1987).

Beer appears to pass more slowly out of the stomach than other alcoholic beverages, and for this reason beer creates lower BALs than the same amount of alcohol consumed in some other beverage. The passage of alcohol through the stomach may also be facilitated by carbonation. Sparkling wines such as champagne and rosé frequently have more "kick" than still wines.

The concentration of the alcohol also contributes to the speed of absorption. Diffusion rates increase with increases in concentration, and therefore the alcohol from beverages with high alcoholic content diffuses into the blood faster than the same amount of alcohol mixed in a weaker concentration. There is, however, an upper limit to this effect because high alcohol concentrations slow down the rate at which the stomach empties its contents into the intestine

and thus can interfere with absorption. It is probably not a coincidence that the most rapid absorption appears to occur at about 40 percent alcohol, the concentration of most hard liquor.

DISTRIBUTION

Alcohol dissolves much more readily in water than in lipids or fat, and so alcohol is distributed almost entirely in body water. Therefore, individuals with different proportions of body fat, even though they may weigh exactly the same, may reach different BALs after drinking identical amounts of alcohol. Males, for example, have a lower percent of body fat than females. Thus, if a man and a woman who weigh exactly the same drink the same amount of alcohol, the woman will have a higher BAL (also assuming similar first pass metabolism). The alcohol she drinks will be more highly concentrated because her body has less water to dilute the alcohol.

Age also makes a difference, at least for males. As males age, the percent of body fat increases slowly. Even though total body weight may not change, the same amount of alcohol will result in higher BALs as men get older. Women show a much smaller change in body composition with age.

It is possible to calculate the BAL for an individual after the consumption of a given amount of alcohol. Box 6–1 shows you how to make these calculations for any individual.

Alcohol is distributed rather evenly throughout body water and crosses the blood-brain barrier as well as the placental barrier without difficulty. Consequently, alcohol levels in most tissues of the body including the brain and the fetus accurately reflect the blood alcohol content of the drinker. Alcohol in the blood circulates through the lungs and vaporizes into the air at a known rate, so it is possible to measure the alcohol level in the blood and the rest of the body by measuring the alcohol vapor in exhaled air using a Breathalyzer, as described earlier.

BOX 6–1 Calculating Blood Alcohol Levels

Calculating the blood alcohol level is relatively simple. You have to know the weight and sex of the individual and the amount of alcohol consumed. To illustrate, let's calculate the BAL of a 175-pound man who has drunk 1 ounce of spirits. Because the BAL is usually given in milligrams per 100 ml of blood, it is easier to do the calculations in metric than in pounds and ounces.

First, we convert the body weight (175 pounds) to kilograms by dividing by 2.2 (1 kg = 2.2 lb). This equals 80 kg. This weight must then be adjusted because not all of the body is capable of absorbing alcohol. The percentage that can absorb alcohol differs slightly between men and women: It is estimated to be 75 percent in men and 66 percent in women. Therefore, an 80-kg man will have 60 kg to absorb alcohol ($80 \times 0.75 = 60$); 60 kg equal 60,000 g or 60,000 ml of fluid because 1 ml of water weighs 1 g.

Next we must convert alcohol to milligrams. One ounce of spirits (100 proof, or 50 percent by volume) will contain 11.2 g of alcohol (0.5 fluid ounce of water weighs 14 g, and alcohol has a specific gravity of 0.8; $14 \times 0.8 = 11.2$); 11.2 g is 11,200 mg.

Now we can divide the 11,200 mg of alcohol by 60,000 ml of body fluid and multiply by 100. This calculation yields the BAL: 18.6 mg per 100 ml. Our 175-pound man will raise his BAL by 18.6 mg per 100 ml of blood with every ounce of spirits.

Beer is usually about 5 percent alcohol by volume and comes in 12-ounce bottles. One such bottle would contain 13.5 g of alcohol, or 13,500 mg. When this is spread around a 60,000-ml body, it gives a concentration of about 22.5 mg per 100 ml. Our 175-pound man would raise his BAL by 22.5 per 100 ml with each beer. The accompanying table gives the alcohol content of various common drinks so you can do the appropriate calculations for different sources of alcohol.

To calculate how each of these drinks would affect you, take your weight in pounds and convert it to kilograms by dividing by 2.2. Next calculate the body weight for your sex that is

EXCRETION

A small amount of alcohol may be eliminated in breath, sweat, tears, urine, and feces, but over 90 percent of all alcohol consumed is metabolized, mostly in the liver. The usual route of metabolism is shown in Figure 1–9. It involves two steps. In the first, alcohol is converted to *acetaldehyde* by the enzyme *alcohol dehydrogenase*. This is the slowest step in alcohol metabolism, and consequently the rate at which this conversion takes place limits the speed of the entire process (it is the *rate-limiting step*). The conversion rate of alcohol to acetaldehyde is determined by the amount of alcohol dehydrogenase available, and it is relatively independent of the concentration of alcohol, and so the metabolism of alcohol, usually takes place at a steady rate throughout most of BALs. This rate may vary between individuals and from species to species.

In the next step, the acetaldehyde is converted into *acetyl-coenzyme A* by several enzymes, the most common of which is *aldehyde dehydrogenase*. Acetyl-coenzyme A is converted mainly into water and carbon dioxide through a series of reactions known as the *citric acid cycle* during

capable of absorbing alcohol: male, 75 percent; female, 66 percent. This figure must then be converted to milligrams (and milliliters) by multiplying by 1,000.

Now calculate the amount of alcohol consumed in milligrams, divide it by your weight in milligrams, and multiply by 100. Remember that the body metabolizes alcohol at a rate of about 15 mg per 100 ml per hour, and so you can subtract 15 mg per 100 ml for each hour that has passed since drinking started. *Caution:* These estimates of your BAL using this technique are just that—estimates. Two factors in this equation are approximations: The percentage of the body that will absorb alcohol and the rate of alcohol metabolism. Both depend on many factors such as age, health, build, experience with alcohol, and even other drugs in your system. The figures given here are population averages that might not apply to you. In general, however, this technique tends to overestimate BAL, so it should be reasonably safe for most people most of the time. It is not recommended, however, that you bet your life or your driver's license on it.

Alcohol Content of Some Beverages

Beverage	Alcohol Content, Percent (volume)	Alcohol Content (mg)
Spirits (1 fl oz*)		
(100 proof)	50	11,200
(89 proof)	43	9,600
(80 proof)	40	8,900
Beer (12 fl. oz.)	5	13,500
Wine (2.5 fl. oz.)	12	8,400

*A shot is 1.25 oz., so that these figures must be increased by 25 percent if "shots" are being used to mix drinks.

which usable energy is released to the body. Acetyl-coenzyme A is also used in a number of bodily processes such as the production of *fatty acids* and *steroids*. As a result, alcohol consumption and its consequent metabolism can alter a great deal of body chemistry.

There are some reports that women metabolize alcohol at a faster rate than men, but many recent studies have not been able to confirm this generalization (Whitfield & Martin, 1994).

Between individuals there is considerable variability in elimination rates. The range found in one study was from 5.9 to 27.9 mg per 100 ml per hour with a standard deviation of 4.5 (Dubowski, 1985). For the majority of individuals, the range is usually accepted to be between 10 and 20 mg per 100 ml per hour with a mean of 15. The rate of metabolism of alcohol also seems to be influenced by drinking experience. Nondrinkers metabolize alcohol at a slightly slower rate (12–14 mg per 100 ml per hour) than light to moderate drinkers (15–17 mg per 100 ml per hour) (L. Goldberg, 1943; Whitfield & Martin, 1994).

Methanol is also metabolized in the liver by alcohol dehydrogenase, but the metabolic by-products are *formaldehyde* and *formic acid*, which are very toxic and metabolize very slowly themselves. Methanol alone is not very toxic, but consumption of methanol can result in severe illness, blindness, and death as a result of accumulation of these toxins in the body. Surprisingly, these toxic effects can sometimes be avoided if a great deal of ethanol is consumed at the same time, because both alcohols use the same enzyme system. Ethanol competes with methanol for the available enzymes and thereby slows down the formation of formaldehyde, so it may never reach toxic levels.

Though most alcohol is handled by the alcohol dehydrogenase system, another system appears to be in operation as well. This is known as the *microsomal ethanol-oxidizing system (MEOS)*. The MEOS normally handles only 5 to 10 percent of the metabolism of alcohol, but its activity increases at higher levels of blood alcohol. The activity of the MEOS may be doubled or even tripled by continuous alcohol consumption. This increase may account for 50 to 65 percent of the increased alcohol metabolism induced by heavy drinking, a change that partly accounts for alcohol tolerance. The MEOS system is important for another reason: It is also responsible for the metabolism of a number of other drugs such as barbiturates. Therefore, if the MEOS system is stimulated by continuous alcohol use, the metabolism of these other drugs will also be speeded, and vice versa (Leiber & DeCarli, 1977; Leiber, 1977). Thus alcoholics usually have a great deal of resistance to the effects of barbiturates and other drugs.

NEUROPHARMACOLOGY

The neuropharmacology of alcohol is complex and involves a number of systems. Even though it has been studied intensively and much is now known, there are still many mysteries. Because there are a number of similarities between the effects of alcohol and the general anesthetics, it is believed that both have a similar mechanism of action and that what has been learned about general anesthetics can tell us much about alcohol.

Whatever that mechanism of action might be, it is clear that neither alcohol nor the general anesthetics produce a direct effect on specific receptor sites. Some of the observations that support this conclusion are that alcohol has many effects on a variety of tissues, relatively large quantities of alcohol are required in order to have an effect, and there are no drugs that act as competitive antagonists to alcohol (more on this shortly).

It has been known for many years that the potency of a particular anesthetic is closely correlated with its lipid solubility. This correlation suggests that the anesthetic may be having its effect by dissolving in the lipid layer of membranes and perturbing some property of the membrane. What exactly this perturbation might be is still a matter of considerable investigation (K. W. Miller, 1993). One suggestion has been that when these drugs are dissolved in membranes, the membranes expand or change state so that they exert pressure on the ion channels embedded in the membrane and interfere with their ability to open and allow ions to pass through. In turn, the ability of the membrane to form resting and action potentials is altered (see Chapter 4). This notion is further supported by the observation that the effects of some anesthetic drugs similar to alcohol can be reversed by high air pressure that mechanically pushes the membranes back into shape.

For example, it has been shown in several parts of the brain that acute doses of alcohol at concentrations achieved by normal drinking depress the functioning of the ion channel controlled by the excitatory neurotransmitter glutamate at a receptor site called the NMDA receptor. It has also been shown that chronic exposure to alcohol causes the brain to "up-regulate" NMDA receptor-ion channel functioning; that is, the brain becomes more sensitive to NMDA (and glutamate) as if to compensate for prolonged depression by alcohol. Such an increase in sensitivity may be responsible for alcohol withdrawal (Sanna & Harris, 1993).

It is also believed that alcohol and other anesthetics alter the characteristics of proteins that act as receptor sites for transmitters either directly or through the perturbation of the membrane in which they are embedded. For example, alcohol stimulates the function of one class of serotonin (5-HT) receptor, the 5-HT$_3$ receptor, which opens ion channels and causes rapid-onset depolarization of the membrane. This appears to be an important step in the release of dopamine in the nucleus accumbens and, consequently, in the reinforcing effect of alcohol. It has been shown, for example, that serotonin antagonists will decrease the reinforcing effects and the discriminative stimulus effects of alcohol.

The GABA-receptor-ionophore complex is also involved in the effect of alcohol, particularly ionophores controlled by the GABA$_A$ receptor. These are inhibitory, and alcohol enhances their inhibition (see Chapter 7).

Alcohol also has a myriad of other neurophysiological effects. It is known to disrupt second messenger systems. For some receptor sites, it inhibits binding to the opiate sigma receptor and alters the functioning of monoamine oxidase, the enzyme responsible for the destruction of monamine neurotransmitters (Tabakoff & Hoffman, 1987). It also has been shown to alter responsiveness of the endogenous opiate system (Froehlich & Li, 1993).

Alcohol Antagonists

For thousands of years people have been searching for a substance that would reverse the effects of alcohol. The ancient Greeks believed that the amethyst, a semiprecious stone, had this property, and the term *amethystics* has been used to describe these agents.

In 1985 researchers at Hoffmann–La Roche reported that they had synthesized a substance called *RO 15–4513* that seemed to be able to an-

tagonize the effects of alcohol. Careful research has shown that the drug antagonizes only some of the effects of alcohol (including self-administration; June et al., 1992) and does so because it appears to change the effect of GABA in a manner directly opposite to the effect of alcohol. It does not, however, act as a competitive antagonist to alcohol; that is, it does not compete with alcohol for a receptor site. In addition, RO 15–4513 appears to antagonize the effects of the barbiturates and the benzodiazepines (see Chapter 7) by working directly on the benzodiazepine receptor site (Lister & Nutt, 1987).

There is little likelihood that RO 15–4513 could have any medical use. While it blocks some of the effects of alcohol, it does not antagonize the lethal effects of alcohol, so it could not be used to treat alcohol overdose. In addition, it seems to possess the ability to cause convulsions, and this would make it unsuitable for treating alcoholism.

As we have seen in the previous section, serotonin blockers are capable of partly blocking the reinforcing and the stimulus properties of alcohol, and it has also been shown that opiate antagonists can block some of alcohol's physiological effects and might also be useful in reducing alcohol consumption and preventing relapse after treatment in alcoholics (Froehlich & Li, 1993).

EFFECTS OF ALCOHOL

Effects on the Body

Alcohol in low and moderate doses causes a dilation of blood vessels in the skin. This is why drinkers sometimes have a flushed face (and heavy drinkers, like W. C. Fields, have a red nose). In addition to causing the skin to turn pink, it also makes the skin feel warm. One of the traditional medical uses of alcohol, therefore, was to treat people who were exposed to cold. Alcoholic beverages, especially brandy, were supposed to warm the body.

By inhibiting the secretion of *antidiuretic hormone*, alcohol causes the loss of body water through increased urination. This occurs only while BAL is steady or falling.

Effects on Sleep

Alcohol, like most depressant drugs, acts as a sedative and induces sleep. Studies of acute effects on normal volunteers have shown that alcohol decreases the time it takes to go to sleep, but it does not have an effect on total sleeping time.

Even at very low BALs, alcohol depresses REM sleep. At low levels this effect is apparent during the first half of a night following drinking and is followed in the second half with an increase in REM so that the total REM times during the night might be unaffected. At larger doses REM is depressed throughout the entire night, but after three nights of alcohol consumption, REM depression shows complete tolerance and REM returns to normal. When alcohol is discontinued after five nights, there is a REM *rebound* on the sixth night; REM rebound is a period when the percentage of REM sleep increases above normal levels, and this causes poor sleep and unpleasant dreams.

When alcoholics stop drinking, they usually have very high percentages of REM sleep, as much as 90 percent, and other disturbances in sleep patterns that may last as long as 200 weeks (W. B. Mendelson, 1979).

Effects on Human Performance

One of the earliest and best reviews of alcohol's effect on human performance may be found in *Actions of Alcohol* by Henrik Wallgren and Herb Barry (1971).

Perception.   Alcohol has a detrimental effect on vision, increasing both absolute and difference thresholds, but usually only at higher doses. A decrease in visual acuity, indicated by a lowering in critical flicker fusion threshold, is caused by a BAL of about 70 mg per 100 ml. There are also decreases in sensitivity to taste and smell at low doses and a decrease in pain sensitivity at BALs of 80 to 100 mg per 100 ml.

Performance.   Alcohol slows reaction time by about 10 percent at BALs of 80 to 100 mg per 100 ml, and large consistent deficits are evident with larger doses. Complex reaction-time tasks that require the subject to scan and integrate stimuli from several sources before responding show that at lower doses both speed and accuracy of performance decrease. Deficits are also seen in hand-eye coordination tasks where the subject is required to maintain a marker over a moving target. In general, the more complex the task, the greater the impairment seen at lower doses. Small deficits occur at doses as low as 10 to 20 mg per 100 ml. Drowsiness caused by alcohol also shows up on vigilance tasks, where impairments are seen at doses as low as 60 mg per 100 ml.

One of the most sensitive tests is the Romberg sway test. The subject is asked to stand with eyes closed and feet together. BALs as low as 60 mg per 100 ml can cause a 40 percent decrease in steadiness as measured by the amount of swaying. This lack of steadiness makes it difficult for a person to stand on one foot with eyes closed. Before the Breathalyzer, the police used this test to detect impairment. At higher BALs this lack of steadiness degenerates into staggering and reeling. It appears that the increase in sway is a result of the effect of alcohol on the sensitive organs of balance in the inner ear and is also responsible for the sensation of the room spinning around that people experience when they lie down after drinking too much. It can also bring on nausea and vomiting (Money & Miles, 1974).

Alcohol decreases performance on standard intelligence tests and tends to alter the ability to judge the passage of time; the passage of five minutes is judged to be eight minutes at the BAL of 50 per 100 ml.

Alcohol is also known to have a detrimental effect on memory. Blackouts sometimes occur in heavy drinkers during periods of heavy consumption. The drinker is unable to remember anything about events that occurred during the period of heavy drinking. Blackouts apparently result because high doses of alcohol prevent memories from being formed. A more common form of alcohol amnesia is the "grayout": The drinker cannot remember events that happened while drunk, but unlike blackouts, where the memories are never laid down, the problem with grayouts is one of recall. The memories can be retrieved when the person drinks again or if reminded of the events. Grayouts are likely to result from dissociation (Overton, 1972); (see Chapter 3). Alcohol-induced dissociation can occur even at rather low levels of consumption where the BAL reaches 80 mg per 100 ml (Lowe, 1982).

Effects on Driving

Studies of the effects of alcohol on driving in simulators and in real cars on closed tracks have generally confirmed that alcohol begins to affect performance at about 50 to 80 mg per 100 ml (Mitchell, 1985). This finding is reflected as well in real-life driving accident statistics. Figure 6–4 shows the relative probability of being responsible for a fatal crash at various BALs. The curve starts to rise between 50 and 100 mg per 100 ml so that at 100 mg per 100 ml the probability of being responsible for a fatal crash is 7 times greater than if the BAL had been 0. After this point, the curve rises sharply so that at a BAL of 200 mg per 100 ml a driver is 100 times more likely to cause a fatal crash (OECD, 1978).

Curves like this establish the rationale for setting legal limits on BAL for driving. In most jurisdictions, the limit is between 80 and 100 mg per 100 ml, the point where the curve starts to rise sharply. It is important to remember, however, that these curves underestimate the risk for young inexperienced drivers, older drivers, and people not used to drinking whose risk of being involved in an accident is considerably elevated even at BALs below the legal limit. Figure 6–5

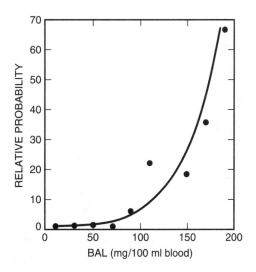

Figure 6–4   The relationship between BAL and the relative risk of being involved in a traffic accident. The risk with a BAL less than 1.0 mg per 100 mL is 1.0. (OECD, 1978.)

Figure 6–5   The relationship between the BAL and the relative risk of being involved in a traffic accident for people of different age groups. (OECD, 1978.)

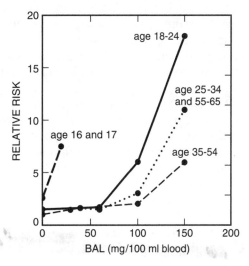

shows similar curves for people of different ages (OECD, 1978).

Effects on Human Behavior

Perhaps an indication of the importance of inebriation in our culture is the vast number of words for being drunk that exist. Back in 1737, Benjamin Franklin compiled 228 terms commonly used for being drunk. He might have missed a few, or drinkers have been actively creating more since his time, because the *American Thesaurus of Slang*, published in 1952, lists almost 900 such terms. What is interesting is that most of these words suggest some sort of violence or damage, such as *crashed, clobbered, bombed, swacked, plastered, tanked, ossified, looped, paralyzed,* and *wiped out,* to cite just a few. Some terms are very old. *Soused,* for example, dates back to sixteenth-century England, and *cut* was used as long ago as 1770 (Levine, 1981).

What does it mean to be *ossified* or *swacked*? The body of literature on this subject dating back to the time of Aristotle is so vast that it is almost impossible to characterize it in this short space. Systematic observation of drinkers has shown that at BALs between 50 and 100 mg per 100 ml, people are more talkative, use a higher pitch of voice, and show mild excitement. At about 100 to 150 mg per 100 ml, subjects appear talkative, cheerful, and often loud and boisterous; later they become sleepy. At BALs above 150 mg per 100 ml, subjects frequently feel nauseous and may vomit. This phase is followed by lethargy and in some cases stupor. At doses as high as 290 mg per 100 ml, subjects are variously sleepy, noisy, and inattentive. Subjective feelings as determined by mood scales generally support these observations. Subjects report that they are more elated, friendly, and vigorous at low BALs when the BAL is rising, but if the blood levels are dropping, they report anger, depression, and fatigue (Babor et al., 1983).

One of the frequently recorded effects of alcohol is *disinhibition*, a term that is generally used to mean that under the influence of alcohol, people do things they normally would not do for fear of adverse consequences. This is most evident in conflict situations where a certain activity has both positive and negative consequences. Alcohol reduces the influence of the negative consequences and appears to release the behavior from inhibition. This was demonstrated in an experiment by Muriel Vogel-Sprott of the University of Waterloo. Subjects made a sequence of responses for which they were given both painful electric shocks and money. The shocks severely depressed the responding of subjects who had been given a placebo but failed to suppress the responding of subjects after they had been given alcohol (BALs of 50 to 80 mg per 100 ml; Vogel-Sprott, 1967). It is interesting that this effect may actually improve performance on tasks where anxiety or conflict are interfering with behavior. A practical example might be someone who is afraid to ask the boss for a raise. Conflict exists because the person wants the raise but is afraid of being fired or making the boss angry. After a few drinks, fear of the boss loosens its control of the behavior, and the task can be performed. Of course, we can only hope that the other effects of alcohol do not interfere and our intoxicated employee does not get fired for being drunk on the job.

It is probably this effect that causes people to do and say things under alcohol that they would never do while sober. For this reason, alcohol is probably the best "truth serum" in the world. This observation has never been demonstrated experimentally, but it is probably true that under some circumstances people are more likely to speak frankly when they are drinking. *In vino veritas.*

In summary, perhaps the best way to characterize the effects of alcohol is to retell the old fable about Saint Martin, the monk who was reputed to have brought grapes to France. At first the vine was hidden in the bone of a bird; then, after outgrowing the bird, it was hidden in the bone of a lion; and finally, in the bone of a donkey. Later, after the vine had grown and wine was made, the monks who drank it showed the characteristics of the animals used in its transportation. After the first bottle, they sang like birds; after the second, they had the courage of lions; but after the third, they behaved like asses.

Effects on Behavior of Nonhumans

Positively Reinforced Behavior. There has not been much research on positively motivated schedules of reinforcement, for two reasons. First, alcohol has an irritating effect when it is injected, and this irritation itself tends to alter behavior. Second, alcohol has caloric value and reduces the motivation levels of animals that have been deprived of food. The studies that have been done tend to show that alcohol has a similar effect on most positively reinforced schedules of reinforcement. On both FI and FR schedules, alcohol increases the rate of responding at low doses and decreases the rate at higher doses.

Adversely Motivated Behavior. It might be expected that a drug that seems to reduce anxiety would also decrease the motivation of an organism to work to avoid shock, and this expectation seems to be borne out. On a continuous avoidance schedule where the animal responds to postpone a programmed shock, low doses increase responding, but higher doses decrease rates and increase the number of shocks received even though they are not high enough to interfere with responding (Heise & Boff, 1962). On this schedule as well, alcohol is similar to the barbiturates.

The effect of alcohol on punished responding is also similar to that of the barbiturates, but not quite as striking. In an early experiment, Conger (1951) trained rats to run down a runway for food and then gave their paws a shock when they began to eat. He adjusted food deprivation and shock levels carefully until the rats were willing to run partway down the runway but not touch the food. He found that alcohol would cause the rats to approach and eat the food immediately, but rats given a placebo took many trials. Since then, several researchers have found that ethanol will increase response rates that are suppressed by contingent shock in an operant task. This result is similar to the finding in humans that alcohol tends to reduce the control of aversive consequences on behavior, as demonstrated by the experiment by Vogel-Sprott described earlier.

Discriminative Stimulus Properties

Animals can be trained very easily to discriminate alcohol from saline in a discrimination task. Overton has shown that at a dose of 3,000 mg/kg, rats will reach criterion discrimination performance in just three trials. Of the drugs tested, the only drugs that were discriminated faster were phenobarbital and pentobarbital (Overton & Batta, 1977; Overton, 1982).

Using the electrified T-maze, Overton found that rats trained to discriminate alcohol from saline generalized the alcohol response when given a barbiturate and vice versa, indicating that the two drugs produce a similar subjective state. However, in a later series of experiments, Overton (1977) was able to show that he could train rats to discriminate between alcohol and barbiturates, showing that although the effects of barbiturates and alcohol are similar, they can be discriminated by rats. It has also been shown that the alcohol response is not generalized to benzodiazepines, meprobamate (Barry, McGuire, & Krimmer, 1982), chlorpromazine, amphetamine, or atropine (Barry & Kubina, 1972).

The stimulus properties of alcohol can be blocked by 5-HT$_3$ receptor blockers, but not by haloperidol, a dopamine D$_2$ blocker, indicating that serotonin rather than dopamine may mediate the subjective effects of alcohol (Grant & Barrett, 1991).

TOLERANCE

Acute Tolerance

Several studies have shown that many of the effects of alcohol are more pronounced while the BAL is rising than later when the BAL is falling.

Figure 6–6 shows this effect for measurements of body sway. Body sway was measured twice, once as the BAL reached 40 mg per 100 ml on the way up and again at the same point as the BAL was falling. As the figure shows, the alcohol-induced increases in body sway had disappeared when the second measure was taken, even though the BAL was exactly the same (M. T. Lee, 1984). The first study of this type was done many years ago when it was shown that while the BAL was rising, subjects appeared intoxicated at 150 mg per 100 ml, but while the BAL was falling, they appeared sober at 200 mg per 100 mg (Mirsky et al., 1945).

Chronic Tolerance

Chronic tolerance appears to develop rapidly to alcohol in both animals and man. The extent and speed of tolerance depend on the species studied and the alcohol effect measured. The maximal tolerance develops in a few weeks in humans and reaches a point where doses have to be increased from 30 to 50 percent to overcome it. Tolerance disappears in rats after two or three weeks of abstinence but develops again more quickly with repeated exposure (Kalant, LeBlanc, & Gibbins, 1971).

Metabolic Tolerance

One effect of heavy drinking is the stimulation of both alcohol dehydrogenase, the major enzyme responsible for the destruction of alcohol, and the MEOS. As described in the section on alcohol metabolism, light to moderate drinkers are able to metabolize alcohol faster than abstainers (Goldberg, 1943; Whitfield & Martin, 1994). Although such changes certainly decrease the effects of alcohol, they cannot account for the extent of tolerance to alcohol described in the literature.

Behavioral Tolerance

Practice seems to be important in the development of tolerance of some of the effects of alcohol. In one experiment, a group of rats was given alcohol and placed on a treadmill. The rats quickly developed tolerance to the disruptive effects of the drug, but those that were given the same number of alcohol injections after the treadmill sessions did not show any tolerance when tested on the treadmill under the influence of alcohol (Wenger et al., 1981).

It has also been demonstrated that rats' tolerance to the hypothermic effect of alcohol (de-

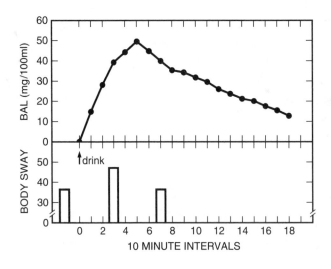

Figure 6–6 Top: Mean BAL of a group of university students taken every 10 minutes after drinking alcohol. Bottom: The effect of the alcohol on body sway. Note that the effect is only seen when the BAL is rising. Sway measures taken at the same BAL during the descending limb of the curve are not different from normal. (Adapted from M. T. Lee, 1984.)

crease in body temperature) is the result of a conditioned hyperthermic effect (increase in body temperature) associated with the specific environment in which the alcohol has been administered (Le, Poulos, & Cappell, 1979). Rats were given alcohol in one environment and saline in another environment. As expected, tolerance developed to the hypothermic effects of the alcohol, but when rats were given the alcohol in the environment where they had previously received only saline, the tolerance was diminished. In addition, rats that were given saline in the alcohol-related environment showed an increase in body temperature. This increase was a conditioned compensatory response to the alcohol effect (see Chapter 3).

WITHDRAWAL

As with most of the depressant drugs, chronic consumption of alcohol can cause withdrawal symptoms. Although the distinction may not always be appropriate, it is customary to think of two separate stages of withdrawal, the *early minor syndrome* and the *late major syndrome*, also known as *delirium tremens*, or the *DTs*. The early minor symptoms usually appear about 8 to 12 hours after the end of a drinking bout, although many aspects of withdrawal may be seen during the latter part of long drinking sessions even while drinking is still going on. Withdrawal starts in the form of agitation and tremors; other symptoms such as muscle cramps, vomiting, nausea, sweating, vivid dreaming, and irregular heartbeats may also be seen. This stage is usually over within 48 hours.

Fewer than 5 percent of patients hospitalized for alcohol withdrawal go on to show the late major withdrawal symptoms. After two days of the minor symptoms, patients show increasing agitation, disorientation, confusion, and hallucinations. Seizures may also occur (Wolfe & Victor, 1972). These major symptoms may last as long as 7 to 10 days. Alcohol withdrawal hallucinations are not usually of the proverbial pink elephant. They frequently involve smaller animals such as rats, bats, or insects and can be quite terrifying.

Late major withdrawal can cause death in a substantial number of cases if the symptoms are not treated. An early report from the beginning of the twentieth century, before treatment techniques had been developed, showed a 37 percent (52/140) mortality from alcohol withdrawal (Boston, 1908). Modern estimates are about 2 percent (Naranjo & Sellers, 1986).

In general, the most effective treatment of alcohol withdrawal is a combination of supportive care and the administration of another depressant drug such as a benzodiazepine like diazepam, which suppresses those withdrawal symptoms and has a long duration of action. Other specific symptoms may also be treated with other drugs; for example, hallucinations can be controlled with haloperidol, an antipsychotic. Effective supportive care consists of measures such as reducing sensory stimulation by placing the patient in a dimly lit, quiet room, providing adequate food and water to prevent dehydration, keeping the patient warm and comfortable, and providing reassurance (Naranjo & Sellers, 1986).

ALCOHOL USE IN POPULATIONS

Rates of Alcohol Consumption

A French mathematician, Sully Ledermann, studied alcohol consumption figures for many countries and populations and proposed that while the mean alcohol consumption in different populations might vary, the distribution curves all have similar characteristics: They are all *logarithmic normal curves*. This theory is known as the *single-distribution theory*. Figure 6–7 is typical of a logarithmic normal distribution curve. It shows the frequency distribution of male drinkers in the province of Ontario, Canada, in 1972. Note that about 12 percent drink no alco-

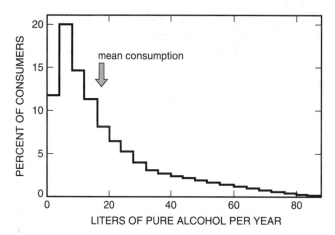

Figure 6–7 Distribution of alcohol consumption of male drinkers in Ontario in 1972. The mean consumption of this population is 17.5 liters per year. This distribution demonstrates Ledermann's log normal distribution. (Adapted from W. Schmidt, 1977, "Cirrhosis and Alcohol Consumption: An Epidemiological Perspective," in *Alcoholism: New Knowledge and New Responses,* ed. G. Edwards & M. Grant, pp. 15–47, London: Croom Helm.)

hol. The curve rises and then tails off rather smoothly without any humps or bumps. Ledermann proposed that distribution curves for all populations have this basic shape, although populations that have a high mean consumption will be shifted a bit more to the right and would not drop off as steeply as populations with lower mean consumption.

If single-distribution theory is correct, it means that the proportion of heavy drinkers in a society will increase as the mean alcohol consumption rate increases and decrease as the mean decreases. In societies that have a low mean consumption, a small percentage of the population will drink beyond a certain high level of consumption, but in a country where the mean consumption is high, the percentage of the population above that level will be high.

To demonstrate the relationship between mean consumption and heavy drinking, researchers have compared mean consumption with the death rate from liver cirrhosis and alcoholism in a number of countries. Since liver cirrhosis is almost exclusively caused by prolonged heavy drinking, it serves as a good index of the number of heavy drinkers in a country. Table 6–1 shows this relationship. Mean consumption is clearly related to the alcoholism and liver cirrhosis death rate.

A practical implication of the single distribution theory is that the number of heavy drinkers in a society can be decreased by any measure that decreases the national average consumption. Politicians and policy makers who want to lower the amount of heavy drinking need not aim programs directly at the population of heavy drinkers. Any measure that will lower the national average, like increasing the price or decreasing its availability, should also lower the rate of excessive consumption.

Availability

Governments have considerable control over availability of alcoholic beverages by a number of means that include legal drinking age, licensing drinking establishments and liquor stores, and regulating their hours of operation. There is considerable research showing that alcohol consumption increases as alcohol becomes easier to obtain and decreases when it is more difficult to get (Single, 1988); that is, it behaves like any other commodity in the marketplace (Popham, Schmidt, & de Lint, 1976; Babor, 1985; Österberg, 1992).

Here are some examples: In 1989, when Iceland ended a 75-year prohibition on beer, the

TABLE 6–1   Annual Rates of Alcohol Consumption, Alcoholism,* and Death from Cirrhosis of the Liver in Various Countries. Based on data collected in 1966 and 1967 for alcohol consumption; death rates are for the year 1963, 1964, or 1965.

Country	Consumption per Drinker (liters of absolute alcohol)	Alcoholism Rate (per million population)	Death Rate from Liver Cirrhosis (per million population)
France	25.9	9,405	45.3
Italy	20.0	5,877	27.3
West Germany	16.0	3,978	26.7
Hungary	12.4	2,952	12.9
United States	12.0	2,189	18.4
Canada	11.1	2,272	10.0
England and Wales	10.9	1,946	3.7
Denmark	9.4	1,884	10.2
Poland	9.0	1,752	8.6
Sweden	8.4	1,515	7.9
Finland	5.9	945	4.6

Source: Adapted from de Lint and Schmidt (1971), p. 428.
*Estimated.

consumption of wine and liquor declined by 25 percent and 18 percent, respectively, but total alcohol consumption from all sources increased by 23 percent (Österberg, 1992). Studies of the effects of permitting wine to be sold in grocery stores in four states—Idaho, Maine, Virginia, and Washington—showed that in three of the four states, the change in law resulted in an overall increase in total alcohol consumption (Macdonald, 1986). For eight months, ten of Finland's liquor monopoly stores were closed on Saturdays on a trial basis. This experiment resulted in a total decrease in alcohol consumption of 3.2 percent and, as well, a decrease in public drunkenness and alcohol-related violence (Säilä as cited in Österberg, 1992).

Price

It can be shown that mean consumption can be altered by changing availability. What effect do changes in price have on consumption?

Figure 6–8 shows the consumption of alcohol, the price (adjusted for cost of living and income),

and the death rate from liver cirrhosis in the province of Ontario from 1933 to 1956 (Seeley, 1960). After the Canadian version of prohibition, the price of alcohol dropped dramatically from 1930 to 1956, and there was a corresponding increase in consumption. This increase in consumption was mirrored about 10 years later by a corresponding increase in deaths from liver cirrhosis. Since it takes about 10 years of heavy drinking to cause cirrhosis, the statistics indicate that the changes in the price influenced alcohol consumption, not only of the general population of drinkers, but also of the heavy drinkers. This outcome was predicted by the single distribution theory.

As pointed out by Gene Heyman of Harvard University (in press), this study only tells half the story because, like most studies that measure effects on both heavy and light drinkers, it only looked at changes in consumption during times when the price of alcohol decreased, not when it increased. In fact, the real price of alcohol (taking income into account) in most Western industrialized societies has dropped over the last two-

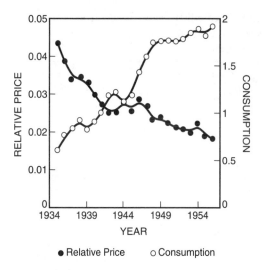

● Relative Price   ○ Consumption

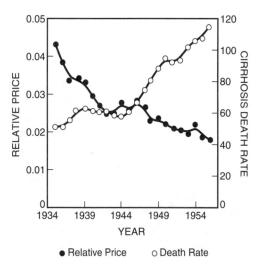

● Relative Price   ○ Death Rate

Figure 6–8 Top: The relationship between the price of alcohol (price of an imperial gallon of alcohol as a percent of average adult disposable income) and the rate of alcohol consumption (imperial gallons of alcohol per adult) in Ontario between 1935 and 1959. Clearly, as the price dropped, consumption increased. Bottom: The price of alcohol is shown in the same manner as the top graph, but the death rate from liver cirrhosis (deaths per million adults) is also shown. It parallels consumption with a lag of a bit more than 10 years. (Data from Seeley, 1960.)

thirds of the twentieth century, and so the opportunities to do such a test have been limited. The issue is complicated by the fact that occasions when prices have increased, such as prohibition, have been accompanied with other legal and practical restrictions on availability.

Heyman has speculated that the change may not be symmetrical. It is possible that low prices may entice more and more people to become heavy drinkers, but once they have been recruited to heavy drinking, increased prices may not have any effect on consumption of these heavy drinkers (Heyman, in press).

Numerous experiments in laboratory settings with both alcoholics and casual drinkers have shown that increases in the cost of alcohol or increases in the work required to get a drink will decrease the amount of alcohol consumed (Mello & Mendelson, 1972). For example, in an experiment by Bigelow and Liebson (1972), two skid row alcoholics were given the opportunity to earn drinks by pulling a lever. At the lowest cost requirement, one consumed the maximum of 24 drinks a day and the other consumed 17. At the highest work requirement, both consumed fewer than four drinks per day.

Elasticity. It seems clear that consumption drops when the price increases, but what is the exact relationship between price and consumption? That is, does the demand for alcohol show elasticity when the price changes?

Studies on Laboratory Animals. Most studies with laboratory animals have shown that the demand for alcohol is elastic. An experiment by Carroll, Rodefer, and Rawleigh (1995) with rhesus monkeys responding for oral ethanol on FRs ranging from 4 to 128 show a coefficient of −2.3, indicating elasticity. (Remember that a coefficient between 0.0 and −1.0 indicates inelasticity, and a coefficient with an absolute negative value greater than −1.0 indicates elasticity; see Chapter 5.) Heyman (in press), however, in a study with rats with a long history of alcohol consumption found a coefficient of 0.09, indicating inelasticity. His rats responded on a VR schedule that ranged from VR 4 to VR 20, and he found inelasticity even though a sucrose substitute was available.

Studies with Humans.   There have been numerous studies of the elasticity of alcoholic beverages in populations using many different techniques and statistics from a variety of sources, and some consistencies have been noted. Beer, for example, has an elasticity coefficient of about −0.30 (inelasticity). This means that if the price of beer were to double, consumption would go down by only 20 percent.

Demand for spirits, on the other hand, has much higher coefficients (ranging from −0.57 to −1.95) indicating elasticity. Elasticity of wine varies depending on the country. In France, where wine is consumed with meals and considered a necessity, it is inelastic (−0.06), but in the United States and Great Britain demand appears to be elastic (−1.65 and −1.23, respectively).

These estimates are based on studies of consumption of national populations, and it remains an interesting question whether the price of alcohol has the same influence on the demand for beverages by different types of drinkers. For example, do price increases alter the consumption of heavy drinkers the same way as moderate drinkers? Personal accounts and anecdotal evidence suggest that price does not alter the consumption of alcoholic drinkers, but remember that the fall in alcohol prices in Ontario (Figure 6–8) was followed by an increase in alcoholic liver disease, suggesting that decreasing prices at least influenced the behavior of heavy drinkers. But, as Heyman has suggested, it has yet to be demonstrated that increasing prices will decrease heavy drinking (Heyman, in press).

Public Policy: Availability or Harm Reduction

The assumptions of single-distribution theory are not as widely accepted in the 1990s as they were previously, and the policy of many governments seems to have shifted from attempts at controlling the average consumption by manipulating price and availability to reduction of harmful drinking. One factor that seems to predict alcohol-related problems better than average consumption is number of heavy drinking occasions. Indeed, the people who suffer most from acute alcohol problems like impaired driving, family dysfunction, and employment difficulties are basically low or moderate drinkers who occasionally drink immoderately. Current research suggests that the most effective approach a government can take is to focus efforts on reducing heavy drinking occasions through education of alcohol consumers and server training programs, and increasing enforcement of drinking and driving legislation (Single, 1995).

SELF-ADMINISTRATION IN HUMANS

Patterns of Consumption

Culture.   Cross-cultural studies in numerous societies where alcohol is consumed have revealed some interesting patterns that appear to be consistent across cultures, even in our own. Alcohol consumption is generally a male activity, practiced socially outside the home among peer groups and not in the company of family members or people of higher status. Drinking is generally more acceptable among warriors and people who must grapple with the environment than among members of a society who are charged with preserving tradition, like priests, mothers, and judges (D. Robinson, 1977, p. 63).

Among individuals and cultures, many drinking patterns have been identified. The spree drinker, common in Finland, binges occasionally but stays relatively sober otherwise. A drinker common in France consumes a large fixed amount of alcohol every day steadily over the course of the day and exhibits few symptoms of intoxication. Such differences in national drinking patterns do not seem to influence certain consequences of consumption, such as rate of alcoholism or alcohol-related diseases. However, the difference may be significant where acute intoxication is important; for example, one beer a day may not ever cause a traffic accident, but the same quantity of beer consumed on one occasion every two weeks could easily be responsible for traffic accidents.

Gender.   Although heavy drinkers are more likely to be male, this fact does not mean that women drink less than men. Studies have shown that women do consume less alcohol than men, but when adjustments are made for differences in body size and ability to absorb alcohol, it turns out that women social drinkers achieve the same blood alcohol levels as men (Vogel-Sprott, 1984; McKim & Quinlan, 1991).

Age.   People tend to drink less when they get older. A number of studies have shown that although people drink just as frequently as they age, they tend to drink less on each occasion (Vogel-Sprott, 1984), and so total consumption declines. Unlike the difference in consumption between genders, this age-related decline in consumption per occasion cannot be explained by changes in body composition with age (McKim & Quinlan, 1991).

Laboratory Studies.   In the laboratory, the pattern of alcohol self-administration when freely available is fairly consistent. Alcohol is consumed at high levels for several days, followed by a self-imposed period of low consumption lasting two or three days during which withdrawal symptoms may appear. Figure 5–3 shows the drinking pattern of alcoholic volunteers who worked on an operant schedule of button pushing to earn drinks. This pattern is very similar to that of a rhesus monkey under similar conditions and to the typical pattern of many chronic alcoholics under natural conditions (Griffiths, Bigelow, & Henningfield, 1980).

Alcoholism

Like the term *dependence, alcoholism* may be used in two different ways, as an explanation or as a description of behavior. Many definitions are purely descriptive; they describe a pattern of behavior and then label it alcoholism. What is confusing is that many descriptions are used as though they were explanations. For example, the DSM-IV defines substance dependence (see Box 5.1). This is the definition of alcoholism where the "substance" is alcohol.

The DSM-IV definition is a *description* of a state of affairs; it is *not* an explanation. Unfortunately, many writers use such descriptions as though they were explanations. For example, it could be said that an individual is an alcoholic because he or she fits the DSM-IV description. This statement is fair enough, but it cannot be said that this individual drinks excessively because he or she is an alcoholic. (This would be a circular argument; we know that person X is an alcoholic because he or she drinks too much, and we know that person X drinks too much because he or she is an alcoholic.) The only way around this circularity is to define the condition of alcoholism in terms other than the behavior of drinking; then the term can legitimately be used as an explanation of the behavior. There have been several attempts to do so. It is possible, for example, to say that alcoholics have an underlying state of physical dependence on alcohol so that the person experiences withdrawal when drinking ceases, and this withdrawal motivates the person to continue drinking. By equating *alcoholism* with physical dependence on alcohol, we can now use the word to *explain* the behavior it describes, and we would be presuming that the physical dependence was the explanatory mechanism. One of the defining characteristics of dependence according to the DSM-IV is physical dependence, but it is possible to meet these criteria without being physically dependent.

As you can see, explaining something is considerably more complicated than describing it.

Explanations take the form of theories, and good theories must withstand the test of scientific investigation. Over the years a great number of theories have been proposed to explain alcoholism. It is beyond the scope of this book to explore them, but other very good accounts are available (Chaudron & Wilkinson, 1988; Pattison, Sobel, & Sobel, 1977).

Here we will briefly discuss two different approaches: (1) the classical disease concept approach, which suggests that alcoholism is a pathology or a disease, and (2) the behavioral approach, which suggest that alcoholism can be explained using the same principles we know to govern other "normal" behavior. Many of these concepts were discussed in Chapter 5 in a more general context.

Disease Model

As described in Chapter 5, excessive and self-destructive alcohol consumption was originally considered to be a moral failing or loss of self-control on the part of the drinker and, consequently, a sin to be dealt with by the law and the penal system or the church. But the social reform movement of the nineteenth century introduced the idea that alcohol abuse was a disease to be treated, rather than a sin to be punished. Consequently, the treatment of alcohol abusers evolved into the domain of the physician. Previously drunkenness was known by such terms as *inebriety* or *intemperance,* but more medical sounding terms were developed including *alcoholism, dipsomania,* and *narcomania. Alcoholism* survived and is now the commonly accepted term (Barrows & Room, 1991).

Even though the notion that alcoholism was a disease had been around for many years previously, it was E. M. Jellinek in the 1950s who first clearly proposed that alcoholism be called a disease. His arguments were published in his book *The Disease Concept of Alcoholism* (Jellinek, 1960). Jellinek was a associated with the Alcoholics Anonymous movement, and it was the in-

creasing prominence of this movement that brought the issue to a head. Now, alcoholism has been declared a disease by both the American Medical Association and the World Health Organization and is included in the DSM-IV, but its status as a disease is still the subject of considerable heated debate.

Not surprisingly, the issue hinges on how "disease" is defined. Maltzman (1994) argues that two characteristics define a disease: (1) there must be a lawful pattern of recurrent observable signs and symptoms, and (2) these signs and symptoms must represent a significant deviation from a norm or a standard of health; that is, they must constitute a serious threat to life and health.

There are few who would argue with the second assumption, but it is the first that defines the nature of the disease and is hotly debated. Jellinek originally described the "lawful pattern of signs and symptoms" in the following manner: Everyone starts drinking in the same way, in a moderate, social manner, but there are some who progress to drink more and more heavily and eventually they enter the "prodromal" phase of alcoholism characterized by frequent blackouts. Many such people are not "alcoholics," they are "problem drinkers" who either stay that way or eventually stop drinking. Some individuals progress to become "gamma alcoholics" (to use Jellinek's term). The change from being a problem drinker to a gamma alcoholic is marked by two symptoms: (1) a loss of control over drinking and (2) physical dependence indicated by high levels of tolerance and withdrawal symptoms such as seizures, hallucinations, and the DTs. Those individuals who go on to "alcoholism" are believed to have some predisposing characteristic that existed even before they started drinking which inevitably led them to this stage. It is worth noting that the distinction between "problem drinkers" and "alcoholics" is the presence or absence of physical dependence and loss of control, not the amount consumed. Problem drinkers may actually consume more than "alcoholics," but they are not considered "alcoholics" and do not have the disease. Any research on the "disease" of alcoholism therefore must be done on "alcoholics" not "problem drinkers." As we shall see, this distinction is responsible for many arguments over data between supporters and opponents of the disease model.

Is There a Syndrome? The debate, then, emphasizes a number of interesting issues. First, is there a syndrome as described by Jellinek? Jellinek's original research on this question has been criticized because it was based on a very small and unsystematically selected sample of AA members. Jellinek's work, however, has been replicated in larger, more scientifically selected samples, even though some of the details have not been confirmed (Schuckit et al., 1993). Other studies that fail to show a consistent progression have been criticized on the grounds that they were not done on "gamma alcoholics."

What Is the Nature of the Disease Process? The main difficulty with the disease model is that the nature of the disease has never been defined. A number of specific theories have been advanced, including allergies to alcohol, genetically determined biochemical deficiencies, psychodynamic disorders, and nutritional deficits, but none has ever been widely accepted. It is surprising that after years of research we are still unable to do more than speculate on what sort of disease processes might be involved in making people drink destructively, but as discussed in Chapter 5, this failure in itself does not mean that there is no disease.

Alcoholics and Prealcoholics: Different from Nonalcoholics?

Are alcoholics different from nonalcoholics even before they start drinking? Some progress has been made in identifying specific factors that distinguish alcoholics and potential alcoholics from nonalcoholics. Two strategies have generally been used in research on this topic. The more common strategy has been to study alcoholics and nonalcoholics and try to identify differences. The second strategy has been to identify people who are known to be at risk of becoming alcoholics and study differences between them and those not at risk.

Many studies have compared alcoholics with nonalcoholics in the hope of identifying characteristics that might provide a cue about the nature of alcoholism. This has not been a fruitful area of research for a number of reasons. One scientist who studied the field concluded, "The investigation of any trait in alcoholics will show that they have either more or less of it" (Keller, 1972, p. 1147).

Demographic Variables. A number of demographic variables appear to be related to consumption. People who live in urban centers drink more than people who live in the country, and some occupations are at more risk than others— waiters, bartenders, longshoremen, and stevedores drink more than other occupations, while farmers and carpenters are at the low end of the scale. Heavy drinkers are more likely to be male by a ratio of about 6 to 1, and about 80 percent of people at first admission to a hospital for alcohol problems are between the ages of 30 and 55 (de Lint & Schmidt, 1971).

It has also been shown that alcoholism and other social and behavioral problems are more likely to occur in people who were raised in broken homes or homes where there was a domineering mother and an openly antagonistic father (McCord, 1972).

Personality. Much research has been conducted on the personalities of alcoholics and other drug users in the hope of identifying an *addictive personality*. No such personality has been found; in general, any type of person can develop drinking problems. Nonetheless, some researchers have noted consistent personality differences between populations of alcoholics and nonalcoholics. One influential theory holds that alcoholics have a preoccupation with personal power (McClelland et al., 1972). They show aggression, thrill-seeking behavior, and antisocial activities, and their main concerns are with power, glory, and dominance over others. The theory holds that the alcoholic feels weak and impotent, and drinking makes him or her feel more powerful. The sort of power that alcoholics want is personal power for its own sake, for personal glory, and not to be used for the benefit of others. As a result, they tend to be gregarious but not belong to groups, exploitative, exhibitionistic, and good at storytelling. Perhaps the best prototype of the alcoholic personality is Willy Loman in Arthur Miller's play *Death of a Salesman.*

Genetics. One of the primary assumptions of the disease model of alcoholism is that people who become alcoholics are an identifiable population even before they start to drink. The factors that make such people drink in an alcoholic manner may be determined genetically. Understanding the genetics may permit us to identify people at a high risk of problem drinking and intervene early before problems develop. One should remember that even if there is clear evidence that genetics are involved in the development of alcoholic drinking, it does not necessarily mean that alcoholism is a disease.

Evidence is clear that the risk of becoming an alcoholic is increased by as much as fourfold if you have a close relative (mother, father, or sibling) who is an alcoholic. Families, however, share both genetics and environment, and the challenge to researchers has been to separate these factors.

It is known, for example, that the amount of drinking of identical twins (who have exactly the same genes) is more similar than the drinking behavior of fraternal twins (who have the same genetic similarity as normal siblings). Thus the closer the genetic makeup, the more similar the drinking pattern. It has also been shown that an adopted person with a biological parent who is an alcoholic has an increased risk of alcoholism, but having an adoptive parent who is alcoholic does

not increase the risk of becoming alcoholic (Schuckit, 1992). Unfortunately, twin studies cannot completely disentangle genetics from environment, and adoption studies have serious conceptual and methodological flaws that make it difficult to draw firm conclusions (Searles, 1988). Nevertheless, there is an overwhelming volume of data supporting the heritability of alcoholism. It seems, though, that heritability varies considerably depending on a number of other factors, including gender, the measure of drinking behavior, the definition of alcoholism, and the population studied (Goldman, 1993).

It is clear that there is no single "alcoholism gene" and that the influence of genetics is modified by environment. A person with an identical twin who is alcoholic only has a 60 percent chance of being alcoholic. Genetics probably controls some aspect or aspects of body chemistry, personality, or brain function that increase the probability that a person will drink in an alcoholic manner in a particular environment. There may be a variety of genetic susceptibilities to alcohol that only cause problems in particular environments. The right combination of environment and genetics may be necessary to make a person drink in an alcoholic manner.

FHP versus FHN. As mentioned, one difficulty in comparing alcoholics with nonalcoholics is that it is quite likely that any differences might be caused by the alcohol rather than the other way around. One way to avoid this difficulty is to study the differences between people who are likely to become alcoholics and those less likely before they start drinking. It is known that people who come from families where there is a history of alcohol problems (family history positive, FHP) are at a greater risk of becoming alcoholic than those who have a family history without alcohol problems (family history negative, FHN). One interesting line of research has attempted to compare high-risk (FHP) and low-risk (FHN) individuals to see if it is possible to detect "markers" that might be able to identify potential alcoholics.

Though early studies were encouraging, there do not appear to be any consistent differences between FHP and FHN individuals in terms of pharmacokinetics and metabolism of alcohol, and no clear-cut differences have been established in cognitive and neuropsychological measures or personality (Searles, 1988). In a choice experiment where subjects were given the opportunity to consume either a placebo or alcohol, no difference was found in alcohol preference, alcohol-liking scores, BALs, or alcohol-induced impairment between FHP and FHN subjects (de Wit, 1989).

One interesting difference has shown up consistently in the EEG. High-risk individuals can be identified because they have a diminished responsiveness in their response to an anticipated stimulus. Normally, when an infrequent but expected stimulus is presented, a distinctive brain wave called the *P300* (or just *P3*) appears about 300 milliseconds after the stimulus. Not only do alcoholics show a diminished P300, but their sons do as well (Schuckit, 1987, p. 1531; Schuckit, 1992; Porjesz & Begleiter, 1987). In addition, there is some evidence that FHP individuals have a decreased percent of slow-wave alpha brain waves (Schuckit, 1992).

Although the result is not found by all researchers, many large scale studies have found an indication that a proportion of young men who are sons of alcoholics are less sensitive to alcohol when measured by subjective feelings of intoxication, some motor performance tests, and some hormonal and electrophysiological responses. Generally, these differences are only found in large-scale studies that give a single acute dose of alcohol equivalent to 3 to 5 drinks. Follow-up studies are currently under way to determine whether the individuals who show less sensitivity to alcohol are the ones who will develop drinking problems later (Schuckit, 1992).

If alcoholics are really different from nonalcoholics, these differences are rather difficult to establish and appear to be limited to subtle changes in the EEG, hormone levels, and subjective sensitivity that require large-scale, carefully controlled experiments to detect. It is still not clear how any of these differences contribute to the development of alcoholic drinking, if they do at all.

Is There Such a Thing as "Loss of Control"?

According to the disease model, one of the defining characteristics of alcoholism is loss of control. This is the assumption that exposure to even one or two drinks of alcohol in the alcoholic will cause an uncontrollable craving to drink more and more. In other words, the alcoholic will lose control of alcohol consumption; that is, one drink equals one drunk. Because of loss of control, it is firmly believed that total abstinence must be the only aim of therapy; social or moderate drinking is not possible for alcoholics.

The disease concept of alcoholism and belief in the loss of control have achieved such prominence that it is important to remember that the idea was first identified by Jellinek, on the basis of a questionnaire designed by members of Alcoholics Anonymous (AA), distributed in the AA magazine *The Grapevine*, and filled out by only 98 AA members (Curson, 1985). (Actually, 158 were returned, but many were eliminated because they were filled out jointly by groups of people or by women.) In fact, Jellinek's explanation of loss of control is quite different from contemporary explanations and is actually very similar to the behavioral theories of alcoholism to be described shortly.

Since the time it was proposed, the loss-of-control theory has never received significant experimental support. In fact, most research has disconfirmed the basic notion (Finagrette, 1988). A number of studies have found many cases of alcoholics who have reverted from excess drinking to moderate social drinking and have maintained that level for years. In 1962, D. L. Davis discovered, almost incidentally, many such controlled drinkers in a follow-up study at the

Maudsley Hospital in London. This discovery was followed by a string of similar findings that culminated in a report compiled by the Rand Corporation, which took on the job of evaluating the treatment outcomes of a network of alcohol treatment centers run by the National Institute on Alcoholism and Alcohol Abuse in the United States. The Rand Report (Armor, Polach, & Stambul, 1978) showed that controlled drinking rather than total abstinence could be a reasonable treatment aim for many alcoholics. Although the Rand report was not the first and only to document controlled drinking in former alcoholics, it received the greatest publicity and caused a storm of controversy. Many alcoholism experts denounced the report as dangerous and unscientific, and there were suggestions that its publication should have been suppressed.

Since the time of the Rand report, research claiming to demonstrate the feasibility of controlled drinking has been attacked on various grounds (Pendrey, Maltzman, & West, 1982). Some argue that most of these studies were done with problem drinkers, not on populations of "gamma alcoholics" as defined by other characteristics such as physical dependence. In addition, it has been argued that most studies purporting to show that alcoholics can return to controlled drinking do not allow a sufficiently long time frame to detect whether controlled drinking is possible (Maltzman, 1994).

In addition to the research with alcoholics in treatment, laboratory studies have repeatedly shown that alcoholics are perfectly capable of moderating their alcohol intake and virtually never lose control (Mello & Mendelson, 1972). Such laboratory studies are also challenged on the grounds that the laboratory is too artificial to be relevant to alcohol use in a natural setting (Maltzman, 1994).

Perhaps related to the concept of loss of control is the phenomenon of *priming*. It was shown some time ago that noncontingent infusion of the drug would reinstate drug self-administration in laboratory animals that had stopped pressing a lever. For example, J. Stewart and de Wit (1987) have shown that bar pressing by rats for cocaine and heroin that has been extinguished by discontinuing the drug injection can be reestablished if the rats are given a free, noncontingent injection of the drug. These researchers have developed a theory of drug self-administration based on the idea that the desire to use a drug can be "induced" by the presence of drug in the body. Their theory suggests that the drug excites certain brain systems and artificially creates the drive for more drug. Additional support comes from other experiments showing that in experienced users of cocaine, craving for cocaine was much greater 15 minutes after an injection of cocaine than it was before the injection (Jaffe et al., 1989).

De Wit and Chutuape (1993) have shown that social drinkers are much more likely to choose an alcoholic drink and report an increased craving for alcohol after they have been given a priming dose of alcohol.

Moral Responsibility of the Drinker. Perhaps the main reason why Jellinek's disease explanation has won such support is that it portrays the alcoholic as a helpless victim of a physiological disorder beyond his or her control, rather than someone with a moral weakness. The implication is that the alcoholic is a person who must be treated rather than punished. The acceptance of the disease concept vastly improved the lot of people with alcohol problems. Rather than finding themselves being thrown in jail, alcoholics found themselves under the care of a physician. Public attitudes changed, and medical research into alcoholism gained credibility and expanded. It also provided alcoholics with a rational context in which they could understand their own behavior and a clearly defined goal, though a difficult one to reach, of achieving sobriety. It is little wonder that the disease concept gained such wide backing from the medical profession, government agencies, and alcoholics themselves, and is so resistant to change.

Although the disease concept of alcoholism was better for alcoholics than the notion of moral weakness and lack of willpower that it replaced, it has one major problem. As described earlier, the nature of the disease of alcoholism has never been established; therefore, the medical profession does not know how to treat it. Though great medical advancements have been made in handling such problems as withdrawal from alcohol and in treating alcohol-related diseases that have a basis in understood physiology, when it comes to the treatment of the disease of alcoholism, the medical profession has traditionally resorted to counseling with perhaps a little pharmacological assistance from tranquilizers. Marlatt calls this the "control paradox." He points out that loss of control is the primary characteristic by which alcoholism is diagnosed, and yet when it comes to treatment, the best that physicians can offer is "moralistic/physiological arguments and descriptions of complications that follow from continued alcohol abuse." In other words, they attempt to "browbeat the alcoholic into self-controlled abstinence" when, by the disease model definition, the alcoholic is incapable of control (W. H. George & Marlatt, 1983, p. 107).

The Behavioral Approach

It is commonly assumed that a rejection of the disease concept would mean a return to the moral weakness model of alcoholism and punishment notions of treatment, but there are alternatives to the disease concept that offer a similarly sympathetic understanding and seem to hold considerably more promise in terms of treatment. These models are based on the idea that excessive drinking is not a result of a disease or a pathological state existing within the organism but rather a result of normal behavioral processes that have, for one reason or another, caused the person to behave in a maladaptive manner. For example, we know that our brains have the ability to protect us from poisons by causing us to dislike the taste of things that have made us sick. Thus if we

eat a poisonous berry for the first time and it makes our stomach sick, we will not like the taste of that berry in the future and probably will not eat anything that tastes like it again. This is called *flavor toxicosis learning,* and it has been demonstrated in a large number of species including humans. Consider, however, this situation: You go on a boat ride and buy a chocolate ice cream cone. Later, a wind comes up, and the motion of the boat makes you seasick. Flavor toxicosis learning will make you dislike the taste of chocolate even though it was not the chocolate that made you sick. Your chocolate aversion may last for many years and cause you to avoid chocolate ice cream even though it is irrational and maladaptive and quite beyond your control, but it is not a disease. It is a result of perfectly natural behavioral process that has been misdirected.

Alcoholism may be a similar phenomenon. It too may be a result of normal healthy (rather than disease) processes that have been misdirected. Alternative theories to the disease model are based on possible explanations derived from what we know about normal behavioral processes and how they might have been misdirected to create behavior that appears to be "abnormal."

Chapter 5 contains a discussion of how drug self-administration can be explained as a general process in which drug administration is considered to act as a positive reinforcer and to control behavior in a manner similar to other positive reinforcers. There is no reason to believe that the self-administration of alcohol is any different from the self-administration of any other substance, and so the positive reinforcer concept should apply to alcohol and alcoholism as it does to cocaine, tobacco, or any other drug.

As explained in Chapter 5, this model can account for the compulsive and self-destructive nature of drinking and can also offer explanations of how different drinking patterns develop in different people. Unlike the disease model, the behavioral approach does not insist that alcoholism is a unitary phenomenon and that alcoholics are in a qualitatively different category from nonalcoholics. It accepts the possibility that alcohol consumption is a graded response varying from abstinence at one extreme to heavy drinking at the other and that an individual can move up or down on this scale at different times. It also suggests the factors that might contribute to where an individual is on the scale at any given time. It does not preclude the possibility that there may be genetic predispositions or biochemical or nutritional deficiencies in some individuals that could make them particularly susceptible to the reinforcing or debilitating effects of alcohol; in fact, it offers a theoretical framework in which such physiological differences could interact with environmental variables to cause alcoholic behavior.

Ironically, Jellinek's explanation of loss of control is a behavioral explanation rather than a disease explanation. Jellinek noticed that alcoholics who had developed physical dependence on alcohol often experienced withdrawal symptoms while they were drinking and showed extensive tolerance to the pleasurable effects of alcohol. He suggested that loss of control was merely excessive drinking in an attempt to alleviate withdrawal symptoms and to achieve euphoria (positive reinforcement):

The inability to stop after one or two glasses . . . seems to be characterized by minor withdrawal symptoms in the presence of alcohol in the blood stream and *the failure to achieve the desired euphoria* for more than a few minutes. These symptoms explain superficially the behavior observed in the so-called loss of control. (Jellinek, 1960, pp. 146–147; italics added)

In addition, Jellinek explained why drinking causes withdrawal symptoms using traditional learning theory: "In the gamma alcoholic who drinks concentrated spirits in a concentrated period of time, the metabolism of nervous tissue becomes conditioned by the 'signal' of the 'first drink'" (p. 149).

Finally, because the behavioral approach offers an explanation of why heavy drinking occurs, it also suggests treatment strategies. The disease model presumes that the drinking behavior of alcoholics is not normal, that it is governed by different rules from other behavior. But as we have already established, the disease model has not been able to define what those rules are and consequently has not been able to come up with a treatment. Because the behavioral approach assumes that ordinary behavioral laws apply to drinking, it has access to a considerable body of knowledge about behavior in general that it can apply to drinking and its control.

SELF-ADMINISTRATION IN NONHUMANS

Oral Self-Administration

When alcohol is freely available to rats and monkeys in conditions where food and water are also freely available, they will drink the alcohol, but not in quantities sufficient to cause obvious intoxication or physical dependence. This type of drinking resembles typical human drinking patterns, but the thrust of this research has been to provide a model of human alcoholism, so there has been considerable research over the years to attempt to find what factors can cause this consumption to increase. Research using oral administration has been hampered because alcohol has a disagreeable taste that most nonhuman species prefer to avoid, and the effects on the CNS are somewhat delayed due to slow absorption from the digestive system (Meisch, 1977).

It has been found that one way to increase these low levels of intake is to subject the animal to a period of forced consumption when its only source of food or water is laced with alcohol. After a rat has been forced to consume the alcohol, its voluntary intake may increase. Animals that have been deprived of either food or water will also drink alcohol. Intake will sometimes remain high even after the food or water is returned. One reason these procedures induce drinking may be that alcohol has some value to the animals as a source of food energy. After a period of exposure, it may acquire reinforcing value because it acts like any other food on the energy requirements of the animals.

Other procedures can increase the consumption of alcohol. One is *schedule-induced polydipsia*. If an animal is given a pellet of food on a regular basis, such as in an FI schedule of reinforcement, it will tend to develop a stable pattern of drinking if water also is available. After the pellet has been consumed, the animal will drink and, in the course of a session, may actually drink many times its usual daily water intake. If the fluid is alcohol, it will drink that as well. In this way the animal can be induced to consume large quantities of alcohol. This consumption is continued even when the inducing schedule is discontinued (Meisch, 1975).

Animals whose ethanol intake has been increased by these measures will learn to press a lever on a reinforcement schedule for access to alcohol. Their pattern of behavior is similar to that induced by any other reinforcer. Although some reports claim that food deprivation and other induction procedures are not necessary, they are generally used.

It has been noted in these studies that physical dependence is not necessary for alcohol consumption and that when physical dependence exists, it does not increase alcohol intake. Animals that have been made physically dependent will sometimes fail to drink alcohol even while experiencing withdrawal symptoms (Hunter, Walker, & Riley, 1974).

Intravenous Self-Administration

Induction procedures are generally not necessary when alcohol is administered through a cannula implanted in the bloodstream. Giving the alcohol this way avoids the problem of bad taste and slow effect on the CNS, and most animals rapidly learn to self-administer alcohol. When alcohol infusions are freely available, the pattern of self-administration is somewhat erratic. There are periods of high-level intake followed by self-imposed abstinence lasting two to four days, when withdrawal symptoms may occur. These periods do not seem to follow any regular pattern like that seen with the stimulants such as cocaine (see Figure 10–2). Figure 5–3 shows the intake of a rhesus monkey pressing a lever for intravenous alcohol over a period of 90 days in the laboratory of Jim Woods and his colleagues. The similarity of this pattern to human alcohol intake has already been noted.

HARMFUL EFFECTS OF AN ACUTE ADMINISTRATION

Alcohol Poisoning

A single dose of alcohol, if large enough, can be lethal. A blood alcohol level of about 300 to 400 mg per 100 ml will usually cause loss of consciousness. In a study of alcohol poisonings, Kaye and Haag (1957) report that without therapy people whose BALs reached 500 mg per 100 ml died within an hour or two. The world record high BAL is probably 1,500 mg per 100 ml reported in a 30-year-old man whose life was saved by vigorous medical intervention. Later he reported that he had drunk 4.23 liters of beer and an undetermined number of bottles of liquor in the space of three hours (O'Neil et al., 1984).

Death by alcohol, as with most depressant drugs, usually results from respiratory failure. Alcohol, then, is a rather toxic substance with the lethal dose uncomfortably close to the usual social dose. A 150-pound male would have to drink 7.5 ounces of liquor to have a BAL of 150 mg per 100 ml: This is at the upper levels of an acceptable social high. Around 25 ounces of liquor would produce a BAL of 500 mg per 100 ml, probably a lethal dose for most people. Thus the therapeutic index for alcohol is about 3.5 (25 ÷ 7.5), not very high.

Fortunately, alcohol has a built-in safety feature: We either vomit or pass out before we have a chance to kill ourselves. People who die from alcohol poisoning usually drink it quickly and in high concentrations, so that they are able to get a lethal dose into their bodies before they lose consciousness.

Hangover

The problem of how to avoid a hangover from alcohol has occupied some of the best minds since Plato, as this passage from *The Dialogues of Plato* illustrates:

They were about to commence drinking, when Pausanias said, "And now, my friends, how can we drink with the least injury to ourselves?" I can assure you that I feel severely the effect of yesterday's potations, and must have time to recover; and I suspect that most of you are in the same predicament, for you were of the party yesterday. Consider then "How can the drinking be made easiest?" (Symposium 176a-b, Jowett translation, 1931)

Like the ancient Greeks, most drinkers have, at one time or another, suffered the next day for having too much the night before. Apart from the puritanical notion that we are getting just what we deserve, there are several explanations for a hangover. These explanations suggest that hangover results from alcohol-produced effects such as low blood-sugar levels, dehydration, and irritation of the lining of the digestive system. There is no doubt that most of these effects of alcohol contribute to discomfort the next day, but it is probably best to think of hangover as a mini-withdrawal from alcohol, a rebound excitation of an alcohol-depressed nervous system. This rebound makes the brain more sensitive to seizures.

No doubt some of the discomfort arises from alcohol-induced disruptions of many of the daily cyclic changes in body physiology known as *circadian rhythms*. These disruptions are similar to those commonly known as "jet lag" experienced by air travelers, and a person who has been drinking can take as long as 48 hours to get back on track.

For most, hangovers are not physiologically serious, but for some, such as those with epilepsy, heart disease, or diabetes, hangovers could have serious medical consequences (Gauvin, Cheng, & Holloway, 1993).

The Greeks never did answer Pausanius's question "How can the drinking be made easiest?" apart from concluding that "drinking deep is a bad practice," but over the centuries a number of cures have been suggested, including eating a spoonful of sugar or drinking lots of water. To the extent that a hangover can be thought of as a withdrawal from alcohol, one cure is to take a "hair of the dog that bit you." Consuming more alcohol relieves the hangover by depressing this rebound excitability in the same way that other depressant drugs are used to treat withdrawal. If the alcohol is taken in small quantities, it might work, but if too much is consumed, it will only postpone withdrawal.

Alcohol-Induced Behavior

Apart from the self-inflicted physical harm that can be done by an acute administration of alcohol, the drug can be responsible for changes in behavior that cause untold social, psychological, financial, and physical harm to the drinker and others. It is not possible to catalog all of these sorts of harm, but most people have experienced them in some form or another. They include accidents caused while drunk or hung over, not only while driving but also in industry and at home; crimes committed under the influence of alcohol; and damage done to families and social relationships. All these effects are difficult to quantify, and some may not be a direct result of alcohol. They are nonetheless real and must be included in any assessment of the harmful effects of alcohol.

Reproduction

A well-known quote from Shakespeare's *Macbeth* states that drink "provokes the desire, but takes away the performance" in matters sexual. The bard's analysis is essentially correct. Acute alcohol consumption may increase interest by diminishing inhibitions, but, at least in higher doses, it reduces sexual arousal in both males and females. In males, alcohol at lower doses (BAL less than 100 mg per 100 ml) may increase the duration of erections and thus provide increased opportunities for fulfillment of the partner. This fact may explain why alcohol is often perceived as enhancing sexual performance (Rubin & Henson, 1976; Mello, 1978).

A study with rats showed that increasing doses of alcohol caused increasing disruptions of copulation of male rats with receptive females. In addition, low doses of alcohol that disrupted copulation with receptive females caused male rats to attempt to copulate with unreceptive females, something they would normally not attempt. These findings support the speculation that low doses of alcohol adversely affect uninhibited sexual performance but can stimulate sexual behavior that is normally inhibited (Pfaus & Pinel, 1988).

HARMFUL EFFECTS OF CHRONIC CONSUMPTION

The Liver

Prolonged drinking of alcohol damages the liver. The damage usually starts with a buildup of fat in the liver. Alcoholics also frequently contract *alcoholic hepatitis*, which usually develops into *cirrhosis*. Cirrhosis is present in 8 percent of chronic alcoholics; among nonalcoholics, the condition affects only 1 percent. Cirrhosis means scarring. The liver becomes filled with scar tissue and is no longer able to function, and the result is frequently fatal, especially if alcohol consumption is not stopped. A review of studies showed that of people who continued drinking after diagnosis of cirrhosis, the five-year survival rate ranged between 35 and 48 percent, but the sur-

vival rate of those who were able to quit ranged from 63 to 77 percent (Williams & Davis, 1977). Women drinkers are more likely to suffer from liver cirrhosis than men.

As a direct result of liver damage, the immune responses of alcoholics are also impaired, leaving them susceptible to a host of other infections (Wands, 1979).

The Nervous System

Alcoholics and heavy drinkers frequently show a cluster of symptoms that include a loss of memory for past events, an inability to remember new material, and disorientation and confusion. These symptoms are collectively known as *Korsakoff's psychosis*. They are a result of damage in certain parts of the brain first noted by Wernicke and called *Wernicke's disease*. The condition seems to be a result of deficiency of *thiamin (vitamin B₁)* that is common among many alcoholics (Victor, Adams, & Collins, 1971). Many of the conditions suffered by alcoholics can be traced to vitamin deficiencies, many of which result because people who drink large quantities of alcohol do not normally have a balanced diet. It is also known that alcohol can damage the digestive system and interfere with the normal absorption of some nutrients.

The Wernicke-Korsakoff syndrome is not the only neurological damage associated with heavy drinking. A number of other disorders of both the central and peripheral nervous systems, such as *epilepsy, cerebellar syndrome*, and *alcoholic dementia*, are attributable either directly or indirectly to excessive alcohol use (Marsden, 1977, p. 189).

Cancer

The use of alcohol is directly related to cancers of the mouth, throat, and liver, the parts of the body directly exposed to high alcohol concentrations and susceptible to alcohol damage. The risk of these cancers is much greater in people who combine smoking and drinking. Though the relationship of these cancers to alcohol consumption can be demonstrated statistically, the actual role of alcohol in the development of cancer is not well understood. Direct exposure to alcohol may change the reactivity of tissue and cause it to become cancerous directly, although it is possible that the real culprit may be something else in the alcoholic beverage that is the *carcinogen* (cancer causer). It is also believed that alcohol augments the cancer-causing effect of tobacco either by acting as a solvent that allows the tobacco carcinogen to get into the tissues of the mouth and throat more easily or by inhibiting salivation and interfering with the rinsing mechanisms that would otherwise decrease the concentrations of the tobacco carcinogens in the mouth (Kissen & Kaley, 1974).

Reproduction

In males chronic alcohol consumption is known to cause impotence, shrinking of the testicles, and a loss of sexual interest. Although there have been few studies of the effects of chronic alcohol consumption in females, there is evidence that it can cause menstrual dysfunctions such as amenorrhea, dysmenorrhea, and premenstrual discomfort (Mellow, 1987, p. 1517).

There are ancient beliefs that alcohol might be teratogenic (responsible for birth defects). In ancient Carthage, drinking on wedding days was forbidden in the belief that it might cause an abnormal child to be born (Jones & Smith, 1975). Aristotle warned against drinking during pregnancy, and later, at the time of the gin epidemic in England, it was noted that there was an increase in infant deaths. Similar effects associated with alcohol consumption have been reported in the medical literature since, but the extent of the problem has only recently been appreciated. It is now recognized that the use of alcohol during pregnancy can harm the developing fetus and may result in a number of behavioral, anatomical, and physiological irregularities that may be known as *fetal alcohol syndrome (FAS)* in their more severe form, or *fetal alcohol effects (FAE)* or *alcohol-related birth defects (ARBD)* if only a few symptoms are present.

Alcohol consumption during pregnancy can result in a variety of outcomes, which include spontaneous abortion, lowered birthweight, congenital facial and urogenital abnormalities, and retarded motor and mental development.

The manifestations of FAS are mental retardation, poor coordination, loss of muscle tone, low birthweight, slow growth, malformation of organ systems, and peculiar facial characteristics such as small eyes, drooping eyelids, and a misshapen mouth that looks like the mouth of a fish. These symptoms do not always appear together, but the chances of any or all of these effects increase with the amount of alcohol drunk during pregnancy.

The worldwide incidence of FAS has been estimated at 1.9 per 1,000 live births. Among alcoholic women and "problem drinkers," however, the incidence has been estimated to be between 24 and 42 per 1,000 live births in the United States and as high as 256 per 1,000 live births in Europe (Abel & Sokol, 1989).

The mechanism by which alcohol affects the developing fetus is not known. It is known that many normal, healthy children are born to women who have drunk heavily during pregnancy. These normal births show that alcohol alone cannot be entirely responsible. As Abel and Sokol (1989) suggest, alcohol is a necessary but not a sufficient condition for FAS or FAE. Other factors that may be involved are not known, but it has been shown that they include (1) having previous children, (2) being black, (3) having a high score on an alcohol screening test, and (4) having a high percent of drinking days. It also seems clear that occasional high levels of consumption do more damage than the same amount of alcohol consumed at chronic low levels (Abel and Sokol, 1989).

There does not appear to be any time during pregnancy when it is safe to drink. Rosett has pointed out that malformations probably are produced by high concentrations during the first three months (trimester) when embryonic development of the central nervous system is taking place. Growth may be most vulnerable to heavy drinking during the second and third trimesters. Behavior disturbance and intellectual impairment may be related to alcohol's effects on the central nervous system early in pregnancy or during the later period of cell division associated with rapid brain growth and functional organization (Rosett, 1979).

An example of functional disruption of organization is in the formation of the cortex. It appears that alcohol is responsible for a disruption of cell migration in the cortex so that only four layers rather than the normal six layers are formed. In addition, these cells may also end up migrating to the wrong layer (Abel, 1989).

It appears that the only way to be certain of avoiding all of these effects is to avoid alcohol completely during pregnancy. If there is any drinking at all, high blood alcohol levels should be avoided.

Heart Disease

A degeneration of the heart muscle known as *alcoholic cardiomyopathy* results directly from the chronic consumption of alcohol. This condition most likely arises from the effect alcohol has on the metabolism of the membrane of the cells of the heart muscle. The result is very similar to cirrhosis of the liver and was once described as "cirrhosis of the heart" (Myerson, 1971, p. 183).

Other Effects

Chronic use of alcohol may also be responsible for a number of other pathologies. These include diseases of the digestive system such as ulcers and cancer, inflammation and other disorders of the pancreas, pneumonia and other diseases of the lungs and respiratory system, abnormalities of the blood, and malnutrition.

It has been observed for some time that alcoholics are more susceptible to many infectious diseases and less responsive to treatment. There are many reasons for this susceptibility including differences in lifestyle, nutrition, and liver functioning, but it has become clear recently that alcohol has an adverse effect on all aspects of the functioning the immune system, thus impairing the body's ability to resist and fight infections (Baker & Jerrells, 1993).

BENEFITS OF ALCOHOL CONSUMPTION

In addition to being a recreational drug, from the time of its invention, alcohol has been used as a medicine. Avicenna, the tenth-century Persian physician, recommended wine for his older patients, although he cautioned his younger patients to drink it in moderation. Arnaud de Villeneuve, who reputedly invented brandy in the thirteenth century, hailed it as the water of immortality and called it *aqua vitae*, "water of life." He was convinced that it would increase longevity and maintain youth (McKim & Mishara, 1987).

More recently, several studies have offered beer and wine to elderly people in a geriatric hospital during a "happy hour." It was found that consumption of these beverages improved sleep, boosted morale, increased participation in activities, relieved depression, and had no detectable ill effects (Mishara & Kastenbaum, 1980).

While it is clear that heavy drinking is very unhealthy, there is also some evidence that moderate alcohol consumption can decrease the probability of death from heart attack. This may be the case, but when all causes of death are taken into account, any benefits from moderate drinking that may be gained by decreased risk of heart attack are made up for by the increases in cancer, stroke, or accidents associated with drinking (Ashley, 1982). Further research has shown that for those under 60, increased alcohol consumption is related to increased risk of dying from any cause, but for those over 60, the relative risk of dying was less for light and moderate drinkers than for heavy drinkers and abstainers. This relationship was the same for both sexes (Rehm & Sempos, 1995). It is not clear what is causing what. It has not been established whether moderate alcohol consumption has a protective effect, or whether healthy people simply feel more like drinking. It is possible that all this was foreseen a thousand years ago by Avicenna, who recommended wine for his older patients.

TREATMENTS

Because there has been little agreement over the years about what alcoholism really is and why people drink, many types of treatments have been developed to help those who want to reduce their alcohol intake. It is usually agreed that the first step must be to eliminate physical dependence if it is present. This is usually done in a hospital or a detoxification center where the alcoholic goes through withdrawal under medical supervision until all withdrawal symptoms are over. Following detoxification comes an active treatment phase that may or may not be followed by a long-term program to prevent the recurrence of drinking, or *relapse* in the language of the physician.

The nature of the therapy and its outcome goal are determined by how the therapist defines alcoholism. In this chapter we have discussed two models of alcoholism, the disease model and the behavioral model.

If alcoholism is considered to be a disease, theoretically it should be possible to cure the underlying disorder, and the excessive drinking, which is a symptom, will disappear. As mentioned earlier, there is little agreement on the nature of the underlying disorder, so this sort of cure is not currently possible. It is widely believed that the underlying disorder is an allergic reaction or a nutritional or biochemical deficiency, or some combination of these factors. Treatments based on the notion have stressed nutritional supplements and dietary changes (Beasley, 1987), but the aim of this intervention

is not to cure the disease. The aim is to help restore normal bodily functioning, which should reduce or eliminate the physiological need and craving for alcohol and make it easier for the individual to stop drinking. Because of loss of control, all treatments based on the disease model stress that the only legitimate outcome of therapy must be total abstinence from alcohol.

The behavioral approach described earlier presumes that excessive drinking is a result of normal behavioral processes interacting in a maladaptive way with the environment, and as a result, treatments should be aimed at reestablishing acceptable behavior patterns. This is done by using the behavioral principles of conditioning and instrumental learning that have been developed to change other sorts of abnormal or undesirable behavior patterns.

In practical terms, there is little difference between the disease model approach and the behavioral approach. Both are aimed at changing the behavior of alcoholics. The disease approach differs from the behavioral approach in two basic ways: (1) The disease approach is more likely to include physical interventions such as nutritional supplements and dietary supplements or the use of other drugs (antidepressants to treat underlying depression, tranquilizers to treat underlying anxiety), and (2) the disease approach insists that because the disease cannot be cured, the aim of all therapy *must* be total abstinence from alcohol.

It is important to note that treatments based on the disease model do not preclude the use of behavioral interventions such as aversion therapy and skills training, and treatments based on the behavioral approach do not necessarily preclude the therapeutic goal of total abstinence for many alcoholics. Consequently, it is not always possible to characterize a particular treatment program as one or the other.

Alcoholics Anonymous

Alcoholics Anonymous was founded in 1935. It grew out of a popular Protestant religious movement, the Oxford Movement. The Oxford Movement consisted of small groups that met weekly for prayer, worship, and discussion, with the aim of self-improvement. One Oxford Group meeting in Akron, Ohio, was attended by an alcoholic stockbroker and an alcoholic physician, both of whom were seriously but unsuccessfully trying to stop drinking. They found that their fellowship and that of the group was able to help them stop drinking. They brought other alcoholics into the group, many with similar success. In fact, helping other alcoholics to stay sober seemed to be making an important contribution to the maintenance of their own sobriety. As the meetings got bigger, new groups were formed, and eventually they broke away from the Oxford Movement and became Alcoholics Anonymous (Alcoholics Anonymous, 1980).

The organization has grown rapidly and spread around the world. It is not known how many members there are because the organization does not keep membership lists, but in 1982 there were 20,000 groups in 100 countries around the world with an estimated world membership of well over 1 million (Maxwell, 1984, p. 2).

Though AA broke away from the Oxford group, it has retained many of the elements that seemed to be responsible for its effectiveness, in-

2. For our group purpose there is but one ultimate authority—a loving God as He may express Himself in our group conscience. Our leaders are but trusted servants; they do not govern.
3. The only requirement for A.A. membership is a desire to stop drinking.
4. Each group should be autonomous except in matters affecting other groups or A.A. as a whole.
5. Each group has but one primary purpose—to carry its message to the alcoholic who still suffers.
6. An A.A. group ought never endorse, finance or lend the A.A. name to any related facility or outside enterprise, lest problems of money, property, and prestige divert us from our primary purpose.
7. Every A.A. group ought to be fully self-supporting, declining outside contributions.
8. Alcoholics Anonymous should remain forever nonprofessional, but our service centers may employ special workers.
9. A.A., as such, ought never to be organized; but we may create service boards or committees directly responsible to those they serve.
10. Alcoholics Anonymous has no opinion on outside issues; hence the A.A. name ought never to be drawn into public controversy.
11. Our public relations policy is based on attraction rather than promotion; we need always maintain personal anonymity at the level of press, radio, and films.
12. Anonymity is the spiritual foundation of all our Traditions, ever reminding us to place principles before personalities.

Source: Reprinted with the permission of Alcoholics Anonymous World Service.

cluding religion, although this aspect can be moderated to suit each individual.

At every meeting of AA, someone reads the 12 steps and the 12 traditions that explain the basic principles and processes the organization has found to be effective over the years. These are presented in Box 6–2. The AA approach, also known as the 12-steps approach, has been adapted to many other support groups for people who have problems controlling behavior like gambling, overeating, and the use of other drugs.

AA is not a temperance organization. The temperance movement is religion based and made up largely of individuals who are not alcoholics and

have never had a drinking problem but wish to impose their view about alcohol on others. AA is made up of alcoholics. AA members are not antiliquor and do not seek to impose their views on anyone else. The organization exists only to help alcoholics who want to achieve sobriety.

The AA approach to alcoholism coincides with the disease model discussed earlier. Most AA members believe that to control drinking, the individual must first admit to being "powerless over alcohol" and unable to control drinking without help. AA members believe that drinking can be controlled only by relying on a greater power, often identified as "God," or "God as we have come to understand Him" (or Her) for people who are uncomfortable with the concept. They feel that there is no cure; there are only alcoholics who drink and alcoholics who do not drink. For this reason, members are expected to attend regular meetings for extended periods of time. It is not unusual for new members to attend more than six meetings a week. (In fact, there is a tradition of new members doing "90 meetings in 90 days.") In addition to attending meetings, members often see each other socially outside of meetings and frequently talk on the phone (Maxwell, 1984). For many people, AA is not a treatment at all; it is a long-term commitment, and for many, it becomes a way of life.

It has been estimated that AA is currently helping as many alcoholics in the United States as all medical facilities combined, and it does so with apparent success.

Treatment with Other Drugs

Antabuse (disulfiram) and *CCC (citrated calcium carbamate)* block the action of the enzyme acetaldehyde dehydrogenase. Drinking alcohol with this enzyme out of commission will cause a buildup of acetaldehyde in the body, which makes a person feel very sick. If alcohol is not consumed, the drug has little effect. Therefore, a person taking the enzyme blocker cannot drink without getting sick. It is frequently prescribed for alcoholics as an adjunct to other therapies, but it can work only if the alcoholic takes it regularly. Some studies with disulfiram show fairly high alcohol abstinence rates among those that take the drug regularly, but properly controlled clinical trials with random assignment to groups fail to show that disulfiram is superior to a placebo (Gorelick, 1993). Antabuse offers some protection from unplanned or spontaneous drinking, but a patient who wants to drink can simply stop taking the drug.

There is another possible difficulty with Antabuse. In our discussion of the neurophysiology of alcohol, it was suggested that the reinforc-

ing and euphoric effects of alcohol may depend on acetaldehyde, and we also know that acetaldehyde can function as a reinforcer. If this is true, enzyme blockers that increase levels of acetaldehyde may well be increasing the reinforcing effects of alcohol in addition to punishing alcohol consumption.

Tranquilizers (barbiturates and benzodiazepines) and antidepressants are frequently prescribed for alcoholics in the belief that these individuals drink because of anxiety or stress or because they are depressed, and the alcohol relieves these unpleasant symptoms. The tranquilizer or the antidepressant should relieve the anxiety or depression and therefore remove the cause of drinking. While tranquilizers frequently appear to reduce alcohol intake, it is probably not because of their effect on stress. Alcohol and the tranquilizers have similar effects, and tranquilizers potentiate the effects of alcohol. Heavy drinkers taking tranquilizers often cut down on their drinking because the pills substitute for the alcohol, not because the pills have relieved any anxiety.

There have been encouraging results using drugs that specifically operate on the serotonin system. The most studied drugs in this regard are serotonin reuptake blockers (SSRIs, see Chapter 13) which increase levels of serotonin in the synapse. A series of studies at the Addiction Research Foundation in Toronto found that fluoxetine and sertraline, drugs normally used as antidepressants, reduced alcohol intake by 9–14 percent and increased the number of abstinent days in volunteer subjects who were described as heavy social drinkers or early problem drinkers. The result has been replicated as well with alcoholics (Gorelick, 1993). A number of other drugs have also been shown to reduce alcohol consumption in both humans and laboratory animals, including drugs that stimulate 5-HT_{A1} receptors (buspirone) and drugs that block either 5-HT_2 (ritanserin) or 5-HT_3 receptors (ondansetron). It seems that the SSRIs reduce all consummatory behavior, but the effect of these drugs seems to be more specific in reducing alcohol consumption (Litten & Allen, 1993).

It is puzzling why both agonists and antagonists of serotonin receptors should show this effect. Many of these drugs are also used clinically as antidepressants, and alcohol abusers are frequently found to be clinically depressed. Interestingly, though, the alcohol-suppressing effect is evident as soon as the drug is taken, but the antidepressant effects usually do not show up for several weeks (see Chapter 13). Clearly serotonin is involved in a complex way with the neurophysiology of alcohol consumption.

There is also evidence that the dopamine D_2 receptor agonist bromocriptine and the opiate receptor blocker naltrexone are effective in reducing alcohol consumption in laboratory animals and in human alcoholics (Litten & Allen, 1993).

Psychoanalysis and Counseling

Psychoanalytic theory holds that drinking is partly a symptom of some deep underlying maladjustment in the functioning of the three components of the self—the id, the ego, and the superego. Alcoholism is believed to be a result of a disturbance during the three stages of psychosexual development. Drinking cannot be controlled until alcoholics achieve insight into the source of their problems and fully understand themselves, their past, and their relationships with others. Psychoanalysis is not widely used, largely because of a lack of research supporting psychoanalytic interpretations of alcoholism (Barry, 1988).

Counseling, by contrast, tends to concern itself with more immediate causes of drinking. It may be attempted on an individual or group basis, and its aim is to provide the drinker with an understanding of his or her behavior through discussion with a trained alcoholism counselor or others with similar problems.

Behavior Therapy

The behavior therapist treats alcohol drinking like any other sort of positively reinforced response and tries to stop drinking either by punishing it or by reinforcing behaviors that are not compatible with drinking (Caddy & Block, 1983).

Aversion Therapy. Some success with alcoholics has been achieved in hospitals where drinking was punished with painful electrical shocks, although this technique is no longer used. A more promising technique was tried by Fred Boland and his colleagues (Boland, Mellor, & Revusky, 1978) at Memorial University in Newfoundland, who gave alcoholics a flavor aversion to the taste of alcohol using the principle of flavor toxicosis learning described earlier. Boland worked with hospitalized alcoholic patients who were permitted to drink their favorite beverage and then were given capsules of lithium carbonate, a drug that causes nausea. After several conditioning trials, many came to dislike the taste of alcohol, and this aversion helped them to refrain from drinking. After training, one former alcoholic even vomited at the smell of booze from another alcoholic who was being admitted. Unfortunately, the effectiveness of this technique is limited because the aversion extinguishes rapidly if the individual decides to return to drinking.

Skills Training and Relapse Prevention. Counselors may also use techniques like role playing, transactional analysis, and assertiveness training to try to teach social and life skills that will help the drinker to handle social situations, especially ones that involve drinking.

It is also known that relapse to drinking is more likely to occur in circumstances where a person (1) feels angry or frustrated with a personal or social situation or (2) is under social pressure to drink. One approach developed by G. A. Marlatt and his associates (George & Marlatt, 1983) stresses the identification of situations that cause a high risk of relapse to excessive drinking and then the training of coping responses to each situation so that the individual will feel in control of the situation and will not need to resort to alcohol.

If competing sources of reinforcement can reduce the use of alcohol, as discussed in Chapter 5, perhaps it might be possible to teach people to take advantage of other sources of reinforcement and reduce their dependence on alcohol. The training of social skills such as how to get and hold a job or more effective ways of relating to people are often incorporated into treatment programs. Because interpersonal relationships and social support are also seen as important, it is becoming more common to incorporate the entire family of the alcoholic into the therapeutic process.

Effectiveness

In spite of the many treatment techniques that have been tried, none stands out as better than any other. There is good evidence that certain types of treatment work better for certain types of people and that success rates could be improved if individuals were *matched* with particular treatments (Finagrette, 1988). At this time, however, much more research needs to be done on which specific characteristics are important to match with which types of treatments, but the outcome aim, abstinence or controlled drinking, seems to be one of the important factors (Annis, 1988).

Without matching, the characteristics of the alcoholic appear generally to be more important for predicting treatment outcome than the characteristics of the treatment (Costello, 1980). Alcoholics most likely to be helped by any treatment are those who have a high socioeconomic status and a stable social situation, are highly motivated to quit, are between ages 40 and 45, and have spouses who help with the treatment (Baekeland, 1977).

There can be no doubt that AA is very effective for many drinkers. In fact, it has been claimed that participation in AA is the most effective treatment, but this is a difficult claim to test, largely because AA does not permit itself to be subjected to the same sorts of close scientific evaluation that other treatment techniques must undergo. In addition, the sorts of persons who try AA and stick with it, those with the characteristics listed in the preceding paragraph, are the best candidates for help no matter what the treatment (Ogbourne & Glaser, 1981). It is quite likely that there is some sort of matching going on with AA. Alcoholics who are most likely to benefit from an association with AA are also the ones who are attracted to it and stick with it. It has been estimated that about 5 percent of all alcoholics are affiliated with AA (Finagrette, 1988, p. 89).

Vaillant has suggested that one reason why AA works is that it provides alternative sources of reinforcement and keeps the alcoholic busily engaged in activities that do not involve alcohol.

AA provides a busy schedule of social and service activities with supportive former drinkers, especially at times of high risk (e.g., holidays). A requirement of AA is that a member "work the program," and . . . AA encourages its members to return again and again to group meetings and to sponsors who provide an external conscience. (Vaillant, 1992, p. 52)

CHAPTER SUMMARY

- *Ethyl alcohol* is created during the *fermentation* of the sugar contained in fruits and grains. Such fermented beverages as wine and beer have a low alcohol content (10 to 15 percent). The concentration of alcohol can be increased by *distillation*. The result is hard liquor, which usually has an alcohol content of 40 to 50 percent.
- Alcohol consumption in the United States has cycled through highs and lows. Currently its use is declining.
- Alcohol levels in the blood can be measured with a Breathalyzer and are usually reported in terms of percentage or milligrams of alcohol in 100 milliliters of blood.

- Alcohol is consumed orally. It is absorbed quickly and distributed evenly in body water. It crosses the blood-brain barrier and the placental barrier easily.

- Most of the alcohol consumed is metabolized by the enzyme *alcohol dehydrogenase* at a constant rate which averages 15 mg per 100 ml of blood per hour.

- One likely mechanism of action of alcohol is that it changes the *fluidity* of the membranes of the nerve cells and alters their ability to generate or conduct nerve impulses. The action of many neurotransmitters, including GABA and serotonin, is altered by alcohol.

- Even at low levels, alcohol disrupts performance and can interfere with complex activities. It generally causes feelings of happiness and reduces the ability of aversive events to control behavior. Higher doses cause loud, vigorous behavior, and even higher doses cause loss of consciousness and finally death. Increasing BAL is associated with an increased risk of being involved in an automobile accident, and the risk is much higher in young, inexperienced drivers.

- The discriminative stimulus effects are similar to the barbiturates and can be blocked by a serotonin receptor blocker.

- Tolerance develops to the effects of alcohol. Alcohol causes physical dependence, and the withdrawal symptoms can be quite severe and even cause death if not treated.

- Frequency of consumption of alcohol in most societies can be described by a *logarithmic normal distribution*, which means that the higher the mean alcohol consumption in a society, the greater the proportion of people who will drink to excess and the more alcohol-related health problems there will be. This is known as the *single-distribution theory,* and it is used to justify government policy aimed at reducing heavy drinking by reducing the average consumption of a population by imposing restrictions on alcohol availability.

- The fact that much of the harm done by alcohol is done by moderate drinkers who occasionally binge has led many governments to adopt a *harm reduction strategy* aimed at education and server training programs rather than restricting availability.

- There are many explanations of excessive drinking or *alcoholism*. The disease model claims that alcoholism is a unitary disorder and that alcoholics are different from nonalcoholics even before they start drinking. In addition, because of "loss of control," alcoholics can never drink in moderation and are unable to control their drinking.

- No disease process has ever been identified that explains alcoholism. Small differences have been found between those with a positive family history of alcoholism (FHP) and those with a negative family history (FHN).

- The behavioral approach maintains that excessive alcohol consumption is a result of normal behavioral processes that have been misdirected and that alcoholics are not different from nonalcoholics.

- Nonhumans in experiments consume alcohol both orally and intravenously, and their patterns of consumption resemble human patterns, especially when the alcohol is administered intravenously.

- Research on laboratory animals shows the demand for alcohol to be elastic in most circumstances, but in some cases it shows inelasticity.

- Alcohol has many harmful effects. Acute effects can cause both industrial and automobile accidents, and continuous use can cause *cirrhosis* of the liver, *Wernicke-Korsakoff syndrome*, and various types of cancer and heart disease. In addition, if taken during pregnancy, it can cause various malformations of the fetus known as *fetal alcohol syndrome*.

Excessive alcohol use, or alcoholism, can be treated, but success rates are low.

- There are numerous treatments for alcoholism including Alcoholics Anonymous, treatment with other drugs, counseling, behavior therapy, and social skills training, but no one appears to be better than any other. The characteristics of the drinker are more likely to contribute to success than characteristics of the treatment unless the alcoholic is matched to a specific treatment program.

7

The Barbiturates and Benzodiazepines

The barbiturates and benzodiazepines are two families of drugs that are sometimes called *tranquilizers* or *sedative-hypnotics*. The term *tranquilizer* or *anxiolytic* is applied to drugs that are used therapeutically to treat agitation and anxiety. The term *sedative-hypnotic* is used to refer to drugs that are used to aid sleep—sleeping pills. Often, as in the case of the benzodiazepines and barbiturates, hypnotic, sedating, and tranquilizing properties are a result of the same neural mechanism, and the medical use of a drug—that is, whether it is prescribed as a tranquilizer or a sedative-hypnotic—is determined by other factors such as the speed of action and the duration of effect.

The barbiturates and benzodiazepines share some properties with alcohol and other substances generally called *depressants* or *general anesthetics*. Alcohol, depressants, and general anesthetics, however, appear to produce their effects by altering the membranes of neurons, while the barbiturates and benzodiazepines work at receptor sites and cause their effects by alter-

ing the functioning of the inhibitory transmitter GABA.

HISTORY

Barbiturates

The barbiturates have been used for a long time. In Germany in 1864, Adolf von Baeyer, a 29-year-old research assistant, successfully synthesized a new substance, malonylurea, by condensing malonic acid and urea (Dundee & McIlroy, 1982). Although the origin of the name is not known for certain, the new substance became known as *barbituric acid*. Barbituric acid is not a behaviorally active drug, but slight modifications of the molecule produce a family of chemicals known as the *barbiturates* that are. The first barbiturate was *barbital*, which was synthesized in 1882 but not marketed until 1903. Later, Emil Fischer (who isolated caffeine) synthesized *phenobarbital*, which was marketed in 1912. Both were therapeutically very useful as sedatives and anticonvulsants and became popular with physicians, who at the time had only chloral hydrate and bromides for this purpose. Over the years thousands of different barbiturates have been synthesized, and about 50 have been marketed. Compounds containing barbiturates have been recommended in the treatment of no less than 77 different disorders ranging from arthritis to bed-wetting (Reinisch & Sanders, 1982). But by the 1990s benzodiazepines replaced barbiturates in almost all their medical uses with a few exceptions. Phenobarbital is still used to prevent seizures. *Butalbital* is also used in combination with drugs such as aspirin, caffeine, acetaminophen, and codeine in analgesic preparations such as Fioronal and Fioricet for headaches, and some very short-acting barbiturates are used as anesthetics.

All the barbiturates have similar effects; they differ only in their speed of action. Some, like *thiopental* and *methohexital*, act very quickly, producing their effect in a matter of seconds. These are used as anesthetics. When these are injected they cause anesthesia almost immediately. Other barbiturates such as *secobarbital* (Seconal) and *amobarbital* (Amytal) act in less than an hour and have been used as sedative-hypnotics. The barbiturates such as *phenobarbital* (Nembutal) that are much slower to take effect and last longer have been used to treat chronic conditions, for example, as tranquilizers for anxiety. Phenobarbital is still used as an anticonvulsant for prevention of epileptic seizures.

In North America it has become a convention to use *al* at the end of the generic name of all barbiturates, although in the United Kingdom the ending *one* is used. Thus barbit*al* and barbit*one* are exactly the same drug.

Barbiturates are sold illicitly on the streets as *downers*. Almost all illicit barbiturates are diverted from medical use, and their names reflect the color of their capsule, for example, *blues* or *blue heavens* for amobarbital, *yellow jackets* for pentobarbital, and *reds, red birds,* or *red devils*

for secobarbital. Other names for barbiturates are *dolls, goofballs,* and *King Kong pills*.

Benzodiazepines

The first synthesis of the benzodiazepines was a combination of good science and good luck. In the 1930s, Leo Sternback synthesized several substances known as *heptoxdiazines* while working on the chemistry of dyes in Krakow, Poland. But it was not until the 1950s, when he was working at the Hoffman–La Roche drug company in the United States, that Sternback and his colleagues did further work with these compounds. Their research was stimulated by an attempt to find a new, safe drug that could be used as a tranquilizer. Their approach was simple; they would pick a class of biologically active chemicals that were simple to make and easy to change and that no one else had studied. They would then make as many derivatives as they could and test them, hoping to discover a useful drug by chance. The heptoxdiazines fitted this description perfectly, so the researchers started to synthesize all sorts of new variations and had them tested for their biological properties.

They found out that none of the derivatives they tested had any biological effect. However, one of these derivatives, called Ro 5–0690, was not tested at that time; it was assumed to be inactive and was set aside. Not until 1957, after it had been taking up needed space on the workbench for two years, was it finally sent for testing. In fact, one story has it that the reason it was sent for testing rather than being thrown out was that it had "such pretty crystals." To everyone's surprise, it was found that the pretty crystals had sedative properties (Sternback, 1973). The researchers finally decided to call Ro 5–0690 *chlordiazepoxide*. After further testing, it was marketed as Librium (Greenblatt & Shader, 1974).

In the years that followed, many more drugs of this type, known as the *benzodiazepines*, were synthesized and tested, and a number were eventually marketed. One of these was *diazepam*

(Valium), which was also developed by Stern-back and marketed in 1963. Although all the benzodiazepines have very similar effects in humans, they differ in their relative potency; some are more potent as sedatives-hypnotics, and some are more potent as tranquilizers. Like the barbiturates, they also differ in their speed of action. Different drugs are marketed for different purposes. Apart from diazepam and chlordiazepoxide, common anxiolytic benzodiazepines are *lorazepam* (Ativan), *chlorazepate* (Trannxene), *alprazolam* (Xanax), and *oxazepam* (Serax). Sedative-hypnotic benzodiazepines are *nitrazepam* (Mogadon), *flurazepam* (Dalmane), *triazolam* (Halcion), and *temazepam* (Restoril). *Clonazepam* (Rivotril) is the only benzodiazepine used as an anticonvulsant.

Recent trends in prescribing show an overall decrease in prescriptions for benzodiazepines since a peak in the mid-1970s (Griffiths & Sannarud, 1987, p. 1536). There has been an increase in the use of short-acting benzodiazepines that do not have active metabolites and a decrease in use of long-acting benzodiazepines such as diazepam that do (Busto, Isaac, & Abraham, 1986).

ROUTE OF ADMINISTRATION AND ABSORPTION

Both barbiturates and benzodiazepines are readily absorbed after oral or parenteral administration. The choice of route depends on the purpose for which the drug is given. If the drug is being used as an anesthetic and a rapid effect is needed, an i.v. injection would be indicated, but if a long-term effect is wanted, as when phenobarbital or diazepam is used to treat anxiety, the oral route is appropriate. Absorption from the digestive system is more rapid than absorption from an intramuscular site, probably because the drugs tend to bind to protein and do so more readily at an injection site than in the digestive system.

All the barbiturates are weak acids with a pKa near 8.0. Consequently, they are almost entirely nonionized at the pHs of the digestive system and are readily absorbed into the blood after oral administration. There is considerable variability in the lipid solubility of barbiturates, and this affects the rate of absorption; highly lipid-soluble drugs are absorbed more quickly than the less lipid-soluble ones.

Benzodiazepines are weak acids that have a pKa of about 5, and they also are readily absorbed from the digestive system. There is a range of lipid solubility in the benzodiazepines and a resulting difference in the speed of absorption of different benzodiazepines. Diazepam is one of the fastest acting benzodiazepines, reaching a peak in about one half to one hour, whereas many others take several hours to peak. There is also a great deal of variability among individuals in the rate of absorption and the peak blood levels obtained by a given dose of a benzodiazepine. A dose of diazepam in one person may cause a blood level 20 times higher than the same dose in another person (Garattini et al., 1973).

Absorption from the digestive system may be greatly increased by the drinking of alcohol. After small amounts of alcohol are drunk, the blood levels of diazepam can be nearly doubled (Laisi et al., 1979).

DISTRIBUTION

Once a barbiturate or benzodiazepine is in the blood, distribution and consequently duration of action are determined by the lipid solubility of the particular drug. The highly lipid-soluble drugs pass through the blood-brain barrier quickly and affect the brain, and their effects are seen quickly. However, the effect can be gone within minutes because their levels in the brain soon fall. This decrease occurs because the drugs become redistributed to areas of the body that contain fat. From these fat deposits the drug is released slowly into the blood and metabolized by the liver. Thus fast-acting drugs also tend to have a short duration of action even though they may still circulate at low levels in the blood for a period of time (Mark, 1971a).

The benzodiazepines and barbiturates also cross the placental barrier easily, and they appear in the milk of nursing mothers.

EXCRETION

With the exception of barbital, which is excreted unchanged, most barbiturates are fully metabolized in several ways before excretion. The barbiturates are metabolized primarily by enzymes in the liver, although some metabolism takes place at other sites in the body. In general, the fast-acting, highly lipid-soluble barbiturates have shorter half-lives.

The enzymes used to deactivate the barbiturates are easily induced, which means that activity can be increased by barbiturate administration. Thus, with repeated administration, the metabolism rate of barbiturates increases. Pretreatment with other drugs also increases the rate of barbiturate metabolism. These other drugs include such dissimilar agents as antipsychotics like chlorpromazine, anesthetics like nitrous oxide, alcohol, antihistamines, and nicotine. (This effect is the reason an anesthetist will ask you whether you smoke or drink before an operation so that the amount of anesthetic can be adjusted.) Similarly, barbiturate administration will stimulate the metabolism of many other drugs by inducing the enzymes that metabolize them. Drugs that are affected in this manner include chlorpromazine, meperidine, morphine, caffeine, general anesthetics like halothane, and local anesthetics like procaine (Parke, 1971). Barbiturate-induced increases in metabolism can also reduce the levels of natural hormones in the body, and as we shall see later, these lowered levels can have adverse consequences in developing organisms.

Because the barbiturates are acids, the efficiency of the kidneys at excreting them can be greatly increased by making the urine basic. Such techniques are used successfully in treating people suffering from overdoses of barbiturates.

The redistribution of the benzodiazepines in body fat creates a two-phase excretion curve. During the first phase there is a rather rapid drop in blood level as the drug is redistributed. This phase has a half-life of 2 to 10 hours. In the second phase the blood level drops more slowly as a result of metabolism. The half-life during this phase varies from 27 to 48 hours (Wilder & Bruni, 1981, p. 109). Once again, there is considerable variability from individual to individual.

The older benzodiazepines like diazepam are usually completely metabolized, and only a small amount of the parent compound is eliminated unchanged. This metabolism can be speeded by enzyme induction brought on by repeated administration. Although the benzodiazepines cause some enzyme induction, they do not do it to the same extent as the barbiturates.

The duration of the effect of the benzodiazepines, however, is not always determined by their half-lives, because the metabolites of some of the older benzodiazepines like diazepam, chlordiazepoxide, and flurazepam are also active and have effects similar to those of the parent compound. These metabolites have even longer half-lives and may have somewhat different effects.

One consideration given to the development of newer benzodiazepines has been the elimination of these active metabolites. The newer benzodiazepines—oxazepam, triazolam, alprazolam, clonazepam, and lorazepam—do not have any active metabolites (Rickels, 1983; American Society of Hospital Pharmacists, 1987, p. 1141).

The metabolism of benzodiazepines can be slowed by the consumption of alcohol. It has been shown that the half-life of chlordiazepoxide is increased by 60 percent after a small drink of alcohol (Desmond et al., 1980).

NEUROPHYSIOLOGY

The neurophysiology of the barbiturates and benzodiazepines is complex and not fully understood, but we do know that many of their effects are mediated by their ability to modify the effects of the inhibitory transmitter GABA (see Chapter 4).

GABA works by interacting with a receptor site that is directly linked with a gated chloride ion channel in a large protein complex known as the *GABA receptor–chloride ionophore complex.* When GABA is released at a synapse, it interacts with the receptor which directly opens the chloride channel. The open channel permits the negatively charged chloride ions to flow into the cell, increasing the resting potential. As a result the membrane becomes more stable; that is, it makes the neuron more difficult to fire. In this way GABA acts as an inhibitory transmitter (see Figure 7–1).

Both the barbiturates and the benzodiazepines increase the ability of GABA to open this ionophore, and thereby they enhance the inhibition caused by GABA in the central nervous system. The barbiturates and benzodiazepines do not modify the effects of GABA by altering the levels of GABA or by interacting with its receptor site. They both enhance the ability of GABA to open the ionophore by interacting with receptor sites of their own on the GABA receptor–ionophore complex (Haefely, 1983).

Barbiturates and benzodiazepines each have their own receptor site, and each enhances the ability of GABA to open the ionophore in a different manner. The benzodiazepines only have the ability to make GABA more effective and do not alter the operation of the ionophore directly. At low doses the barbiturates have the same effect, but at higher doses barbiturates seem to be able to open the ionophore directly by themselves.

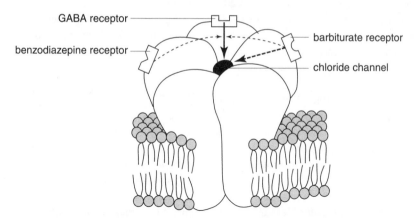

Figure 7–1   A schematic drawing of the GABA receptor–chloride ionophore complex. Three receptor sites are shown: a GABA receptor, a barbiturate receptor, and a benzodiazepine receptor. The solid arrow indicates that the GABA receptor can open the ionophore when it is occupied. The dark, dashed arrow indicates that the barbiturate receptor can also open the ionophore, but only at high doses. The two light, dashed arrows indicate that both the benzodiazepine and the barbiturate receptors can enhance the ability of GABA to open the ionophore. When the ionophore is open, it permits chloride ions (Cl⁻) into the cell and causes inhibition.

GABA is a universal inhibitory transmitter, and its receptors are found all over the central nervous system. Increasing the effectiveness of GABA increases the *inhibitory tone* of the brain; that is, it decreases excitability and depresses activity in many parts of the brain. In lower doses, this depression has the effect of reducing arousal and anxiety and seems to be the basis of the sedating and tranquilizing effect of barbiturates and benzodiazepines. The increased inhibitory tone can also block seizures by making it more difficult for excitatory synapses to make neurons fire repeatedly. Higher levels of inhibition can be caused only by barbiturates because they have the direct ability to open the ionophore. High doses of barbiturates produce unconsciousness and anesthesia (Richards, 1980) and depress breathing by inhibiting the autonomic centers on the brain stem. The respiratory depression caused by barbiturates is similar to the depression caused by alcohol. Barbiturates cause slow, shallow breathing and at high doses may stop breathing altogether. This depression of breathing and a similar depression of the cardiovascular system is a disadvantage of barbiturate anesthesia and is also the main cause of death in cases of barbiturate overdose.

The difference in the potential to cause lethal overdose effects is the major difference between the barbiturates and the benzodiazepines and is the reason why the benzodiazepines have replaced the barbiturates for use as tranquilizers and sedative-hypnotics.

Why would the brain have receptor sites for barbiturates and benzodiazepines? It is more than likely that the body has endogenous substances that use these receptors. The search is under way to find an endogenous benzodiazepine. It is thought that such a substance might be responsible for modulating anxiety. In fact, it has been demonstrated that there is an enhancement in the receptivity of benzodiazepine receptors immediately following periods of stress in laboratory animals. Such an increase in "inhibitory tone" would make the organism less sensitive to the

physiological and possibly cognitive effects of the stress and distress (Hommer, Skolnick, & Paul, 1987, p. 982).

Actually, there might be two endogenous substances, one that decreases anxiety and one that increases anxiety. It has been shown that the benzodiazepine receptor works both ways. There are some benzodiazepine-like drugs called *inverse agonists* that have the opposite of the usual benzodiazepine effect; they decrease GABA's ability to open the ionophore, and they increase feelings of tension, anxiety, and panic (Squires & Braestrup, 1977; Stephenson, 1987; Carvalho et al., 1983). Likewise, there are barbiturates that induce seizures (Ticku & Olsen, 1978).

Even though many of the effects of the benzodiazepines and barbiturates can be understood in terms of their effects on GABA, their neurophysiology is complex, and other transmitters and neuromodulators may be involved. For example, the benzodiazepines also enhance the effects of adenosine, another inhibitory transmitter, by blocking its reuptake and permitting its accumulation (Phillis & O'Regan, 1988).

EFFECTS OF BENZODIAZEPINES

Effects on the Body

Apart from a depression in respiration and a slight drop in blood pressure, there are few physiological effects of low doses of barbiturates in most individuals. Unlike the barbiturates, the benzodiazepines do not produce significant depression or respiration in healthy individuals, even at high doses. They also have little effect on heart rate or blood pressure. The benzodiazepines are also reported to increase appetite, and weight gain is sometimes a consequence of continuous use (Greenblatt & Shader, 1974, p. 5).

The benzodiazepines have very few effects outside the CNS. They have muscle-relaxant properties that are clinically useful and appear to be a result of the effect of the drug on the brain rather than on the muscles themselves. They also suppress some polysynaptic reflexes, but this suppression does not appear to affect behavior at usual clinical doses (Greenblatt & Shader, 1974, p. 106). These properties have made benzodiazepines useful in treating increased muscle tone caused by multiple sclerosis, Parkinson's disease, and brain injury. The benzodiazepines are also reported to be useful in the treatment of backache and muscle strain.

The benzodiazepines have anticonvulsant properties and may be more useful in treating petit mal seizures and infantile spasms than other anticonvulsants such as the barbiturates, but for long-term control of epilepsy, the benzodiazepines are not likely to replace the barbiturate and barbiturate-like drugs now commonly in use.

Effects on Sleep

One of the most popular uses of the short- and intermediate-acting barbiturates has been as sleeping pills. There can be no doubt that these drugs decrease the time required to fall asleep and increase sleeping time, but careful studies of brain activity during sleep have revealed that the sleep induced by barbiturates is not the same as normal sleep. The barbiturates reduce the amount of time spent in REM sleep. As with other drugs that have this effect, the reduction shows tolerance after about a week, and the amount of REM sleep returns to normal, about 20 percent. When the drug is discontinued, however, there is a *REM rebound*, a period of several days when REM increases to as high as 40 percent of sleep time and may remain elevated above normal for several weeks. In addition, there are other disruptions in sleep, including increases in the time taken to fall asleep and more frequent wakening during the night (Freemon, 1975).

The benzodiazepines are also effective in treating insomnia; flurazepam is used in the United States, and in Europe nitrazepam is used for this purpose. The benzodiazepines decrease latency to fall asleep, decrease wakings during the night, and increase total sleeping. These effects do not appear to develop tolerance, so doses need not be increased with continued use. Unfortunately, like the barbiturates, the benzodiazepines decrease the percentage of time spent in REM as well as stage 3 and stage 4 sleep. As with the barbiturates, this effect diminishes with continued use, and when the drug is discontinued after as little as two weeks, there is a withdrawal rebound (Griffiths & Sannerud, 1987, p. 1539). With nitrazepam, this rebound reaches a peak about 10 days after the drug is stopped and may last for several weeks. With the increase in REM comes an increase in bizarre dreaming and restlessness and wakings during the night (Ozwald et al., 1973) and the desire to resume taking the drug to get a good night's sleep.

This rebound appears to be a withdrawal symptom that can be eliminated simply by returning to the use of the sleeping pill. As a result, it is difficult for people to stop using sedative-hypnotics for sleep once they have started. After periods as short as a week, they find that they cannot get a good night's sleep without their pill, and every time they try to stop, the same thing happens. They do not realize that they must go through a period, sometimes as long as a month, of poor sleep before they can sleep well without their pill.

EFFECTS ON THE BEHAVIOR AND PERFORMANCE OF HUMANS

Effects on Mood

Both the barbiturates and the benzodiazepines have similar effects on mood. Many (although not all) studies have shown that subjects report euphoria and liking along with sedation and fatigue (de Wit & Griffiths, 1991). In one experiment, diazepam and a placebo were given to volunteers who were asked to fill out the Profile of Mood States at that time and one, three, and six hours later. The scale provides a profile of mood on four dimensions: vigor, fatigue, confusion, and arousal. Compared with a placebo, doses of 5 mg and 10 mg of diazepam caused a decrease in feelings of arousal and vigor and an increase in fatigue and confusion. These effects were seen only at one hour with the low dose but were generally seen for up to three hours with the high dose. These feelings were considered unpleasant by the subjects, few of whom voluntarily took the drug again when they were given the chance (Johanson & Uhlenhuth, 1980).

Feelings of confusion and fatigue may also be seen when the barbiturates are given therapeutically. These effects are more common at higher doses and in older patients.

The benzodiazepines appear to be effective *anxiolytics* (they decrease anxiety), and this is one of their chief medical uses, but it has been demonstrated that these effects do not occur in individuals with normal levels of anxiety. The anxiolytic effects are seen only in people with high levels of anxiety to begin with (Barrett & DiMascio, 1966).

Effects on Performance

The barbiturates have no effect on the acuity of hearing, but there is a decrease in critical flicker fusion (CFF) threshold, which indicates a decrease in visual acuity (Landis & Zubin, 1951). Barbiturates also cause an overestimation of the passage of time; a period of time will seem longer than it really is (Goldstone, Boardman, & Lhamon, 1958).

Like alcohol, pentobarbital causes a decrease in standing steadiness and an increase in body sway detectable even at low doses. Also impaired are the ability of the eye to track a moving pendulum and the ability to perform a task that requires divided attention. These abilities are more impaired while the blood level of the barbiturate is rising than when it is falling (Ellenwood et al., 1981). In another experiment, 100 mg of secobarbital impaired the athletic performance of competitive swimmers. Under the influence of

the drug, however, they believed that their performance had improved (G. M. Smith & Beecher, 1960).

At the phenobarbital doses used to treat epilepsy, about 100 mg per day, it has been demonstrated that a slight impairment of short-term recall develops after a week of continuous use. Long-term memory is not affected (MacLeod, Dekaban, & Hunt, 1978).

The benzodiazepines are like the barbiturates in that they decrease the CFF threshold, indicating a decrease in visual acuity. Some studies have also reported that auditory flicker fusion threshold is also diminished by the benzodiazepines (Vogel, 1979).

While simple reaction time appears to be slowed slightly by the benzodiazepines, finger-tapping speed is not affected, and there does not appear to be any effect on the choice reaction time task. Tasks that are affected by the benzodiazepines are tracing a figure in a mirror, sorting cards into piles, and canceling or marking designated letters on a page of print. In most of these studies, the adverse effects were found only at the higher therapeutic doses, suggesting, perhaps, that the benzodiazepines at lower doses might not have any adverse performance effects. Several other tasks do not appear to be affected at all. These include short-term memory as measured by the digit span test and tasks that involve counting and discriminating stimuli (Vogel, 1979).

The benzodiazepines have a clear effect on the ability to acquire new information. Acquisition of both verbal and visual information has been shown to be reduced by as much as 66 percent. The benzodiazepines, however, do not appear to alter the ability to recall information acquired prior to their administration (Taylor & Tinklenberg, 1987).

These effects may start as soon as one hour after oral administration for diazepam or three hours for lorazepam. The duration of the impairment will vary, depending on the dose, but can last 24 hours. The time course of the impairment does not reflect the concentration in the blood, and shorter-acting benzodiazepines may actually cause a longer-lasting effect than long-acting benzodiazepines. The degree of impairment is also not always evident to the individual, who will frequently report that he or she feels fine (Taylor & Tinklenberg, 1987; Roache & Griffiths, 1987).

Most of these studies looked at single rather than chronic doses. It is clear that most impairments show considerable rapid tolerance when the drug is repeated.

In some cases it was noted that the benzodiazepines actually improved performance in some people. Improvements were usually seen in individuals who were highly anxious or in difficult and stressful situations where anxiety might be expected to interfere with performance (Janke & DeBus, 1968).

Hangover Effects

Barbiturates and benzodiazepines are widely used at bedtime to induce sleep, but they have such a long half-life that they are still in the body for some time the next day. Because sleeping pill users may drive to work, operate equipment, and engage in other activities that might be impaired by the drug, it is important to determine whether these residual levels of the drug can affect performance the next day. Research has shown that barbiturate-induced performance deficits can be detected the next morning in simple reaction time and in tasks such as tapping rate, but choice reaction time is not impaired. There is even an improvement in performance on a pursuit rotor task. Impairments in body steadiness are still evident after as long as 18 hours (Bixler et al., 1975). Most of these hangover effects are not severe, but they also are not generally detected by individuals, who are unaware of their reduced functioning.

Like the barbiturates, the benzodiazepines also have hangover effects. Studies show that EEG changes can be detected 12 hours after administration of flurazepam, and disruptions of performance and mood changes are still evident at 12

hours. The effect of benzodiazepine seems to last longer than the effect of barbiturates (Bond & Lader, 1973). The benzodiazepine hangover also greatly enhances the effect of a single drink of alcohol (Saario & Linnoila, 1976).

Effects on Driving

Barbiturates can severely impair driving ability. A 200-mg dose of secobarbital, even when spread out over a day, causes an impairment on a simulated driving task equivalent to that caused by a BAL of 150 mg per 100 ml (Loomis & West, 1958), almost twice the legal blood alcohol limit in many jurisdictions.

Some studies have failed to find impairment in driving and simulated driving tasks caused by a single low dose of benzodiazepines. However, one study (Betts, Clayton, & MacKay, 1972) showed that if a 50-mg dose of chlordiazepoxide was divided and given over 36 hours, it would cause significant driving impairment. Extensive research by a group at the University of Helsinki in Finland has also shown that a 10-mg dose of diazepam will increase collisions in a simulated driving task. This impairment is also greatly increased by alcohol (Linnoila & Hakkinen, 1974). In general, there is good evidence that there is a considerable risk of an automobile accident in first-time users of benzodiazepines. The risk is probably amplified by the fact that the individual is often not able to detect the impairment (Taylor & Tinklenberg, 1987).

EFFECTS ON THE BEHAVIOR OF NONHUMANS

Unconditioned Behavior

One might expect that a "depressant" like a barbiturate would decrease activity, but a number of studies of both unconditioned and conditioned behavior have shown that this assumption does not seem to be true. In a study by Hannah Steinberg and her colleagues (Steinberg, Rushton, &

Tinton, 1961) at University College in London, amobarbital was given to rats who were then placed in a Y-maze. This maze had three similar arms, and the number of entries into the arms was counted as a measure of activity. In this experiment there were two conditions: One group of rats was exposed to the apparatus 32 times before testing, and the other group was not exposed to the maze at all. The researchers found that the barbiturate increased the activity of the unexposed rats but decreased the behavior of the rats that had been exposed to the maze. The authors concluded that the barbiturate decreased the anxiety of the rats placed in the apparatus for the first time, and the lessened anxiety increased their exploratory behavior. This experiment serves as an elegant demonstration of how the effect of a drug can depend on the history of the organism.

The effect of a dose of benzodiazepine on spontaneous motor activity appears to be first an increase and then a decrease, although some studies have not reported an increase and others have found, as with the barbiturates, that the increase depends on whether the animal is in a novel environment (Greenblatt & Shader, 1974, p. 45). The benzodiazepines also seem to stimulate eating, but again, this effect is not always evident (p. 44).

One of the first effects noticed in the early screening tests of the benzodiazepines was a "taming" effect. The research animals became more placid, and fighting behavior induced by electric shocks was reduced. It has since been demonstrated that chlordiazepoxide and diazepam are effective in reducing only defensive aggression—aggression that is induced by an attack or provoked by a painful stimulus like a shock. Unprovoked aggression or attack behavior does not seem to be altered at lower than toxic doses (DiMascio, 1973). It has been suggested that this change in provoked aggression is a result of the ability of the benzodiazepines to diminish anxiety, since defensive aggression is presumably a result of anxiety or fear caused by being attacked. Attack itself is not motivated by anxiety (Hoffmeister & Wuttke, 1969).

Positively Reinforced Behavior

In a classical experiment, Peter Dews (1955) of Harvard Medical School demonstrated that increasing doses of pentobarbital would increase and then decrease response rates of a pigeon responding for food. What was fascinating about this experiment was that at low doses, the drug increased the pigeon's key pecking when the response was reinforced on an FR schedule but decreased the frequency of responding when an FI schedule was in effect. Like the Steinberg experiment just described, this experiment generated considerable interest because it showed that a "depressant" could either increase or decrease behavior in the same animal; in this instance, the result depended on the schedule of reinforcement in effect. These behavior changes were produced by drug doses so low that they had no other apparent effect on the animal.

Both the Dews and Steinberg experiments demonstrated clearly that it is not proper to characterize the effects of the barbiturates as "depressant" and that drugs in this class are just as likely to stimulate as to depress behavior.

It is not surprising that there is a great similarity between these effects of the benzodiazepines and the effect of the barbiturates. The benzodiazepines increase responding on FI and VI schedules at low doses and decrease response rates at high doses in most species. Although increases in FR rates are reported by some researchers, FR rates are generally decreased by low doses in rats and monkeys (Sanger & Blackman, 1981). Responding on DRL schedules is usually increased, with a consequent reduction in reinforcements.

Aversively Motivated Behavior

Because the barbiturates are used in humans to treat anxiety, it would be reasonable to expect that they would have a specific effect on anxiety-motivated behavior in nonhumans. The traditional way of evaluating this effect is by using an avoidance task. Not surprisingly, barbiturates such as phenobarbital and hexobarbital are selectively able to decrease responding motivated by fear of electric shock without interfering with escape from the shock. This effect is not as powerful with the barbiturates as it is with the benzodiazepines, antipsychotics, or even morphine (Heise & Boff, 1962).

The barbiturates have a spectacular effect on behavior suppressed by punishment: They cause a drastic increase in punished behavior at doses that have little effect on positively motivated behavior (Hanson, Witloslawski, & Campbell, 1967). Animals injected with barbiturates continue to make responses that are punished by electric shock at normal, unpunished rates. The reason for their unchanged behavior does not appear to be that they no longer feel the shock; they jump and flinch when it happens, but they nevertheless continue to make the punished response. It also appears that the barbiturates increase responding that is suppressed by noncontingent electric shocks in the CER paradigm (Kelleher & Morse, 1964).

The effect of the benzodiazepines on shock-motivated behavior is similar to that of the barbiturates but more pronounced. Heise and Boff (1962) have shown that doses of benzodiazepine that decrease avoidance responses are one-fourth to one-sixth the size of doses that have any effect on escape responding. The barbiturates can also depress avoidance without interfering with escape, but they are much less selective. With the barbiturates, avoidance responding is affected at doses only about half the size of those that impair escape behavior.

As with the barbiturates, the most spectacular effect of the benzodiazepines on the behavior of nonhumans is on punishment-suppressed responding. Behavior that has been reduced to a low rate by response-contingent electric shock is generally increased by the benzodiazepines.

DISSOCIATION

The very first experiment showing that drugs were discriminable stimuli was done with pentobarbital at McGill University by Donald Overton (1964), a graduate student at the time. Overton also showed that dissociation could be caused by pentobarbital. In his experiment, he trained rats to turn to one side in a T-maze to escape electric shock after an injection of pentobarbital. Later, when the drug had worn off, these rats showed no evidence of being able to remember the task. This inability to remember worked the other way around as well: Rats that learned the task while sober were unable to remember it when tested after an injection of pentobarbital. The two states had become *dissociated;* what the rats learned in one state they could not transfer to the other (see Chapter 3).

DISCRIMINATIVE STIMULUS PROPERTIES

Animals trained to discriminate pentobarbital from saline generalize the pentobarbital response to other members of the depressant class of drugs, including other barbiturates, alcohol, meprobamate, chloral hydrate, and paraldehyde, but not to amphetamine or LSD.

If proper adjustments are made for dose levels, animals cannot be trained to discriminate one barbiturate from another. They can, however, be trained to discriminate alcohol from a barbiturate (Overton, 1977), indicating that although the subjective effects of alcohol and barbiturates are similar, differences can be detected.

The discriminative stimulus properties of the benzodiazepines were investigated in a comprehensive series of experiments by Frances Colpaert of the Janssen Pharmaceutical Laboratories in Beerse, Belgium. He found that the chlordiazepoxide response would generalize to all other benzodiazepines and to barbiturates but not to the antipsychotics chlorpromazine or haloperidol. No tolerance developed to the discriminative stimulus properties of the benzodiazepines even though tolerance did develop to the toxic effects.

Colpaert also found that stimulant drugs like amphetamine, caffeine, cocaine, and the hallucinogen mescaline would not antagonize the chlordiazepoxide cue, but high doses of both nicotine and the convulsant bemegride were able to block the cue (Colpaert, 1977). In this regard the benzodiazepines are different from the barbiturates because bemegride will block the barbiturate cue, but nicotine will not.

Although Colpaert found that the benzodiazepine cue would generalize to the barbiturates, it has been shown that rats can be trained to discriminate chlordiazepoxide from barbiturates and alcohol but not from diazepam. This finding shows that there are qualitative differences between the subject effects of all these drugs, even though they are similar enough to generalize to each other (Barry, McGuire, & Krimmer, 1982).

TOLERANCE

Acute Tolerance

Tolerance can develop to the effects of a barbiturate during a single administration. Studies have shown that the drug has a more powerful effect at a given concentration as the blood level is rising than at the same blood level on the descending limb of the curve (Ellenwood et al., 1981).

Chronic Tolerance

A considerable amount of tolerance can develop to the barbiturates. In a nontolerant individual, a dose of 150 mg can cause loss of coordination and some intellectual impairment, but in one report a highly tolerant individual was capable of taking 2,200 mg of secobarbital a day and could still talk coherently and walk without staggering (Fraser, 1957).

Tolerance develops at different rates to the different effects of barbiturates and disappears at different rates as well. For example, the antiepileptic effects show no tolerance, even after years of use. But other effects disappear rapidly. In one experiment, 400 mg (a rather large dose)

was given to volunteers for 90 days. Reaction time and hand-eye coordination were severely impaired for the first three days but were nearly normal within a week. Total sleeping time increased by more than 1½ hours a day at first but was normal by day 70 (Fraser, 1957).

In a series of experiments (Cannizzaro et al., 1972) it was shown that tolerance develops first to the depressant effects of flurazepam. When the depressant effects wear off, the antianxiety or disinhibitory effect on suppressed behavior becomes more and more prominent. This differential rate of tolerance development may be responsible for the increased hostility in some humans who continue use; at first there is drowsiness and a general slowing of all reactions. As this wears off, it permits the expression of behaviors that had been suppressed by fear or anxiety. In some people these take the form of aggression (see "Harmful Effects"; "Aggression and Violence").

In time even the antianxiety effects show tolerance. Tolerance develops in rats to the disruptive effects of chlordiazepoxide on avoidance when the drug is administered every day for six weeks (Masuki & Iwamoto, 1966). Tolerance also develops slowly to the anticonvulsant effects of the benzodiazepines as well as to the drowsiness that is seen sometimes at therapeutic doses. A number of long-term studies have failed to show the development of tolerance to the sleep-producing properties of the benzodiazepines (National Academy of Sciences, 1979, p. 179), although the REM suppression effects do exhibit tolerance.

Cross-Tolerance

The barbiturates are completely cross-tolerant with each other and show considerable cross-tolerance with all other drugs in the depressant category including alcohol and the general anesthetics. There is some cross-tolerance between the barbiturates and all drugs with metabolizing enzymes that can be induced by the barbiturates.

There is also cross-tolerance between the benzodiazepines and other depressant drugs. The drowsiness sometimes produced by higher therapeutic doses of the benzodiazepines is less often seen in people who have a recent history of barbiturate and alcohol abuse (Greenblatt & Shader, 1974, p. 232).

WITHDRAWAL

Barbiturates

Barbiturate withdrawal was first described in the medical literature in 1905, two years after the introduction of the first barbiturate into medical practice. In spite of this early report, the medical literature on barbiturate withdrawal was contradictory until the 1930s, when the weight of evidence could no longer be denied. Part of the problem was that the nature of the withdrawal varies with different individuals and patterns of barbiturate administration. If doses are kept low, the only withdrawal symptom may be something as subtle as REM rebound and may be reflected in mild sleep disturbances, but at higher doses, withdrawal can be medically serious. Withdrawal may begin from 12 to 24 hours after the final dose of the drug, although it can be as long as 48 to 72 hours for the longer-acting barbiturates. The symptoms are similar to alcohol withdrawal and can include tremors, anxiety, insomnia, nausea, delirium, and seizures. The seizures may occur anywhere from the second to the eighth day. They are seizures of the grand mal type, and in severe cases, if left untreated, these may cause death.

The delirium is usually evident after two to four days and may last as long as 10 days. There are usually vivid auditory and visual hallucinations, disorientation, agitation, confusion, and fear. As with alcohol, it has been suggested that these hallucinations are a manifestation of the rebound of suppressed REM dreaming that intrudes into waking thought (Aston, 1972, p. 41). Improvement in all these symptoms is gradual; they are usually gone within two weeks, but a weakness may last as long as 12 weeks.

As with tolerance, individuals vary tremendously in their responses to sudden withdrawal from barbiturates. Severe withdrawal symptoms of this nature do not occur after doses of less than 400 mg per day. At 400 mg per day only minor symptoms are experienced. At 600 mg the symptoms are more intense and convulsions may occur, and at 800 mg convulsions and delirium may result (Fraser, 1957; Aston, 1972). For most medical uses, the usual daily dose of barbiturates is 100 mg. Severe withdrawal, therefore, seldom results from therapeutic doses, but more subtle withdrawal effects such as REM rebound are likely to be encountered at these doses.

Benzodiazepines

The benzodiazepines have been used widely in medical practice since the early 1960s, but like the barbiturates it took years before their ability to cause physical dependence at therapeutic doses become widely acknowledged. It has been known for some time that withdrawal from relatively high doses of benzodiazepines taken for a long time will cause symptoms similar to those of barbiturates and alcohol. These symptoms include agitation, depression, abdominal pain, delirium tremens, insomnia, and seizures (Greenblatt & Shader, 1974; L. B. Hollister, Motzenbecker, & Degan, 1961). Such dependence was believed to be rare, and most physicians were confident that there was no chance of physical dependence in their patients who received low therapeutic doses. An early study estimated that physical dependence occurred in only 1 percent of patients receiving diazepam for various emotional disorders (Bows, 1965). In fact, physical dependence was considered so unlikely that some researchers concluded, "It is time to dispel the myth that the unsuspecting housewife must be protected from the careless prescribing of dangerous drugs likely to produce lifelong addiction" (Rickels, Downing, & Winokur, 1978, p. 403). Box 7–1 gives an account of an "unsuspecting housewife" whose ex-

BOX 7–1   Benzodiazepine Dependence: A Case Study

Here is an account from a British medical journal of one woman's experience with Valium. This account is not typical of all Valium users, but it is representative of the sort of experience reported by those who develop a physical dependence on the drug and are able to overcome it (Ashton, 1984, pp. 1135–1136).

I am 39 years old, married, with two children aged 18 and 14 years. The younger was a very active baby, and when he was 18 months old I mentioned to the doctor that he was sleeping very little and though he did not seem tired in any way, I certainly was! After a course of vitamins I still felt worn out and this was when I was first prescribed Valium.

This was 1971; I was then 27 years old. I remember instantly feeling a lot better—all the irritability and tiredness seemed to disappear and I became a lot more relaxed and content. The next three years seemed to fly over; the eldest child began school, my husband gained promotion, and we bought a new house. Any problems which cropped up during this time could always be wiped out just by taking a Valium. Life was pretty good! Moving house also meant changing doctors and this doctor was not very keen on repeating the monthly prescription on which I had come to depend. "You must cut them down," she said; "three years is far too long." I agreed wholeheartedly. "Why not," I thought, "I don't need them now." . . . The youngest was at school and slept soundly—in fact had done for a long time. I started reducing the tablets and can honestly say I felt no ill effects.

During this time my life hit an emotional crisis but this time, unlike in the past, I did not have the pills to cover it up. In January 1975 I suffered a miscarriage and after this, together with the conflict in my personal life, I visited the doctor in tears. She immediately put me back on Valium, this time increasing the dosage. Although the world was not as rosy as it was before, at least it was bearable, I did not realise then that this was the beginning of a new road to despair, mental and physical pain, and nearly complete disaster.

My problem did not go away like in the early days on the pills—they seemed greater. I started to become withdrawn, insecure, and confused and suffered bouts of depression together with uncontrollable outbursts of rage. One day I could cope no longer and the doctor recommended a top psychiatrist. This seemed the most logical solution at the time, so I agreed. It was diagnosed as endogenous depression and acute anxiety. During the following months I was prescribed many different forms of antidepressants, hypnotics, and tranquillizers to take with the Valium. None of these had any lasting good effects; in fact I gradually became

perience with benzodiazepines is typical of many others.

In a study by Cosmo Hallstrom and Malcolm Lader (1981), four patients were gradually weaned from a high (average of 135 mg) daily dose of diazepam, and six patients were weaned from a low daily dose (average of 20 mg per day). After the drug was withdrawn, patients in both groups showed symptoms that included anxiety, sleep disturbances, intolerance to bright lights and loud noises, weight loss, unsteady gait, and numbness or tingling feelings. There were also

worse instead of better. I saw a young doctor who told me it was not the pills I needed but psychotherapy. The pills were only covering up the mental turmoil.

The next year involved extensive analysis and although at times this was mentally distressing, it seemed to help. During the weekly sessions it was suggested I drop my dose of Valium so I quickly agreed; at first it was easy—a bit jumpy when I dropped 1 mg—but then things became much worse. My confidence began to wane dramatically—I could not go out or be left on my own. My husband finally had to give up his job, as I spent most of the time begging him to come home as I was frightened. I started to feel very ill, and even going to the shops was a mammoth task. My doctor advised me not to drop the Valium any more (I was down from 15 mg to 4 mg) as I was suffering from chronic anxiety and needed some form of sedation. What both of us did not realized was—I was in tranquillizer withdrawal.

In July this year I begged the doctor to help me—I could not go on any more like this—it was like a "living death." He suggested another form of tranquillizer and took the remaining Valium away—I thought I had gone mad. In sheer desperation I remembered a newspaper article about a group of people who suffered from tranquillizer side effects and withdrawal. I made a phone call, which was the most important call of my life; I was on the verge of madness and could they help?

That was nine weeks ago and during that time I have not touched a tablet. This brought on a series of symptoms that I had experienced only mildly before. Noises jarred every fibre in my body and my eyes seemed to shun the light of day. I shook from head to foot and enormous panic attacks would sweep through my body, leaving me exhausted and totally afraid. Complete fatigue took over the feeling of tiredness and sleep no longer came with the night. Many times I thought it would be best to die.

I am lucky to have found somewhere where sufferers can be encouraged and supported through withdrawal. I have found many new friends, who, like me, were caught up in the web of addiction. Also I have the good fortune to have a very caring and warm doctor to help me through this withdrawal. It has not been easy—it has been one of the hardest jobs of my life and it is not finished yet. In the early days I began to think I had gone mad, but gradually a new world is emerging. A world that is not covered over with pills. It can be a very frightening place until my mind becomes adjusted to its colours, noises, and pictures once more. (pp. 1135–1136)

changes in EEG activity and an increase in the electrical activity of the cortex that follows a loud noise (auditory evoked potential). These changes were similar in both the high- and the low-benzodiazepine subjects. Most of the symptoms peaked in intensity after five days and were gone within two weeks. Other researchers have found similar withdrawal effects at therapeutic doses (Petursson & Lader, 1981; Crawford, 1981). Clearly, therapeutic doses were causing problems.

David E. Smith of the Haight-Ashbury Free Medical Clinic and Donald R. Wesson (1983) have suggested on the basis of extensive clinical experience that there are actually two types of withdrawal from benzodiazepines, each with a different set of symptoms (Griffiths & Sannerud, 1987). Each type has a different time course, and the occurrence of both types of withdrawal may overlap. The first type of withdrawal symptoms, which they call the *sedative-hypnotic type,* involves tremors, delirium, cramps, and possibly convulsions. These are similar to the symptoms of barbiturate withdrawal (described earlier) and alcohol withdrawal (described in Chapter 6), and they are the symptoms described in studies where high doses of benzodiazepines were given. Sedative-hypnotic withdrawal can be expected in people who have taken the drug in higher than recommended therapeutic doses for at least a month. Generally, the withdrawal symptoms start within a few days of abstinence and are gone within about 10 days. These withdrawal symptoms are more likely to be seen with benzodiazepines that have short half-lives because blood levels of these drugs fall more rapidly than the longer-acting drugs.

The second type of withdrawal is called *low-dose withdrawal.* Its symptoms are seen in some individuals after low therapeutic doses that have been taken for longer than six months. They emerge more slowly and include anxiety, panic, irregular heartbeat, increased blood pressure, impairment of memory and concentration, feelings of unreality, muscle spasm, and a sensitivity to lights and sounds. Patients consistently report feeling as though walking on cotton wool, in a mist, or wearing a veil over their eyes. There are also frequent reports of perceptual distortions such as walls or floors sloping and distortion of reality and self-perception: "Everything feels unreal or distant"; "I feel I'm not really me"; "My head feels like a huge balloon" (Ashton, 1984, p. 1138).

Very often these feelings come in cycles or waves with varying frequency with each symptom (Ashton, 1984). Smith and Wesson suggest that many symptoms cycle every 10 days.

There are no consistent data on the duration of these symptoms. They have been reported to last as little as two weeks (Owen & Tyrer, 1983) or as long as a year (Smith & Wesson, 1983; Ashton, 1984). It is also not clear how many users of benzodiazepines at therapeutic doses have with-

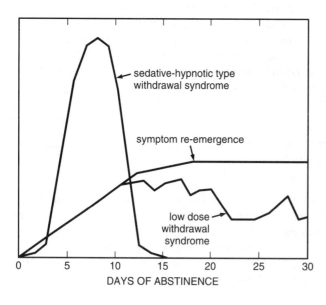

sedative-hypnotic type
withdrawal syndrome

symptom re-emergence

low dose
withdrawal
syndrome

DAYS OF ABSTINENCE

Figure 7–2 These curves represent two types of withdrawal symptoms that may be seen after use of the benzodiazepines. The sedative-hypnotic type of withdrawal has severe symptoms but lasts only a few days. The low-dose benzodiazepine withdrawal symptoms are less intense but last much longer and seem to come and go in cycles. Also shown is the reemergence of symptoms that were there before the benzodiazepine was started and may reappear causing more distress. (Adapted from D. E. Smith & Wesson, 1983, p. 89.)

drawal symptoms, although estimates range from 15 to 44 percent (Higgitt, Lader, & Fonagy, 1985). It is also not clear whether there are certain people who are more susceptible than others.

As with most withdrawal symptoms, both the sedative-hypnotic type and the low-dose type of symptoms disappear quickly when the withdrawn drug is resumed. The low-dose withdrawal symptoms are especially sensitive to resumption of treatment and can be controlled with only a few milligrams of benzodiazepine.

Individuals who have taken high doses of benzodiazepines for longer than six months may well experience both types of withdrawal. Figure 7–2 shows these two types of withdrawal. This figure also shows that other changes may occur when the benzodiazepines are stopped. These are due to *symptom reemergence,* the expression of symptoms that were present before the drug was started and were suppressed while the drug was being used. Such reemerged symptoms are not really withdrawal symptoms, but their presence contributes to and complicates benzodiazepine withdrawal.

SELF-ADMINISTRATION IN HUMANS

Laboratory Studies

Choice Experiments. In a study using normal human subjects that has been replicated several times, Johanson and Uhlenhuth (1980) gave people a choice between capsules of different colors. In an earlier part of the experiment, subjects had been given each of the capsules twice, so they knew what effect each colored capsule would have, even though they did not know what each capsule contained. In this experiment the subjects chose capsules containing amphetamine much more often than a placebo, but did not choose diazepam more often than a placebo (Griffiths, Bigelow, & Henningfield, 1980). It has been shown using a similar procedure that

lorazepam is not chosen more often than a placebo either. In fact, at higher doses, subjects chose a placebo more frequently than lorazepam or diazepam (de Wit, Johanson, & Uhlenhuth, 1984, Johanson & Uhlenhuth, 1980).

In a similar study subjects were selected for high anxiety levels and given the choice between diazepam and a placebo. While the highly anxious subjects reported that the capsules containing the diazepam reduced their anxiety, they did not choose the diazepam capsule more frequently than a placebo. This finding suggests that relief from anxiety is not a motivation for benzodiazepine self-administration and that highly anxious people are not particularly at risk for benzodiazepine abuse (de Wit & Johanson, 1987).

Choice of benzodiazepines over a placebo has been demonstrated in two experiments, however. In one, it was shown that people with a history of sedative-hypnotic and alcohol abuse would chose benzodiazepines (de Wit & Griffiths, 1991). In another, people would choose benzodiazepines when the choice was reliably followed by a task that involved relaxation (Silverman, Kirby, & Griffiths, 1994).

Also, choice experiments have not found evidence for the reinforcing effects of barbiturates in normal populations. Pentobarbital is not chosen more often than the placebo even though the subjects report that the drug is having classical sedative effects (de Wit, Perri, & Johanson, 1989; de Wit & Griffiths, 1991).

Self-Administration. In a study conducted by Roland Griffiths and his colleagues (Griffiths, Bigelow, & Lieberson, 1979) at the Johns Hopkins University School of Medicine, pentobarbital was made available to male volunteers in an experimental hospital ward setting. The subjects, all of whom had a history of sedative drug abuse, could earn an administration of a drug by riding an exercise bicycle for 15 minutes. They found that 5 of the 7 subjects continued to self-administer doses of 90 mg pentobarbital over the 10 days of the experiment at a high level, indicating that the drug acted as a positive reinforcer in humans. The same experiment also showed that subjects would not self-administer a placebo. Diazepam was self-administered by some subjects, but not as frequently or as reliably as the barbiturate.

Outside the Laboratory

Outside the laboratory, humans show two patterns of barbiturate or benzodiazepine self-administration apart from use for legitimate medical conditions. In the legal or *iatrogenic* (physician-caused) pattern, the drug is prescribed for its effects as an aid to sleep or anxiety problems and is then continued unnecessarily or the dose escalated. In the street use pattern, the drugs are obtained illegally and are taken either orally or by injection at high doses. Of these two patterns, the first is more common.

Iatrogenic Use. Barbiturates and now benzodiazepines are widely prescribed for a variety of symptoms, and in many cases the prescribing and use are entirely consistent with appropriate treatment of medical conditions; however, the use of these drugs often changes in nature and may cause problems for the patient in a couple of different ways. As we have seen, if they are prescribed at too high a dose or for too long, they can cause physical dependence and require special treatment to avoid withdrawal when the drug is discontinued. In addition, patient use may also become motivated by the reinforcing effects of the drug and may start exhibiting an inappropriate amount of behavior toward obtaining the drug in increasing amounts. Such patients may learn exactly how to tailor a medical history so that a physician will predictably prescribe the drug they want and go "doctor shopping" to find a compliant physician. Such patients may refuse to stop taking a drug and not consider alternative therapies even though the drug is causing adverse side effects or the doctor recommends stopping. Other signs include a tendency to escalate doses, requests for early refills of the prescription because the prescription was "lost," and so on.

Even though many people take benzodiazepines each day, the extent to which they are "abused" is difficult to determine. In a survey conducted in the United States in 1979, Balter and his colleagues concluded that about 12 percent of the adult population had used a benzodiazepine during the previous year and about 15 percent of those, or 1.6 percent of all adults in the United States, used benzodiazepines every day for at least one year before the time of the interview (Uhlenhuth et al., 1988). According to the popular stereotype, the typical Valium user is a well-educated, middle-class, suburban housewife denied personal or professional fulfillment by husband and family. In fact, this does not appear to be the case. The Balter survey found that typical long-term users of anxiolytic benzodiazepines tended to be over 50, female, and suffering from substantial anxiety and some significant chronic health problem such as heart disease or arthritis. This type of survey has shown that, in general, most of the people who are receiving long-term benzodiazepines are receiving them for legitimate medical reasons, usually anxiety. Mellinger, Balter, and Uhlenhuth (1984) showed that at least half of long-term users suffered from high levels of psychic distress (anxiety).

Surveys have shown that large numbers of people who report severe symptoms of anxiety do not report the use of benzodiazepines. On the basis of this information, some have concluded that benzodiazepines are underused rather than overused, since there appear to be many people who could benefit from benzodiazepine use but are not receiving benzodiazepine treatment (Uhlenhuth et al., 1988).

The extent of abuse or misuse of the benzodiazepines is not well understood. In one study of 176 people referred for assessment of benzodiazepine abuse to an outpatient clinic, 56 percent used benzodiazepines at clinically appropriate doses, but did so longer than recommended by their physician. Others who took doses larger than prescribed did so in combination with other substances such as alcohol, opiates, and cannabis

(Juergens, 1993). In another study of 136 people who were found to be benzodiazepine abusers in a clinic, very few, less than 0.5 percent, abused benzodiazepines alone. Most were well-educated Caucasian females more than 30 years old, and they received their benzodiazepines legally from a physician. Diazepam was the preferred benzodiazepine, particularly by primary cocaine and opiate users (Malcolm et al., 1993). The use of alprazolam and diazepam is a particular problem for many on methadone maintenance (Sellers et al., 1993).

Street Use. The illegal or street use of barbiturates follows a somewhat different pattern from the iatrogenic habit. To begin with, barbiturates are used in higher doses and are taken in binges rather than continuously. They are also frequently combined with other drugs. Among young people and casual drug users, barbiturates are used as an alcohol substitute or in combination with alcohol to enhance its effects. This type of use is episodic and usually restricted to weekends or when the drug is available.

Among more serious drug users, the barbiturates are frequently injected and combined with heroin or amphetamines. When the contents of a secobarbital or amobarbital capsule are dissolved and injected intravenously, the user can experience a rush similar to that caused by heroin. This rush does not occur after oral administration. This fact is probably one reason why heroin users frequently inject barbiturates, especially if their heroin supply is low. It is also common to find the barbiturates taken in conjunction with cocaine or amphetamine. The barbiturates are used to reduce or "smooth" some of the unpleasant side effects of the stimulant.

When used for recreational purposes, the benzodiazepines are most often used in conjunction with some other drug. This is often alcohol, but surprisingly, it has been reported that 60 to 70 percent of patients on methadone maintenance use benzodiazepines. They often report that the benzodiazepines boost the effects of the metha-done. Laboratory data also support the claim that diazepam will enhance the subjective and physiological effects of opiates (Griffiths & Sannerud, 1987, p. 1537), although one study showed that diazepam did not alter the blood levels of methadone, and vice versa (Preston et al., 1986).

National surveys in the United States show that the illicit use of barbiturates steadily declined from 1975 to 1988 and has remained steady at a low rate of 1.9 percent of young adults reporting use. A similar pattern has been reported for the benzodiazepines (Johnston, O'Malley, & Bachman, 1994), although this pattern may be changing. *Flunitrazepam* is a very short-acting benzodiazepine sold in Europe, Mexico, and South America under the name of Rohypnol, but it is not marketed in the United States. It is smuggled from Mexico to the Southern states and by 1995 it was used quite extensively by young people—especially in conjunction with alcohol. It is known as "Mexican Valium," "roaches," or "roofies."

SELF-ADMINISTRATION IN NONHUMANS

Barbiturates

Like humans, rats and monkeys will readily work to give themselves infusions of all types of barbiturates, although it appears that the short-acting barbiturates may maintain higher rates of responding than the longer-acting barbiturates (Winger, Stitzer, & Woods, 1975). Responding maintained by barbiturates on FI and FR schedules is similar to typical response patterns maintained by other reinforcers and takes place at doses that do not appear to cause physical dependence (Kelleher, 1976), indicating that barbiturate infusions act as positive reinforcers in nonhumans.

In one study (Griffiths et al., 1981), baboons were trained to self-administer intravenous infusions of cocaine. When responding was stable, different barbiturates were substituted for cocaine. It was found that amobarbital, pentobarbital, and secobarbital all maintain responding at the same rate as cocaine. Following each injection, the researchers noted that the barbiturate infusion caused surgical anesthesia lasting from several minutes to an hour. In the same experiment, the monkeys were also free to respond for food pellets. They found that overall responding for food was not affected by the concurrent self-administration of barbiturates.

When barbiturates are freely available to monkeys on a continuous basis, consumption increases every day until it stabilizes after five or six weeks. After this initial period, the amount administered every day remains fairly constant, and there are no periods of self-imposed abstinence as with ethanol or the stimulants (Griffiths, Bigelow, & Henningfield, 1980). This finding is somewhat surprising because in most other respects the barbiturates resemble alcohol. In fact, the pattern of barbiturate self-administration in nonhumans is more similar to the pattern for opiates than for alcohol.

Benzodiazepines

Early self-administration research with benzodiazepines had difficulty demonstrating that benzodiazepines were reinforcing, but later research has shown that laboratory animals will self-administer this class of drugs both intravenously and orally (B. S. Stewart et al., 1994). The problem may have been that early research used benzodiazepines with rather slow onset and long duration of action. In general, drugs with these properties are difficult to establish as reinforcers. Currently there are many demonstrations of self-administration of both short- and long-acting benzodiazepines (Griffiths et al., 1991), although short-acting benzodiazepines like triazolam maintain higher rates of responding than long-acting benzodiazepines (Griffiths et al., 1981). Where comparisons have been made, the positive reinforcing effect of benzodiazepine is not as robust as that of barbiturates (Griffiths et al., 1991).

The reinforcing effects of the benzodiazepines, even long-acting ones, can be enhanced by a period of exposure to the drug or other barbiturates or benzodiazepines. In one study, Harris, Glaghorn, and Schooler (1968) gave rats a choice between drinking a solution of chlordiazepoxide and drinking pure water. The rats always chose water. Then for 25 days the rats had to drink the chlordiazepoxide in order to obtain food. After this period of forced consumption, the rats showed a preference for the chlordiazepoxide when given the choice between it and water. Other research has shown that the effect of prior exposure does not depend on the development of physical dependence (Ator & Griffiths, 1992).

Taken together with the human choice and self-administration laboratory studies that show reinforcing effects in people with a history of sedative-hypnotic abuse, it appears that, at least for the longer-acting benzodiazepines administered orally, a period of forced consumption greatly enhances the reinforcing effect of the drug. In this respect benzodiazepines are very different from the barbiturates, which are very powerful reinforcers right from the start in humans and nonhumans.

HARMFUL EFFECTS

Reproduction

The barbiturates readily cross the placental barrier and circulate in the body of the fetus, and it is now well established that these drugs can cause birth defects. In one survey it was shown that 6 percent of babies born to epileptic mothers being treated with an anticonvulsant during pregnancy showed malformations. The rate was only 2.7 percent in nonepileptic women and 4.2 percent in untreated epileptic women. Barbiturates are only one class of drugs used to treat epilepsy, but it seems to make no difference which drug is used. The most common of these abnormalities are cleft lip and palate and abnormalities of the heart, skeleton, and CNS (Wilder & Bruni, 1981, p. 168). There is also an increase in malformations of the male genitals.

Numerous studies on nonhumans have shown that barbiturates administered during pregnancy have severe effects on fetus brain weight and the neurological development of certain parts of the brain. In addition, such prenatal exposure also specifically interferes with development in the brains of males and seems to diminish male sexual behavior later in life. On the basis of these studies, it has been predicted that "prenatal exposure to these potent substances [barbiturates] in human subjects may lead to learning disabilities, decreased IQ, performance deficits, increased incidence of psychosocial maladjustment, and demasculinization of gender identity and sex role behavior in males" (Reinisch & Sanders, 1982, p. 381). The demasculinization arises from a direct effect of the drug on the brain, but it is also an indirect effect of the fact that the barbiturates stimulate enzymes that metabolize steroid hormones. As a result, the steroid hormone testosterone, which must be present to stimulate sexual differentiation in males, is metabolized and may not be present in sufficient quantities.

When the mother is physically dependent on barbiturates, the newborn must go through barbiturate withdrawal after birth. Because the baby's liver metabolizes the barbiturate slowly, the withdrawal symptoms may not appear until the infant has left the hospital. The median time of onset is seven days. The neonatal withdrawal symptoms are similar to withdrawal in adults. Some of the symptoms are sleep disturbances, a high-pitched cry, tremors, diarrhea, vomiting, delirium, and even seizures (Wesson & Smith, 1977, p. 100).

Initially it was thought that the benzodiazepines interfered with the menstrual cycle and fertility in women, but such concerns have not been substantiated. In males, chlordiazepoxide has been reported to cause a failure to ejaculate, but this does not appear to be a common problem (Greenblatt & Shader, 1974, p. 231). In fact, there have been reports that the benzodiazepines improve reproductive success in previously infertile couples.

Although the research is not conclusive, evidence has been accumulating that benzodiazepines can cause birth defects in humans. One study conducted in Atlanta, Georgia, found that mothers of babies born with a cleft lip were four times more likely to have taken diazepam during the first three months of pregnancy than mothers of children with other deformities (Safra & Oakley, 1975). This report caused considerable concern, but it was followed by a number of studies that failed to find any effect (Jick, 1988). In the late 1980s, however, researchers in Sweden reported a fetal benzodiazepine syndrome similar to the fetal alcohol syndrome (see Chapter 6) in babies whose mothers had used either diazepam or oxazepam during pregnancy. They reported that the baby's face is malformed and expressionless and that there is poor muscle tone, delayed hand-eye coordination, tremors, delayed mental development, and learning disabilities (Laegried et al., 1987).

Unfortunately, the studies showing teratogenic effects in humans have problems with their methodology and cannot be considered conclusive. This is an area that will need considerably more research (Jick, 1988).

In one study with rats, it was shown that pups born to mothers injected with diazepam during the third week of gestation showed an absence of locomotion responses and acoustic startle responses seen in normal rats (Kellogg et al., 1980). In fact, it appears that exposure to benzodiazepines in the uterus has effects on the reaction of animals to various stressors, and these effects may be different at different developmental stages throughout the life span, even extending into old age (Kellogg, 1988).

Withdrawal symptoms have been reported in infants when the mothers used normal therapeutic doses of diazepam during pregnancy. The withdrawal symptoms are tremors, irritability, and hyperactivity, which are similar to withdrawal from opiates. They start 2½ to 6 hours after delivery and can be treated with barbiturates (Rementiria & Bhatt, 1977). Even benzodiazepines given during labor have been reported to affect the newborn infant by depressing respiration, creating a reluctance to feed, and decreasing the ability to maintain normal body temperature. Apgar scorers (ratings of cardiac and respiratory functioning at birth) are also depressed. The drug has been detected in the blood of the baby for as long as eight days after delivery (Cree, Meyer, & Hailey, 1973).

As with most drugs, it is probably unwise to take benzodiazepines at any time during pregnancy or even if pregnancy is possible. This could be a serious problem, since women tend to be prescribed benzodiazepines much more frequently than men.

Aggression and Violence

Although the benzodiazepines appear to reduce tension and to have a taming effect on laboratory animals, a number of clinicians and researchers have noted that these drugs can cause an increase in human hostility and aggression. This has been called by a number of names including rage reaction, paroxysmal excitement, and behavioral or aggressive dyscontrol. The increase in hostile behavior takes time to develop. One researcher describes the phenomenon this way:

Many of the patients receiving [diazepam] displayed a progressive development of dislikes or hates. The patients themselves deliberately used the term "hate." This hatefulness at first involved nonsignificant figures in the patient's environment, progressed from there to the involvement of key figure such as aides, nurses, and physicians and went on to the involvement of important figures such as parents and spouses. The phenomenon was progressive and in some instances, culminated in overt acts of violence. (Feldman, 1962)

This benzodiazepine-induced hostility has been studied more systematically. In one experiment using volunteers, chlordiazepoxide and placebos were given for a week, and hostility was rated by the individuals themselves and by observers who did not know which subjects were getting the placebo and which were getting the drug. It was found that the drug group showed more hostile feelings and behavior than the placebo subjects (Saltzman et al., 1969). Other studies, however, have not shown any increases in aggression, and some have shown a decrease in aggression (Dietch & Jennings, 1988).

In rare instances this increase in hostility develops into violence or even what has been described as rage (Dietch & Jennings, 1988). Box 7–2 gives an example of a case of benzodiazepine-induced violence.

Overdose

The major danger from barbiturates is overdose, either accidental or deliberate. The lethal dose of barbiturates does not show the same degree of tolerance as the dose required for intoxication. Since the barbiturates have a low TI anyway, there is always the danger of accidental overdose. (The estimated lethal dose in humans is 4,000 to 6,000 mg; Moeschlin, 1971.) This danger is intensified by the similarity in effect of the barbiturates and any other depressant drug, especially alcohol. When barbiturates are taken with another of these drugs, the effects are additive, and the danger of overdose is greatly increased. For example, a BAL of 100 mg per 100 ml in combination with a secobarbital level of 0.5 mg per 100 ml of blood can be fatal. By themselves, blood alcohol levels are lethal over 400 mg per 100 ml, and lethal secobarbital levels range from 1.1 to 6 mg per 100 ml (Gupta & Koefed, 1966).

One of the major reasons why barbiturates have experienced such a drastic decline in use is their potential for being used to commit suicide. At one time more than 15,000 deaths per year in

BOX 7–2   Benzodiazepine-Induced Aggression: A Case Study

Here is a case study of benzodiazepine-induced aggression as reported by Greenblatt and Shader in The Benzodiazepines in Clinical Practice *(1974).*

A 39-year-old tree worker was placed on diazepam (20 mg) by his family physician following an accident at work in which he injured his back. Three days after starting on this regimen, he began to be argumentative at home. He thought that this was related to being at home, so he returned to work on the fifth day on diazepam. At work he was also argumentative and got into a physical fight with a co-worker. Since this behavior seemed extreme for him (he hadn't had a fight since high school), his wife insisted that he seek psychiatric consulation. In the evaluation it became clear that this patient had a considerable amount of unexpressed resentment which he had previously contained by passive-aggressive behavior. Diazepam was discontinued immediately and the argumentativeness subsided within two days. He was referred for counseling to a good mental health clinic where he was supported and encouraged to examine and ventilate some of his long-standing resentments. (pp. 83–84)

the United States resulted from barbiturate overdose, and without doubt, the majority of these were suicides.

In cases of barbiturate poisoning, the higher toxic doses cause a loss of consciousness, a depression in heart rate and blood pressure, and a reduction in motility of the intestines, and blisters may appear on the skin. There is a decrease in urine flow as a result of both lowered blood pressure and increased levels of antidiuretic hormone. There may also be a loss in the ability of the body to regulate temperature, and hypothermia may result in cases of exposure. In addition to all this, of course, there is severe respiratory depression (Beveridge, 1971).

There is little doubt that benzodiazepine overdoses are not as dangerous as barbiturate overdoses. About 12 percent of drug overdose emergencies involve the benzodiazepines, but the outcomes of benzodiazepine overdoses are seldom fatal, and there seem to be no lasting effects. Doses as high as 2,250 mg of chlordiazepoxide have been tolerated with symptoms of sleep and drowsiness. There is no deep coma or severe respiratory depression, and the victims can usually be awakened (Greenblatt & Shader, 1974, p. 251). Most symptoms disappear within 48 hours.

Although the benzodiazepines are safe by themselves, they intensify the effect of other depressants such as alcohol and the barbiturates. The benzodiazepines can be—and frequently are—fatal when combined with alcohol (Torry, 1976).

TREATMENT

Anyone wishing to discontinue using the benzodiazepines after a long period of use should not attempt it alone because the withdrawal can be severe and involve convulsions, which require medical treatment. Withdrawal should be done under medical supervision with the aid of a physician who appreciates the problem. Although withdrawal can usually be accomplished on an outpatient basis, hospitalization may be necessary in some cases, especially for patients with a history of seizures, psychotic episodes, or high doses of the drug (Higgitt, Lader, & Fonagy, 1985).

The approach to detoxification from a benzodiazepine is similar to detoxification from other sedative drugs and alcohol. If only the low-dose benzodiazepine withdrawal symptoms are anticipated, the best way to proceed is gradually to reduce the daily dose of the benzodiazepine. This is most successfully done in conjunction with counseling and careful monitoring of the patient's withdrawal symptoms. It is important that the patient be told exactly what symptoms to expect and how long they will last. It is sometimes helpful to seek social support from self-help groups and members of the family. The patient should also be taught various strategies for coping, not only with the withdrawal but also with the reemergence of the symptoms for which the benzodiazepine was prescribed in the first place (Colvin, 1983). The most intense withdrawal and the greatest anxiety and panic are experienced while the last few milligrams of the drug are being withdrawn (D. E. Smith & Wesson, 1983). Treatment of iatrogenic physical dependence is usually successful, with 88 to 100 percent of patients stopping their benzodiazepine intake (Higgitt, Lader, & Fonagy, 1985).

Once withdrawal has been managed, various therapies may be attempted, but it is important to match the patient with an appropriate therapeutic strategy. Such therapies could involve group therapies with people with similar problems, education, family involvement, 12-step programs similar to Alcoholics Anonymous where participants are encouraged to "work" a program of recovery, and the support of peer groups (such as that described in Box 7–1) and a physician who understands the process.

The illegal user seldom abuses barbiturates and benzodiazepines except as an adjunct to some other addiction such as alcohol, heroin, or amphetamine, and treatments usually focus on the primary addiction. The first step in treatment is the elimination of physical dependence if it exists. This can be dangerous and should not be attempted without medical supervision. As pointed out earlier, withdrawal from the barbiturates can have very serious medical complications and can be fatal if attempted abruptly. One method is to substitute phenobarbital for the barbiturate (or other depressant, including alcohol) being used. Phenobarbital has the advantage of being a long-acting drug, and blood levels can be controlled more easily over a longer period. Once a stabilizing dose of phenobarbital is established, it can be reduced by a small amount every day to prevent dangerous withdrawal symptoms (Wesson & Smith, 1977, p. 97). Of course, counseling and other support are also necessary for the treatment of the low-dose benzodiazepine withdrawal, which will continue for some time after the sedative-hypnotic type withdrawal is over.

After detoxification, there is no established form of treatment for the barbiturate user. In some cases antidepressants are beneficial, and there has been some success with nonpharmacological treatments such as transcendental meditation and biofeedback (Wesson & Smith, 1977, p. 104).

CHAPTER SUMMARY

- The barbiturates are a large class of drugs that have been used medically since the turn of the twentieth century. Most barbiturates have similar effects but differ from each other primarily in their speed of action.

- The benzodiazepines are a class of drugs that were developed in the 1950s and became popular during the 1960s and 1970s for the control of anxiety and insomnia. Benzodiazepines replaced the barbiturates because they are much safer.

- Barbiturates and benzodiazepines are absorbed readily after oral administration and may also be injected, depending on the medical reason the drug is being used. Their speed of absorption depends on their *lipid solubility*. Highly lipid-soluble barbiturates and benzodiazepines are redistributed into body fat.

- Barbiturates and benzodiazepines enhance the action of *GABA*, an inhibitory transmitter found widely throughout the brain. They both act at their own receptors located near the GABA receptor on the *GABA receptor–ionophore complex*. This action potentiates the ability of GABA to stabilize the cell membrane. At higher doses, barbiturates, but not benzodiazepines, are able to open the ion channel directly.

- The effects of the barbiturates on human performance are similar to those of alcohol. Some of these effects are still evident the day following the use of barbiturates as sleeping pills, although the individual may not be aware of them. High doses cause death from respiratory depression, which results from a depression of the respiratory centers in the medulla.

- In low doses the benzodiazepines cause decreases in arousal and vigor and increases in *fatigue* and *confusion*. They also decrease feelings of anxiety, their chief medical use. Reaction time is slowed, and the drug impairs other skills, including driving. Some of these effects can be seen as long as 12 hours after a single dose of the drug is taken.

- There have been ample demonstration that the barbiturates and benzodiazepines increase behaviors suppressed by punishment. This effect in nonhumans predicts the *antianxiety* effect of these drugs in humans.

- Tolerance develops to many of the effects of the barbiturates and benzodiazepines.

- Withdrawal from large doses of barbiturates can cause serious, life-threatening symptoms.

- There are two separate withdrawal symptoms to the benzodiazepines: The *sedative-hypnotic* type, similar to withdrawal from alcohol and the barbiturates, and *low-dose benzodiazepine* withdrawal, which emerges slowly after therapeutic doses have been stopped. The symptoms of anxiety, panic, irregular heartbeat, and memory impairments come and go in cycles of about 10 days and may last for six months to a year.

- The barbiturates and benzodiazepines have reinforcing properties in both humans and nonhumans and are readily self-administered. In humans there are two patterns of use: *iatrogenic* or physician-caused use and illegal *street use*. The illegal pattern is characterized by episodic binges. Barbiturates are frequently used in conjunction with other drugs such as heroin, cocaine, or alcohol.

- Because of their lethal effects, the barbiturates have caused many accidental poisonings and have been a favorite drug used for *suicide*. For this reason the barbiturates are being replaced by the safer benzodiazepines in medical practice.

- A serious side effect of the barbiturates is that they can cause many *birth defects* if taken during pregnancy. Some of these include malformations of facial features, CNS, heart, and skeleton.

8

Tobacco

TOBACCO AND NICOTINE

Tobacco is the only known natural source of nicotine, and it is now clear that nicotine is the active ingredient in tobacco. The tobacco plant belongs to the genus *Nicotiana*, of which there are two subgenera, *rustica* and *tabacum*, used for their nicotine content. Both subgenera contain many species and varieties that differ quite widely in physical characteristics. By far the principal source of tobacco today is *Nicotiana tabacum*, which is cultivated in temperate climates all over the world. Species of *rustica* are grown only in Russia and India. It is interesting to note that cultivated strains of tobacco have a much higher nicotine content that any wild members of the same genus. These facts suggest that the presence of nicotine in tobacco is much more than mere coincidence. The actual nicotine content of the cured tobacco leaf may reach as much as 6.17 percent.

Although some scholars have claimed that to-bacco originated in Africa or Asia, it is now certain that its origins are exclusively American and that the aboriginal peoples of North and South America were the first and only users of the drug at the time of the European discovery of the New World. The earliest known illustration of smoking is reproduced in Figure 8–1. It is a stone carving from a Mayan temple showing a priest smoking what appears to be a cigar or a reed cigarette.

The plants of *N. tabacum* are usually about 2 meters tall and have long, broad, pointed leaves that are harvested two or three at a time from the bottom of the plant as they mature, although for some types of curing the entire plant is cut at one time.

In 1809 a French chemist, Louis Nicolas Vauquelin, claimed to have discovered the active ingredient in tobacco, but his extracts were not pure. He called it *nicotianine*. It was not until 1828 that pure nicotine was isolated by L. Posselt and F. A. Reimann.

cessed and flavored. Tobacco snuff is made by drying the leaves, grinding them to a very fine powder, and mixing it with various aromatic and flavoring agents. While the vast bulk of tobacco is consumed as cigarettes or cigars and in pipes, there has been a resurgence in oral consumption of tobacco, or what is now commonly called smokeless tobacco. This is either the traditional form of chewing tobacco or something called moist snuff, which is not chewed, but tucked between the cheek and the gum. Frequent spitting is not required. Smokeless tobacco has the advantage that it can be used in places where smoking is banned, and can be used when both hands are busy, for example, when playing baseball.

HISTORY

One aspect of the life of the native peoples of North America commented on by every early European explorer from Columbus on was the use of tobacco. At San Salvador, the site of Columbus's first landfall in 1492, the local inhabitants presented him with some "dry leaves," which Columbus concluded "must be a thing much appreciated among them." Later, members of his expedition went ashore in search of the Great Khan. They found no Khan, but they did observe the natives smoking cigars, something that they did not appreciate or understand. They reported that the natives were "perfuming themselves" and that they "drink smoke." One of these men, Rodrego de Jerez, was later to become all too familiar with the significance of the activity; he took up smoking and was imprisoned by the court of the Inquisition for this "devilish habit."

Jean Nicot, the French ambassador to Portugal, became convinced of the medical usefulness of the plant and sent seeds to the royal family in France. Because of his great interest in this plant, Nicot's name was given to the genus *Nicotiana* and subsequently to the alkaloid *nicotine*.

Tobacco use spread as a wonder cure, but it did not take long to catch on as a recreation, al-

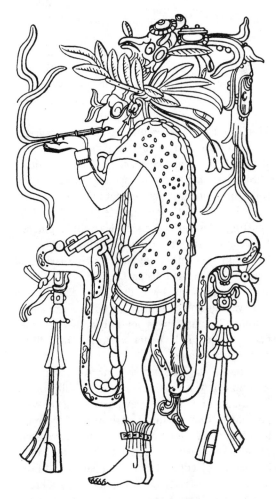

Figure 8–1 Carving found in a Mayan temple of a priest smoking a cigar or reed pipe. Native American priests and shamans took tobacco in large quantities in order to foretell the future and cure illness. (From Dunhill, 1954, p. 4.)

PREPARATIONS

The leaves of the tobacco plant are cured and prepared in different ways depending on the use to which the tobacco is to be put. Tobacco for burning is made into cigars, cigarettes, or pipe tobacco. Tobacco for chewing is specially pro-

though many users were quick to point out that they were really using it to prevent such diseases as the plague. When Samuel Pepys, the British diarist, encountered houses where victims of the Great Plague had perished, he felt "an ill conception of myself and my smell, so that I was forced to buy some roll-tobacco to smell and to chew, which took away the apprehension" (Brooks, 1952, p. 40). This association of tobacco with healing lasted into the Victorian era.

The English were among the last Europeans to take up tobacco. In the late sixteenth century, British sailors and sea captains, among them Hawkins, Drake, and Raleigh, carried the habit home from the West Indies. Raleigh's name has long been associated with tobacco, not only because he is credited with the introduction of smoking to the English court but also because he founded the colony at Virginia that was later to owe its survival and prosperity to tobacco cultivation.

Though the British were late to take to the drug, they made up for their tardiness in the popularity tobacco acquired. By the end of the sixteenth century, the demand for the leaf was beginning to cause concern in some quarters. In 1604, King James I published an antitobacco essay titled "A Counterblaste to Tobacco" in which he refuted all the arguments claiming medical benefits from smoking. As a matter of fact, James I anticipated most of the modern antismoking campaigns even to claiming that smoking affects "the inward parts of man, soiling and infecting them with a vicious and oily kind of Soote, as hath been found in some great tobacco takers, that hath after their death opened" (Arber, 1895, p. 111).

The tobacco that the English were smoking all this time and that so angered the king was imported from Spain at great expense, but the English colony at Virginia was to change all that. The colonists under John Rolfe had gotten off to a very bad start, suffering shipwreck and starvation, and were on the point of quitting when Rolfe decided to try growing some Spanish tobacco seeds (*Nicotiana tabacum*) in the soil of Virginia. The experiment was a great success. The plants prospered, and in 1616 a shipload of Virginia tobacco was sent to Britain. At first the English were skeptical, but the quality of Virginia tobacco was obvious, and within a decade it had replaced the Spanish imports. In spite of the king's taxes and other attempts to discourage the tobacco trade, the colony flourished and secured the English colonial presence in North America.

Smoking has been the primary means of administering tobacco throughout most of its European history, but for a time it was eclipsed by snuffing. Powdered tobacco was either pinched between the fingers or placed on the back of the hand and then sniffed into the nostrils. The result was usually a vigorous sneeze. The early use of snuff was associated with the clergy (Pope Urban VII was an ardent snuffer), who preferred it to smoking because it was not outlawed in churches and its use could be better concealed from disapproving parishioners.

Tobacco chewing was a North American contribution. It was first observed as a habit of the American Indian, but chewing was never very popular in Europe. In the early part of the nineteenth century, however, there was a strong nationalist sentiment in the new United States and a deliberate rejection of European habits and fashions; snuff was rejected and chewing tobacco was adopted with patriotic fervor. Chewing was democratic, while snuff was aristocratic; snuff and the pipe had "filtered down from the leaders of fashion to the common folk, while chewing was a practice which . . . seeped from the common man upward into the higher ranks of society" (Robert, 1967, p. 103). The popularity of chewing prompted one Englishman, Charles MacKay, to suggest that the national emblem of the United States be a spittoon rather than an eagle.

Like tobacco chewing, cigarette smoking had its beginnings in America. Early Spanish explorers report that Mexican Indians smoked tobacco through "reeds." These were hollow canes filled with tobacco and lighted so that they "burned themselves out without causing a flame." For centuries cigarette smoking was confined to the Spanish and Portuguese empires and even there accounted for only a small part of tobacco use. Quite suddenly, in the 1840s, it became very popular in France, especially among French ladies, and it was chiefly the enthusiasm women showed for this means of smoking that stimulated its general acceptance. It was also about this time that flue-cured, or "bright," tobacco was discovered in North Carolina. This low-nicotine, sweet, mild smoke was perfectly suited to the cigarette. Some people considered cigarettes a novelty, a fad that would soon pass, but they were wrong.

Tobacco smoking persisted unabated until the 1960s, when tobacco was dealt a severe but not fatal blow. This blow was the U.S. Surgeon General's Report of 1964, which for the first time definitely linked smoking to cancer and other diseases. This was followed in 1971 by a similar report of the Royal College of Physicians of London. The truth could no longer be hidden or ignored: Tobacco smoking was unhealthy. These statements combined with the environmentalist and naturalist movements were actually able to stop the growth of smoking and start a popular decline.

The 1993 National Household Survey in the United States showed the rate of current smokers to be 24 percent, down from 31 percent in 1985. This decline is evident in all age categories, but it now appears that smoking rates in the youngest category, 12–17-year-olds, are stabilizing at about 10 percent. Males generally smoke more than females, but the decline in smoking rates has been highest in males, so that there is now very little difference between the genders, especially in the younger age categories (see Figure 8–2).

While use of tobacco in the industrialized nations is declining, tobacco consumption has been rising in the developing countries of the world. Per capita consumption increased by 32 percent in developing countries in Africa and by 224 per-

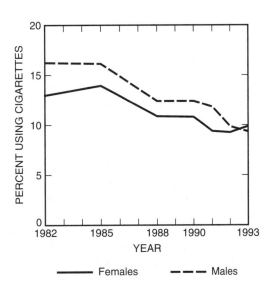

Figure 8–2   Cigarette use in one month reported by 12–17-year-olds in the 1993 U.S. National Household Survey. Smoking rates of males have declined faster than those of females, and by the early 1990s there was no significant difference between the sexes.

cent in South America between 1973 and 1983. It appears that tobacco manufacturers, discouraged by the shrinking of their traditional market, have turned their attention to populations not so well educated about the health risks of smoking (Fielding, 1985b).

A new chapter in the history of tobacco is unfolding. Even though tobacco contains an active ingredient, nicotine, for various political and economic reasons tobacco has never been treated as a drug or medicine, and it is not regulated by governments in Western industrialized countries. In fact, tobacco is not even classed as a "consumer product" for purposes of regulation by the U.S. Consumer Product Safety Commission.

In the United Kingdom tobacco is not governed by the Medicines Act, and until recently, in the United States nicotine tobacco products were not regulated by the Food and Drug Administration (FDA). The FDA is entitled to regulate drugs in the United States, and a drug is defined as a substance intended by its makers to affect the structure or functions of the body or intended for use in the diagnosis, cure, mitigation, treatment, or prevention of disease. The tobacco industry had escaped FDA control by claiming that they sold their products for smoking pleasure only and not for the effect of nicotine.

In February 1994, after years of planning, the commissioner of the FDA formally requested that the FDA regulate cigarettes as drugs. This request led to a series of hearings before a subcommittee of the U.S. House of Representatives. In the course of the hearings the commissioner outlined the arguments that nicotine was addicting and presented evidence that cigarette manufacturers knowingly manipulated nicotine delivery of tobacco products (Kozlowski & Henningfield, 1995; Schwartz, 1994) and that, in fact, cigarettes were "nicotine delivery systems." The FDA won its case, and it will now regulate nicotine in tobacco products, but the implications of such regulation are not clear. The FDA is entitled to place an outright ban on all tobacco products, but it has decided to try to control tobacco use by pursuing a policy that will discourage young smokers from taking up the habit by regulating lifestyle images in advertising, and controlling availability of tobacco to teenagers.

ROUTE OF ADMINISTRATION

Unlike cocaine from the coca leaf or morphine from opium, nicotine from tobacco was virtually never self-administered in its pure form. The main reason is probably that nicotine is a highly toxic poison and doses must be controlled precisely; too high a dose will have quite unpleasant effects. Because of its dilute concentration in tobacco, precise control over dose can more easily be achieved when the nicotine is in its natural form.

When tobacco is chewed, the nicotine is absorbed through the membranes of the mouth.

Usually, the tobacco juice is spit out and not swallowed, so this process does not represent the usual form of oral administration. Nicotine is only rarely swallowed. Nicotine is a weak base with a pKa of about 8 so it will not have many lipid-soluble molecules when dissolved in solutions with a pH lower than 6. Consequently, nicotine is not quickly absorbed from the acidic digestive system. Oral administration of nicotine has another disadvantage because the blood from the capillaries of the digestive tract must pass through the liver before it achieves general circulation throughout the body. The metabolism of nicotine is rather fast in the liver, so much of the nicotine taken orally is metabolized during this *first pass* before it can get to the body. Although nicotine is not normally self-administered orally, there are a large number of poisonings each year involving children who eat tobacco. Fortunately, in this type of situation, the nicotine that gets into the blood induces vomiting, and the swallowed tobacco is frequently expelled before the nicotine reaches toxic levels.

Tobacco taken in the form of snuff is sniffed into the nostrils. With this route of administration, most of the nicotine is absorbed through the mucous membranes of the nasal cavity, although some tobacco eventually gets into the stomach and lungs.

When tobacco is burned, nicotine vaporizes and can be found in the smoke and particles of ash that dissolve in the mucous membranes of the inside surface of the lungs. About 90 percent of inhaled nicotine is absorbed into the blood in this way (Pierce, 1941). Studies have shown that the major determinant of nicotine absorption is the volume of smoke inhaled and that increasing the duration of the inhalation does not significantly increase nicotine absorption (Zacny et al., 1987).

Nicotine from tobacco smoke may be absorbed through membranes of the mouth in a similar fashion, but this route is more readily influenced by changes in the pH of saliva. In general, cigarettes are made from flue-cured tobacco, which has an acidic smoke, and this lowers the pH of saliva to about 5.3. In acidic saliva, nicotine is ionized, and absorption is reduced. To be absorbed, the nicotine from cigarette smoke must therefore be inhaled into the lungs, which are so efficient that pH has no effect on absorption. By contrast, pipe and cigar tobacco is usually air-cured, and this process results in a more basic or alkaline smoke. Its pH of about 8.5 is well into the range where ionization of nicotine is less than 50 percent, and absorption is facilitated. Consequently, nicotine in the smoke from cigars and pipes can be absorbed from the mouth, and inhalation is not necessary (Armitage, 1973; R. Jones, 1987).

Nicotine absorbed from the lungs is carried directly to the heart, and from there much of the blood containing the nicotine goes straight to the brain. Because of this direct route, the nicotine does not get a chance to dissipate, so the high concentration in the lungs after a puff or rapid inhalation of smoke tends to remain in the blood as a *nicotine bolus* until it reaches the brain (M. A. H. Russell, 1976). Because nicotine is absorbed much more slowly from the capillaries of the mouth and nose, no such bolus occurs if the smoke is not inhaled. The role of the nicotine bolus in nicotine self-administration and dependence will be discussed later in this chapter.

The average cigarette contains 8 to 9 mg of nicotine, of which a typical smoker absorbs 1 mg in the course of taking 10 puffs per cigarette (R. Jones, 1987, p. 1592). The amount of nicotine actually delivered to the smoker is determined to a greater extent by the way the cigarette is smoked than by the actual nicotine content of the cigarette and can vary between 0.3 mg and 3.2 mg per cigarette (Benowitz & Henningfield, 1994).

More recently, several newer forms of nicotine administration have been developed as a means of avoiding nicotine withdrawal in people who have given up smoking. Nicotine chewing gum was the first of these. The fact that nicotine can be absorbed transdermally (through the skin) allowed for the development of *"the patch"*; nicotine-containing patches are placed on the skin and release nicotine in various concentrations for a period of time. Most recently, a nicotine nasal spray has been tested.

The patch causes a slow buildup of nicotine in the blood and maintains it at a constant level for hours with no fluctuations. The gum will cause rises and falls in blood nicotine levels in response to its use; as a result, it causes patterns in blood nicotine that more closely resemble those caused by smoking, although peak levels reach only one-third that of smoking (Keenan, Henningfield, & Jarvik, 1995). The nasal spray causes the most cigarette-like changes in blood levels. Within 2.5 minutes of administration nicotine reaches 85 percent of peak levels in the blood (Sutherland et al., 1992).

DISTRIBUTION

The patterns of nicotine distribution in the body depend on route of administration and time after administration. When initial high concentrations circulate in the blood, as after inhalation, a high concentration is apparently retained in the brain. After about 30 minutes the nicotine leaves the brain and is concentrated in the liver, kidneys, salivary glands, and stomach (Schmiterlow & Hanson, 1965).

Nicotine crosses most barriers, including the placenta, and may be found in sweat, saliva, and the milk of nursing women.

EXCRETION

The amount of nicotine excreted by the kidneys depends on the pH of the urine, as described in Chapter 1. Acidic urine (pH < 7) tends to ionize nicotine and reduce its reabsorption through the nephron wall. Consequently, as much as 30 to 40 percent of administered nicotine may be eliminated in the urine. Reduced ionization at an alkaline pH increases reabsorption into the blood, and the efficiency of the kidneys is reduced, thereby shifting the load of excretion to the enzymes of the liver.

Nicotine is metabolized by two pathways in the liver to two inactive metabolites, *cotenine* and *nicotine-l'-N-oxide* (Beckett, Gorrod, & Jenner, 1971a). There is evidence that smokers are able to metabolize nicotine faster than nonsmokers and that among nonsmokers there may be a difference in nicotine metabolism between males and females (Beckett, Gorrod, & Jenner, 1971b). The half-life of nicotine is variable but is estimated to be about 30 minutes. While nicotine will accumulate in the body of a smoker over the course of a day, elimination is sufficiently rapid that there will be no day-to-day accumulation (Issac & Rand, 1972). Figure 8–3 shows typical blood nicotine levels for smokers smoking five cigarettes in the space of 3½ hours.

As this figure shows, there is an initial steep drop in blood nicotine levels after finishing a cigarette. This is due to the absorption of the nicotine from the blood into other body tissues. After this phase is complete, metabolism of nicotine and excretion by the kidneys are responsible for the decline in blood levels (R. Jones, 1987).

NEUROPHYSIOLOGICAL EFFECTS

There are two basic types of cholinergic receptor sites: *muscarinic* and *nicotinic*. Muscarinic receptors are stimulated by *muscarine* and blocked by anticholinergics such as *atropine* (see Chapter 4). Nicotinic receptors may be stimulated by *nicotine* and blocked by *curare*, a poison used by South American Indian tribes on the tips of their spears and arrows. Another drug that blocks nicotinic receptors but does not appear to have toxic effects in effective doses is *mecamylamine*. This drug is useful in research with nicotine because if a nicotine effect can be blocked by giving mecamylamine, it is reasonable to conclude that the nicotine effect was a result of its effect on ACh receptors.

Since nicotine occupies and activates nicotinic cholinergic receptor sites, it has traditionally been classified as a nicotinic cholinergic stimulant, but nicotine has a biphasic effect on cholinergic transmission. In low doses it stimulates these receptors, but it can also block them at higher doses, so it is more accurate to think of nicotine as both a stimulant and a blocker of cholinergic transmission.

What we know about cholinergic receptors is a result of research on the peripheral nervous sys-

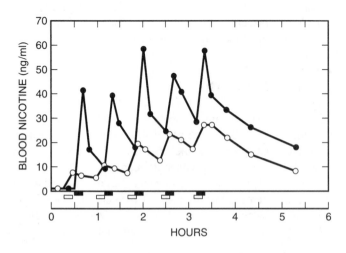

Figure 8–3 The rise and fall in blood levels of nicotine during the course of smoking five cigarettes with 30 minutes between each. Data from two subjects are presented. The times of the cigarettes are indicated by the solid and open bars below the horizontal axis, and these correspond to the solid and open circles on the graph. (From Issac & Rand, 1972, p. 310.)

tem. Though muscarinic receptors have been known to exist in the central nervous system for many years, it was not until 1980 that nicotinic receptors were discovered in the brain (Romano & Goldstein, 1980). This research showed that these receptors are part of cholinergic synapses in the brain and are similar to nicotinic cholinergic receptors in the peripheral nervous system. In addition, many nicotinic receptors are found in the synapses and cell bodies of cells in the brain that use DA and NE, and when they are stimulated, they cause a release of DA and NE. Nicotinic receptors of this nature are found in the cortex, the basal ganglia, the ventral tegmental area, and the nucleus accumbens (Levin, 1992; Balfour, 1991).

In addition to its effect on acetylcholine and the catecholamines, nicotine causes the release of serotonin, beta-endorphin, and numerous hormones such as vasopressin, growth hormone, and prolactin, all known to have effects on behavior (Pomerleau & Pomerleau, 1984).

EFFECTS OF TOBACCO

Effects on the Body

Peripheral Nervous System. In the peripheral nervous system, nicotinic receptor sites are located primarily in the neuromuscular junctions of striated or voluntary muscles. The poisonous effects of curare result because the drug blocks these junctions and the muscles become paralyzed; the victim can no longer breathe and dies of suffocation. The fact that nicotine stimulates these receptors results in muscular tremors. One British surgeon, H. J. Johnson (1965), was motivated to quit smoking when he noticed that an extra cigarette before surgery caused a fine hand tremor. In addition, there may be an inhibition of some reflexes. There is a decrease in the *patellar reflex* (knee jerk) after a cigarette. This effect is due to a lowering in the tone of voluntary muscles and appears to be a direct result of stimula-

tion of inhibitory cells in the motor pools in the spinal cord (E. F. Domino, 1973).

The biphasic effect of nicotine on cholinergic transmission is reflected in the ability of nicotine to stimulate and then block transmission in autonomic ganglia. These two effects, however, are modified because nicotine causes the release of other neurotransmitters that affect the peripheral nervous system. One such neurotransmitter is epinephrine, which produces sympathetic stimulation of its own. When this is combined with neuromuscular and parasympathetic stimulation and blocking, the result is a very complicated array of peripheral nervous system changes.

In general, at doses encountered in tobacco smoking, nicotine produces increases in heart rate and blood pressure and causes a constriction of blood vessels in the skin. This constriction causes a drop in skin temperature and is probably responsible for the cold touch that smokers have and the reason that the skin of smokers tends to wrinkle and age faster than that of nonsmokers (Daniell, 1971). The reduced blood flow to the skin also explains why smokers do not blush easily. This lack of skin color prompted one judge in the 1930s to accuse cigarettes of "deadening the sense of shame" and corrupting the morals of young people.

Nicotine also inhibits stomach secretions and stimulates activity of the bowel. For this reason, especially for someone with little tobacco tolerance, a cigarette can act as a good laxative.

Central Nervous System. The effects of nicotine in the CNS are complicated. Apart from its direct effects on synapses, nicotine also stimulates the release of epinephrine from various sites, including the adrenal glands. This causes a CNS arousal reflected in a decrease in alpha activity as shown in the EEG. Arousal is also produced by direct stimulation of the reticular activating system. Respiration is increased because of both direct and indirect stimulation of the medullary respiration centers. Respiratory arrest caused by an overdose of nicotine results from a block of these centers as well as at the neuromuscular junctions that control the muscles used in breathing.

Another brain stem center that is stimulated both directly and indirectly by nicotine is the vomiting center. This effect is most noticeable in naive smokers who have no tolerance and do not have the experience to control dosage appropriately. The initial experience of most young people with tobacco makes them nauseous and "green about the gills." This effect is subject to tolerance, but even experienced smokers can feel a bit "green" if they consume more than their accustomed amount of tobacco.

Higher in the brain, nicotine causes the release of NE and DA and the activation of systems that use these transmitters. One of these systems is the mesolimbic dopamine system, which has synapses in the nucleus accumbens. This is the reward system, and its activation is most likely responsible for the reinforcing effects of nicotine (Balfour, 1991). Increased activity in this system may also contribute to the ability to handle stress (Balfour, 1991).

Serotonin systems are also altered by nicotine, particularly the system that runs from the Raphé system to the cortex. This system is the primary site of action of the antidepressant drugs (Chapter 13), and nicotine appears to have a similar effect to the antidepressants (Balfour, 1991).

It has also become clear that cholinergic systems, both muscarinic and nicotinic, are important in cognitive functioning. In a later section in this chapter the cognition-enhancing effects of nicotine are discussed.

Effects on Sleep

There is some evidence that intravenous infusions of nicotine may cause REM sleep in cats (E. F. Domino & Yamamoto, 1965), but nicotine given intravenously before bedtime did not have any effect on sleep stages in healthy humans (E. F. Domino, 1967).

In another study, withdrawal from tobacco did disrupt sleep. Smokers undergoing withdrawal were shown to have a moderate increase in REM sleep time. This increase was accompanied by subjective reports of an increase in dreaming and in the vividness of dreams (Kales et al., 1970).

EFFECTS ON THE BEHAVIOR AND PERFORMANCE OF HUMANS

Effects on Mood

In most studies nicotine appears to cause an arousal in brain wave activity and a release of epinephrine that arouses the sympathetic nervous system, yet most smokers report that they smoke because smoking a cigarette relaxes them. Even people who have given up smoking for a long time report that they feel the need for a smoke during moments of stress. This unexpected observation has been called *Nesbitt's paradox* by one researcher (Schachter, 1973) after a man who first studied it, and it has been the object of considerable research.

There are a number of explanations of Nesbitt's paradox, and all are related to the question of why people smoke. It may be that lighting and holding a cigarette gives people something to do with their hands, and this act calms the nerves, as pressing worry beads does. In fact, one study showed that the act of smoking causes increases in alpha waves indicating relaxation, but the nicotine causes arousal (Murphree, Pfeiffer, & Price, 1967). It is also possible that the calmness is a result of relief from nicotine withdrawal symptoms that smokers may experience in a mild form between cigarettes, or it may be that stimulation is caused by low doses and relaxation by high doses, and the smoker can control the effect desired by altering inhalation of the smoke (Pomerleau & Pomerleau, 1984; Stepney, 1982). One study showed that the effect of smoking on arousal can depend on the stressfulness of the circumstances in which the cigarette is smoked. When subjects were stressed by noise, smoking reduced arousal as measured by the EEG, but under conditions of low arousal, smoking had an activating effect on EEG (Mangan & Golding, 1978). Another study showed that subjective arousal (although not arousal measured by blood pressure and heart rate) was related to baseline arousal levels. It was found that nicotine nasal spray and cigarette smoking increased arousal in people who had low baseline levels, but had little effect on those whose arousal levels were already high (Perkins et al., 1992).

Whether nicotine relaxes or stimulates, it is a pleasurable experience for many smokers. In one study, nicotine was administered either by tobacco smoke inhalation or by intravenous infusion to volunteers, and their subjective responses were measured using the Addiction Research Center Inventory. Smokers reported increased liking scores and reported subjective effects similar to those caused by morphine and amphetamine. These effects peaked about one minute after administration and were gone within a few minutes. Nonsmokers did not enjoy the experience (Henningfield, Miyasato, & Jasinski, 1985; Jasinski, Johnson, & Henningfield, 1984). These subjective effects were blocked by mecamylamine (Henningfield et al., 1983). In another experiment, smokers were given cigarettes with different levels of nicotine in the morning after being deprived of smoking since the previous evening. They were permitted to smoke the cigarettes themselves and were asked to push a button when they experienced a "rush, a buzz, or a high." Nineteen of 22 subjects experienced at least one such sensation. Frequency and duration of sensations were related to blood nicotine levels. These sensations lasted for about 11 seconds and occurred with a delay of about 30 seconds after a puff (Pomerleau & Pomerleau, 1992).

As we shall see later, one theory of why people smoke is that they are using the nicotine in tobacco to control their response to stress and to create a positive mood. There are, in fact, few data to support this. A survey in the United Kingdom has shown that smokers have lower levels of psychological well-being than nonsmokers and ex-smokers (West, 1993). In addition, even though it is typically found that mood worsens when a person stops smoking, it slowly returns to the normal smoking level after three or four weeks. What's more, it then continues to improve even further over the following 10 weeks so that mood becomes even better than it was during smoking (Hughes, Higgins & Hatsukami, 1990).

Effects on Performance

There have been many studies of the effects of nicotine on human performance, and the results have not been entirely consistent. The data are further complicated by the fact that the effects of nicotine appear to be different in smokers and nonsmokers. In general, the major effect of smoking is to improve the performance of regular smokers whose behavior has been degraded by withdrawal from nicotine. In a simulated driving task, for example, it was found that the performance of nonsmokers and smokers who were allowed to smoke was equal, but an impairment in vigilance and tracking was detected in smokers deprived of nicotine (Heimstra, Bancroft, & De Kock, 1967). Other studies, however, have shown that smoking enhances performance, even beyond the performance of nonsmokers on tasks such as driving which require vigilance and sustained attention (Tarriere & Hartemann, 1964; Wesnes & Warburton, 1983). In an extensive review of nicotine and human performance, Wesnes and Warburton (1983) concluded that smoking does help sustain performance on monotonous tasks and improves both the speed and accuracy of information processing.

In addition to speeded information processing, faster motor reaction speeds produced by nicotine have also been reported for both cigarette smoking and chewing nicotine gum (Sherwood, Kerr, & Hindmarch, 1992; Pritchard, Robinson, & Guy, 1992).

Smoking can also improve performance on learning tasks. The effects of smoking one cigarette on serial anticipation learning of a list of nonsense syllables was determined in an experiment by Anderson (1975). She showed that the effects of the cigarette were similar to any arousing stimulus—the learning of the list was impaired, but recall of the list 45 minutes later was improved. She suggested that this outcome reflects the fact that arousal at the time of learning causes poor immediate recall because of the interfering effect of an increase in nonspecific activity. The increased arousal, however, aids the process of consolidation and improves recall of the list at a later time. Similar effects on consolidation have also been reported in studies on nonhumans, as we shall see.

Other improvements in memory have also been reported, and it has now been demonstrated that some of these effects are not attributable to relief of smoking withdrawal in regular smokers (Warburton, 1992).

Interestingly, nicotine has been shown to improve various aspects of cognitive functioning in patients with Alzheimer's disease and in aging laboratory rats and monkeys (Levin, 1992).

In spite of the fact that there are demonstrations that nicotine can improve performance and learning, there are many more reports that it has no effect or may even interfere with cognitive and performance variables (R. West, 1993). These divergent findings have led to a rather heated debate among researchers that was reviewed in a 1993 issue of the journal *Addiction* (1993, vol. 88, pp. 591–600). This debate is particularly interesting because, as we shall see later, one theory of why people smoke is that they find it improves their performance. This theory is advanced as an alternative to the theory that smoking can be considered similar to "addiction" to other drugs (Robinson & Pritchard, 1992).

EFFECTS ON THE BEHAVIOR OF NONHUMANS

Unconditioned Behavior

Spontaneous motor activity (SMA) of rats is initially depressed by 0.8 mg/kg of nicotine, but after seven days of testing this dosage produces an increase in SMA, which on repeated testing gets greater until the increase is similar to that produced by 0.8 mg/kg of amphetamine. It is believed that the initial depression is a result of increased ACh levels in the brain, an effect that disappears with tolerance after a few days. Once the ACh levels drop, the increases in epinephrine cause an increase in SMA in a manner similar to amphetamine (Morrison & Stephenson, 1972b; Stolerman, Fink, & Jarvik, 1973).

Effects of Positively Reinforced Behavior

Nicotine usually produces a suppression in operant behavior for about 15 minutes after injection, depending on the dosage. Following this depression, some researchers report an increase in FI and VI response rates. Response rates on FR schedules, however, are generally reduced in a manner similar to those for amphetamine. With an FI, the increases appear largely due to a decrease in the duration of the pause after reinforcement and an increase in low rates. Nicotine is similar to amphetamine in that the effect is dependent on control rate; high rates are depressed while low rates are increased (Pradhan, 1970; Morrison, 1967).

Effects on Negatively Reinforced Behavior

The effects of nicotine on aversively motivated behavior are also similar to those of amphetamine. Nicotine does not appear to increase responses that have been suppressed by response-contingent shock (Morrison & Stephenson, 1972a). Nicotine in low doses will improve the performance of rats on a Sidman avoidance schedule by increasing response rates and decreasing shocks, but high doses slow response rates and increase the number of shocks received. It has also been shown that withdrawal from 0.4 mg/kg of nicotine can disrupt the ability of rats to avoid a shock in the same manner that nicotine withdrawal can interfere with the behavior of humans (Morrison, 1974).

This great similarity between the effects of nicotine and amphetamine on operant behavior suggests that many of these effects are likely brought about by a similar mechanism. Since amphetamine increases activity at catecholamine synapses (see Chapter 10) and nicotine causes the general release of epinephrine and stimulates DA and NE synapses, it is possible that many of these behavioral effects of nicotine are a result of the release of catecholamines (Pradhan, 1970). This increase in catecholamine activity, however, depends on the action of nicotine at its receptor sites because most of these behavioral effects can be blocked by pretreating the animal with mecamylamine, a drug that blocks nicotinic receptor sites (Morrison, 1967).

DRUG STATE DISCRIMINATION

Nicotine is an effective cue in a drug state discrimination task in a dosage range similar to one that alters operant behavior. It has been shown that 0.2 mg/kg nicotine can be used as a cue and will not generalize to various doses of epinephrine, pentobarbital, physostigmine, chlordiazepoxide, or caffeine. The cuing effect of nicotine can be blocked by mecamylamine, the same cholinergic blocker that prevents other behavior effects of nicotine including self-administration (Morrison & Stephenson, 1969; Stolerman, Pratt, & Garcha, 1982).

Although it cannot be found consistently, there is some evidence of partial generalization between nicotine and d-amphetamine, and animals trained to discriminate cocaine will sometimes generalize the cocaine response to nicotine (Stolerman, 1987). This finding corresponds to the observation made earlier that humans sometimes describe the effect of intravenous nicotine as being similar to that of cocaine.

It has been shown that humans can discriminate between identical cigarettes that are different only in nicotine content (Kallman et al., 1982), although it is not known whether this is done by taste or through a central mechanism.

WITHDRAWAL SYMPTOMS

When most tobacco users attempt to give up their habit, they experience withdrawal symptoms in varying degrees of intensity. If you have ever attempted to quit smoking or have suffered along with someone going through tobacco withdrawal, you will be familiar with the symptoms. Withdrawal from nicotine is not as severe physically as withdrawal from heroin, but it is just as stressful psychologically. Indeed, many ex-heroin addicts who have also quit smoking report that they found it harder to give up tobacco than heroin.

Systematic studies of nicotine withdrawal in regular smokers reliably show the following symptoms: decreased heart rate, increased eating causing weight gain, an inability to concentrate, increased awakenings during sleep, craving for cigarettes, and anxiety, anger, aggression, and depression (Hughes, Higgins, & Bickel, 1994; Hughes et al., 1991). Other symptoms that have been reported are nervousness, drowsiness, lightheadedness, headaches, dizziness, tremor, and nausea (Jarvik, 1979, p. 27). Most of these symptoms except for weight gain and craving are over within a month. For about 25 percent of people, these symptoms persist, but are usually gone by six months, although there are reports that craving may continue as long as nine years (Fletcher & Doll, 1969).

Withdrawal symptoms can be relieved by the administration of substitute nicotine from other sources such as nicotine gum and transdermal patches. However, unlike withdrawal from many other drugs, the administration of the receptor blocker for nicotine, mecamylamine, does not induce withdrawal in nicotine-dependent smokers (Hughes, Higgins, & Bickel, 1994). Symptoms of nicotine withdrawal can also be reduced, at least temporarily, by the taste and smell of tobacco or the act of smoking itself. One study showed that tobacco withdrawal symptoms were relieved if smokers were allowed to smoke a denicotinized cigarette that delivered no nicotine at all to the smoker (Butschky et al., 1994).

For a time, nicotine withdrawal can interfere with performance on various cognitive and motor tasks. As we have already seen, nicotine withdrawal also interferes with rats' shock avoidance (Morrison, 1974).

Unlike most other drugs that cause physical dependence, withdrawal severity does not seem to be related to dose; heavy and light smokers report equally severe withdrawal. Nor is withdrawal severity related to length of time smoking, previous attempts at quitting, sex, age, education or alcohol and caffeine use (Hughes et al., 1991).

SELF-ADMINISTRATION IN NONHUMANS

Since self-administration of nicotine in humans is so persistent and widespread, it is surprising that accounts of animal self-administration are rare. There are some anecdotal accounts of tame monkeys smoking. Indeed, Charles Darwin in *The Descent of Man* (1882) claims to have seem monkeys "smoke tobacco with pleasure" (p. 7). Darwin used these observations to support his contention that the sense of taste and the nervous systems of man and monkeys are similar. Surprisingly, however, systematic research from laboratories has found monkeys to be reluctant smokers (Jarvik, 1973, p. 296). Monkeys have been taught to inhale cigarette smoke, but the procedure involved a period of forced consumption in which the monkeys were reinforced with drinking water for sucking on a tube through which they received tobacco smoke. After this training, some animals seemed to prefer sucking on a tube that delivered tobacco smoke over one that delivered only air. It is doubtful whether this procedure represents a situation similar to human tobacco use. Animals do not normally initiate smoking on their own (Jarvik, 1973).

There are few accounts of animals that will work for intravenous infusions of nicotine. Most of these studies show that if nicotine is self-administered, responding is not robust and rather slow (Stolerman, 1987). In one study (Deneau & Inoki, 1967), monkeys were given the opportunity to self-administer nicotine through an intravenous cannula. After being given hourly infusions of nicotine for two to five days, some animals reliably responded for nicotine, but response rates were low, and the pattern was not consistent from day to day. In a later study, Goldberg, Spealman, and Goldberg (1981) were able to demonstrate reliable intravenous self-administration in monkeys. Using a procedure called a *second-order schedule*, they found that if the nicotine infusion was preceded by a colored light, monkeys would respond at a high rate for the light alone, even if it was paired with the nicotine infusion only occasionally. It appears that the stimuli associated with the delivery of nicotine make a very important contribution to the effectiveness of nicotine as a reinforcer. Goldberg and his associates also demonstrated that injections of the nicotine antagonist mecamylamine reduced responding to saline control levels.

In another study, Risner and Goldberg (1983) demonstrated that dogs would self-administer nicotine on an FR 10 schedule when a four-minute time-out was imposed after each infusion. Progressive ratio schedules showed that some nicotine doses would support ratios as high as 510 responses per infusion, much higher than saline but considerably lower than cocaine.

It appears, then, that nicotine infusions do have reinforcing properties in laboratory animals under a restricted range of conditions. Conditions that support nicotine infusion are a period of forced consumption, stimuli paired with the infusion, and a fixed interval or second-order schedule that imposes an abstinence period between opportunities to self-administer.

Intravenous nicotine can also serve as a punisher. In one study, food-reinforced behavior of monkeys was suppressed if it was followed by an infusion of nicotine (Goldberg & Spealman, 1983). This suppression occurred at the same dose that served as a positive reinforcer for monkeys in other experiments conducted in the same laboratory. It is not clear what should make nicotine a reinforcer under some circumstances and a punisher in others.

SELF-ADMINISTRATION IN HUMANS

Hallucinogenic Use

There appear to be two distinct patterns of nicotine self-administration. The pattern we are most familiar with involves more or less continuous use throughout waking hours, but this is not the only way that nicotine has been used. If nicotine is taken infrequently and in large doses, it produces a highly intoxicating effect and can act as a hallucinogen. It appears that American Native people, the first users of tobacco, frequently used the drug in this way. Monardes, a seventeenth-century medical historian, gives us the following account:

Tobacco smoke is received by the nose, and in smoking the priest receives the smoke through little tubes or canes, and after they tumble as in ecstasy. Upon recovering, they related what they had conversed about the evil spirits, and gave ambiguous replies to their followers. In addition to this the people take the smoke both by the mouth and by the nose for pleasure when they desire to see the future in their dreams. (G. A. West, 1970, p. 84)

Although this type of tobacco use is rare, it still survives today in some remote areas (Welbert, 1972).

Low-Dose Pattern

Most cigarette smokers space cigarettes out fairly evenly throughout waking hours, but a careful analysis shows that there is a regular daily pattern. Smoking is usually greatest in the early afternoon right after lunch and after supper between 7 and 10 P.M. Throughout the course of a week, Wednesday and Sunday are the lightest smoking days and Saturday is the heaviest (Meade & Wald, 1977).

Although the pattern of cigarette smoking is fairly regular over the course of a day and a week for any individual, there are factors that can increase cigarette intake in particular circumstances. One such factor is the presence of cigarettes or other smokers. Experiments have shown that if smokers are asked to wait in a room, they will light up a cigarette much sooner if other people in the room are smoking (Glad & Adesso, 1976). People are also more likely to smoke if a pack of cigarettes is left in a conspicuous place in the room (Herman, 1974).

Tobacco Chippers.   As with other drugs, the amount consumed varies considerably among individuals. The average regular smoker consumes about 25 cigarettes a day and shows signs of physical dependence on nicotine, but about 10 percent of regular smokers consume fewer than five cigarettes a day and are clearly not physically dependent. These smokers have been called tobacco "chippers" because this pattern of occasional use without physical dependence resembles a pattern of heroin use called "chipping" (Shiffman, 1989) (see Chapter 11).

Who Smokes?

As with other drugs, tobacco is not used by everyone. Studies of smokers and nonsmokers have revealed some interesting differences. Like drinking, smoking appears to have a genetic component. Studies of twins have shown that identical twins are more likely to have similar smoking habits than fraternal twins. Even when they are not reared together, the smoking behavior of identical twins is highly correlated (Eysenck & Eaves, 1980; Hughes, 1986).

Smokers are more likely than nonsmokers to use other drugs such as coffee and especially alcohol. In addition, smokers are more likely to change their jobs, get married and divorced, have more traffic accidents, be more rebellious, achieve less academically, and be more sexually active than nonsmokers (Ashton & Stepney, 1982, p. 121; Jarvis, 1994).

Before the middle of the twentieth century when smoking rates were near 80 percent, there was no relation between social class, education, and smoking, but now that smoking rates have fallen, a distinct effect of social class and economics has become apparent. People who are unemployed, work in unskilled and manual labor jobs, and have less than a high school education are much more likely to smoke than people who work at professional jobs and have a college degree.

Typically people start to smoke when they are teenagers. At this stage, social class does not seem to have an effect; however, having smoking parents, a boy or girl friend, and poor academic achievement do weakly predict who will start smoking. Few people become smokers after the age of 20.

Smokeless tobacco is currently used primarily by males. In the 1993 National Household Survey in the United States, 2.9 percent report use of smokeless tobacco. The rate is as high as 20 percent in Sweden (Jarvis, 1994).

Behavioral Economics

Numerous attempts have been made over the years to determine the price elasticity of cigarettes. Estimates range from −0.4 to −1.3, but the figure is generally accepted to be about −0.7. This indicates a relatively inelastic demand. Further analyses, however, have shown that this inelasticity is not the same for different segments of the population or for different measures of demand. Teenage smokers are more susceptible than older smokers to price increases both in terms of the number of cigarettes smoked and in terms of the number of smokers. The elasticity index for participation (number of smokers) was shown to be −1.20 for smokers 12–17 years old in the United States, and the quantity (cigarette smoked per smoker) was −0.25, with a combined elasticity of −1.40. In this study the combined

elasticity for smokers over 20 was −0.42. What these figures indicate is that demand in young smokers is elastic—that is, increasing the price of cigarettes will have a considerable impact on the initiation rate of young smokers—but it may not have a large effect on the smoking behavior of older, established smokers. Since most people become smokers before the age of 20, price increases will have a considerable effect not only at the time they are put into effect, but will decrease cigarette consumption far into the future (Lewitt, 1989).

Another study of demand elasticity for cigarettes has shown that elasticities are greater if long-term effects are measured. This study of cigarette prices in the United States from 1955 to 1985 found that a permanent increase of 10 percent in price had an immediate effect of reducing consumption by 4 percent. In the long term, however, there was a decrease in consumption of 7.5 percent. In addition, it was found that elasticities were much smaller if the price increase was temporary than if the increase was permanent (G. S. Becker, Grossman, & Murphy, 1988).

Compulsion to Smoke

Perhaps one of the most tragic examples of the strength of the tobacco habit is the case of the founder of psychoanalysis, Sigmund Freud. Freud smoked cigars most of his life in spite of the fact that he suffered from heart pains and cancer of the mouth as a direct result, and toward the end of his life he was in constant pain after undergoing 33 operations for his cancer yet was still unable to quit. One report concludes:

Freud died of cancer in 1939, at the age of eighty-three. His efforts over a forty-five-year period to stop smoking, his repeated inability to stop, his suffering when he tried to stop, and the persistence of his craving and suffering even after fourteen continuous months of abstinence—a "torture . . . beyond human power to bear"—make him the tragic prototype of [the tobacco addict]. (Brecher & editors of Consumer Reports, 1972, p. 215)

Freud, of course, is not alone. In his Statement on Nicotine-Containing Cigarettes before the House Subcommittee on Health and the Environment, David Kessler, the commissioner of the Food and Drug Administration (FDA), made the following points: (1) Two-thirds of adults who smoke say that they wish they could quit. (2) Seventeen million try to quit each year, but fewer than one out of ten succeed. Three out of four adult smokers say they are addicted. By some estimates, as many as 74 to 90 percent are. Eight out of ten smokers say they wish they had never started.

Explanations of Nicotine Self-Administration

The hallucinogenic pattern has not been extensively studied and is virtually unknown in industrialized cultures, but the pattern of continuous low-dose use has been the subject of considerable research.

It has been demonstrated that nicotine by itself can function as a reinforcer in humans. Studies carried out with human volunteers show that intravenous infusions of nicotine serve as a reinforcer. One experiment showed that responding on a lever that produced nicotine gradually increased over sessions and stopped when saline was substituted for nicotine infusions. Other research showed that 3 out of 4 smokers make more presses on a lever that produced nicotine fusions than on a lever that caused an infusion of saline. When doses were reduced, responding increased to compensate in a manner typical of psychomotor stimulant drugs such as cocaine. However, some subjects in these experiments, even if they were smokers, found the nicotine infusions unpleasant and actually worked to avoid infusions (Henningfield, Lucas, & Bigelow, 1986).

Nicotine Titration

For some time it had not clearly been established that nicotine is really the ingredient in tobacco responsible for tobacco consumption. To show that it is, researchers used the strategy of changing the nicotine content of cigarettes and seeing if the amount of smoking changed as a consequence; that is, they sought to demonstrate the *titration* of nicotine dose. This approach was based on the assumption that smokers adjust their nicotine intake to keep the levels from getting too high or too low. It assumes that in order to avoid withdrawal the smoker starts smoking when the nicotine blood level falls below a certain point, and stops smoking when blood levels get too high in order to avoid unpleasant toxic effects.

Early studies had trouble demonstrating titration when they simply counted the number of high- and low-nicotine cigarettes a person smoked. They soon found out that people control nicotine intake not by changing the number of cigarettes they smoke, but by changing their smoking behavior; that is, they compensate for low-nicotine cigarettes by taking deeper and more frequent puffs on the cigarette. It is possible to measure these variables precisely by having subjects smoke through a special cigarette holder connected to a computer that monitors total smoke inhalation. Using these techniques, it has been demonstrated that smokers will compensate for increased or reduced doses by increasing and decreasing their puffing behavior, but the compensation is not as complete as when intravenous infusions are used.

One of the predictions of the nicotine titration theory is that the first few puffs on a cigarette will be rapid and deep as the smoker tries to raise blood nicotine levels that have fallen between cigarettes. As nicotine level increases, the puff rate will decrease, and fewer puffs will be taken near the end of the cigarette. This change in puff rate has been recorded by several researchers and can easily be demonstrated. Box 8–1 describes a project on this effect that you can do. In addition, the theory predicts that people will be highly motivated to smoke when the blood levels are low, and the lowest levels occur after a night of sleeping. A British study showed that 14 percent of smokers light up within 5 minutes of waking in the morning and 50 percent do so within 30 minutes.

BOX 8–1   Measuring Nicotine Titration

One of the predictions of the nicotine titration hypothesis is that smokers will compensate for low blood nicotine levels by attempting to increase nicotine intake during the early part of a cigarette. Smokers can increase the amount of nicotine they get from a single cigarette by increasing the depth and frequency of puffs on a cigarette. You would predict, then, that early puffs on a cigarette when nicotine blood levels are low would be more frequent than later puffs; that is, the first few puffs on a cigarette will have shorter *interpuff intervals* (time between puffs) than later puffs.

An experiment by L. D. Chait and R. R. Griffiths of Johns Hopkins Medical School confirmed this prediction. Chait and Griffiths (1982) used computer technology to measure puff frequency, but you can replicate their findings with the aid of a simple stopwatch or a timer that is accurate to within a second. One advantage of using simple technology is that you are not tied to the laboratory. You can conduct your experiment in the real world and determine if what Chait and Griffiths found in the lab is also true in the field.

You could do this project on someone you know, such as your roommate or a member of your family, but you should be careful that the subject is not aware of what you are up to. People are likely to change their behavior when they know that they are being observed. Another way of gathering data is to go to a public place where people are smoking and unobtrusively observe their behavior.

What you will need to do is measure the length of time from the lighting of a cigarette to the first puff and between all successive puffs until the cigarette is stubbed out. If you are collecting all your data from a single individual, you should have enough information after 10 or 15 cigarettes, but if you are collecting from a number of different people, you may need as many as 20 observations.

The best way to plot the data is to make a graph with puff number on the horizontal axis and mean interpuff interval—the length of time between one puff and the next—on the vertical axis. For example, for the third puff, find the average length of time between the second and the third puffs for all the cigarettes you observed. Not all cigarettes will have the same number of puffs. Such differences can create some difficulties when you get to higher puff numbers because then each data point will be based on a decreasing number of observations. For this reason, plot only for the number of puffs you have complete data for; for example, if the smallest number of puffs on a cigarette is eight, plot only the first eight puffs on all cigarettes.

What you should see when your graph is complete is that interpuff intervals get longer with the higher puff numbers. See if you can find the original article by Chait and Griffiths and compare your findings with theirs.

In an elaboration of the titration theory, Stanley Schachter of Columbia University has suggested why smoking increases in times of stress. He points out that during stress, the urine becomes acidic. Because nicotine is a weak base, it becomes highly ionized in the acidic urine and consequently cannot be reabsorbed into the blood. As a result, the kidneys are very efficient in excreting nicotine, and the blood levels drop rapidly. Schachter (1978) suggests that this rapid drop in blood nicotine is the signal that another cigarette is necessary. In other words, "The smoker's mind is in the bladder." Consequently, smoking increases in times of stress.

One difficulty with the titration theory is that compensation for changes in nicotine is far from complete; smokers do make adjustments for the amount of nicotine delivered by their cigarette, but they are unable to compensate completely, allowing their blood levels to become higher than normal when nicotine content is increased and lower than normal when it is decreased. In addition, increasing blood nicotine levels with nicotine chewing gum to high levels will decrease smoking but does not eliminate it.

Nicotine titration is a description of the way people smoke. It presumes that the motivation for smoking is the avoidance of withdrawal at low blood levels and the avoidance of toxic effects at high blood levels, but titration can exist even if smoking is motivated by other factors.

Nicotine as a "Psychological Tool"

Another explanation of smoking is related to Nesbitt's paradox, described earlier. It suggests that the smoker uses nicotine to help cope with daily tasks by manipulating levels of arousal and other psychological functions. As we have seen, nicotine can subjectively both increase and decrease levels of arousal, depending on dose and circumstances. *Psychological tool* theories suggest that the smoker uses smoking as a tool to decrease arousal in times of stress and increase arousal during fatigue and boredom, and thus is able to maintain an optimal level of arousal. Changing arousal levels allows performance on tasks to be enhanced as well. These factors together increase the psychological comfort of the smoker and provide the motivation for smoking (Hutchison & Emley, 1973; Balfour, 1982; Stepney, 1982, pp. 193–196; Robinson & Pritchard, 1992).

This idea has considerable intuitive appeal, and there is some evidence to support it. Most of this evidence, however, is indirect. Though it has been shown that nicotine can enhance performance on some tasks and can reduce the effects of stress, these effects are disputed and not easily replicated. Additionally, it is difficult to show that these effects, even if they do occur, are responsible for nicotine self-administration. Recent studies with amphetamine and sedatives have shown that people will sometimes choose to use a drug that either stimulates them or sedates them depending on the demands of a task they will be performing (Silverman, Kirby, & Griffiths, 1994), but many other studies described in Chapter 5 indicate that in general, drugs are seldom self-administered for their therapeutic effects. Though we know that smoking does increase in times of stress, this observation can be explained more simply by other mechanisms, as Schachter has done. In addition, stress-reducing agents such as the benzodiazepines (Librium and Valium) do not appear to be effective in helping people to stop smoking (Jaffe, 1987).

Nicotine Bolus Theory

The *nicotine bolus theory* has been proposed by M. A. H. Russell of the Maudsley Hospital in London to explain other aspects of smoking behavior. Careful observation of a cigarette smoker will show that when smoke is inhaled into the lungs, it is frequently done with one rapid inhalation rather than gradually as with a normal breath. This sudden filling of the lungs with smoke tends to saturate the blood in the capillaries of the lungs with nicotine at the moment of inhalation. This concentration of nicotine in the blood, known as the *nicotine bolus*, stays together as the blood returns to the heart and is pumped to the brain. This theory suggests that it is the sudden high level of nicotine in the brain that acts as a positive reinforcer and keeps the smoker smoking. Because the bolus is so pleasurable, it is responsible for the intense craving for tobacco (M. A. H. Russell, 1976). A similar theory has been proposed to explain the addicting nature of intravenous injections of heroin (Dole, 1980).

Since a nicotine bolus can be achieved only by smoking, this theory explains why the craving for the drug is worse in smokers than in those who take tobacco by other means, but it cannot account for the great popularity of tobacco in its other forms throughout history.

Comparing Theories

The nicotine bolus theory, the titration theory, and the psychological tool theory are not mutually exclusive. It is possible that they may all be correct to some extent. Clearly, nicotine can act as a positive reinforcer. Constant blood levels may well be reinforcing, and so may the nicotine bolus and the ability to alter arousal and performance. Smokers may be trying to achieve any one, or all three, and, in addition, trying to avoid some of the unpleasant effects of withdrawal at the same time. A combination of all ideas can explain more of the data than either theory alone. It is also possible that one theory may not be appropriate for all smokers. Different people may smoke for different reasons. Clearly, tobacco smoking is a complicated activity.

The nicotine bolus theory, the titration theory, and the psychological tool theory all predict that a smoker who switches to low-nicotine cigarettes will increase the frequency and depth of each puff in an attempt to create a larger nicotine bolus or maintain optimal blood levels. The result will be an increase in smoke inhalation. The theories, however, make differential predictions concerning the effectiveness of nicotine gum and the nicotine patch in the treatment of smoking. While the titration theory predicts that the patch and the gum will be effective, the nicotine bolus theory predicts that taking nicotine in the form of a patch will be ineffective, since these will not create a bolus and consequently will not reduce the craving. Gum does not cause nicotine boluses as smoking does, but it does create a more "smoking-like" effect on blood levels. Interestingly, a combination of nicotine gum and a nicotine patch is more effective in helping people stop smoking than either alone (Fagerström, Schneider, & Lunell, 1993).

The debate on the nature of smoking has taken on a political significance since the 1988 U.S. surgeon general's report and the 1994 U.S. House of Representatives hearings on whether the tobacco industry in the United States should be regulated by the U.S. FDA. The FDA and the surgeon general argue that smoking is addicting in the same sense that cocaine and heroin are; that is, it stimulates reward centers in the brain and is reinforcing. Defenders of the tobacco industry claim that this is not the case: Smoking is motivated by a desire to control mood and performance; that is, it is a behavior enhancer (Robinson & Pritchard, 1992). The debate has not been settled on either the scientific or the political front, but the behavior enhancer argument seems to be losing ground on both fronts (Kozlowski & Henningfield, 1995).

TREATMENTS

Clearly, tobacco smoking can be a difficult habit to break. Nevertheless, up to 95 percent of former tobacco smokers quit without the benefit of any treatment. For those who need help, however, a great variety of therapies are available.

Behavior Therapy

Behavior therapies assume that smoking is a learned response that is established by some form of positive reinforcement, although the origin of the reinforcement is usually not important to the therapy. Attempts are made to eliminate this learned response through punishment, positive reinforcement, or extinction. One widely used technique is to administer an electric shock every time the smoker reaches for or lights a cigarette. Another variation of the process is to have the smoker puff rapidly on each cigarette and administer an aversive overdose of nicotine. Smoke has the advantage of being a more natural and available aversive stimulus. Electric shock is normally available only in the laboratory, whereas cigarette smoke always accompanies smoking.

Positive reinforcement has been used by providing the smoker with rewards for increasingly long periods of abstinence.

Other techniques make assumptions concerning the motivation for smoking. If it is assumed that the function of smoking is to relieve stress, it would follow that relaxation training would have the same effect and reduce the need for smoking.

One traditional method of self-control is to teach the person to imagine vividly either the disastrous consequences of smoking or the benefits of abstinence when considering whether or not to light up a cigarette. Contracting is also used as means of self-control. The smoker may enter into a contract with the therapist or someone else to forfeit a sum of money if he or she relapses. Thus there is an additional incentive to refrain from smoking during moments of weakness.

Behavior therapies seem to be effective in the short term but not for maintenance of abstinence, although recent developments in the technique are encouraging (Singh & Leung, 1988).

Substitution Therapy

One treatment that appears to be effective for some smokers is based on the same strategy as methadone maintenance with heroin addicts (Chapter 11). It assumes that smoking is diffi-cult to stop because the withdrawal symptoms are so unpleasant. Nicotine chewing gum is substituted for cigarettes in order to block withdrawal from nicotine and reduce the compulsion to smoke. Reports on the use of nicotine gum show that it significantly reduces cigarette consumption more than a placebo over a period of two to three weeks. Other reports show that the gum is effective in reducing smoking for a much longer period of time provided that the smoker continues to use the gum. In addition, it appears that the gum may be more effective for heavy smokers than for light smokers (Stepney, 1982, p. 201).

Gum, however, has the disadvantage that it is difficult to maintain an adequate dose. It is necessary to chew 20 to 30 pieces of gum a day to achieve one half of the nicotine dose of cigarette smoking (Keenan, Henningfield, & Jarvik, 1995). The transdermal patch does not have this problem and is also effective, but a combination of the patch and the gum is better than either alone (Fagerström, Schneider, & Lunell, 1993). A nicotine nasal spray has been developed that has been shown to mimic the blood-nicotine effects of smoking more accurately (Sutherland et al., 1992).

Nicotine substitution therapy should continue for several months with a gradual weaning of dose, and occasionally it may be necessary to revert to use of the gum or patch in circumstances where relapse is likely.

Substitution may not always lead to smoking cessation, but even if substitution only succeeds in reducing the number of cigarettes, as it often does, it will have achieved partial success (Keenan, Henningfield, & Jarvik, 1995).

One meta-analysis of nicotine replacement therapies showed that people receiving any form of replacement therapy were 1.7 times more likely to be abstinent from smoking after six months than control subjects. Nasal spray and inhaled nicotine were the most effective followed by the patch. Gum was the least effective (Silagy et al., 1994).

Relapse and Quitting

As with most drugs that are self-administered continuously, once the behavior is established, it is very difficult to stop. Fewer than 25 percent of all successful participants in smoking therapy programs are still nonsmokers after a year, and fewer than 15 percent of all smokers are able to stop smoking permanently. This success rate is similar to the sort of success rates achieved in alcoholism and heroin addiction programs. Though some therapies appear to work better for some types of smoker, overall no particular type of therapy has a higher success rate than any other, but the success rate is higher among smokers who participate in therapy than among those who quit on their own (Raw, 1978).

Smokers who are most likely to be able to quit successfully are those who have a low overall level of consumption, have smoked for a short time, and do not report inhaling (Cherry & Kernan, 1976). Quitters are seldom able to stop on the first try. It often takes a number of attempts before a permanent cure is achieved.

Interestingly, the severity of withdrawal does not reliably predict relapse to smoking. Relapse, however, is related to weight gain; those who gain weight are more likely to be successful quitters. It is not clear why this is so, but it may be related to the finding by Carroll (Carroll & Meish, 1984) that hunger increases the reinforcing effect of drugs. Quitters who reduce food intake to counter weight gain may also be increasing the reinforcing effect of nicotine by increasing their hunger (Hughes, Higgins, & Bickel, 1994).

Health warnings in the media may be effective in motivating some individuals to change their behavior, but with others it appears that a more personal reminder is required. Among those who have successfully quit smoking, the most frequently given reason for stopping is that the smoker experienced some symptom of disease caused by smoking, frequently a cough (Fletcher & Doll, 1969). It may be beneficial to think of the choice to smoke in terms of the discussion of choice in Chapter 5. Clearly, if matching law is governing the choice to smoke, short-term benefits will determine the behavior and the decision will be to smoke, but if a longer time period is involved in the bookkeeping, delayed harmful effects will be incorporated into the decision, and the choice may be not to smoke. A cough or some other health symptom may well act as a stimulus reminding the smoker that he or she may experience harmful effects from the cigarette. Similarly, this principle may also be illustrated by the man who successfully controlled smoking by putting a picture of his granddaughter on his pack of cigarettes to remind him of some of the long-term benefits of not lighting up.

Even though some people respond to subtle health signs, many others do not. Forty percent of smokers who suffer a heart attack resume smoking before they leave the hospital; the majority of these do so within 2 days of leaving intensive care. After undergoing surgery for lung cancer, 50 percent of those who survive resume smoking (Jarvis, 1994).

HARMFUL EFFECTS

There can be little doubt that tobacco smoking increases the risk of many diseases and premature death. The following summary of deaths caused by smoking was given in 1977 by Dr. William Pollin of the U.S. National Institute on Drug Abuse.

In 1977 it was estimated that more than 37 million people (one of every six Americans) die from cigarette smoking years before they otherwise would (Pollin, 1977). This means that 350,000 Americans die prematurely each year because of tobacco (Fielding, 1985a). If tobacco-related deaths were eliminated, there would be 170,000, or 30 percent, fewer deaths from coronary heart disease; 125,000, or 30 percent, fewer deaths from all cancers and 80 percent fewer from lung cancer; and 62,000 fewer deaths from bronchitis and emphysema. In addition, smoking is responsible for 25 percent of all deaths caused by fires, accounting for the loss of more than 1,500 lives and for more than 4,000 fire-related injuries every year.

Heart Disease

Heart disease caused by tobacco smoke appears to be due largely to the combined action of nicotine and carbon monoxide; the nicotine increases the workload of the heart, and the carbon monoxide reduces the oxygen-carrying capacity of the blood and consequently the oxygen supply to the heart itself. These effects are further complicated by the fact that other constituents in the smoke reduce the lungs' ability to absorb oxygen, so the heart must work even harder pumping more blood through the lungs to satisfy the oxygen needs of the body. In addition, there is a relationship between *atherosclerosis* and the number of cigarettes smoked per day. Atherosclerosis is a disease wherein plaques, or deposits, build up in blood vessels and eventually stop the circulation of blood. When the blood flow to the heart itself is stopped in this manner, the heart muscle dies, and a heart attack results. Atherosclerosis is caused in part by high cholesterol levels in the blood, but smoking doubles the risk of heart attack both in people who have normal cholesterol levels and blood pressure and in those with raised cholesterol and high blood pressure. Figure 8–4 summarizes how smoking cigarettes contributes to heart disease.

Lung Disease

When tobacco smoke is inhaled, the ash and tars are deposited on the moist membranes on the inside surface of the lung through which oxygen and carbon dioxide must pass to and from the blood. Normally, particles are cleared from the lungs by small hairs called *cilia* that agitate and work the pollutants upward until they are ejected by coughing. Another line of defense against inhaled particles is the action of *phagocytes*. The phagocytes attack, surround, and destroy foreign matter in the lungs. Smoking reduces the actions of both the cilia and the phagocytes, leaving the lungs more vulnerable to the toxic effects of inhaled pollutants and infections by bacteria and viruses. As a result, smokers are more susceptible to chronic bronchitis and emphysema.

Cancer

The causal link between smoking and cancer is less well established. It is known that smoking greatly increases the risk of cancers of the mouth, lungs, and bladder, but the mechanism by which tobacco smoke actually causes cancer is not entirely understood. There are a number of substances in tobacco smoke that could produce cancerous cells by altering the DNA in normal body cells, but whether this process is what actually takes place in humans has not been conclusively demonstrated. What is known is that smoking greatly increases the risk of cancers produced by other known carcinogens such as pollutants, asbestos, and alcohol. For example, the risk of smokers getting cancer of the mouth and pharynx is two to six times greater in heavy drinkers than in nondrinkers (Rothman & Keller, 1972).

The risk of lung cancer can be greatly decreased by quitting, and the risk lessens considerably over time after a person stops as shown in Table 8–1.

Reproduction

There is some debate whether women who smoke are more likely to be infertile than nonsmokers, but the bulk of evidence to date suggests that they are and that the effect is dose related. Women who smoke more than 20 cigarettes per day are 1.7 to 3.2 times more likely to be infertile than nonsmokers. It also appears that the effect is reversible and that fertility returns to normal after cessation of smoking (Baird, 1992).

There is now some evidence that smoking during pregnancy may cause birth defects. Such defects are associated with smoking of both the

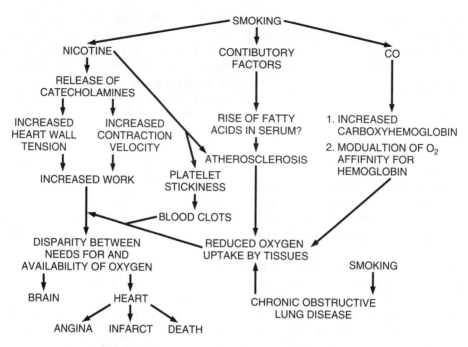

Figure 8–4 The mechanisms by which smoking contributes to heart disease are shown in this diagram. Smoking increases the demand on the heart by increasing its workload while at the same time decreasing the oxygen the heart muscle receives by increasing carboxyhemoglobin and causing atherosclerosis and lung diseases. (From Van Lancker, 1977, p. 252.)

mother and father (U.S. DHHS, 1990a). In addition, many years of research have clearly established that babies born to women who smoke during pregnancy are likely to be anywhere from 150 to 200 grams lighter at birth than babies born to nonsmoking mothers. This effect is dose dependent and is estimated to be a loss of birthweight of 11 grams per cigarette smoked per day by the mother. The weight loss may occur because smokers do not put on as much weight during pregnancy as nonsmokers do and therefore their babies would be lighter. Another possibility might be that the developing fetus receives less oxygen from the body of a smoking mother because of the reduced oxygen-carrying capacity of her blood (C. S. Russell, Taylor, & Law, 1968).

In any case, women who smoke during pregnancy are more likely to spontaneously abort and have babies prematurely, and their children are also more likely to be ill and die (Kramer, 1987; U.S. DHHS, 1989; U.S. DHHS, 1990b).

Further research has shown that the effects of maternal smoking can last for some time. At 7 years of age, the children of mothers who smoked during pregnancy have lower spelling and reading scores, have shorter attention spans, and are more often hyperactive than children of mothers who did not smoke during pregnancy (Naeye & Peters, 1984). It is not clear, however, whether these effects are due entirely to smoking or to some other factor that correlates with smoking.

Table 8–1   The Relative Risk of Lung Cancer in Ex-Smoking Women by the Number of Years since Quitting

Cigarettes per day	1–20	20+
Never smoked	1.0	1.0
Current smokers	10.3	21.2
Years Since Quitting:		
less than 2	13.6	32.4*
3–5	8.4	20.3
6–10	3.3	11.4
11–15	3.0	4.1
16+	1.0	4.0

Source: Garfinkle and Silverberg, 1991.

*Read: The risk of getting lung cancer of a woman who smoked more than 20 cigarettes a day and has quit for less than two years is 32.4 times greater than a woman who never smoked.

It has been estimated that if maternal smoking could be eliminated altogether, the overall infant death rate could be reduced by 10 percent (Haglund & Cnattingius, 1990).

Environmental Tobacco Smoke

Smoking is unhealthy not only for smokers, but also for those who work and live with them. In 1992, the U.S. Environmental Protection Agency (U.S. EPA, 1992), released a document reviewing what was known at that time about the dangers of being exposed to environmental tobacco smoke (ETS).

ETS comes from two sources, *mainstream smoke* (MS), smoke that the smoker inhales and then breathes back out into the atmosphere, and *sidestream smoke* (SS), smoke that issues from a burning cigarette between puffs. Mainstream smoke is created when the smoker draws air through the cigarette, and so the flame that creates MS smoke is 200 to 300 degrees hotter than the flame that creates SS smoke. While both types of smoke contain the same carcinogens and toxic substances, the combustion differences mean that the concentration of these substances is much higher in SS smoke than MS smoke. For example, the concentration of one carcinogen, *4-ABP*, is 30 times greater in SS than MS smoke. Levels of 4-APB in the blood of nonsmokers have been measured at 10 to 20 percent that of smokers even though the smoke they inhale is much less concentrated (U.S. EPA, 1992).

The EPA report concluded that in the United States carcinogens in ETS are responsible for 3,000 lung cancer deaths per year among nonsmokers. Even though the health dangers of ETS are present for all age groups, children are particularly vulnerable. The report also concludes that ETS is responsible for between 150,000 and 300,000 cases of bronchitis and pneumonia in infants up to 18 months of age, and that ETS exposure worsens the severity of symptoms of between 200,000 to 1 million asthmatic children per year (U.S. EPA, 1992; Spitzer et al., 1990). The report also finds a strong link between ETS and sudden infant death syndrome (SIDS, infants dying suddenly and unexpectedly between the ages of 1 month and one year of age). The risk of dying of SIDS is between 1.6 and 7.7 times greater for babies of smoking mothers than for babies of nonsmokers. The risk is also dose dependent, higher for babies in homes where the mother smokes more than 20 cigarettes per day (U.S. EPA, 1992; Nicholl & O'Cathain, 1992). It has been estimated that there would be a 27 percent decrease in SIDS if maternal smoking were eliminated (Haglund & Cnattingius (1990).

The low birthweights created by smoking while pregnant can also occur in nonsmoking women if they are exposed to several hours of ETS daily (U.S. EPA, 1992).

CHAPTER SUMMARY

- Nicotine is a drug found exclusively in the tobacco plant, which is consumed in various forms. It may also be administered in the form of a transdermal patch or nicotine chewing gum.

- Nicotine is absorbed best from the lungs and is distributed rapidly throughout the body. It is both excreted unchanged by the kidneys and metabolized by the liver. It has a half-life of about 30 minutes.

- Even though nicotine increases arousal level in the brain, smokers report that nicotine causes a feeling of relaxation. Some studies have shown that nicotine has little effect on performance, but others have concluded that nicotine at certain levels can enhance performance on some tasks.

- Intravenous and smoked nicotine are reported to cause brief euphoric episodes, or *rushes*.

- Nicotine has unpleasant withdrawal symptoms, which include irritability, weight gain, and sleep disturbances. Withdrawal can interfere with performance.

- Although nicotine is not self-administered by nonhumans as readily as many other drugs, tobacco is a powerful reinforcer for humans. One possible source of the reinforcing effect of nicotine is the sudden high concentration of nicotine that the brain receives after a puff on a cigarette; this is the *nicotine bolus* theory. Another theory, the *psychological tool* theory, claims that smokers use nicotine to increase and decrease level of arousal so as to enhance performance.

- Population studies show that the *demand for cigarettes is inelastic* in established smokers, but in young smokers, price increases are effective in decreasing the number of smokers and the number of cigarettes they smoke.

- Those who are able to quit usually do so for health reasons, motivated by experiencing a symptom of smoking-related disease. The *transdermal patch* and *nicotine gum,* which relieve the unpleasant effects of withdrawal, are effective aids to quitting.

- Smoking is not healthy. Tobacco smoking has been linked to heart disease, lung diseases such as emphysema and lung cancer, and cancer of the mouth and bladder. Smoking during pregnancy causes increases in the rate of stillbirths and illness in the newborn.

- *Environmental tobacco smoke (ETS)* from *mainstream smoke* (smoke inhaled and expelled by smokers) and *sidestream smoke* (uninhaled smoke from a burning cigarette) have also been shown to present a health hazard to nonsmokers.

9

Caffeine and the Methylxanthines

Coffee is useless since it serveth neither Nourishment nor Debauchery.

—Anonymous, 1650 (Austin, 1985, p. 236)

Caffeine is the best-known member of a family of drugs known as the *xanthine stimulants* or the *methylxanthines*. Although there are many methylxanthines besides caffeine, only two others occur naturally and are widely self-administered. These are *theophylline* and *theobromine*. The three have similar molecular structures and similar behavioral and physiological effects. The methylxanthines occur naturally in a number of species of plants belonging to 28 genera and over 17 families, but its most common sources are coffee, tea, and chocolate. Caffeine is also typically added to cola beverages and is an ingredient in many over-the-counter painkillers, cold remedies, and stimulants.

Caffeine was first isolated from coffee in 1820 by Ferdinand Runge, a German chemist, who called it *Kaffeebase*. It has been suggested that Runge's interest in coffee was stimulated by Wolfgang von Goethe, the author of *Faust*, who was a close friend of Runge's and a great coffee lover. No one is sure where the name *caffeine* came from, but a medical dictionary first used the term in 1823. Theobromine was isolated in 1842 and theophylline in 1888. Most of the basic chemistry of the methylxanthines was worked out and published in 1907 in a book by the Nobel Prize–winning organic chemist Emil Fischer.

SOURCES OF METHYLXANTHINES

Caffeine is available to us from a wide variety of sources. Table 9–1 gives a summary of some of these sources and an estimate of the amount of caffeine and other methylxanthines they contain.

Coffee

Coffee is made from the fruit of a bush or small tree of the genus *Coffea*. The two most common species are the *arabica* and the *canephora* (also called *robusta*) which together account for 99 percent of the world's coffee.

Table 9-1   Sources of Methylxanthines

Source	CAFFEINE (MG)		Other Methylxanthines
	Mean	Range	
Coffee (5-oz. cup)			
Instant	60	40–108	
Percolated	85	64–124	
Drip	112	56–176	
Decaffeinated	5	2–5	
Tea (5-oz. cup)			
Bag	40	28–48	Theophylline
Instant	30	24–31	Theophylline
Cola beverages (12 oz.)			
Coca-Cola	45		
Pepsi-Cola	30		
Chocolate (1 oz.)			
Milk	6	1–15	
Sweet	20	5–35	
Baking (bittersweet)	35	18–118	150–300* mg
Chocolate milk (8 oz.)	5	2–7	75–100* mg
Chocolate bar (40–50 g)	—	40–50	86–240* mg
Over-the-counter analgesics (1 tablet)			
Anacin	32		
Dristan	16		
Excedrin	65		
Pre-Mens	66		
Vanquish	32		
Over-the-counter stimulants (1 tablet)			
Wake Ups	100		
No-Dōz	100		
Ban Drowz	100		
Vivarin	200		

Source: Gilbert (1976); Syed (1976); Barone and Roberts (1984); Mumford et al. (1994).
*Theobromine.

They are native to Ethiopia but now widely cultivated in Africa and South America and in tropical climates all over the world. The coffee bean is a seed kernel of the coffee berry (or cherry), which grows in clumps along the branches. Each berry contains two seeds within its pulp. Usually the berry is picked and dried briefly in the sun before the seeds are removed from inside the pulp.

In preparation for making coffee, the beans are roasted. Roasting serves no function other than to enhance the flavor. The roasted beans are then crushed or ground and mixed with boiling water. The caffeine content of a cup of coffee may vary considerably because of a number of factors, including the caffeine concentration in the coffee beans (*robusta* has about twice the caffeine content of *arabica*), method of brewing (most brewing methods extract nearly all the available caffeine), and the size of the cup. Actual surveys have shown that the caffeine content of a cup of coffee may range between 40 and 176 mg, but the mean is closer to 85 mg (Barone & Roberts, 1984). However, this estimate is based on a cup size of 5 oz. (150 ml) of coffee. This size may be generally found in restaurants and hospitals, but actual measurements of "typical" cups used in the home and at work are closer to 7.5 oz. (225 ml). Table 9–1 shows typical sources of caffeine, but this table assumes the 5-oz. cup size. These figures can be increased by 50 percent. For the sake of convenience, it is usually presumed that a regular cup of coffee contains 100 mg of caffeine.

In order to decaffeinate coffee, it is brewed and mixed with a solvent that absorbs the caffeine. The solvent is then removed along with the caffeine, and the remaining coffee is dried and prepared in the same manner as ordinary coffee.

Tea

Tea is made from the leaves of *Camellia sinensis*, which in its natural form is a large tree but in its commercial cultivated form is more like a bush. For the best-quality teas, only the bud and the first two leaves of each twig are plucked. Inferior-quality teas are made from the third and fourth leaves. Caffeine content, as well as quality, decreases the farther the leaf is from the bud.

A drink may be made from the raw green leaves, but such concoctions are rather bitter. Most of the tea consumed outside of Asia is black or *fermented tea* (the process is not really fermentation but *oxidation*). The green leaves are dried slightly and then crushed and left to oxidize. The crushing or rolling breaks the membrane and releases enzymes that cause the oxidation. This turns the leaf black and gives it a particular taste. In semifermented or *oolong* tea, the oxidation process is stopped by roasting before it is completed. In *green Chinese tea* or *unfermented tea,* the leaves are steamed soon after picking and before drying to prevent oxidation. Consequently, green tea has quite a different taste from black tea. In the Orient, teas are frequently scented with flower petals. Jasmine tea is an example.

The amount of caffeine in a cup of tea is variable, but it is probably less than in a cup of coffee. One study showed a median of 27 mg per 5-oz. cup with a range of 8 to 91 mg. In addition to caffeine, tea also contains theophylline and theobromine (Gilbert, 1976; Graham, 1984).

Cocoa

Cocoa is made from seeds found in the seedpods of the cacao tree, *Theobroma cacao*, which is native to the dense, tropical Amazon rain forest. It is cultivated now mainly in Central and South America, the West Indies, and West Africa. The mature tree grows seedpods from the trunk and main branches. These pods are about 6 to 10 inches long and 3 to 4 inches in diameter and contain 20 to 40 seeds surrounded by pulp. The seeds are removed and put in boxes or piles for fermentation. During this process, which lasts five to six days, the pulp ferments, becomes very watery, and separates from the seed; fermentation heats the beans, which causes them to germinate and then kills them. The beans are then dried in the sun or in commercial driers. All these things are done on the plantation.

At this stage the dried beans are shipped to manufacturing plants for further processing. The beans are roasted for enhanced flavor and then crushed, and the husks of the shells are removed. The result is sold as *unsweetened chocolate*, a product that has a high fat content and is not very appealing. In 1828 a Dutchman named Van Houten invented a press that could remove most of the fat, or cocoa butter. This turned out to be a major breakthrough in the processing of cocoa. In addition to inventing the press, the Dutch also learned to *alkalize* cocoa, which gives it a stronger flavor and a darker color and makes the powder disperse better in water. (The name *cacao* refers to the tree and its seeds; the term *cocoa* is used to refer to the processed products of the bean. Care should be taken not to confuse either of these terms with *coca*, the bush that is the source of cocaine; see Chapter 10.)

In the production of cocoa powder, the unsweetened chocolate is pressed into cakes.

This process removes a large part of the cocoa butter. The cakes are then ground to produce the dry cocoa powder. Chocolate is made by mixing the roasted, alkalized, and refined beans with sugar and cocoa butter and, in the case of milk chocolate, with milk or milk solids. The details of the mixing process are complicated and vary according to the type of chocolate being produced and its proposed use (Minifie, 1970).

Chocolate contains both caffeine and theobromine in varying concentrations. It has been estimated that an ounce of sweet chocolate may contain between 75 and 150 mg of combined methylxanthines, and a cup of hot chocolate or chocolate milk may contain 150 to 300 mg.

Other Natural Sources of Methylxanthines

Other natural sources of caffeine are the *ilex* plant of the Amazon region of South America and the *cassina* of North America. The ilex plant, *Ilex paraguayensis*, is a holly (related to the Christmas holly) that contains between 1 and 2 percent caffeine. A tealike drink called *maté* is made from the leaves and is popular in South America. Each morning men of the Peruvian Achuar Jivaro tribe are reported to drink a strong herbal tea made from the ilex that contains the caffeine equivalent of 5 cups of coffee, after which they vomit in order to avoid overdose symptoms. It is considered to be part of a macho ritual passed down through the ages (*Science News*, 1992).

Cassina is another type of holly, *Ilex vomitoria*, from which a beverage known as *youpon, cassina tea,* or *black drink* is made. Youpon is not used today, but at one time it was widely consumed by native peoples of the southeastern United States. It was considered a noble beverage, and its use was restricted to great men and chiefs. Cassina tea enjoyed a revival during the American Civil War and World War I when coffee and tea were either not available or very expensive.

Guarana is a paste made from the seeds of *Paullaina cupana*, which, at 2 to 6 percent caffeine, is the most potent of the natural sources of caffeine. The plant grows in the regions of the Amazon, Orinoco, and Negro rivers in South America. The paste is moulded into sticks or bars, or even sculptures, and dried in the sun. For use, it is powdered and mixed with water. Because it has an acrid taste, like chocolate, it is usually sweetened with sugar.

There are a number of species of the genus *Cola*, a small evergreen tree native to southern Nigeria, whose nuts are edible and contain caffeine and theobromine. Kola trees are now cultivated all over western Africa, and chewing the nut is a widespread habit. The nut is sold commercially to the United States, where it is used to flavor cola beverages such as Coca-Cola and Pepsi-Cola. Most of the caffeine in these beverages, however, does not come from the kola nut but is added later.

Medicines and Food Additives

In addition to being added to cola beverages, caffeine is also added in small quantities for flavor to pudding mixes, baked goods, dairy desserts, and candy (Barone & Roberts, 1984).

Caffeine can be found in hundreds of prescription and over-the-counter medicines. Table 9–1 shows a few of these. They include common analgesics such as Anacin, weight control aids, allergy relief compounds, and stimulants.

Both theophylline and caffeine are used as a respiratory stimulant for newborn babies and people suffering from asthma.

HISTORY OF METHYLXANTHINE USE

Coffee

The coffee bush is native to Ethiopia. Its properties were discovered sometime between the twelfth and fifteenth centuries. From there its use spread across Arabia, Egypt, and North Africa, around the Mediterranean into Turkey, and then to Europe.

William Harvey, the first person to describe the circulation of the blood, was one of the first coffee drinkers in England, and he promoted the beverage for its therapeutic benefits. Two of his students believed that it was a cure for drunkenness (Austin, 1985). The first English coffeehouse opened in Oxford in 1650, and the concept soon spread throughout England. The coffeehouses were referred to as "schools of the cultured," and coffee was "the milk of chess players and thinkers." Along with coffee, this intellectual tradition associated with coffeehouses soon spread throughout Europe.

At one time coffee drinking gained such popularity in England the consumption of alcoholic beverages, particulary cheap gin, started to decline. Coffee remained popular throughout Europe, as it still is today, but in Great Britain it was eventually replaced by tea.

Though tea was the preferred drink in colonial America, coffeehouses were as common as in England and filled the same social function—a meeting place for intellectual and political discussion. Boston coffeehouses such as the Brown, the North End Coffee-House, and the Exchange served as headquarters for Whigs and Tories and were the scenes of much plotting and fighting. One famous coffeehouse, the Green Dragon, is still marked by a plaque at the site where "such adventurous and ardent patriots as Otis, Joseph Warren, John Adams, Samuel Adams, Cushing, Pitts, Molyneux, and Paul Revere met nightly to discuss public affairs" (Cheney, 1925, p. 233).

Tea

There are many legends about the origins of tea. One tale credits the discovery of the beverage to the Chinese emperor Chen Nung. It is known that tea was cultivated and sold commercially in China by A.D. 780 when the book *Ch'a Ching*, or *Tea Classic*, was written. The book was sponsored by a group of merchants, and its purpose was to promote tea drinking (D. Forrest, 1973, p. 16).

Tea was first mentioned in print in Europe in 1559, but it was not until 1606 that the Dutch actually shipped some to Europe. In the 1630s the Dutch started shipping tea on a regular basis to satisfy a growing demand in their country as well as Germany and France. Tea was also becoming popular in Portugal, which had an extensive Oriental trade of its own. In the 1640s and 1650s tea enjoyed a brief phase of popularity in France, but this was short-lived, and the French turned to coffee in the 1660s.

All this time, tea was not extensively used in England. It did not become fashionable until Charles II married the Infanta Catherine, who brought tea drinking with her from Portugal in 1662. Tea also became popular in the 13 colonies of North America. In fact, by 1760 tea was the third-largest export from England to the colonies, and this figure represented only a quarter of the total tea imported; the rest was smuggled. The reason for this smuggling was the tea tax the English Parliament at Westminster imposed on all tea imported into Britain. When this tea was later shipped to America, the price included this import tax. In 1767 this indirect tax was removed and a direct tax imposed. These taxes angered the colonists, and when the British East India Company tried to export a tea surplus to the colonies in 1773, the angry colonists dumped it into Boston harbor. This "tea party" was the first of many and set the stage for the American Revolution.

Cocoa

The Mayas of the Yucatán Peninsula, the Aztecs of Mexico, and the Incas of Peru cultivated the cacao tree long before the European discovery of North America. They believed it to be a gift of the gods. This belief is the origin of the genus name of the cacao bush, *Theobroma*, which is Greek for "food of the gods." Among the Central American Indian tribes, chocolate was a food generally reserved for the wealthy and powerful. It was believed to be an aphrodisiac and was used at wedding feasts and by wealthy noblemen who could afford to support and had to satisfy many wives. It has been reported that Montezuma, emperor of the Aztecs at the time of Cortés, consumed 50 golden goblets full a day. He called it *chocolatl*, but what he downed must have been quite different from modern chocolate. The Aztecs' concoction included maize and spices such as peppers but no sugar or milk.

Cortés introduced the drink to the Spanish court in 1520 with the addition of vanilla and sugar, and this sweetened form eventually gained popularity all over Europe. The Spanish managed to keep the source of chocolate secret for 100 years, but eventually the Dutch introduced the plant into the Philippines and Ceylon (now Sri Lanka).

Chocolate was introduced into Europe before coffee and tea and enjoyed a brief popularity, but because it was expensive, its use was restricted to the wealthy and the nobility. In every case it was displaced by coffee, which remains the most popular xanthine-containing beverage today. (The exception is in England, where coffee was replaced by tea.) In time chocolate did become cheaper and more readily available, but not until too late. The first chocolate factory in England was founded by S. J. Fry in 1728 when chocolate became more plentiful, but by that time tea was the indisputable beverage of the people.

Even though chocolate did not make it as a popular drink, with the development of better processing techniques it did make it as a confection.

Today the bulk of the world's supply of cocoa comes from West Africa rather than South America. It is also grown commercially in Indonesia and Sri Lanka. It is perhaps ironic that cocoa, which is native to South America, is now a more profitable crop in Africa. The South Americans,

however, have had their revenge many times over, since coffee, which is a native African plant, is now grown primarily in South America.

ROUTE OF ADMINISTRATION

When consumed in natural products, the methylxanthines are normally taken orally without difficulty, but when given for medical reasons, the purified drugs sometimes cause nausea and gastric irritation, especially in children. In such cases the drugs may be given in the form of a rectal suppository, or by intramuscular or intravenous routes.

Absorption

Although the methylxanthines are absorbed from the stomach, they are absorbed much more rapidly through the walls of the intestine. Factors that decrease stomach-emptying time, such as the presence of food, will slow methylxanthine absorption. The methylxanthines are bases, and consequently when they are dissolved in the acidic environment of the digestive system, you might expect them to be highly ionized and not lipid soluble. However, these drugs have a very low pKa, about 0.5. Consequently, at the pH of the digestive system, and any other pH encountered in the body, the methylxanthines will not be ionized at all and will be free to dissolve in any tissue in accordance with their lipid solubility. The methylxanthines are quite lipid soluble and dissolve poorly in water.

The caffeine in coffee, tea, and chocolate exists and is consumed in its alkaloid form, but for medicinal purposes the methylxanthines are usually given as salts. In this form they are absorbed much more readily. *Aminophylline* is the most widely used methylxanthine preparation. It is a mixture of theophylline and *methylenediamine*. This latter substance is considered therapeutically inert, but it increases the amount of dissolved theophylline 20 times and thereby speeds absorption. *Oxtriphylline (Choledyl* or *choline theophylline)* is also widely used.

After drinking coffee or tea, a person completely absorbs caffeine from the digestive system, and peak blood levels of caffeine are reached between 30 and 60 minutes later (Marks & Kelly, 1973; Axelrod & Reisenthal, 1953; Arnaud, 1994), although peak absorption may vary between 15 to 120 minutes depending on the amount of caffeine swallowed and ingestion of other foods. There is also considerable individual variability in peak blood levels, with the same dose producing a sixfold variation in peak blood levels in different individuals (Dews, 1984). There is no significant first pass metabolism.

There is some evidence that caffeine in cola beverages is absorbed more slowly than caffeine from coffee and tea and reaches a peak after one or two hours.

DISTRIBUTION

Caffeine crosses the blood-brain and placental barriers without difficulty and reaches all body organs, although the rates of entering and leaving these organs may vary. About 10 to 30 percent of caffeine in the blood becomes bound to protein and trapped in the circulatory system (Axelrod & Reisenthal, 1953; Arnaud, 1994). Caffeine is present in all body fluids including breast milk.

EXCRETION

In humans, less than 2 percent of caffeine is excreted in the urine unchanged (Arnaud, 1993), and the remainder is converted to various metabolites (Burg, 1975; Bonati & Garattini, 1984). For a given individual, the half-life of caffeine is fairly constant, but this may vary from 2½ to more than 4½ hours in different individuals, with a mean of 3½ hours. In spite of this long half-life,

it has been shown that caffeine does not appear to accumulate in the bodies of normal individuals over days if caffeine is not consumed after 6 P.M. (Axelrod & Reisenthal, 1953). In nonhumans the half-life varies considerably, from 11 to 12 hours in the pig and squirrel monkey to 2 hours in the rat (Kihlman, 1977, pp. 20–21).

Caffeine metabolism is slowed by alcohol and speeded by broccoli (yes, it is good for you), and smokers eliminate caffeine twice as fast as nonsmokers (Parsons & Neims, 1978; J. J. James, 1991). Women metabolize caffeine 20 to 30 percent faster than men, but in women, rate of elimination is closely related to hormone levels. The caffeine half-life in women is longer during the luteal phase (after ovulation) than the follicular phase (before ovulation) of the menstrual cycle (Arnaud, 1993), and the half-life in women taking oral contraceptive steroids is twice that of women ovulating regularly (Callahan et al., 1983). Caffeine elimination is also slowed during pregnancy (Neims, Bailey, & Aldrich, 1979). These changes appear to be due to alterations in enzyme levels.

It has also been shown that newborns cannot metabolize caffeine well and excrete about 85 percent of it unchanged in the urine, with the result that the half-life is about four days. The adult pattern of caffeine metabolism is not developed until 7 to 9 months of age (Aldrich, Aranda, & Neims, 1979).

Caffeine is metabolized into numerous metabolites, but no other species metabolizes caffeine the way that humans do. For this reason one must always approach nonhuman studies of the methylxanthines with caution because some metabolites created in other species may be more active or toxic than those created in humans (Stavric & Gilbert, 1990). Even in humans, there are differences in metabolic pathways between infants and adults. Not only do newborn babies metabolize methylxanthines more slowly, but they also create different metabolites (Aldrich, Aranda, & Neims, 1979).

NEUROPHYSIOLOGICAL EFFECTS

The effects of methylxanthines on neural functioning are not well understood, but there are a number of interesting theories based on known physiological actions of caffeine.

One promising explanation involves the effect of methylxanthines on *adenosine* receptors. Adenosine functions as a neuromodulator and works presynaptically by blocking the release of many neurotransmitters, and it reduces the rate of spontaneous firing of neurons. Its general effect is to inhibit the firing of many neurons in the brain. It may also act postsynaptically as a neurotransmitter, but this possibility has not been established. The methylxanthines compete with adenosine for its receptor and block it, thus preventing adenosine's inhibitory action and causing stimulation (Snyder, 1981, 1984; Nehlig, Daval, & Debry, 1992).

In addition to its effect on adenosine, caffeine and the methylxanthines are also known to block benzodiazepine receptors, but this effect seems to require higher doses of caffeine than those that normally cause behavioral effects. At the dose equivalent of 10 cups of coffee, as many as 20 percent of benzodiazepine receptors are blocked (Paul et al., 1980). Among the methylxanthines, however, there does not seem to be a correlation between the ability to block benzodiazepine receptors and most of the methylxanthine's effects (Snyder, 1984), but it is possible that some of the effects of caffeine, particularly the increases in anxiety seen at high doses, are mediated by the ability of the drug to block benzodiazepine receptors.

Caffeine also appears to cause the release of epinephrine and other catecholamines from brain tissues and from the adrenal gland at usual doses. These indirect effects may also contribute to the stimulating effects of the drug. It is also known that large doses, in the range of 500 mg taken all at once, cause a response similar to the body's reaction to acute stress: The levels of some hormones drop, and corticosteroid and internal opiate (beta-endorphin) levels increase (Spindel & Wurtman, 1984). It is not known whether this effect is mediated by adenosine or benzodiazepine receptors.

EFFECTS OF CAFFEINE AND THE METHYLXANTHINES

Effects on the Body

Since the methylxanthines cause the release of epinephrine from the adrenal gland, there is a resultant stimulation of the sympathetic nervous system. However, much of caffeine's effect outside the CNS is due to its direct effect on the muscles; smooth muscles tend to relax, and striated muscles are strengthened.

The smooth muscle relaxation results in a dilation of the bronchi of the lungs, which decreases airway resistance. Theophylline is the most potent methylxanthine in producing this effect, and as a result it is used clinically in the treatment of asthma. Methylxanthines also reduce the susceptibility of striated (voluntary) muscles to fatigue. The mechanism of this change is probably related to caffeine-caused increases in fatty acids that the muscles can use as fuel (Nehlig & Debry, 1994). Possibly related to this effect is a decrease in hand steadiness (Dews, 1984).

Caffeine has different effects on blood flow in different parts of the body: It causes a constriction of blood vessels in the brain but dilation in the rest of the body. By constricting the blood flow to the brain, caffeine is able to reduce headaches caused by high blood pressure, and for this reason caffeine is found in many over-the-counter headache remedies.

High levels of caffeine stimulate the spinal cord. This is first manifested as an increase in excitability of spinal reflexes. Higher doses lead to convulsions, which are sometimes the cause of death at lethal doses. The regulatory centers of the medulla are also stimulated at high doses, producing an increase in the rate and depth of breathing. This ability of methylxanthines to stimulate respiration makes them useful in the treatment of babies born with breathing difficulties.

Many books suggest that the primary effect of caffeine on the brain is a stimulation of the cortex, but there is little evidence of this effect. Most of the evidence is indirect and based on behavioral studies (Gilbert, 1976).

Effects on Human Performance and Behavior

Textbooks usually give a standard account of the effects of caffeine at low doses (100 to 200 mg). Typically, the following sorts of effects are listed: "greater sustained intellectual effort and a more perfect association of ideas," "a keener appreciation of sensory stimuli" (Ritchie, 1975, p. 367). In reality, there is very little hard evidence that changes of this nature take place. No doubt such accounts are based on subjective experience and the intellectual tradition associated with coffee. Although subjective accounts can be useful in understanding drugs, they must be interpreted with great caution (see Chapter 2). In an early experiment by Goldstein, Kaizer, and Warren (1965), subjects were asked to rate the effects of caffeine on their alertness, physical activity, and wakefulness. Then they were given caffeine and tested on their ability to detect a number in an array of numbers flashed on a screen for $\frac{1}{32}$ second. They were also tested on coordination in a line-drawing task. The subjects' assessment of their alertness and physical activeness did not correlate with their real abilities as measured by these various tasks; though all subjects thought they were doing better, caffeine produced no improvement.

There are reports that moderate doses of caffeine can significantly increase visual sensitivity to light, increase the speed of auditory reaction time (Dews, 1984), improve some aspects of driving involving reaction time, and improve performance in a flight simulator (Nehlig, Daval, & Debry, 1992). Unfortunately, not all laboratories can replicate these effects, and some find decrements. It seems that the effects of caffeine depend upon many factors that include individual susceptibility, dose, time of consumption, and the nature of the task (James, 1991).

In an extensive review by Weiss and Laties (1962) and another review by Dews (1984), the effects of caffeine on human performance were evaluated. Both reviews concluded that performance on a wide range of activities, with the exception of intellectual tasks, could be enhanced by caffeine. These included athletic activities (see the next section) and perceptual tasks such as monitoring a visual array. It appears, however, that most reports of improved performance occur only if performance had been degraded by fatigue. The main effect of caffeine was to reduce the effect of drowsiness and boredom. Weiss and Laties also noticed that caffeine caused an improvement in the mood of subjects and in their attitude toward their task, but they were not able to determine whether this improvement in performance caused the mood change. In any case, it appears that coffee breaks may be beneficial, especially for people doing repetitive jobs.

Effects on Athletic Performance

It is still a matter of some controversy, but caffeine has been shown to improve performance on some types of athletic performance in doses of about 10 mg/kg (700 mg in a 155-lb. person). It does not seem to improve performance in events that require muscle strength such as weight lifting, nor does it improve performance that requires intense output over a short duration, for example, sprinting and throwing. It does, however, improve performance in tasks that require submaximal output for an extended period of time such as cross-country skiing, running, or cycling (Nehlig, Daval, & Debry, 1992). However, even in these events, results are far from consistent, and the effect is moderated by other factors such as body composition. It is not entirely clear how caffeine improves performance, but the most likely reason is that caffeine increases blood levels of fatty acids that can be used as fuel by the muscles. As a result, the muscles use less glycogen, their normal fuel, and keep it in reserve so that muscles are not fatigued as fast in endurance events. These effects are subject to tolerance, and there is a delay between maximal blood levels of fatty acids and caffeine blood levels. For this reason, athletes wanting to take advantage of this effect should abstain from taking caffeine for 4 days before the event and should consume caffeine 3 to 4 hours before the event (Nehlig & Debry, 1994).

Because of the possibility that caffeine is an athletic performance enhancer, caffeine is a drug controlled by the International Olympic Committee (Lombardo, 1986). Caffeine in concentrations in the urine higher than 15 mg/l is considered a disqualifying factor. One rough method of estimating blood caffeine concentrations (and consequently urine concentrations) is to assume that, on average, one cup of coffee increases blood level by 1 mg/l. Therefore, it would be necessary to drink 15 cups of coffee at one sitting to achieve this level. One study concluded that this concentration could not be reached by normal social consumption of caffeine-containing beverages and could only be achieved by deliberate doping. Nevertheless, bearing in mind the considerable individual variation in caffeine pharmacokinetics and the ubiquitous nature of caffeine in foods, soft drinks, and medicines, athletes required to submit urine samples for testing should be cautious. Only one athlete has ever been disqualified from Olympic completion for exceeding the caffeine limit, a member of the Australian pentathlon team in the 1988 Seoul Olympics (Janes, 1991).

Effects on Sleep

There is little doubt that the methylxanthines can produce insomnia (Goldstein, 1964). Their effect seems to be in increasing the "stability of wakefulness" by increasing the length of time it takes to fall asleep and reducing total sleeping time. In one study, 300 mg of caffeine caused an increase in the latency of sleep onset, normally 18 minutes, to 66 minutes, and reduced total sleeping time from 475 minutes to 350 minutes, compared to control subjects (Brenesova, Ozwald, & Loudon, 1975). As can be seen in Table 9–1, caffeine is the major ingredient in many over-the-counter stimulant pills. Most such tablets contain 100 mg of caffeine.

Though caffeine does not alter the frequency or duration of REM sleep, it does increase the percent of time spent in light sleep (stage 2) and decreases deep-sleep time (stages 3 and 4). In general, people who take caffeine before going to bed report sleeping less soundly and are less rested. Caffeine also lowers the acoustic arousal threshold while sleeping; that is, people wake up more easily in response to a sound in the night. This effect is variable between individuals, with habitual coffee drinkers being less affected than coffee abstainers. Recently it has been shown that this difference is probably due to tolerance rather than a preexisting difference between coffee drinkers and abstainers. After seven days of exposure to a 400-mg dose it was shown that measures such as total sleep time and awakenings had returned to baseline levels (Bonnet & Arand, 1992).

It has also been demonstrated that caffeine can counteract the sleep-inducing effects of pentobarbital. A usual sleep-inducing dose of pentobarbital, 100 mg, when given in combination with 250 mg of caffeine, produces the same effect on sleep as a placebo (Forrest, Bellville, & Brown, 1972).

Effect on Behavior of Nonhumans

Unconditioned Behavior. Caffeine will increase spontaneous motor activity of mice in an open field with maximum increases at 20 to 40 mg/kg. A dose of 80 mg/kg will greatly decrease spontaneous motor activity. Increases in activity are also produced by theophylline at similar doses, but there is some evidence that theophylline may be slightly more potent than caffeine (Scott & Chen, 1944).

The LD$_{50}$ of caffeine for both rats and mice is in the neighborhood of 250 mg/kg i.p. (Barnes & Elthrington, 1973). Death may be due to convulsions, but sometimes animals die at lower doses from bleeding as a result of attacking themselves. *Automutilation* has been observed in rats when caffeine was given at a dose of 185 mg/kg for 14 days. The rats bit their tails and paws even though they seemed to retain their normal sense of pain. When a ball of wire was placed in their cage, they temporarily attacked it but soon returned to biting themselves. When picked up, they did not bite the hand of the experimenter, but they did attack other rats placed with them in a cage (Peters, 1967).

Positively Motivated Behavior. The first person to experiment with the effects of caffeine on conditioned behavior was Pavlov (1927). He showed that the drug could disrupt conditioned discriminations by increasing responses to the negative stimulus. After ingesting caffeine, the animals responded to stimuli that did not signal food in the same way that they responded to stimuli that did signal food. He concluded that the drug produced "an increase in excitability of the Central Nervous System."

The methylxanthines are similar to amphetamine in that they will increase responding on an FI schedule and then depress it at higher doses. In mice the maximum increases are produced by 10 mg/kg of caffeine and 30 mg/kg of theophylline. The methylxanthines are different from amphetamine because they do not depress responding on an FR schedule at the same dose that also increases FI response rates (McKim, 1980).

Effects on Aversively Motivated Behavior. There is some evidence that caffeine at 30 mg/kg in the rat will increase food-reinforced responding that has been suppressed by being punished with an electric shock (Morrison, 1969). If this observation is true, it makes this effect of caf-

feine more similar to the barbiturates than to amphetamine.

In general, caffeine appears to increase avoidance responding. Increases were seen on nondiscriminated avoidance responding of squirrel monkeys at a dosage of 1 to 30 mg/kg of caffeine; these increases were almost as great as those seen with amphetamine (Davis, Kensler, & Dews, 1973). Doses of 10 and 15 mg/kg of caffeine also decreased response latencies of rats on a discriminated avoidance task (Battig & Grandjean, 1957).

Although the effects of caffeine and the other methylxanthines on conditioned animal behavior have not been extensively investigated, it appears that they are very different from the effects of amphetamine on some types of behavior and very similar to amphetamine on others. These data clearly show that caffeine cannot be thought of as a mild amphetamine; its behavioral properties are quite distinctive and difficult to classify with any other category of drug.

DISCRIMINATIVE STIMULUS PROPERTIES

At a dose of 32 mg/kg, rats can be trained to discriminate between caffeine and saline in a two-lever Skinner box. Rats generalize the state produced by caffeine to lower doses of caffeine and higher doses of theophylline, but there is no generalization to a range of doses of amphetamine, methylphenidate, or nicotine (Modrow, Holloway, & Carney, 1981). There is, however, partial generalization to cocaine, and caffeine will increase discriminative effects of low doses of cocaine.

For some time there has been a concern over what are known as *look-alike* or *turkey* drugs. These are preparations that look in all regards like a controlled psychoactive drug, such as amphetamine, but instead contain a drug or a combination of drugs that are not prescribed or controlled substances. Turkey drugs designed to mimic amphetamine or cocaine often contain caffeine in combination with other substances such as ephedrine and phenylpropanolamine. One study has shown that in rats, at least, this combination of drugs can mimic the discriminative stimulus effects of 10 mg/kg of cocaine (Gauvin et al., 1989).

Although there is considerable individual variability, humans can discriminate the presence of caffeine in capsules in very low doses. In one experiment a dose of 1.8 mg of caffeine was detected by one subject, although two others detected a dose of 10 mg and one subject needed 178 mg. In the same experiment, the same subject who was able to detect 1.8 mg of caffeine detected a dose of 100 mg theobromine, but two subjects out of seven were unable to discriminate 1,000 mg of theobromine (Mumford et al., 1994).

SUBJECTIVE EFFECTS

Early studies on the subjective effects of caffeine were confusing. In some studies subjects reported increased anxiety, jitteriness, and nervousness, and other studies reported no subjective effects at all. Recent studies, however, have found increasingly that subjects experience an array of positive effects such as increases in feelings of well-being, alertness, energy, motivation for work, and self-confidence. Griffiths and Mumford (1995; Rush, Sullivan, & Griffiths, 1995) report that positive effects are more reliably detected under a restricted set of conditions. First, they are seen when caffeine is administered to people who are not caffeine users, or caffeine users who have been deprived at least overnight. The fact that positive effects are seen in coffee abstainers indicates that these effects are not simply a matter of alleviating caffeine withdrawal. Second, positive effects are more likely to be seen at low doses of from 20 to 200 mg. The higher the dose, the more likely it is that unpleasant effects will be reported. Finally, positive effects are most likely to be reported by individuals

for whom caffeine acts as a positive reinforcer (see the next section).

In a study by Mumford and associates (1994) subjects were given 178 mg of caffeine, and responses to a mood scale were determined at various times afterward. The drug caused increases in well-being, magnitude of drug effect, energy, affection for loved ones, motivation to work, self-confidence, social disposition, alertness, and concentration, and decreases in "sleepy" and "muzzy" feelings. These changes were evident within 30 minutes and remained higher than placebo levels for at least eight hours.

The same study also examined the subjective effects of theobromine. A dose of 100 mg produced positive changes in energy, motivation to work and alertness, but to a much smaller extent than caffeine. The time course for these changes was similar to caffeine, but five to ten hours after ingestion subjects reported unpleasant effects such as headache and lethargy.

In another experiment, subjects with experience with street drug use including cocaine were given intravenous doses of caffeine, and subjective effects were measured. There was a dose-related increase in ratings of "liking," "drug effect," "high," and "good effects." These occurred two minutes after injection and decreased over the following 60 minutes. At high doses, caffeine was identified as "a stimulant (like cocaine or amphetamine)." Most subjects were reasonably certain that they had been given cocaine (Rush, Sullivan, & Griffiths, 1995).

TOLERANCE

Studies of adenosine receptors have shown that chronic administration of caffeine causes an increase in the number of adenosine receptors, presumably an attempt to restore the influence of adenosine prior to caffeine (Hirsh, 1984).

Tolerance to the behavior effects of caffeine has been shown to develop in rats. One study (Wayner et al., 1976) showed that bar pressing on an FI schedule could be depressed to about 40 percent saline control rates by a 100 mg/kg injection of caffeine. After eight injections of caffeine this dose could only depress responding to 75 percent of baseline. It has also been demonstrated in a study of operant responding in rats that chronic treatment with caffeine shifted the caffeine DRC to the right by a factor of 6. This means that after exposure to caffeine, a sixfold increase in dose was required to produce the same effect as before the exposure (Carney, 1982).

A number of studies using human subjects show that caffeine has less effect on heavy drinkers of coffee than on nondrinkers of coffee. In one experiment (Goldstein, Kaizer, & Whitby, 1969), it was shown that 150 to 300 mg of caffeine produced complaints of jitteriness, nervousness, and upset stomach in nonusers, but users reported increased alertness, decreased irritability, and a feeling of contentedness. It should be pointed out that studies like these, while probably demonstrating tolerance, may simply be showing that individuals who are resistant to the effects of caffeine are the ones who become heavy coffee drinkers.

To demonstrate tolerance to a drug effect, an experimenter must give the drug to one group of subjects and a placebo to a second group for a period of time. The effect must diminish in the drug-exposed group. Furthermore, the placebo group must show the effect when switched to the drug. Tolerance to several effects of caffeine has been demonstrated using this design. Different effects of caffeine at normal doses show tolerance at different rates; for example, cardiovascular effects fade within 2–5 days, but caffeine-induced increases in urination may take considerably longer or never show complete tolerance. Similarly, tolerance to various physiological effects has also been demonstrated (Griffiths & Mumford, 1995). We have seen that the sleep-disrupting effects of 400 mg caffeine show tolerance within seven days. Subjective effects of 300 mg tolerate within 4 days (Evans & Griffiths, 1992). In general, many effects of caffeine seem to disappear within a week at usual levels of consumption.

WITHDRAWAL

Laboratory animals appear to suffer from caffeine withdrawal, although the main symptom is a decrease in locomotor activity and a disruption of ongoing operant responding. In humans there have been a number of documented cases of caffeine withdrawal dating back to 1833. The most common symptom is a headache. In addition, people report drowsiness, decreased energy, and fatigue that can be described as weakness, letdown, or lethargy. People also report decreased motivation for work and impaired concentration, decreased feelings of well-being and self-confidence, increased irritability, and flulike feelings such as aches and muscle stiffness, hot and cold spells, heavy feelings in the limbs, and nausea (Griffiths & Mumford, 1995). The severity of symptoms is directly related to dose.

Doses as high as 600 mg per day can cause physical dependence after only 6 to 14 days of exposure. Withdrawal symptoms can also be seen at daily exposures of as little as 100 mg per day over a longer period of time (Griffiths & Mumford, 1995).

Withdrawal symptoms usually start within 12 to 24 hours of the last coffee intake, peak at 20 to 48 hours, and last as long as a week (Griffiths & Woodson, 1988; Griffiths & Mumford, 1995). Figure 9–1 shows the time-course incidence of headache and scores on an "energy/active" scale of subjects maintained on 100 mg of caffeine and switched to a placebo. As you can see, it took nearly two weeks for these scores to return to normal (Griffiths & Mumford, 1995).

Studies have shown that among coffee consumers in the United States who have gone without coffee for 24 hours, 27 to 52 percent report experiencing headaches. Estimates of the number of people who are exposed to caffeine with-

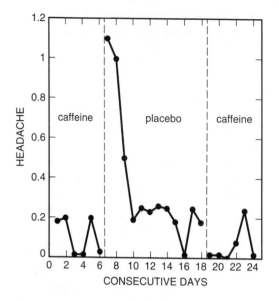

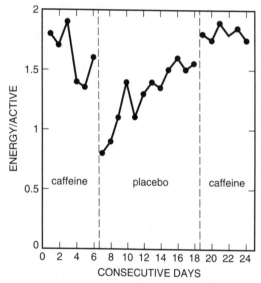

Figure 9–1 Changes in frequency of reported headaches and scores on an "energy/active" scale of subjects for 24 days while they were consuming 100 mg caffeine capsules and then a placebo, and then switched back to caffeine. Caffeine withdrawal caused increases in reported headaches and a decrease in energy and activity that lasted as long as a week. (From Griffiths, et al. 1990.)

drawal—that is, the number who consume more than 100 mg a day—is enormous. Caffeine withdrawal is often overlooked as a possible diagnosis when people report headache, fatigue, and mood disturbances in circumstances where normal diet, including caffeine, is disrupted. Such circumstances might include fasting before various laboratory tests, operations, or procedures such as endoscopies.

On a more mundane level, caffeine withdrawal may well be responsible for the behavior of people who are grouchy and impossible to get along with until they have had their first cup of coffee in the morning. It is probably also responsible for illnesses and headaches that occur during holidays or weekends or when people interrupt normal routines that include coffee drinking.

SELF-ADMINISTRATION IN NONHUMANS

In laboratory animals, caffeine is not a robust reinforcer. It can serve as a reinforcer, but only in a limited number of circumstances, and it does not seem to be able to support a lot of behavior. In one study where bar pressing delivered an i.v. caffeine infusion, only 2 out of 6 monkeys self-administered the caffeine spontaneously. The four monkeys that did not give themselves caffeine were then given automatic infusions of caffeine for a period of time. This procedure succeeded in establishing caffeine as a reinforcer in 3 of the 4 remaining monkeys (Deneau, Yanagita, & Seevers, 1969). The pattern of self-administration was irregular, with periods of voluntary abstinence. There was no tendency to increase dose over time. Other researchers have also demonstrated modest reinforcing effects with caffeine, but they were limited to specific doses and particular animals (Griffiths, Bigelow, & Lieberson, 1979). Other studies have not been able to demonstrate reinforcing effects of caffeine at all, although these studies used only one dose of caffeine or tested for only a short time (Hoffmeister & Wuttke, 1973).

Figure 9–2 shows the pattern of caffeine self-administration in a baboon (Griffiths & Mumford, 1995). This animal is typical of most. Caffeine is administered erratically, and irregular periods of abstinence occur. The reinforcing nature of caffeine is demonstrated, however, because rates of responding decline to near zero when a placebo is substituted.

Similar results have been found with rats given the opportunity to consume caffeine orally. Few spontaneously consume caffeine orally. Usually some period of forced consumption is required before caffeine is self-administered (Vitiello & Woods, 1975).

Even though it may not be a robust reinforcer on its own, caffeine has been shown to potentiate the reinforcing effects of cocaine (Horger et al., 1994), and it will act as a *primer* for cocaine; that is, an injection of caffeine will reinstate previously extinguished cocaine self-administration in rats (Worley, Valdez, & Schenk, 1994).

SELF-ADMINISTRATION IN HUMANS

A number of human self-administration preference studies have shown that both caffeinated coffee and capsules containing caffeine will serve as reinforcers in humans. These studies have shown that the preference for caffeine is partly determined by the state of physical dependence on caffeine. People who have been permitted to consume caffeine freely for one week be-

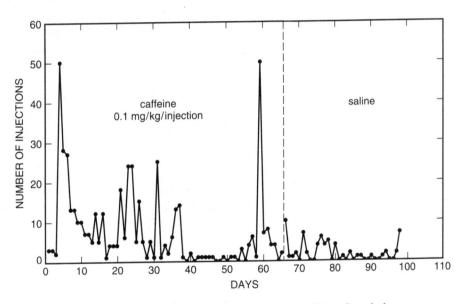

Figure 9–2 Intravenous self-injection rates of caffeine for a baboon with a history of self-administering numerous sedative and stimulant drugs. Caffeine was available on an FR2 schedule, and a maximum of 50 administrations were available each session. The dotted line indicates that a saline placebo injection was substituted for the caffeine. (From Griffiths & Mumford, 1995.)

fore the test reliably preferred caffeinated coffee, but people who were not permitted to have any caffeine for one week and were presumably not physically dependent on caffeine showed considerable individual variation in caffeine preference (Griffiths & Woodson, 1988). In later research, people who were not selected for heavy coffee consumption were given a choice between capsules containing caffeine and a placebo. Of 12 subjects, 4 showed a clear-cut preference for caffeine. Coffee consumption prior to the experiment did not seem to be related to caffeine preference (Griffiths & Woodson, 1988).

Another study conducted with moderate coffee drinkers showed that there was a distinct preference for caffeinated coffee over decaffeinated coffee. This preference could be detected in some people at doses as low as 25 mg per cup and was greatest when the subjects reported caffeine withdrawal (Hughs et al., 1987; Hughs et al., 1989).

In both humans and nonhumans, it seems that the reinforcing properties of caffeine vary considerably from individual to individual, and several factors have been identified as contributing to choosing caffeine. Being physically dependent is one. Another is that the people who usually report positive subjective effects from caffeine also show a caffeine preference, and people who report adverse effects usually avoid it (Griffiths & Woodson, 1988). But these characteristics are not essential. In one experiment, a person who was otherwise a coffee abstainer showed a definite preference for caffeine over a placebo (Griffiths & Mumford, 1995).

Higher doses are not as reinforcing as lower doses. Increasing doses beyond 100 mg usually decreases rate of self-administration, and doses in the 400 to 600 range are usually avoided.

Recent studies have also shown that caffeine preference may also be related to task requirements after ingestion. All subjects in an experiment where they were required to participate in a computer vigilance task after taking a capsule showed a preference for caffeine-containing cap-

sules, but only two of seven subjects had a preference for caffeine when the capsule was followed by a relaxation activity (Silverman, Mumford, & Griffiths, 1994).

Caffeine Dependence Syndrome?

In Chapter 5 the criteria for "substance dependence" used by the DSM-IV were discussed. These criteria are used to make the clinical diagnosis of dependence on a variety of drugs such as cocaine and heroin. Is it possible to be clinically diagnosed "dependent" on caffeine? Evidence from case histories suggests that it is. One study published in the *Journal of the American Medical Association* in 1995 reported on clinical interviews with a number of people recruited through newspaper notices who thought that they were dependent on caffeine. These people were interviewed using a structured clinical interview by a psychiatrist, and 16 were identified as meeting the DSM-IV criteria of caffeine "dependence." Of these 16, 94 percent reported withdrawal, 94 percent reported use continuing despite knowledge of persistent or recurrent physical or psychological problems likely to have been caused or exacerbated by caffeine use, 81 percent reported persistent desire or unsuccessful attempts to cut down or control use, and 75 percent reported tolerance. These people reported daily doses of caffeine that ranged between 129 and 2,548 mg per day, and three people diagnosed as dependent had daily doses less than the average daily consumption in the United States. Seven of the 16 primarily consumed soft drinks, one drank tea, and the remainder drank coffee (Strain et al., 1995).

Behavioral Economics

In a laboratory study, coffee and cigarettes were made available to subjects on an FR schedule of 100, and then FR requirement was increased to 1,000 and 2,500 independently for each reinforcer. Coffee demand was relatively inelastic (elasticity index 0.26 and 0.51) meaning that coffee consumption did not decrease in proportion to the price increases. As the price of cigarettes increased, the consumption of both coffee and cigarettes decreased, but as the price of coffee increased and coffee consumption fell, the consumption of cigarettes did not change. This finding suggests that changes in smoking behavior can influence coffee consumption, but people will smoke whether they are drinking coffee or not (Bickel et al., 1992); that is, coffee and cigarettes are *complements*, but the relationship is not symmetrical.

Population Studies

It is surprising that nonhumans are reluctant caffeine consumers and that humans do not show a more avid and compelling preference in the laboratory because caffeine and the other methylxanthines are probably the most widely self-administered drugs in the world. After oil, coffee is the world's most valuable traded commodity.

The Scandinavian countries, where per capita consumption is about twice that in the United States, have the world's greatest partakers of coffee. Canada ranks quite a bit below the United States, and countries such as Iraq, the Sudan, and Japan are at the bottom of the list of coffee consumers. Where tea is concerned, Ireland and Great Britain outconsume Canada by about 4 to 1 and the United States by about 12 to 1. European countries including the Scandinavian countries are at the bottom of the tea list.

The average caffeine consumption of the world's population is about 70 mg per person per day, 90 percent of which is consumed in the form of coffee and tea. North American consumption is probably over 200 mg per person per day (Barone & Roberts, 1984). About 60 percent of caffeine consumption is in the form of coffee, 16 percent as tea, 16 percent in soft drinks, and less than 2 percent as chocolate (Gilbert, 1984). Elsewhere it is estimated that the total consumption of methylxanthines in the United States is more than 230 mg per day, with caffeine accounting for 84 percent; theobromine, 17 percent; and theophylline, less than 1 percent (Hirsh, 1984).

HARMFUL EFFECTS

Reproduction

At high enough levels, caffeine will damage chromosomes, but it appears that such effects do not occur at the concentrations normally found in the human body, and caffeine is generally considered safe in this regard, although there is some speculation that it might enhance the chromosome-damaging activity of other agents such as X rays (Kihlman, 1977, pp. 414–415). Even though it does not damage chromosomes, caffeine can affect the fetus by other mechanisms. For example, caffeine raises the levels of circulating catecholamines, which could affect the unborn child by reducing blood flow to the fetus. Studies in animals have shown that low levels of caffeine retard both embryonic and neonatal growth in animals (Dunlop & Court, 1981). There is now some evidence that caffeine consumption does retard fetal growth and lowers birthweight in humans, especially if caffeine consumption exceeds 300 mg per day. In addition, it has been shown that caffeine will potentiate the effect that smoking has on reducing birthweight (see Chapter 8). For a review see E. M. McKim (1991). Remember that rate of caffeine metabolism is considerably delayed during pregnancy, and women who maintain usual consumption will experience higher and higher blood levels of caffeine as their pregnancy progresses.

Methylxanthines are also found in considerable concentrations in breast milk. Considering that the rate of methylxanthine metabolism in newborns is extremely slow, even small amounts acquired in breast milk will accumulate, possibly to toxic levels.

Some claim that there is no reason why pregnant women should be concerned about caffeine consumption during pregnancy, but the majority of expert opinion suggests that, until a safe level of consumption can be established, it is probably wiser for pregnant women (and nursing mothers) to abstain from caffeine-containing beverages and medicines (James, 1991).

Cardiac Disease

Even though it is clear that caffeine has direct effects on cardiac functioning, increasing blood pressure and causing irregularities in heartbeat, the epidemiological evidence linking caffeine consumption to heart disease is still not unequivocally established. In the early 1970s, the Boston Collaborative Drug Surveillance Program published two studies that showed that drinking more than six cups of coffee a day doubled the risk of heart attack. Since that time, numerous studies have failed to replicate the finding. One difficulty with epidemiological studies in this area is that exposure to caffeine is usually not measured accurately and as a result risk is consistently underestimated (James, 1991). Even though many have assumed coffee consumption is not a risk factor in heart disease (Robertson & Curatolo, 1984), the issue is far from settled.

Cancer

Studies with caffeine in laboratory animals have failed to show clearly that caffeine causes cancer. Some studies have found that caffeine may enhance the effect of other cancer-causing agents by inhibiting the ability of the cell to repair damaged DNA. Other studies have actually found that caffeine may inhibit some cancers (James, 1991).

Epidemiological studies have suffered from the same problems as described for cardiac disease; that is, the ability to measure exposure to caffeine is imprecise. Many studies find increased cancer risk for coffee users as opposed to nonusers, but no difference in risk between those who use different amounts of caffeine. Some have suggested that this failure to find a dose ef-

fect means that the link between coffee and cancers is circumstantial rather than causal. Nevertheless, it has been pointed out that studies may be examining the wrong measure of coffee exposure. In one study, it was found that the risk of ovarian cancer was 3.4 times greater in women who had drunk coffee for more than 40 years than in women who had never drunk coffee. Among those who did drink coffee the risk of cancer remained the same no matter how much was consumed. Possibly the crucial variable is duration of use rather than amount of use—a measure seldom taken in epidemiological studies.

A study in the early 1980s claimed to have found an association between caffeine and pancreatic cancer. This caused considerable concern, but there were methodological flaws in the study, and the effect cannot be consistently replicated. Nevertheless, recent work seems to indicate that caffeine may interact with smoking in causing pancreatic cancer; that is, the risk of cancer for smokers is increased by the consumption of coffee, but coffee has no effect in nonsmokers. Interestingly, the cancer risk for smokers was increased by both regular coffee and decaffeinated coffee. This finding may mean that the important agent was not caffeine, or it may indicate that current drinkers of decaffeinated coffee may have been regular coffee users in the past (James, 1991).

Inconsistent associations have also been reported between caffeine use and kidney cancer, bladder cancer, testicular cancer, fibrocystic breast disease, and breast cancer (James, 1991).

Abnormal Behavior

At doses of 5 to 10 cups per day, caffeine can cause sensory disturbances such as ringing in the ears and flashes of light as well as mild delirium and excitement. These are symptoms of a disorder called *caffeinism*, which is very similar to anxiety neurosis and is frequently diagnosed as such. Caffeinism is usually seen at doses above

1,000 mg per day. Patients report a low-grade fever of about 100°F, which is a result of the drug's action on the body's heat-regulating mechanism in the hypothalamus. Other symptoms include flushing, chilliness, insomnia, irritability, irregular heartbeat, and loss of appetite. Unlike anxiety neurosis, these symptoms do not respond to treatment with tranquilizers. The only cure is to eliminate caffeine from the diet (Greden, 1974).

The psychological basis for these effects appears to lie in the fact that at high doses, caffeine blocks benzodiazepine receptors. The benzodiazepines are the family of tranquilizers to which chlordiazepoxide (Librium) and diazepam (Valium) belong (see Chapter 7). The benzodiazepines act at a particular type of receptor in the brain which appears to be the site of action of an endogenous form of benzodiazepine that has similar antianxiety properties. The reason caffeine produces anxiety-like symptoms at higher doses is that it blocks these benzodiazepine receptors, and the body's natural benzodiazepine cannot function. When these receptors are blocked, the therapeutic effectiveness of an administered benzodiazepine is also diminished. There is also evidence that caffeine reduces the effectiveness of the major family of antipsychotic drugs, the phenothiazines, including chlorpromazine (Kulhanek, Linde, & Meisenberg, 1979).

Not only does caffeine interfere with the effectiveness of many psychotherapeutic drugs, but it also seems to make the symptoms of both neurotic and psychotic patients worse (Greden et al., 1978). In one experiment (De Freitas & Schwartz, 1979), patients in a psychiatric hospital were switched to decaffeinated coffee for three weeks without their knowledge. The ward staff, also unaware of the switch, rated all patients on a number of psychiatric symptoms. It was found that there was a decrease in anxiety, hostility, irritability, tension, and psychotic symptoms. There was an increase in scores reflecting social competence and personal neatness.

During a three-week period after caffeine was restored, all the improvements were reversed.

Studies such as this prompted an editorial in the *Canadian Medical Association Journal* that recommended that tea and coffee should not be served in mental institutions; labels should be placed on bottles of psychotherapeutic drugs warning about excessive caffeine intake; psychiatric patients should be informed about the effects of caffeine-containing beverages on their medication; and drugs that contain therapeutically useless caffeine should be removed from hospital pharmacies (Bezchilbnyk & Jeffries, 1981).

At higher doses, 1,800 mg or more, psychotic symptoms may result. These include mania, disorientation, screaming, violence, and finally, exhaustion and collapse (McMammy & Schube, 1936).

Lethal Effects

Six deaths due to caffeine overdose have been reported (Syed, 1976). The lethal dose in humans has been estimated at between 3 and 8 g (30 to 80 cups of coffee or stay-awake pills) taken orally. Death results from convulsions and respiratory collapse.

EPILOGUE

What Do We Really Know about Caffeine?

Caffeine is big business—even bigger than the tobacco business. You can be sure that any threat to the profits of such an economic interest of the coffee industry would be met with the same resources as the tobacco industry has put forward in defending itself against the increasing public awareness of the dangers of smoking. Perhaps it already has.

In a recent editorial in the British journal *Addiction*, one of the world's foremost caffeine researchers, Jack James of La Trobe University in Bundoora, Australia, has warned that the coffee industry has been subtly directing caffeine research away from areas of health problems and manipulating the dissemination of health information about caffeine for many years (James, 1994). The coffee industry established something called the International Life Sciences Institute (ILSI). This sounds as though it should be a scholarly organization with lofty aims, but in reality it was established to make sure that caffeine retained its status as "generally recognized as safe" by the United States Food and Drug Administration. In this regard it has been successful. Despite increasing numbers of studies that have provided reason to doubt it, caffeine is still considered a "safe" food additive.

How does ILSI work? Its influence may be seen in the pages of this book. According to James, the ILSI sponsors international conferences attended by prominent scholars by invitation only, then publishes the results. According to James, however, in the publications that deal with the health hazards of caffeine "evidence is consistently interpreted in a way that is favourable to the interests of the book's sponsors." This approach is given credibility because other publications that do not deal with health issues are balanced, erudite, and scholarly.

In addition, the caffeine industry sponsors research, but is careful to sponsor research in "safe" areas such as the study of compounds in coffee other than caffeine. As James says, "Under the guise of public interest, the industry actively supports continuing research on noncaffeine constituents of coffee, knowing fully that nothing untoward (and nothing of particular interest to the public) is likely to be revealed" (James, 1994, p. 1579).

CHAPTER SUMMARY

- The three commonly used methylxanthine drugs are *caffeine*, found mainly in *coffee*; *theophylline*, found in tea; and *theobromine*, found in chocolate. Caffeine is also added to some cola beverages, headache medications, and over-the-counter stimulants.

- Beverages that contain methylxanthines have been used in Europe and North America since the 1600s, and their popularity has made them important commodities. Their trading and taxation have played an important role in commerce and history.

- The methylxanthines are readily absorbed orally and distributed throughout the body. After its oral administration, caffeine reaches peak blood levels in 30 to 60 minutes. It is metabolized in the liver and eliminated slowly, with a half-life of about 3½ hours.

- These drugs have many effects on neural activity, but it is believed that their behavioral effects are a result of their blocking of the inhibitory neuromodulator adenosine.

- Caffeine can delay sleep and increase the ability to perform boring and tiring tasks, but it does not seem to be able to improve mental performance. There are some circumstances where caffeine can improve athletic performance in endurance events.

- Caffeine appears to be one of the few drugs that do not interfere with REM sleep, but sleep after caffeine is lighter, and people are more easily awakened.

- In nonhumans, caffeine stimulates spontaneous activity and can cause *automutilation* at larger doses. Operant analysis of the effects of caffeine has shown that its effects are similar to those of amphetamine, with some important differences.

- Caffeine can act as a discriminative stimulus and will generalize partially to cocaine. Humans can also detect the presence of caffeine in low concentrations.

- Doses of 100 to 200 mg of caffeine administered to people who are not tolerant to caffeine are experienced as pleasant, and when it is given intravenously, people report a "high" similar to cocaine.

- Tolerance develops to many of the effects of caffeine in both humans and nonhumans. Withdrawal symptoms, consisting of headaches and restlessness, have been reported at doses as low as 100 mg a day. Withdrawal peaks between 20 and 48 hours and may last as long as a week.

- Though humans consume vast quantities of caffeine, it is not a robust reinforcer in laboratory animals. It usually requires a period of forced administration before it will serve as a reinforcer. Humans will choose beverages and capsules containing caffeine if they report pleasant subjective effects and are physically dependent on caffeine.

- It is possible to meet the criteria for "substance abuse" of the DSM-IV with caffeine.

- The average caffeine consumption in North America is over 200 mg per person per day. Most caffeine is consumed in the form of coffee.

- There is evidence of a detrimental effect of caffeine on reproduction, and an association with heart disease and cancer. It has not yet been clearly established that there is a link because of difficulties with measuring caffeine consumption and separating its effects from the use of other drugs such as tobacco. At higher doses (10 to 15 cups a day), the drug can cause *caffeinism*, whose symptoms are indistinguishable from anxiety neurosis. Even at low doses, caffeine will also worsen the symptoms of neurosis and psychosis. Hence caffeine-containing beverages and medications should not be used in mental hospitals.

10

Psychomotor Stimulants

The drugs known as psychomotor stimulants have one effect in common: They stimulate transmission at synapses that use epinephrine (E), norepinephrine (NE), dopamine (DA), or serotonin (5-HT) as a transmitter. These transmitters are called *monoamines (MAs)* or *biogenic amines*. The first three—E, NE, and DA—are very similar. In fact, the body manufactures E from NE in one chemical step, and NE is made by changing the structure of DA slightly. Together these three are called *catecholamines (CAs)*. The odd monoamine is 5-HT. It is an *indoleamine*, which is chemically different from the CAs but is influenced by many of the same drugs and destroyed by many of the same enzymes (see Chapter 4).

You will sometimes see the term *sympathomimetic* used to refer to this class of drugs. This term is used because epinephrine is the primary transmitter in the sympathetic nervous system, and these drugs stimulate sympathetic synapses to some extent and mimic sympathetic arousal.

SOURCES

Some psychomotor stimulants occur naturally and have been used for centuries, and some are very new synthetic drugs. The amphetamines are synthetic and do not occur naturally. There is *d-amphetamine* (dextro-amphetamine, or dex-amphetamine) and *l-amphetamine* (levo-amphetamine). These have exactly the same chemical structure, but the molecules are mirror images of each other (technically, they are called *optical isomers*). In the case of amphetamine, the *d-* isomer is more potent than the *l-* isomer for most central effects. When the term *dl-amphetamine* or just *amphetamine* is used, it refers to a mixture of the two isomers. The most common trade name of *dl*-amphetamine was Benzedrine, but neither Benzedrine nor *dl*-amphetamine is currently in use in the United States or Canada. Dexedrine is a common trade name of *d*-amphetamine. Another similar drug is *methamphetamine*, which differs slightly in structure and effect from the other two. It is sold as Methedrine or Desoxyn and is known on the street as *meth* or *speed*. There are recent reports of a crystallized form of methamphetamine called "ice." Collectively these products are known on the street by a number of names including "speed," "bennies," "black beauties," "crystal," "dexies," and "uppers."

Only slightly different chemically from the amphetamines are two synthetic drugs, *methylphenidate* (Ritalin) and *pipradrol*.

Also included in this group is a naturally occurring drug, ephedrine. Ephedrine comes from the herb *ma huang (Ephedra vulgaris)*, which has been used as a medicine in China for centuries. There are also North American varieties of *Ephedra*.

Another psychomotor stimulant is cocaine. Cocaine is extracted from the leaf of a small tree known as the coca *(Erythroxylum coca)*, which is native to South America. It prefers high elevations and thrives on the slopes of the Andes Mountains. It grows in both wild and cultivated forms from northwestern Argentina to Ecuador.

Cathinone is another naturally occurring cocainelike drug found in the leaves and shoots of *Catha edulis*, a shrublike plant that grows in the countries of eastern Africa and southern Arabia. It is called *khat* in Yemen (also spelled *quat* or *qat* and pronounced "cat"). It is also known as *tscaht* in Ethiopia and *miraa* in Kenya (Kalix, 1994). Cathinone is not stable and degrades shortly after the plant is harvested. For this reason the plant is used primarily in the area where it is grown and is not exported for use elsewhere like cocaine (United Nations, 1980). However, *methcathinone* (the cathinone equivalent of methamphetamine), is an established abused drug in some countries. In Russia it is known as "ephedrone" or referred to as "jeff," "Jee-cocktail," or "cosmos," and has been an abuse problem since the early 1980s. In the early 1990s it appeared in the illicit drug market and was found in clandestine labs in the United States as "cat." In 1992 it was classified as a Schedule 1 substance (the highest restriction a drug can receive) under the Emergency Scheduling Act (Glennon et al., 1994).

HISTORY

Cocaine

For centuries coca leaves have been chewed by various Indian tribes in South America. No one knows how long the coca plant has been used, but it is of great antiquity. Legends of some tribes of Colombian Indians tell how their people came from the Milky Way in a canoe drawn by an anaconda. In addition to a man and a woman, the canoe contained several psychoactive plants including coca (Schultes, 1987, p. 229). Coca leaves have been found in burial middens in Peru that date back to 2500 B.C. Large stone monolithic idols found in Colombia and dating to 500 B.C. have the puffed-out cheeks of the coca chewer. The Incas started to use the plant when they conquered the region in about the tenth century. Under the Incas, coca became sacred. It was used primarily by the priests and nobility for special ceremonies and was not consumed daily by the common folk.

When the Spanish conquered the Incas, at first they banned coca use, considering it to be idolatrous and pagan, but they were not long in changing their minds when they found out how useful it could be to them. The Spanish did not use coca themselves, but they soon learned that it had great value in paying for labor in the gold and silver mines in the Andes. In addition to finding coca an item of commerce, the Spanish realized that the Indians could work harder and longer and required less food if they were given coca.

As the Spanish grew more interested in the plant, attempts were made to classify it. In 1749 samples were sent to Europe, where Linnaeus gave the plant its own family, Erythroxylaceae, and Lamarck named the most important species

Erythroxylon coca in 1786 (Aldrich & Baker, 1976).

Europeans remained unaware of either the medicinal or the psychological effects of the plant, probably because samples sent from South America had deteriorated from age. It is also likely that Europeans were averse to chewing the leaves in the manner of the South Americans. It was not until the form of the drug was changed that they showed any interest in coca. The first change involved identifying the active ingredient. Earlier attempts had been made with partial success, but the credit for isolating and naming cocaine goes to Albert Niemann of the German university town of Göttingen, who published his results in 1860.

For several years cocaine was a drug without a medical use until Sigmund Freud became interested. These events took place before Freud had done any of his work on psychoanalysis. At the time he was an impoverished 28-year-old Viennese neurologist eager to make a name for himself. He obtained some of the drug and tried it on himself with the most pleasing results. It cheered him up, and he found that it "turned the bad mood he was in into cheerfulness, gave him the feeling of having dined well 'so there was nothing at all one need bother about'" (E. Jones, 1953, p. 88). Freud tried the drug on just about everyone he knew, including his fiancée and his sisters, and was convinced he had discovered the cure to nearly all the woes of mankind. He published papers making extravagant claims, including the assertion that cocaine cured morphine addiction and alcoholism. It was one of his associates, Karl Koller, however, who discovered the only real medical use of cocaine—it was the world's first local anesthetic. Freud was later forced to abandon his advocacy of cocaine when its harmful effect became apparent.

The isolation of cocaine not only stimulated a search for medical uses for the drug, but also made it available in an acceptable form that the upper middle class could inject along with morphine, which was also popular at the time (see Chapter 11). Around the turn of the twentieth century, it gained favor with writers and intellectuals. Robert Louis Stevenson is reported to have written *The Strange Case of Dr. Jekyll and Mr. Hyde* with the aid of cocaine. Sherlock Homes, the fictional detective created by Arthur Conan Doyle, was a prototype of the intellectual cocaine user of the time. Over the cautions and objections of the good Dr. Watson, he injected the drug to keep his keen mind stimulated.

In 1863, Angelo Mariani, a Corsican chemist, patented a wine containing coca that became exceedingly popular and made Mariani a very wealthy man. Among its users were Thomas Edison, the czar of Russia, the prince of Wales, Jules Verne, Emile Zola, and Henrik Ibsen. Pope Leo XIII always carried a flask on his belt and was so impressed that he gave Mariani a gold medal. It was probably Mariani's success that inspired a Georgia pharmacist, John S. Pemberton, to produce an American version called "French Wine of Cola, Ideal Tonic." Later, in 1886, he removed the alcohol and replaced it with a kola nut extract, added soda water, and called it Coca-Cola. In its early days Coca-Cola was promoted as a remedy and a health drink, and it is probably for this reason that soda fountains developed in drugstores in the United States. In 1906 the Pure Food and Drug Act outlawed cocaine, and it was removed from the drink. To this day, Coca-Cola is made from coca leaves from which the cocaine has been removed.

The passage of the Pure Food and Drug Act, which removed the cocaine from Coca-Cola, was a manifestation of a growing backlash against cocaine and other drugs in the early part of the twentieth century in the United States. While cocaine was being injected by white professionals and intellectuals, the drug was associated with corruption and crime in the popular mind. It is little wonder that cocaine was included with morphine and opium in the Harrison Narcotic Act of 1914, which effectively banned its use. As a result of this inclusion of cocaine in the U.S. law and the influence of the United States on the development of international narcotics control, cocaine was also included with morphine in all international treaties aimed at the control of narcotics and in the internal legislation of many other countries—all of this in spite of the fact that cocaine is in no way a narcotic and is very dissimilar from the opiates both pharmacologically and behaviorally.

The Harrison Act drove cocaine underground, where it was used by the "unconventional rich and the unconventional poor": party-going, decadent, wealthy whites and gamblers, musicians, and artists of all colors. Cocaine was not a part of the lives of the vast majority of the population of the United States. In the 1960s things started to change. The use of cocaine started to increase for a number of reasons. To begin with, World War II had earlier introduced everyone to amphetamines, and so the idea of the stimulant and the "upper" was no longer new and foreign, but many other changes were taking place as well. One book lists them as follows:

The loss of respect for established institutions and moral attitudes among important parts of the middle class, the bohemianization of middle class youth (the hippie rebellion and its camp followers), the introduction of psychedelics and the spread of marijuana use, with the attendant drug ideologies . . . (Grinspoon & Bakalar, 1976, p. 49).

Amphetamines

Ephedrine, in the herb *ma huang*, has been used in China for more than 5,000 years. Legend has it that its medicinal properties were first identified by the emperor Chen Nung, who was also credited with the discovery of tea. Ephedrine was isolated from the herb in the 1880s, but not until 1924 were its properties investigated by two Americans, Ko Kuei Chen and C. F. Schmidt. They pointed out that the structure and actions of ephedrine were similar to those of the neurotransmitter epinephrine, which was known to be a stimulant of the sympathetic nervous system. Epinephrine was used at the time to treat asthma

because one of its effects was to dilate the airways in the lungs and make breathing easier. Epinephrine, however, was very unstable; it had to be administered by injection, and its effects were very brief. Ephedrine was far superior because it could be taken in pill form, had a longer duration of action, and was less toxic. The use of ephedrine became so widespread that there were fears that supplies would run out, and a search was begun for a synthetic substitute. As it happened, such a substitute had already been discovered, but no one knew it. Many years earlier, in 1887, L. Edealeno had synthesized what we now know as amphetamine, but he had failed to explore its properties, and it remained untested until 1910, when G. Barger and Sir H. H. Dale (the proposer of Dale's principle; see Chapter 4) published a technical paper showing the effects of amphetamine and other sympathomimetic drugs on the body. The significance of Barger and Dale's paper was not grasped until 1927, when Gordon Alles, a young chemist at a research laboratory in Los Angeles, suggested that amphetamine would probably be the best and cheapest substitute for ephedrine.

In 1937 the American Medical Association sanctioned the use of amphetamine for the treatment of the sleep disorder narcolepsy and as a mild "pick-me-up" or stimulant for depression. By 1943 at least half of the sales of the drug were prescribed for weight reduction and diet control, antidepressant or stimulant effects, or extended periods of alertness. Amphetamine was also marketed in inhalers for treatment of asthma and sold over the counter without prescription. The pharmaceutical company of Smith, Kline, and French held the patents of amphetamine and was doing so well that other companies wanted some of the market too. It was not long before the Ciba company started marketing methylphenidate as a "nonamphetamine" stimulant (Grinspoon & Hedblom, 1975).

Physicians, however, were not the only source of amphetamines. A substantial proportion of the legally manufactured amphetamines were diverted into the black market because of slack control and poor recordkeeping. In addition, much amphetamine and methamphetamine could be made in illicit labs and at home. The production of amphetamine is so simple that step-by-step formulas for manufacturing the drug at home with the minimum of equipment could (and still can) be bought on the street (Grinspoon & Hedblom, 1975).

To limit the indiscriminate prescribing of amphetamines by physicians, most countries now limit the medical conditions for which amphetamines may be prescribed. These conditions are narcolepsy and the treatment of hyperactivity in children and do not include obesity or the need to stay awake. The production and marketing of amphetamines is now carefully monitored. Apart from some illegally manufactured methamphetamine, most stimulant abuse in Western countries is confined to cocaine.

Cathinone

Khat use has been known since antiquity. Alexander the Great sent khat to General Harrar to cure his melancholia, and it has been mentioned repeatedly by Arab physicians as a remedy for a variety of disorders. Amda Sion, a fourteenth-century ruler of Ethiopia, was the first recorded case of khat addiction. It has been known in Europe since the early 1600s, but has only recently been used there because of difficulties transporting the leaf.

The first case of khat psychosis in the United States was reported in 1982, and since that time cases have been reported in the United Kingdom (Giannini, Miller, & Turner, 1992), Europe, and Canada (Kalix, 1994). Public awareness of khat has increased as a result of reports emanating from the United Nations Mission in Somalia. Some have expressed concern that U.S. soldiers may have been exposed to khat use because of the interdiction of alcohol in Muslim countries and brought the habit back to the United States. There are, however, no reports of such cases.

ROUTES OF ADMINISTRATION AND ABSORPTION

The amphetamines are weak bases and have a pKa of between 9 and 10. When taken orally, they tend to be ionized in the digestive system, slowing the rate of absorption. The drug is more potent when administered by injection or inhalation. When given for medicinal purposes or to prevent sleep and fatigue, amphetamines are always taken orally, and the decrease in potency can be compensated for by increasing the dose. The oral route has the advantage that blood levels may be kept fairly constant without too much variation over time. When amphetamines are taken for the rush they produce, they are administered by injection, which causes the sudden high blood levels required for this effect.

The same is true for cocaine, which has a pKa of 8.7. Traditionally, the Indians of the Andes rolled coca leaves into a ball, stuck a wad in the cheek, and sucked it. It is also common for those who take coca in this manner to mix the leaves with lime in the form of wood ashes (Schultes, 1987, p. 225) or ground shells; this practice raises the pH of the saliva and the digestive system and consequently reduces ionization and increases absorption. It is very unusual for pure cocaine to be taken orally. It is nearly always injected or sniffed to improve absorption, but recently it has become popular to smoke cocaine, both as a hydrochloride salt and as a freebase.

Most of the cocaine sold in the United States is the salt cocaine hydrochloride (cocaine HCl). It may contain various impurities from the refining process and be deliberately diluted, or "cut." One method that was used to determine the purity of this drug was to place some of the powder on a sheet of tinfoil and heat it until it vaporized; pure cocaine HCl leaves little residue. It soon became apparent to those who performed this test that inhaled cocaine has an effect similar to injected cocaine. Soon this method of smoking, called "tooting," became popular, as did other methods such as mixing cocaine with tobacco or marijuana.

Freebasing is a process that separates the cocaine molecule from the HCl. It is a rather risky process that involves heating highly combustible chemicals. The freebase vapor that is produced has a much stronger effect than the cocaine HCl because of the increased lipid solubility of the freebase form of the drug. Freebasing became extremely popular. The practice was greatly facilitated by the advertising and sale of special pipes and chemical kits for converting the cocaine HCl into the freebase (R. K. Siegel, 1982b).

A more recent development in the cocaine technology is *crack*, which is cocaine HCl mixed with a solution of baking soda (sodium bicarbonate). The water is evaporated, leaving crystalline chunks or "rocks" that are heated in pipes or other devices, and the vapors are inhaled. This process accomplishes the same thing as freebasing and is considerably cheaper and safer.

After oral administration of amphetamines, the absorption rate is determined by factors such as the presence of food in the stomach and degree of physical activity. Peak blood levels may be reached in 30 minutes to three hours (Vree & Henderson, 1980). After intranasal administration (sniffing) of cocaine, peak blood levels are achieved in 10 to 20 minutes (Javid et al., 1983). The rate of absorption of vaporized cocaine HCl and cocaine from vaporized freebase or crack has not been studied, but it is likely extremely rapid because both processes release the cocaine molecule in un-ionized form making it highly lipid soluble. In fact, crack is a variation on the ancient technique used by the Incas, who mixed coca leaves with lime. This made the saliva basic and enhanced the absorption of the cocaine from the coca leaves using the same chemical principle.

Traditionally, cathinone is taken orally by chewing the leaves of the khat plant in much the same manner as the natives of the Andes have used coca. In Russia, methcathinone is usually administered by injection, but in the United States, sniffing of methcathinone powder seems to be preferred (Glennon et al., 1994).

DISTRIBUTION

The amphetamines, cocaine, and other drugs in this class cross the blood-brain barrier and are concentrated in the spleen, kidneys, and brain.

EXCRETION

The excretion of the amphetamines depends to a very great extent on the pH of the urine. Because it is ionized at acid pHs, amphetamine is not reabsorbed from the nephron in acid urine, but as the urine becomes more basic, more of the drug is reabsorbed and more of the burden of excretion is carried by metabolism in the liver. The half-life of amphetamine may be as short as 7 to 14 hours when the urine is acidic. When the urine is basic, excretion is shifted to metabolic processes, and the half-life may be 16 to 34 hours (Creasey, 1979, p. 180). Amphetamine is also excreted in sweat and saliva (Vree & Henderson, 1980; Britton et al., 1978).

Amphetamines that are not excreted unchanged are metabolized through a variety of routes that use a variety of enzymes. Many of the metabolites are also behaviorally active and have very long half-lives (Brookes, 1985, p. 265).

Cocaine is excreted much faster than the amphetamines. It has a half-life of about 40 minutes (Javid et al., 1983), although this also depends on the pH of the urine. Cathinone has a half-life of about one and a half hours, intermediate between cocaine and amphetamine (Kalix, 1994).

NEUROPHYSIOLOGY

All of the drugs in this chapter are grouped together because they have a common effect on synapses that use a monoamine (MA) as a transmitter, but the mechanisms by which they stimulate these synapses differ. (It may be useful at this point to review the discussion of monoamine synapses in Chapter 4.)

The amphetamines, cathinone, and methcathinone primarily affect synapses that use serotonin and the catecholamines (CAs)—epinephrine (E), norepinephrine (NE), and dopamine (DA)—as transmitters or modulators. They have a threefold effect on these synapses. First, they cause the transmitter to leak spontaneously out of the synaptic vesicles into the synaptic cleft. Second, they increase the amount of transmitter released in response to the arrival of an action potential at the synapse. And third, they block the reuptake of the transmitter into the presynaptic cells and prolong the duration and intensity of their effect. All of these actions greatly stimulate the synapse (Carlsson, 1969; Glennon et al., 1994).

Cocaine doesn't produce the first two of amphetamine's effects, but it is a reuptake blocker and stimulates the synapse this way (Groppetti & Di Giulio, 1976; Wolverton & Johnson, 1992).

In the peripheral nervous system, these drugs stimulate E, the transmitter in the sympathetic nervous system, and cause sympathetic arousal, the fight/flight response.

In the central nervous system, several systems are known to be affected by the psychomotor stimulants. These include several DA systems (shown in Figure 12–2). One is the *nigrastriatal system* between the substantia nigra and the striatum (basal ganglia), which are important in the control of motor activity. Another important DA system, the *mesolimbic system*, is associated with reward and pleasure centers and is also linked with psychotic behavior (see Chapter 12). Amphetamine and cathinone are known to increase the release of dopamine in the nucleus accumbens, an important center for this reward pathway (Kalix, 1994). Another system exerts some control over the secretions of the *pituitary gland*. This DA system inhibits the secretion of *prolactin*, a hormone that controls the release of milk during breast-feeding and also suppresses male sexual activity.

In addition to its abilities as an MA stimulant, cocaine also has the ability to block sodium ion channels in membranes. This blocks the conduction of action potentials along nerve axons, and is the basis of its ability to act as a *local anesthetic*. The local anesthetic action, however, has nothing to do with the MA-stimulating effect of the drug and requires much higher concentrations. Cocaine is seldom used for this purpose today. *Procaine* (novocaine), a synthetic substitute that has the local anesthetic action of cocaine without its stimulant properties, was developed for this purpose. Even though procaine lacks the stimulant properties of cocaine, it nevertheless acts as a positive reinforcer in rats and monkeys (Yokel, 1987; Ford & Ralster, 1977).

The influence of cocaine is still felt in the naming of local anesthetic drugs. It is common to use the ending *-caine* in the formulation of generic and trade names to indicate that the drug has local anesthetic action.

EFFECTS OF PSYCHOMOTOR STIMULANTS

Effects on the Body

Because the psychomotor stimulants activate the sympathetic nervous system, they cause an increase in heart rate and blood pressure and a dilation of the blood vessels (*vasodilation*) and the air passages in the lungs (*bronchodilation*). Bronchodilation is medically useful for people suffering from asthma. This was the primary motivation for the invention and development of the amphetamines in the first place. However, most of the sympathetic effects are not considered pleasant by people who inject amphetamines for psychological effects. They generally prefer methamphetamine, which has stronger CNS effects and fewer peripheral effects than *d-* or *l-*amphetamine.

Some patients receiving amphetamines for medical reasons report headaches, dry mouth, stomach disturbances, and weight loss due to depression of appetite. Overdose symptoms include dizziness, confusion, tremor, hallucinations, panic states, heartbeat irregularities, and circulatory collapse. Large overdoses sometimes result in convulsions and coma.

Effects on Sleep

One reason for the widespread use of the amphetamines during World War II and in the 1950s was that they prevented sleep. Amphetamine was used by truck drivers on long trips and students staying awake to cram for exams. Systematic studies have shown that amphetamine use does cause insomnia.

The amphetamines, cocaine, and methylphenidate all suppress REM sleep when sleep does occur. As with other drugs that have this effect, tolerance develops after a while, and there is a REM rebound during withdrawal from the drug. This is characterized by an increased percentage of REM sleep for a period of one to two months (Oswald & Thacore, 1963).

EFFECTS ON THE BEHAVIOR AND PERFORMANCE OF HUMANS

Effects on Mood

When given intravenously, the effects of cocaine and amphetamine are indistinguishable (Fischman et al., 1976).

One of the most noticeable effects of the amphetamines is that they make people feel good; they improve the mood. From the earliest occasions when amphetamines were given to humans, positive mood changes were recorded. There were reports that the drug caused "a sense of well-being and exhilaration," feelings of "high spirits," and "bubbling inside." Most subjects felt a decrease in fatigue and an increase in energy, a clear, organized mind, and a desire to get to work and accomplish things (Grinspoon & Hedblom, 1975, p. 62). Later, systematic double-blind studies confirmed these reports. Figure 10–1 shows

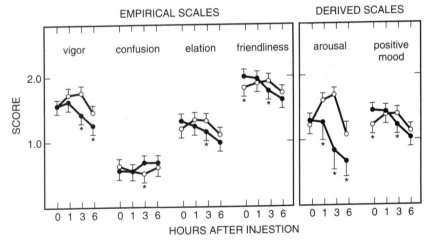

Figure 10–1   Changes in mood after 5 mg of amphetamine. Subjects were given the amphetamine orally and then filled out the POMS after 0, 1, 3, and 6 hours. Statistically significant differences between the drug (open circles) and a placebo (solid circles) are indicated with an asterisk (*). (Adapted from Johanson & Uhlenhuth, 1980, p. 277.)

the results of such a study. Subjects were given a low dose (5 mg) of *d*-amphetamine or a placebo and were asked to fill out the Profile of Mood States (POMS) questionnaire. They filled in the POMS again one, three, and six hours after the drug was taken. As can be seen in Figure 10–1, the drug caused an increase in vigor, friendliness, elation, and positive mood (Johanson & Uhlenhuth, 1980). These effects were greatest three hours after administration, and some of these mood changes lasted as long as six hours. These euphoric feelings were followed several hours later by a feeling of depression (Gunne & Anggard, 1972).

Higher acute doses produce a more intense subjective effect, but acute tolerance to pleasurable effects occurs with repeated doses within a single session. In one study, humans were permitted to administer cocaine intravenously every 10 minutes for one hour. Feelings of positive mood increased after the first infusion but did not increase throughout the session even though the blood levels of cocaine rose steadily with repeated infusions (Fischman & Schuster, 1982).

In addition to making people feel good, amphetamine at high doses after intravenous or intranasal administration produces intense feelings of euphoria and pleasure called *rushes*. Rushes are not exclusive to intravenous administration, but this route is extremely efficient at delivering high drug levels to the brain and increasing their intensity. The rush has been described as "being lifted into the air with feelings of extreme happiness." Another account claims "The heart starts beating at a terrible speed and his respiration is very rapid. Then he feels as if he was ascending in to the cosmos, every fiber of his body trembling with happiness." Many people report that the rush has a strong sexual component. "The shot goes straight from the head to the scrotum," as one user put it (Rylander, 1969, p. 254).

The effects of cocaine are similar but shorter-acting. Within a couple of minutes after cocaine is snorted, there is a numbing sensation called the *freeze*, which is followed after five minutes by a feeling of exhilaration and well-being. As with amphetamine, there is a feeling of energy and the sensation of clear thoughts and perceptions. This lasts for 20 to 30 minutes and is followed by a mild depression called the *comedown* or *letdown*. When cocaine is injected, there is also a rush that may be felt within seconds and lasts about 45 seconds.

This rush is almost universally described in sexual terms, namely the orgasm. Unlike snorting, the effects are far from subtle and gradual, but take hold of the user immediately. . . . The experience is so intense that it tends to encompass and engross the shooter totally and cuts him off from other people who might be nearby. (Waldorf et al., 1977, p. 35)

Recent research has shown that cocaine-produced rushes show rapid tolerance. When a series of i.v. injections of cocaine were given 70 minutes apart, reports of rushes disappeared over the session, but other measures such as "feeling good" were unchanged (Kumor et al., 1988).

There is considerable evidence that feelings of pleasure and euphoria and rushes are a result of the direct effects of these drugs on the dopamine mesolimbic reinforcement system, that is, the pleasure centers of the brain. Direct stimulation of this system is also responsible for the powerful reinforcing effects of the psychomotor stimulants (Wolverton & Johanson, 1984).

This area of the brain is also known to control motivational states such as hunger and thirst. This system is stimulated by activities such as eating, drinking, and copulation that are beneficial to the survival of the organism, causing repetition of the behaviors that led up to these activities. If these reward centers are activated artificially with electrical stimulation or by drugs such as the psychomotor stimulants, we experience the same sort of pleasure (Wise, 1981; see Chapter 5). As Freud said, cocaine made him feel satisfied, like he had just eaten a good meal. This involvement of the pleasure centers may also explain why rushes are described as sexual.

Stereotyped Behavior

In 1965 a Swedish psychiatrist, Gosta Rylander, described a peculiar behavior shown by high-dosage users of *phenmetrazine*, an amphetamine-like drug used for weight reduction. These users ground up phenmetrazine pills and injected them intravenously to experience the rush. The behavior Rylander noticed was what the users called *punding*, the repetitive performance of some useless act for an extended period. Such an act might be taking apart and putting together a watch or a telephone, sorting and resorting things in a handbag, or cleaning an apartment. When users are punding, they will usually not eat or drink or even go to the bathroom, and they become annoyed if the activity is interrupted (Rylander, 1969). This sort of behavior is common among amphetamine users as well. Punding is considered the human equivalent of stereotyped behavior seen in laboratory animals after high-dose injections of amphetamines. Stereotyped behavior of nonhumans will be described in detail shortly.

It is quite likely that both punding and stereotyped behavior are caused by stimulation of the nigrastriatal DA system, which has input into the extrapyramidal motor system; see Chapter 4.

Amphetamine Psychosis

High doses of the amphetamines can cause psychotic behavior in otherwise normal people (Bowers, 1987, p. 820). The psychosis is virtually indistinguishable from true, full-blown paranoid schizophrenia. The symptoms of amphetamine psychosis include auditory and visual hallucinations, delusions of persecution, delusions of grandeur, and sometimes hostility and violence triggered by the paranoid belief that danger is imminent. A case history of amphetamine psychosis is given in Box 10–1.

Amphetamine psychosis can occur in individuals without any history of psychotic behavior. It usually clears in several days without residual effects (Angrist & Sudilovsky, 1978).

Cocaine and cathinone are also capable of causing psychotic episodes at high doses. Such a cocaine-induced psychosis convinced Sigmund Freud that cocaine was not a wonder drug after all. Freud had been giving cocaine to his friend Dr. von Fleischl-Marxow to treat pain from neural tumors. During the course of treatment, Fleischl found it necessary to increase the dose to high levels, and he started showing the signs that are now known to be typical of a psychosis caused by both cocaine and amphetamines. One of the most distressing symptoms Fleischl experienced was the feeling of creatures, in his case white snakes, crawling over him. Others have described the feeling as bugs crawling around just under the skin (Brecher & the editors of Consumer Reports, 1972, p. 275). These are known as *cocaine bugs*, or *crank bugs* if they are caused by amphetamine. This phenomenon is formally called *formication*, from the Latin *formica*, "ant."

Schizophrenia is thought to be, at least in part, a result of excessive DA functioning in the mesolimbic system (see Chapter 12). Drugs such as amphetamine worsen the psychotic symptoms of schizophrenics and create psychotic symptoms in normal persons. We also know that the effectiveness of drugs that reduce the symptoms of psychosis, the antipsychotics, appear to arise from their ability to block DA receptors (Post et al., 1981). Antipsychotics also diminish psychotic behavior caused by excessive amphetamine.

Violence. Violent behavior has been associated with continued amphetamine use. The violent behavior usually results from changes in the user's personality, which becomes hostile, paranoid, and defensive. Though violent episodes are not especially frequent, they are unpredictable and sudden. Rylander (1969) described one such case:

One addict who had just taken a shot stopped his car in a street, not feeling well, leaned backwards and put his feet up on the instrument panel. A bypasser asked if he

BOX 10–1   Amphetamine Psychosis: A Case Study

This is a case history of a fairly typical amphetamine-induced psychotic episode from the files of two widely published researchers in the area, Angrist and Gershon (1969). After reading it, have a look at Box 12–2, which gives an account of a person with schizophrenia. Compare the two accounts. Can you find any similarities?

The 18-year-old had been in a reformatory because of chronic truancy and arrested for the possession of marijuana and petty larceny. At the time of his hospitalization, a trial was still pending for possession of a loaded pistol. He had sniffed glue at ages 12 and 13, had drunk heavily from 13 to 15, and had used amphetamine orally (5 or 10 capsules per day) and intravenously from age 16 onward. He had used heroin for three or four months between the ages of 17 and 18. He left high school in the eleventh grade and thereafter worked at a pizza stand, in bicycle stores, and as a messenger, but no job had lasted more than six months.

  In the two weeks prior to admission, he stayed at his brother and sister-in-law's apartment and had taken three to seven injections per day of powder of unknown purity that he was told was methamphetamine. During this time he heard his brother tell his sister-in-law that the brother had killed their mother and planned to kill him (the patient) as well. He panicked and, in an attempt to escape, ran into the street without shoes or shirt and jumped on the rear fender of a passing mail truck. This led to his being taken to Bellevue Psychiatric Hospital by the police. In the hospital he was frightened and apprehensive, and he felt that the staff and the other patients were implying that "he knew something" that he refused to tell. When he was seen by the research staff, two days after admission, he showed flattened emotions that were sometimes inappropriate to the situation. After being transferred to the research ward, he became frightened and tearful, fearing that this was a place where patients were sent to be punished and perhaps even killed. He displayed a formal thought disorder; for example, on the day of his transfer, speaking of his brother's drug use, he said, "My brother has been playing with the fires of hell." On the same day, when asked what "A stitch in time saves nine" meant, he said, "Hurry up with that date and don't be late. *(laugh)* Make that first stitch right and the rest will follow." On the next day, the delusions of persecution had diminished and were replaced by less specific ideas that the other patients in the ward were looking at him peculiarly. His emotions were still shallow and not appropriate to what he was talking about. On the third day in the research ward, the fifth in the hospital, he responded to the proverb "People who live in glass houses shouldn't throw stones" thusly: "If you throw stones, you risk your whole being." He was apprehensive about a female patient in the ward that he referred to as "the girl I call Bonnie" (after the criminal in the movie *Bonnie and Clyde*). After that, his thinking cleared rapidly.

was sick and offered his help. The addict drew a knife, got out and chased the helpful man. He stumbled and fell just when the addict tried to slash his back. (p. 263)

Sensory Effects

Amphetamines have been reported to raise the CFF threshold, indicating an increase in visual acuity (Simonson & Brozek, 1952). Slight improvements have been reported in auditory flicker fusion as well (Besser, 1967). The passage of time is underestimated; one second seems longer than it really is (Goldstone, Boardman, & Lhamon, 1958).

Effects on Performance

The Spanish conquistadores may not have believed the claims of the South American Indians that coca made them stronger, but there seems to be little doubt that amphetamines and cocaine can improve performance on a number of tasks and skills. Most of the early work of this nature was done by the armed forces of several countries during World War II. They found that endurance could be increased and the effects of fatigue could be diminished by amphetamines.

Though it does not appear that amphetamine will improve reaction time under normal circumstances, it has been demonstrated many times that the drug will eliminate the effects of fatigue on reaction time, restoring it to normal. This finding also appears to be true for most measures of motor coordination and control. Improvements are more likely to be seen in complex motor tasks than in simple tasks.

Amphetamine has the ability to improve performance in tasks that require vigilance or prolonged attention. One measure of vigilance is the clock test. In this test, the subject faces a large dial around which a pointer moves in discrete steps. Every once in a while the pointer moves two steps rather than one, and the task of the subject is to detect when such events occur. Over a period of two hours, the performance of normal subjects deteriorates from 95 percent to 80 percent accuracy. Subjects given 10 mg of amphetamine prior to this test show no deterioration at all in accuracy over the two-hour period (Weiss, 1969). Amphetamine can also overcome deterioration in performance caused by other factors such as decreased oxygen levels.

Not only does amphetamine return performance to normal levels, but other studies have shown that there are situations where amphetamine can actually improve performance over normal levels. In a simplified simulated flying task, where subjects are required to move a joystick in order to keep dials from moving off center, it was found that the performance of subjects given a placebo deteriorated over a four-hour period, but the scores of subjects given 5 mg of amphetamine actually stayed above their normal levels for the test (Weiss, 1969). Although these drugs can improve performance, this improvement may be limited to overlearned and overpracticed tasks. Some investigators have suggested that stimulants may actually impair performance requiring flexibility and the ability to adopt new strategies (Judd et al., 1987, p. 1471).

Athletic Performance

In one early study, G. M. Smith and H. K. Beecher (1959) gave amphetamine to competitive swimmers who were then timed while performing in the event for which they were training. They found that amphetamine could produce a 1 percent improvement in their best drug-free times. Though 1 percent does not sound like much, in the highly competitive sport of swimming, athletes may train many months to reduce their times by 1 percent. Similar improvements have been seen in such track events as the 600- and 1,000-yard runs and the mile, and in such field events as putting the shot.

Because the psychomotor stimulants improve athletic performance, their use by athletes is banned by most national sports federations, and urine samples supplied by athletes at sporting events are screened for these drugs. As mentioned earlier, ephedrine is a psychomotor stimulant closely related to amphetamine. Ephedrine and similar drugs act as bronchodilators and are found in many cold preparations, cough syrups, and decongestants. Athletes undergoing such testing should be aware of the contents of these medicines before they take them because they could make their urine test positive for a banned substance. Some banned substances found in cold medicines include norpseudoephedrine, methoxphenamine, isoprenaline, isoproterenol, and methylephedrine.

EFFECTS ON THE BEHAVIOR OF NONHUMANS

Unconditioned Behavior

At low and intermediate doses, amphetamines increase spontaneous locomotor and exploratory activity in rats. At higher doses there is an increase in locomotion at first, but after about an hour the animals start to show increased sniffing and a variety of *stereotyped behavior*. Stereotyped behavior is usually some simple, short act with no particular function that is repeated over and over to the exclusion of other behavior. In rodents, it may take the form of bobbing the head up and down, sniffing in a corner, rearing on the hind legs, or gnawing and biting.

In monkeys there is a decrease in locomotor activity, and the stereotyped behavior is generally more complex than in rodents. It is also different in different subjects. One monkey may examine its hands, while another may move sideways. These behaviors will reappear in the same animals when the drug is given at a later date. In humans, stereotyped behaviors are even more complex and were described earlier as punding.

After high doses of amphetamines and cocaine, it is common for both rodents and monkeys to chew and bite at their own bodies. This self-directed biting is called *automutilation,* and animals may sometimes bite off their fingers, toes, or paws. It is likely that automutilation is a form of stereotyped behavior because it appears to be repetitious, but it may also be a result of formication. As we have seen, this sensation of bugs crawling under or on the skin is a symptom of amphetamine or cocaine psychosis in humans and may result in picking at or cutting the skin in order to let the bugs out.

Even at low doses, amphetamines and cocaine decrease consumption of both food and water in most species. This is probably a combination of the effect of the drug on the part of the brain controlling appetite and of the fact that the drug increases other behavior sequences and reduces the time available for eating and drinking. We know that appetite suppression is not related to the reinforcing effects of these drugs because a drug very similar to amphetamine called fenfluramine is very effective in suppressing appetite but does not appear to have any reinforcing effects at all (Brady et al., 1987).

For an excellent description of the effects of amphetamines on both conditioned and unconditioned behavior, see the review by Melvin Lyon and Trevor Robbins (1975).

Positively Reinforced Behavior

One of the earliest experiments on the effects of amphetamines on operant behavior was by Peter Dews (1958), who gave methamphetamine to pigeons responding on several schedules of reinforcement for food. Dews found that the drug increased responding on the FI but decreased FR responding at exactly the same dose. It was in this paper that Dews first demonstrated a relationship between the effect of amphetamine and the rate at which the pigeon was responding. He noticed that methamphetamine increased the rate of responding if it was low, as in the FI, but slowed responding that was normally fast, as in the FR. This effect became known as the *rate dependency effect*. It has since been demonstrated that this rule applies across all amphetamine-type drugs and many others, across many species, and across many types of behavior and schedules of reinforcement (Dews & Wenger, 1977). The significance of this observation cannot be overestimated because it was one of the first demonstrations that a drug interacts dynamically with ongoing behavior. It also showed that it was not appropriate to understand the effect a drug might have by simply classifying it as a "psychomotor stimulant" as we have done. Whether the drug stimulates or depresses motor activity is a result of the behavior being observed and not entirely determined by the properties of the drug alone.

The effects of cocaine are similar to those of amphetamine, but the rate-increasing effects of cocaine are not as great (C. G. Smith, 1964).

Effects on Negatively Reinforced Behavior

The rate dependency principle also appears to apply to avoidance behavior. Kelleher and Morse (1964) conducted an experiment in which monkeys responded both for food and to avoid a stimulus associated with shock on exactly the same schedules, FI 30, FR 10. Amphetamine had exactly the same effect on both the positively and the negatively reinforced behavior: The low FI rates were increased, and the high FR rates were decreased. In cases where avoidance has been decreased by amphetamines, escape responding is also affected at the same dose. This finding suggests that the decrease was probably due to a disruption in all responding. In this regard amphetamines are quite different from the barbiturates and the benzodiazepines.

One place where the rate dependency principle appears not to apply to amphetamine is in behavior that has been suppressed by punishment. Punishment-suppressed behavior usually occurs at a low rate, but most amphetamines and cocaine do not increase these low rates.

DISSOCIATION AND DRUG STATE DISCRIMINATION

It has been demonstrated that amphetamine causes dissociation; animals trained under the influence of amphetamine cannot completely remember what they learned when the amphetamine has worn off. This may be bad news for people who use amphetamines to help them stay awake and cram for exams (Roffman & Lal, 1972).

Rats can learn to discriminate amphetamine and cocaine from saline with moderate ease, although they are not as easily discriminable as barbiturates or benzodiazepines (Overton, 1982). Animals trained to make this discrimination will generalize the amphetamine response to cocaine, methylphenidate, and some MAO inhibitors (Huang & Ho, 1974; Porsolt, Pawelec, & Jalfre, 1982). In rats, amphetamine responses do not generalize to caffeine, nicotine, the barbiturates, chlorpromazine, atropine, or any of the common hallucinogens (Seiden & Dykstra, 1977, p. 416). Humans can also readily learn to discriminate amphetamine from a placebo (Chait, Uhlenhuth, & Johanson, 1986).

Cathinone is as potent as amphetamine in its ability to act as a discriminative stimulus. Rats trained to discriminate cathinone will generalize the response to amphetamine, methamphetamine, and cocaine (Glennon, 1987, p. 1630; Schechter & Glennon, 1985; Glennon et al., 1994).

TOLERANCE

Acute Tolerance

With continuous use of cocaine, sniffing every 20 or 30 minutes for 10 or 12 hours, cocaine quickly loses its ability to cause rushes and gradually loses its ability to improve mood. This phenomenon is sometimes known as a *coke-out* and is usually why runs come to an end (see the discussion of self-administration of cocaine). This acute tolerance dissipates rapidly and may be gone within 24 hours (Waldorf et al., 1977).

Chronic Tolerance

Some effects of cocaine and amphetamines develop tolerance with repeated administration. The appetite-suppressing effect usually disappears with humans in about two weeks, and the effects on the heart and blood pressure also diminish. The lethal effects also show tolerance, and chronic amphetamine users are able to increase their dose to extremely high levels. In one such case, 15,000 mg of amphetamine was administered in a 24-hour period, 1,000 times the normal therapeutic dose and several times the estimated LD_{50} for nontolerant humans. Some effects, such as the blocking of sleep, show no tolerance.

For other effects, reverse tolerance or sensitization takes place. Stereotyped behavior and psychotic behavior appear more frequently after repeated doses in humans. In rats, chronic administration of cocaine lowers the threshold for convulsions, and some electrical activity within the brain increases with continued use (Stripling & Ellinwood, 1976). With continued administration of cocaine, stereotyped behavior and spontaneous motor activity also increase in frequency and intensity (Post et al., 1987). It is unlikely that this increased sensitivity is a result of a buildup of the drug in the body because cocaine has a short half-life that does not appear to change with repeated administration. It is possible that this increased sensitivity is the result of changes in the levels of MA transmitters or in the sensitivity of receptor sites in the brain.

Behavioral tolerance can develop to some effects of amphetamine. In one experiment (Schuster, Dockens, & Woods, 1966), rats responding to a number of schedules were given repeated doses of amphetamine. As expected, the drug increased the low response rates on FI and DRL schedules. Tolerance quickly developed to the effect on the DRL but not to the effect on the FI. Schuster concluded that the increase in rates on the DRL was causing the animals to lose reinforcement, and so they learned to compensate for the effect of the drug on that schedule. The drug-induced increases on the FI, however, did not interfere with reinforcement frequency, and so the rats did not develop tolerance.

WITHDRAWAL

Amphetamine and cocaine are not associated with a severe or medically serious withdrawal when use is discontinued. Depression seems to be the most prominent characteristic of psychomotor stimulant withdrawal.

After a single dose of amphetamine or cocaine, the high is usually followed by a *letdown*, a period of depression and lethargy that can be thought of as a withdrawal symptom. The depression is immediately relieved by another administration of the drug. This letdown occurs within half an hour with cocaine, but with amphetamines its appearance is delayed for a number of hours. The severity of the depression is related to the dose and the duration of the intake period. If the intake period has been long enough to interfere with sleep and eating, there will also be a compensatory increase in sleeping and eating. The nature of the sleep will also change, since there will be a rebound of REM sleep that the drug suppressed.

After continuous long-term use of cocaine, a permanent depression in mood may arise from changes in the functioning of the monoamine systems in the brain. These changes appear to be similar to the changes associated with depression and can be treated with antidepressant drugs (Gawin & Kleber, 1987).

When high levels of amphetamine have been continuously used for an extended *run*, the depression that results may be quite severe and may be accompanied by suicidal thoughts and suicide attempts. The amphetamine withdrawal depression is similar to psychiatric depression except that the latter is characterized by insomnia and decreased appetite, whereas the opposite is true for the amphetamine-induced depression (Angrist & Sudilovsky, 1978).

SELF-ADMINISTRATION IN HUMANS

Cocaine

Cocaine has a long history of self-administration, starting with the native people of South America, who consumed the drug orally. They would insert the wad of leaves into their cheek, where they would chew and suck on it. When taken this way, the pattern of use is very different from the modern North American patterns of self-administration of pure cocaine or amphetamines. With pure cocaine, such continuous use is rare. When snorted or injected, cocaine is usually taken in large quantities for a brief period of time, followed by periods of abstinence. It is usually consumed at parties and in social settings with some ceremony and ritual.

Cocaine is often taken in conjunction with other drugs. The most usual combination is the *speed ball*, a combination of cocaine (or amphetamine) and heroin. Users claim that the heroin reduces the jitteriness caused by the sympathetic nervous system arousal of cocaine and that the cocaine diminishes the sleepiness or *nod* caused by heroin. Cocaine is also regularly mixed with depressants such as barbiturates or methaqualone for the same reason.

Amphetamines

Like cocaine, amphetamines are self-administered sporadically rather than continuously, but the pattern may depend on the effect for which the drug is taken. Because it is longer-lasting than cocaine, amphetamine allows constant blood levels to be maintained for an extended period of time more easily—for example, when the

drug is used to enhance behavior or prevent sleep, as in the case of truck drivers or students cramming for finals. When the need is over, the drug is usually discontinued, and the person then recovers by making up for the lost sleep.

When amphetamines are used for their euphoric effects, usually much higher doses are taken, and the administration is frequently intravenous. The 1960s saw the beginning of this type of use characterized by the *peak user* or *speed freak*. Speed freaks typically inject amphetamine every few hours for days at a time. During this run they do not sleep, they eat very little, and they may show symptoms of amphetamine psychosis such as punding and paranoia. Eventually, when they are too exhausted to continue or run out of drug, they *crash*—they sleep for an extended period, 24 to 48 hours. When they wake up, they are very hungry and eat ravenously before going out to search for more drugs in order to begin another run. This pattern of amphetamine use has virtually disappeared. Amphetamine is being replaced with crack cocaine.

Trends in Use

While the number of frequent cocaine users (once a week during the past year) has remained stable between 1985 and 1993, the National Household Survey in the United States reports that there has been a considerable decline in the number of casual users (less than once a month) over that period. The number of people reporting use within the past month has also declined considerably. Among 12–17-year-olds this rate declined from 1.4 percent in 1985 to 0.4 percent. For 18–25-year-olds the rate declined from 7.5 percent to 1.5 percent, and for 26–34-year-olds the rates were 5.9 percent and 1.0 percent.

In spite of the decline in use, there has been a considerable increase in emergency room incidents involving cocaine. In 1978 cocaine accounted for 1.0 percent of incidents reported by the Drug Abuse Warning Network (DAWN). In 1993 it accounted for 26 percent. Much of this increase took place between 1990 and 1992. Most of these emergency room visits in 1993 were from people seeking detoxification or having an unexpected reaction.

SELF-ADMINISTRATION IN NONHUMANS

In 1968, Roy Pickens and Travis Thompson, then at the University of Minnesota, published the first detailed account of cocaine self-administration in nonhumans. (The first cocaine self-administration experiments were actually done by G. A. Deneau and his colleagues at the University of Michigan, but these were not published until 1969.) Pickens and Thompson used two rats implanted with intravenous catheters and showed that the rats would bar-press on an FR schedule for cocaine. (This experiment is described in Chapter 5.) This was an important milestone for several reasons. To begin with, this was the first demonstration of self-administration of a drug other than morphine, and it established that a drug with no apparent withdrawal symptoms could be a reinforcer, confirming that the reinforcing effect of drugs was not a result of fear of withdrawal. Since the time of this experiment, there have been many demonstrations of cocaine self-administration in many species.

In fact, it appears that cocaine may have a more robust reinforcing effect than almost any other drug. Animals learn to self-administer cocaine more easily than any other drug and work harder for it. In an experiment reported by Yanagita (1975), the reinforcing potency of cocaine was compared with that of a number of other drugs, using the *progressive ratio* procedure. In this procedure, monkeys self-administer a drug on an FR 50 schedule. With every reinforcement, the schedule is progressively in-creased by 50 until the demand becomes so large that responding stops. Presumably, the more reinforcing a drug is, the higher the ratio will get before responding steps. In 4 of 6 monkeys, cocaine was the most reinforcing drug tested. (One monkey worked the ratio up to 6,400 before stopping.) Cocaine tied for first in a fifth monkey, and the sixth found amphetamine more reinforcing than cocaine.

Figure 10–2 shows data published by Deneau, Yanagita, and Seevers in 1969 and demonstrates the erratic pattern of cocaine self-administration in monkeys when the drug is freely available 24 hours a day. The monkey learns quickly to give itself the drug and is soon administering the drug at levels high enough to cause convulsions. The record shows that there is considerable fluctuation from day to day; on some days no drug is taken, but on others massive quantities are infused. In fact, some monkeys given unlimited access to the drug will administer to the point of killing themselves (Bozarth & Wise, 1985).

Figure 10–2 also shows the typical *run-abstinence cycle* characteristic of human stimulant use. In this case, the monkey actually stopped responding for a 28-hour period on day 17 before resuming injections on day 18.

The pattern of self-administration is quite different when access to cocaine is limited to only several hours a day. Under these conditions, laboratory animals self-administer cocaine in a steady and regular manner, precisely controlling the amount of drug they receive on any given day. If the animal is required to work harder for each infusion, it increases its output to exactly the right extent to keep its daily dose constant. This compensation for changes in schedule demand is not usually seen with other classes of drugs (Goldberg et al., 1971).

If the amount of drug per infusion is changed, the animal titrates the dose very accurately; that is, it will either increase or decrease its rate of responding to compensate. The animal appears to

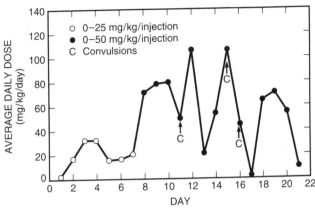

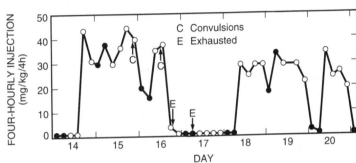

Figure 10–2 The pattern of cocaine self-administration in the monkey. Top: Daily intake for 21 days. Bottom: Intake in 4-hour periods from day 14 to 21, illustrating the cycles of intake and abstinence. (Adapted from Deneau, Yanagita, & Seevers, 1969.)

be motivated to respond for more amphetamine only when the level of drug in the blood falls below a certain point (Yokel, 1987, p. 15).

Nonhumans readily self-administer all the psychomotor stimulants including methylphenidate. Patterns and rates are similar to cocaine. The self-administration of amphetamine can be blocked by pretreatment with AMPT in the same way that the stimulus properties can be blocked by AMPT, indicating that the reinforcing effect of amphetamine is mediated by the CAs, NE, and DA (Schuster, 1975).

Cathinone and methcathinone are also readily self-administered intravenously by monkeys in a manner similar to amphetamine (Kaminski & Griffiths, 1994; Wolverton & Johanson, 1984). When it is available continuously, the same sort of binge-abstinence cycle seen with amphetamine and cocaine is reported (United Nations, 1980, p. 89).

HARMFUL EFFECTS

When methylphenidate is given chronically at low levels in the treatment of hyperactivity in children, it sometimes causes a reduction in growth velocity (Brookes, 1985, p. 267).

There are reports that the Andean Indians who chew the coca leaf regularly seem to have few health problems as a result. It has been noted, however, that these and other regular users of cocaine have a sallow or yellowish complexion, which may be attributable to mild jaundice caused by liver disease. Chronic cocaine use has also been shown to damage the livers of experimental animals (Caldwell, 1976). Chronic cocaine sniffing can also cause inflammation and ulceration of the mucous membranes in the nose. This damage can even progress to the extent that openings appear in the *septum* (the membrane separating the nostrils). Because cocaine is a local anesthetic, this discomfort in the nose will be relieved by sniffing more cocaine, and in this way it will contribute to the motivation to continue sniffing the drug.

Cocaine sniffing, smoking, and injection can lead to an intense compulsion to continue until the drug runs out or the user becomes exhausted. During such runs it is not unusual for vast sums to be spent on the drug (R. K. Siegel, 1982a). The price of a gram of powdered cocaine can range from $30 to over $120 in some U.S. cities. The cost of a rock of crack can range from $5 to $50. People have been known to sell their houses and cars to finance such bingeing. Not only do such binges damage the finances, but many users report disturbing physiological and psychological symptoms as well. Some of the symptoms reported by freebasers include paranoid feelings (62 percent), visual hallucinations (50 percent), cravings (46 percent), antisocial behavior (40 percent), attention and concentration problems (37 percent), blurred vision (34 percent), coughing with black spit (34 percent), muscle pains (34 percent), dry skin (28 percent), tremors (28 percent), and weight loss (28 percent).

The use of oral amphetamine for short periods to stay awake while driving or studying can have harmful effects that include restlessness, excessive talking, confusion, and dizziness. If use is continued for too long, paranoid psychotic behavior starts to appear, which is complicated by the lack of sleep. Punding and irrational thinking may also emerge, and these are not likely to improve driving or studying. In susceptible individuals, the increased blood pressure can cause strokes (Rumbaugh et al., 1971). In addition, when the drug is stopped, there is the period of recovery characterized by depression with suici-

dal tendencies and lethargy, and the REM rebound will cause sleep disturbances.

High-level chronic use, especially associated with intravenous administration, is potentially quite harmful. The harmful effects are both direct and indirect. Amphetamines have a strong direct effect on the heart and circulatory system, causing irregular heartbeat and increased blood pressure that can result in internal bleeding and strokes (Grinspoon & Bakalar, 1979a). Irreversible brain damage has also been reported as a result of deterioration and rupturing of small blood vessels in the brain (Rumbaugh et al., 1971).

As with so many drugs used excessively, many of the harmful effects of amphetamine are indirect and arise from the lifestyle. Because intravenous users rarely use sterile injection apparatus, they frequently contract diseases, particularly hepatitis and AIDS. Their ability to fight diseases is reduced by the poor diet caused by the appetite-suppressing effects of the drug and the fact that they seldom sleep. Coupled with these problems, the high-dose amphetamine user is suspicious, antisocial, and prone to violence (Rylander, 1969). The death rate among intravenous amphetamine users is much higher than expected in the general population, but it is about the same as in chronic alcoholics and heroin addicts of the same age group (Kalant & Kalant, 1979).

Reproduction

Both amphetamine and cocaine have been used to enhance sexual activity. It has been reported that low doses prolong erections and delay ejaculation in males and enhance desire and enjoyment of orgasms in females. These changes, along with a decrease in sexual inhibitions caused by the drug, sometimes lead to changes in sexual orientation and practices while taking these drugs. People who would not normally do such things sometimes engage in marathon sexual acts, group sex, and homosexuality (D. E. Smith, Buxton, & Dammann, 1979). Continuous high doses of cocaine either by inhalation of crack or freebase or by injection often lead to a disruption in sexual activity in males and periods of disinterest in sex (R. K. Siegel, 1982a).

Like cocaine, khat initially increases sex drive in males, but continued use can cause decreased sexual interest and impotency (Giannini et al., 1986). It can also inhibit milk production in nursing mothers who continuously abuse the plant.

There have been some studies of the effects of amphetamine-like drugs on fetal abnormalities. Most of these studies were done on women who used these drugs to control appetite during pregnancy. They provided some evidence linking this chronic, oral, low-dose use with a higher than average incidence of birth abnormalities. Evidence from animal studies also indicates that amphetamine used during pregnancy can cause behavioral and physical problems in offspring (Grinspoon & Hedblom, 1975, pp. 146–147).

While there is mounting evidence that cocaine use by pregnant women is detrimental to the fetus, it appears that the picture presented by the media of "crack babies" was somewhat of an exaggeration. Many studies have found that maternal cocaine use does retard fetal growth, and babies are smaller and possibly more likely to be premature (Zuckerman & Frank, 1994). Other studies, however, have found that babies born to mothers who reported using cocaine while pregnant were not more likely to be born prematurely or have smaller birth weights, but were almost 10 times more likely to have *abruptio placentae* (the placenta detaches prematurely) (Shiono et al., 1995). The existence of long-term developmental and behavioral effects of prenatal cocaine exposure have not been clearly established, although there is some evidence that it may be associated with a diminished IQ at three years of age. These studies are plagued with methodological difficulties, not the least of which is accurately measuring cocaine exposure and separating its effect from other concurrent factors such as the use of other drugs and quality of pre- and postnatal care (Zuckerman & Frank, 1994).

Overdose

Cocaine users who take large doses commonly experience muscle weakness and respiratory depression. The user may be unable to stand up and may collapse but not lose consciousness (Crowley, 1987, p. 202).

The lethal dose of cocaine depends to a large extent on the route of administration. Individuals vary greatly, but the LD_{50} in a 150-pound man is about 500 mg. When the drug is taken intranasally, the LD_{50} may be as low as 30 mg. The absolute dose may not be the important variable in determining the lethality; rather, what seems to be important is the sudden increase in drug levels in the brain.

The cocaine-related deaths of several prominent athletes have emphasized that cocaine has intense cardiovascular effects that can be fatal when the drug is injected or inhaled in concentrated form, the *cocaine sudden death syndrome*. As noted earlier, it is not unusual for laboratory animals to self-administer lethal doses of cocaine. Recently, George and Goldberg (1989) have shown that there is considerable variability between individual strains of rats and mice in sensitivity to various effects of cocaine. One strain of rats, for example, seemed insensitive to the reinforcing effects of usual doses of cocaine but was very sensitive to the lethal effects of cocaine on the heart. If there are similar genetic variations in humans, it is possible that certain individuals might be highly resistant to the euphoric effects of the drug. Such people would be at a considerable risk from cocaine because attempts to reach euphoric doses could easily drive blood levels into the lethal range. Such genetically related variations in sensitivity may account for the cocaine sudden death syndrome (George & Goldberg, 1989).

The cocaine overdose or *caine reaction* has two phases: Initially there is excitement followed by severe headache, nausea, vomiting, and then severe convulsions. This phase is followed by a loss of consciousness, with respiratory depression and cardiac failure causing death. Death may be very rapid, within two to three minutes, or it may take as long as 30 minutes. Someone who survives the first three hours is likely to recover, but if breathing has been depressed long enough, there may be brain damage from loss of oxygen (Gay & Inaba, 1976).

Seizures caused by cocaine overdose can be treated with diazepam, and respiratory depression or arrest can be treated with artificial respiration. Chlorpromazine, the antipsychotic, is also very effective as an antagonist of the toxic effects of cocaine (Crowley, 1987, p. 203).

In a survey of six recorded deaths from amphetamine overdose, the lethal dose ranged from 5 to 630 mg (Kalant, 1973, p. 30).

TREATMENT

The first stage in the treatment of the cocaine abuser involves a period of detoxification during which the direct effects of cocaine are treated. Treatment of cocaine overdose or the caine reaction is done in hospital. The Haight-Ashbury Free Medical Clinic in San Francisco (Gay & Inaba, 1976) has developed a procedure whereby the acute toxic effects of cocaine are treated directly until the patient is out of danger and then, for the next 3 to 12 days, depressant drugs are given and are slowly tapered off. For the less seriously involved, a period of hospitalization may not be essential.

Following detoxication, or for users wishing to stop who are not under the influence of the drug, there are a number of possible long-term treatments. Some of these depend on treatment with other drugs, and some do not.

The initial concern with cocaine abusers seeking treatment is that they will resume using the drug very quickly before any treatment has had a chance to have any effect. It is particularly important to prevent the patient from using cocaine again, even once, since it has been shown that the craving for cocaine increases considerably 15

minutes after single cocaine injection (Jaffee et al., 1989). This fact makes a relapse extremely likely. One strategy used to control this possibility is contracting: The user contracts with the therapist to provide drug-free urine samples for a period of time, often three months. If the urine samples show that the user does not remain abstinent for the period of the contract, or if the user fails to provide a sample, the person must suffer an aversive consequence of cocaine use. Such a consequence might involve sending a letter with the details of the patient's cocaine use to an employer. Contracting is usually very effective in stopping cocaine use during the period of the contract (Crowley, 1987).

This approach has its problems, not the least of which is a reluctance of the user to consent to participate. A newer approach makes use of positive reinforcement in the form of a monetary reward for providing clean urine samples. This reward increases with each succeeding drug-free test. In addition to the money, a relative, spouse, or friend is involved in the program and participates in some previously agreed on enjoyable activity. These incentives are combined with counseling the user to avoid situations where there is a risk of relapse, employment counseling, and encouragement to pursue educational or recreational goals. In a test of this strategy, 11 of 13 cocaine users admitted for outpatient treatment remained drug free for a 12-week period of treatment. Only five of 12 patients in a control group that were offered a 12-steps counseling remained drug free for the 12 weeks (Higgins et al., 1991).

In addition to these treatments, some drugs, primarily the tricyclic antidepressants, have been found to be helpful. There is some evidence that a period of prolonged cocaine use will cause permanent biochemical changes in the brain that are similar to the biochemical changes associated with depression (see Chapter 13). This depression may be responsible for the craving ex–cocaine users have for the drug. Relieving the depression with antidepressant drugs could also diminish the craving. In fact, antidepressants have been reported to diminish the craving for cocaine in ex-users with a delay of about two weeks after beginning treatment. This is, in fact, the same delay that is often seen with the tricyclic antidepressants in their therapeutic effect on depression (Gawin & Kleber, 1987).

Attempts to use methylphenidate and phenmetrazine (an appetite suppressant) as a maintenance drug for cocaine abusers in the same way as methadone is used with heroin users (see Chapter 11) were unsuccessful. A similar technique was tried with amphetamine abusers in the 1960s, but this failed as well (Bergsman & Jarpe, 1969; Gawin & Kleber, 1987, p. 175; Gorelick, 1995).

Unfortunately, few controlled studies have been conducted on the effectiveness of any of these treatments. This is not the fault of the scientists in the field but reflects the fact that this is a difficult area to research. Patients seek treatment at a time of crisis and tend to drop out early. They are often agitated and suspicious and do not want to sign consent forms; nor do they like the possibility that they might be assigned to a control group (Crowley, 1987).

For the chronic, low-dose amphetamine user, there is no standard treatment beyond easing the withdrawal symptoms by tapering off from the drug and then making it unavailable. This approach seems to be sufficient for the majority of iatrogenic amphetamine users. A difficulty arises when the motivation for stopping the amphetamine comes from the physician who is reluctant to continue supplying the drug after several years. The user may not see any reason for stopping and may not be motivated to work within a treatment program (Wesson & Smith, 1979).

CHAPTER SUMMARY

- All the drugs covered in this chapter—amphetamines, ephedrine, cocaine, and cathinone—have a similar effect on the nervous system; they all increase activity at synapses that use a *monoamine (MA)* or an *indoleamine* as a transmitter.

- Amphetamine and cocaine are weak bases. Although they can be absorbed from the digestive system, they are much more effective when injected, sniffed, or smoked and inhaled. They are easily distributed throughout the body and are extensively metabolized by the liver and excreted in the urine. Cocaine has a much shorter half-life than the amphetamines.

- The amphetamines and cathinone increase activity at MA synapses by stimulating leakage of the transmitter, increasing the amount of transmitter released, and blocking reuptake of the transmitter. Cocaine works by blocking uptake of the transmitter.

- MA systems in the brain are closely related to the *pleasure centers* of the *mesolimbic system* and the basal ganglia of the *nigrastriatal system*, which regulate body movement.

- The psychomotor stimulants improve mood. When amphetamine and cocaine are taken in high doses by inhaling or i.v. injection, they cause intense feelings of pleasure called *rushes*. After the effects of the psychomotor stimulants have worn off, a period of depression usually ensues.

- When taken continuously at high doses in both humans and nonhumans, the psychomotor stimulants cause *stereotyped behavior*, the senseless repetition of a meaningless act. In humans, high doses may also cause paranoid behavior and psychosis.

- At low doses, the amphetamines and cocaine can improve performance in certain activities and can eliminate the effect of fatigue on most cognitive and perceptual tasks and on athletic activity.

- The amphetamines can cause dissociation and are readily discriminated from saline. All the psychomotor stimulants and antidepressants will generalize to each other but do not generalize to any other type of drug.

- The psychomotor stimulants are readily self-administered by both humans and nonhumans, and the pattern of self-administration is similar in most species. It consists of a run of self-administration lasting for days or hours during which there is very little eating or sleeping, followed by a period of abstinence and recovery. This period is followed by another run.
- Cocaine is expensive and can be unhealthy. When injected it can contribute to the spread of AIDS. It can make people paranoid and psychotic, injures the health of unborn children, and can cause sudden death in susceptible individuals.
- Treatments for cocaine and psychomotor stimulant abuse are being developed that involve other drugs to reduce craving and withdrawal depression. Behavior therapy is being used successfully to keep the user in treatment long enough for other therapies to have an effect.

CHAPTER

11

The Opiates

The patience of a poppy.
He who has smoked will smoke.
Opium knows how to wait.

—Cocteau (1968, p. 36)

ORIGINS AND SOURCES OF OPIATES

The term *opiate* or *opioid* refers to any drug, either natural or synthetic in origin, that has properties similar to *opium* or its main active ingredient, *morphine*. (Technically, the term *opiate* should be used only to refer to drugs of natural origin, and *opioid* should be used in reference to all opiate-like drugs, but this distinction will not be made here.) This family of drugs is also frequently referred to as *narcotic analgesics* or *narcotics*. A narcotic is a drug that causes sleep. The narcotic analgesics produce analgesia (loss of sensitivity to pain) and make a person sleepy. This name was used to distinguish these drugs

from nonnarcotic analgesics such as aspirin, which do not cause sleep. One difficulty with the word *narcotic* is that over the years it has acquired a new meaning. The word *narcotic* is now commonly used to refer to the habit-forming property of a drug. It has also developed a distasteful connotation; calling a drug a "narcotic" immediately conjures up visions of degenerate and depraved addicts who are slaves to the drug and its suppliers.

This misuse of the term *narcotic* has been given legal sanction, further increasing confusion. In the United States, the Harrison Narcotic Act defined both marijuana and cocaine as narcotics along with opiates. The same is true in Canada, where a so-called Narcotic Control Act regulates the use of many habit-forming drugs, some of which, like marijuana, are not narcotics at all in the sleep-production sense, but in a legal sense they have become "narcotics."

Because there are so many meanings for the term, *narcotic* will be avoided here, and the term *opiate* will be used instead.

Natural and Semisynthetic Opiates

The main natural source of *opium* is a poppy with a white flower (*Papaver somniferum*). This poppy has its origins in Asia Minor but is now grown in countries with similar climates throughout the world. On only 10 days in its life cycle, the plant manufactures the drug, which must be gathered then. Opium is the sap that exudes out of scratches made in the seedpods of the poppy after the petals have fallen off. The scratches are made one day, and the next day the sap is scraped off and compressed into cakes. This is opium.

There are several active ingredients in opium. The two main ones are *morphine,* which accounts for 10 percent of the weight of opium, and *codeine,* which makes up only 0.5 percent. Morphine was first isolated from opium by the German chemist Frederick Sertürner. He called it *morphium* after Morpheus, the Greek god of dreams, and published his findings in 1803. The significance of the finding was not immediately recognized, but in 1831 he was awarded a prize by the Institute of France for his discovery. Also in the 1830s morphine was first manufactured and sold commercially. Codeine was isolated in 1821 by Robiquet while he was experimenting with a new process for isolating morphine.

Heroin is a semisynthetic opiate made by adding two acetyl groups to the morphine molecule (diacetylmorphine). It was first made by the German drug company Bayer in 1898 and sold as having all the good medicinal qualities of morphine and codeine but being free of all their habit-forming properties and other side effects. Heroin is about 10 times more lipid-soluble and gets to the brain faster and in higher concentrations.

Morphine is widely used in medicine and is usually sold as a salt by its generic name, *morphine sulfate.* In the United States, morphine and codeine are legally available only on prescription. In Canada the same is true for morphine, but codeine is available in small quantities in some over-the-counter painkillers and cough medicines without a prescription. Heroin is illegal and cannot be prescribed or used in the United States. For some restricted purposes it may be used in Canada on an experimental basis. It may also be prescribed in the United Kingdom under certain conditions.

Synthetic Opiates

A number of drugs bear little chemical resemblance to morphine but appear to have nearly identical pharmacological and behavioral effects. The best known of these is *meperidine* (Demerol), which is similar to morphine but shorter-acting. *Methadone* (Dolophine) and *LAAM* (*l-alpha-acetylmethadol*) have a much longer duration of action than morphine and are much more effective when given orally. Other synthetics are *levorphanol* (Levo-Dromoran), *pentazocine* (Talwin), *phenazocine* (Narphen), and *propoxyphine* (Darvon). All these drugs are available only on prescription.

Opiate Antagonists

Several synthetic drugs act as antagonists to opiates. One, *naloxone,* is a pure antagonist that will block the action of any other opiate. Others, such as *nalorphine* and *cyclazocine,* have some opiatelike activity of their own but will antagonize other opiates. (We will return to the neurophysiology of opiates later.)

HISTORY OF OPIATE USE

It is believed that the opium poppy was being cultivated in the west Mediterranean region in the sixth millennium B.C., and opium capsules were found in grass bags in Neolithic burial sites in northern Spain dated to about 4200 B.C. (Rudgley, 1995). The earliest written reference to opium is a Sumerian idiogram that is translated as "joy plant." The use of this symbol has been dated to about 4000 B.C. Opium is also mentioned frequently in Assyrian medical tablets dating from the seventh century B.C. These tablets are probably copies of earlier manuscripts. Originally wild, the opium poppy was being cultivated in Assyria and Babylon by the second century B.C. By this time as well, opium use had spread throughout the Middle East and North Africa. It was mentioned in the *Ebers Papyri*, early Egyptian medical scrolls dating to 1550 B.C. In these early writings, the poppy is mentioned primarily as a medicine, but the nonmedical properties of the plant were certainly appreciated.

The ancient Greeks knew of opium as well. The Greek physician Hippocrates recommended the use of opium for a number of conditions, as did the Roman physicians Pliny and Galen and the Arabian physician Avicenna, who recommended it for diseases of the eye and diarrhea.

The use of opium spread from the Middle East in every direction with the expansion of the Islamic religion. It was carried east to India by Arab traders in the ninth century and then from India to China, where it was used primarily as a medicine and taken orally. Later, when tobacco smoking was banned by a Chinese emperor in 1644, the Chinese filled their pipes with opium and invented the practice of opium smoking, a very efficient drug delivery system that assured the popularity of the drug in that country.

The Arabs traded opium along with spices and other goods with the merchants of Venice. In the early part of the sixteenth century, Europeans became aware of opium primarily through the efforts of traveling physicians such as the Swiss doctor known as Paracelsus. Paracelsus traveled throughout Europe carrying opium in the pommel of his saddle and called it "the stone of immortality." Other physicians quickly adopted the drug and prescribed it in various forms to their patients, with great success. John Sydenham, an English physician, wrote in 1680, "Among the remedies it has pleased Almighty God to give to man to relieve his sufferings, none is so universal or so efficacious as opium."

Throughout the seventeenth and eighteenth centuries, the popular use of opiates grew steadily, but in the nineteenth century there was a drastic increase in the British consumption of opium. In 1825 the opium consumption rate was between 1 and 2 pounds per 1,000 population, but at its peak in 1875 the rate was greater than 10 pounds per 1,000 population. Opium was available in many formulations from food stores, pubs, even peddlers on the streets. The most popular form in which opium was sold was tincture of opium, or *laudanum,* which was opium dissolved in alcohol.

It was also about this time that morphine became available. Morphine, however, remained more under the control of the medical profession and was never widely sold in shops like opium. This restriction did not hinder its popularity, as physicians generally prescribed it when requested. For this reason, morphine was more commonly used by the middle and upper classes, since the lower classes seldom saw a doctor.

Though many people were openly addicted to the drug, it was not perceived as a medical or social problem at the beginning of the nineteenth century. Not until the 1830s did all this opium use generate any concern, and not until 1868 was any legislative effort made to control it. This change was brought about by the development of social and political ideas rather than medical research or theory. One contributing factor to this change in perception was the social reform movements of the time, not the least of which was the temperance movement. It has been noted that most of the public concern over opiates was directed at the use of opiates among the lower classes of society. Among the chief concerns of the reformers were the practice of drugging children and the high suicide and accidental poisoning rates associated with opium. While children of all classes were regularly "soothed" with opiate medications, it was believed that working women in the industrial towns doped their babies regularly while they were out of their houses working in the factories. Although it was not as widespread as generally believed, this practice caused great concern among the upper classes. It was also becoming apparent at this time that the drug was not being used by the masses for medical reasons alone but as a source of pleasure, a cheap substitute for liquor. The upper classes could have their addictions, but not the working classes, who, it was believed, must be protected from themselves.

It was recognized that the main problem was the availability of the drug. In 1868, Parliament passed the *Pharmacy Act,* which restricted the sale of opiates to pharmacists' shops. This made it harder for the masses to get the drug but had little effect on upper-class use. This was the first of several laws that slowly brought the use of opiates under the control of the medical profession and out of the hands of the people. It also marked the start of the belief that addiction was a medical problem and should be handled by physicians; this was a new idea at the time.

This designation of opiate use as a medical problem encouraged the perception of addiction as a disease and forced it into a disease model, that of a physiologically based disorder that should be treated by some sort of medical intervention such as admission to an asylum or administration of drugs. The British approach to addictions is basically the same today: In what is known as the *British system,* addicts are given prescriptions for heroin by physicians to treat their "disease."

The story of opiate use in the United States is somewhat different. Americans were just as fond of opiates as the British. In 1870, when British consumption peaked at over 10 pounds per 1,000 population, American consumption rates were greater than 13 pounds per 1,000. Some of this was consumed orally in the form of patent medicines; the majority was refined into morphine and injected by means of the recently developed hypodermic syringe. This route of administration may have become popular because of the wide use of morphine during the Civil War, when morphine addiction became known as the *army disease.* As in Britain, addiction was being defined as a medical problem, but the medical profession was not asked to solve the problem. The American solution to the drug problem was to make opiates illegal. In 1914, Congress passed the Harrison Narcotics Act, which, in effect, made it illegal to be an addict and illegal for physicians to prescribe opiates to addicts.

The Harrison Act banned opium, morphine, and cocaine, but there was one giant omission: heroin. Heroin was invented in 1898 by Heinrich Dreser and marketed by the Bayer company of Germany. Dreser was the inventor of aspirin. He had discovered that if he took salicylic acid, an effective but corrosive painkiller, and added an acetyl group to the basic molecule, he could reduce its corrosive properties. The result was *acetylsalicylic acid* (ASA, originally trademarked as Aspirin). Having made a great deal of money with aspirin, Dreser thought he might try the same trick with the morphine molecule and made *diacetylmorphine,* which the Bayer company marketed as Heroin. The name was derived from the German *heroisch,* meaning "heroic," to imply concentrated power. Early tests showed that heroin was more effective as an analgesic than morphine but did not cause as much nausea and vomiting. It was advertised in newspapers and magazines and sold freely as sort of a superior aspirin. Bayer also claimed that heroin was not addictive and, surprisingly, was believed by the medical profession for many years. This belief was responsible for the omission of heroin from the Harrison Act.

When the Harrison Act was passed, it did not take long for the morphine users to discover heroin. They soon found that heroin could be sniffed into the nostrils and did not always require injections. This fact and the relative lack of nausea must have enhanced its appeal to casual users. By the 1920s it had become obvious to everyone that heroin was indeed as habit-forming as morphine. At this time as well, the newspapers associated heroin with crime, industrial unrest, and a series of Bolshevik bombings, so when heroin was banned by Congress in 1924, it was banned totally. It became illegal for doctors to prescribe it for any reason. This law and the Harrison Act are still in effect today in the United States.

The use of heroin was greatly decreased but never eliminated by these measures. In fact, heroin use has drastically increased in recent years. Estimates suggest that 5 in every 10,000 of the U.S. population were heroin users in 1967. By 1972 this figure had increased to 15, and it reached 23 by 1978 (Wikler, 1980, p. 2). This increase is probably related to the rise in acceptance of drugs by the so-called drug subculture, which was expanding at the same time.

Excellent sources of information on the fascinating history of opiates are J. M. Scott (1969), Latimer and Goldberg (1981), and Berridge and Edwards (1981).

ROUTES OF ADMINISTRATION

Morphine is a base with a pKa of about 8. Consequently, it is not rapidly absorbed from the digestive system, since most of its molecules are ionized in acid pHs. Even though opium eating (or drinking) is common and morphine is frequently given in oral medications, opiates given by the oral route are much less effective than the same dose given parenterally. In addition to slow absorption, morphine when given orally is subject to significant metabolism on its *first pass* through the liver before it can get to the brain (Goth, 1984). Because opiates are frequently given as analgesics, the slowness of the absorption from the digestive system is an advantage because it is easier to maintain constant drug levels in the blood using this route (Melzack, 1990).

When the drug is administered for its subjective effects, most users prefer parenteral routes which cause sudden high levels that appear to be the most reinforcing. Heroin, but not morphine, can be taken intranasally in the form of snuff. Many years ago the Chinese developed a method of smoking opium in a pipe. More recently, the AIDS epidemic has made many people reluctant to use needles, and a newer form of smoking has been developed called *chasing the dragon*. Oil-rich, relatively pure heroin is heated on metal foil till it vaporizes. The user then inhales it through a tube, chasing the smoke so as not to miss any (Schuckit, 1993).

The two most important opiate antagonists, nalorphine and naloxone, are poorly absorbed from the digestive system and are usually administered parenterally. Maximum brain levels are reached in 15 to 60 minutes.

DISTRIBUTION

After absorption into the blood, most opiates are concentrated in the lungs, liver, and spleen, and a large percentage is bound to blood proteins. Though opiates readily pass through the placental barrier into the fetus, they have difficulty getting through the blood-brain barrier because they have poor lipid solubility.

Even though heroin is about 10 times more potent than morphine, the heroin molecule is inactive in the brain. The reason for its potency lies in a combination of its high lipid solubility and its metabolites. Because heroin is highly lipid-soluble, it is absorbed rapidly from its site of administration and then converted rapidly to monoacetylmorphine, which is very potent. The monoacetylmorphine is then converted to morphine (Inturrisi et al., 1983). Codeine also appears to have little direct action on receptors in the brain but has its effect through metabolites, the main one being morphine.

It also appears that the brain is able to eliminate opiates by an active transport mechanism. These two factors combine to keep brain levels of opiate low relative to the levels in other body tissues. Within the brain, opiates are concentrated in the basal ganglia, amygdala, and the periaqueductal gray, an area closely associated with the sensation of pain. The opiate antagonists enter the brain much more quickly than morphine and reach higher concentrations there.

EXCRETION

About 10 percent of morphine is excreted in the urine unchanged, and the remainder is turned into various metabolites, which are eliminated in the urine and in the feces through concentration in the bile. The half-life of morphine is about two hours, and the half-life of codeine is longer, about three to six hours. Ninety percent of morphine is eliminated within 24 hours of administration (Creasey, 1979).

Meperidine is extensively metabolized in the liver, and the metabolites are eliminated by the kidneys. It has a half-life of 3½ hours. Methadone is not completely metabolized; about 10 percent is eliminated unchanged in the urine. It has an extremely long half-life compared to other opiates, 10 to 25 hours, because methadone becomes bound extensively to blood proteins and is not available for metabolism. This long duration of action makes methadone ideal for maintenance therapies. At low doses, methadone is primarily excreted in the feces, but at higher doses, more and more methadone is found in the urine. An even longer half-life has been reported for another synthetic opiate, *l-alpha-acetylmethadol (LAAM)*. Actually, LAAM itself is not active, but two of its metabolites are.

Naloxone and nalorphine are completely metabolized in the liver and have a half-life of about 1½ hours.

NEUROPHYSIOLOGY

Scientists had been certain for many years that opiates worked at receptor sites because their activity seemed to be related to their molecular configuration, and there was competitive antagonism of their effects. But until the early 1970s, no one had ever found an opiate receptor in the body, nor had any endogenous substance been found in the brain that might work as an opiate receptor. In 1973, however, three laboratories independently identified specific receptors for opiates in the brains of rats. This discovery stimulated considerable research, and there has been a veritable explosion of data on opiate receptors since that time. Opiate receptors have now been found in the brains of most vertebrates, from hagfish to humans.

If the brain is equipped with receptors for opiates, it is likely that the brain has opiate-like substances of its own. A search for such a substance was begun. Within two years of the discovery of opiate receptors, six naturally occurring opiates had been isolated from the brains of several different species of animals, including man. One of the researchers, Eric J. Simon (1981), proposed the name *endorphins* for these substances. He derived this name from the words *endogenous* and *morphine*. The endogenous opiates are derived from what chemists call a *polypeptide:* a string of large amino acid molecules. Two of these opiate-acting polypeptides are short strings, five amino acids long, called the *enkephalins.* The longer chains are 16 to 30 amino acids long and are more properly referred to as the endorphins. Many more endorphins have now been isolated, and their molecular structure is now understood (Snyder, 1977). All of these strings of amino acids have been identified as segments of a large molecule called *beta-lipotropin,* 91 amino acids long, which is secreted by the pituitary gland.

In general, endorphins are found in the areas of the brain rich in opiate receptors and are known to be stored in synaptic vesicles, so it might be reasonable to suppose that endorphins are neurotransmitters, but other roles have been postulated for them as well. It is known that the presence of an endorphin interferes with the release of other neurotransmitters such as norepinephrine, dopamine, and acetylcholine and that opiate receptors are located on presynaptic membranes. These discoveries raise the possibility that the endorphins might work as *neuromodulators* by influencing the presynaptic membranes of other synapses. It is also known that endorphins are released into the blood by the pituitary gland for general distribution around the body like other pituitary hormones. Opiate receptors are known to exist outside the nervous system in areas such as the intestine; these might be the targets for the endorphins acting as hormones.

Reviews of the complex neurophysiology and chemistry of endorphins have been written by Teschemacher (1978) and Simon (1981).

Opiate Receptors

There appear to be at least three types of opiate receptors in the brain, referred to as *mu, kappa,* and *sigma*. The one responsible for most of the effects of morphine and the drugs described in this chapter is the mu receptor. Solomon Snyder and his colleagues have demonstrated that not all opiates bind to mu receptors with the same affinity; some have a strong attraction for the receptor, and some have a much weaker attraction. In general, those with the weakest attraction at the receptor have the greatest effect on the receptor. Morphine, for example, does not have a strong attachment to opiate receptors but has a strong effect when it binds with them. In contrast, nalorphine has only a weak effect on the receptor but is bound strongly to it. When these two drugs are mixed together, the nalorphine will be the one to have an effect because it will displace the morphine from the receptor. Since the effect of the nalorphine is only slight, there will be little opiate effect, even though morphine is present. Thus the nalorphine acts as a competitive antagonist to the morphine, turning off the effect of the morphine and substituting its own mild effect. In this sense, it acts as an antagonist because it blocks the morphine, but it is also an agonist because it stimulates the receptor in a mild but morphinelike way. An opiate with both these properties is known as a *mixed opiate agonist/antagonist*. Nalorphine, pentazocine, and cyclazocine belong to this category. They will terminate the activity of more potent agonist drugs and at the same time have a milder effect of their own (Snyder, 1977).

Naloxone is a pure antagonist. It will displace any other opiate from the mu receptor but has no opiate effect of its own. It is used to treat victims of opiate overdoses because it will immediately terminate the action of all agonists. If naloxone is given to an individual who is physically dependent on opiates, it will immediately cause withdrawal symptoms. Opiate antagonists are used in some forms of treatment of opiate addiction. Naloxone is very important in opiate research because it provides a simple way of making sure that the effect of a drug is due to its interaction with mu receptors. This can be established simply by giving naloxone and seeing if the effect is blocked (Garfield, 1983).

The sigma receptor is stimulated by mixed opiate agonist-antagonists such as cyclazocine and pentazocine but is not affected by opiate agonists such as morphine and is only partially blocked by pure antagonists such as naloxone. The sigma receptor is interesting because it appears to be responsible for the unpleasant and psychotic effects produced by higher doses of the mixed agonist-antagonist drugs. The sigma receptor is also stimulated by *phencyclidine (PCP),* a dissociated anesthetic (Martin et al., 1976; see Chapter 15).

Sites of Action in the CNS

The opiates appear to produce their analgesic effects by several mechanisms. They affect areas of the spinal cord that transmit dull burning pain, and it is believed that they block this incoming sensory information. The *periaqueductal* or *central gray* is an area of the brain known to be important in the perception of pain and rich in opiate receptors. When the body undergoes stress and pain, this system is activated, and the sensation of pain is reduced. It is believed that opiates cause their analgesic effects by stimulating the opiate receptors in this part of the brain. Pain is a complicated phenomenon; not only does it have a sensory component, but it has emotional aspects as well. Opiates also reduce the aversive emotion associated with pain. This effect may be mediated through opiate receptors located in various areas of the limbic system such as the amygdala. It is also likely that the reinforcing properties of opiates are also mediated through their effect on limbic system structures. It is believed that in addition to these lower centers, there are opiate systems in the frontal cortex through which opiates relieve pain.

Opiates depress three important centers in the brain stem. They depress the respiratory center and cause slow, shallow breathing. Death from opiate overdose is usually a result of respiratory depression. The vomiting center is also depressed, and so is the center that causes us to cough. This suppression of the cough center is one reason why opiates have been included in cough medicines for centuries. At one time most over-the-counter cough medicines contained codeine, but now they contain *dextromethorphan,* a synthetic opiate without any analgesic effects (Atweh & Kuhar, 1983).

As discussed in Chapter 5, specific sites in the brain are responsible for the reinforcing effects of the opiates. Laboratory animals will readily learn to press a lever to deliver minute quantities of morphine to the ventral tegmental area (VTA; see Figure 5–5), which appears to be part of a pleasure system in the brain. In addition, repeated injection of morphine into the periventricular gray (PVG) will cause the development of physical dependence (Bozarth & Wise, 1984).

EFFECTS OF OPIATES

Effects on the Body

When opiates are first administered, two of their most notable effects are nausea and vomiting. These are caused by the stimulation of an area of the brain known as the *chemoreceptor trigger zone (CTZ),* which detects impurities in the blood and stimulates a center that causes vomiting. Opiates also depress this vomiting center, and this action blocks vomiting. The result of these two effects is that nausea and vomiting are usually seen only after the first administration of the drug. With continuing doses, these symptoms decrease.

Opiates also cause a constriction of the pupils of the eye, so many opiate users have small pupils; this effect diminishes only slightly with tolerance. Pinpoint pupils are also a symptom of opiate overdose. Opiates have little effect on the functioning of the heart, but there is some lowering of blood pressure due to dilation of the peripheral blood vessels. This dilation causes the face and neck to become flushed and warm and may cause sweating. Sweating is one of the unpleasant side effects of methadone.

One of the first medical uses to which opium was put was the treatment of diarrhea and dysentery, and it is still used for this purpose. Opiates do not decrease the overall action of the stomach and intestines, but they seem to disrupt the coordination of digestive activity, with the result that food passes very slowly through the system. This effect stops diarrhea but produces constipation under normal circumstances, and it is probably the most serious medical complication of opiate addiction. Opiates also interfere with urination by causing contractions of the bladder sphincter, making it difficult to pass urine.

Opiate use is known to decrease the level of sex hormones in both sexes, and this lowered hormone level is thought to be responsible for males' difficulty in maintaining erection and reduced sex drive and diminished fertility of both male and female opiate users. Heavy use may even cause atrophy of secondary sex characteristics in males and stop menstruation in women (Cushman, 1981). It has been suggested that opiate addiction is common among prostitutes because they have historically used opiates as a birth control measure.

Effects on Sleep

In spite of the fact that morphine is named after Morpheus, the god of dreams, opiates do not increase sleep. They cause a sleepy sensation and nodding under normal circumstances, but acute administration of morphine and heroin actually causes insomnia and does not increase sleeping time (Belleville et al., 1971). The user may doze off but soon waken with a startle and not feel rested. When subjects do sleep, they show increased muscular tension and spend more time in the lighter sleep stages with a decrease in slow-wave and REM sleep (Kay, Eisenstein, & Jasinski, 1969). However, opiates are useful in causing sleep in people who are kept awake by pain.

Effects on Human Behavior and Performance

Subjective Effects. Many literary figures were known to be users of opium. One of the first people to write about the effects was the English essayist, critic, and writer Thomas De Quincey, who wrote the now famous *Confessions of an English Opium-Eater,* published in 1821. De Quincey used opium for much of his life and wrote about its effects on his mind and on his life in *Confessions.* Like most people in the nineteenth century, he first took opium as a medicine but quickly appreciated its euphoric effects. After his first dose,

In an hour, O heavens! What a revulsion! What a resurrection from its lowest depths, of the inner spirit! . . . That my pains had vanished was now a trifle in my eyes; this negative effect was swallowed up in the immensity of those positive effects which had opened before me, in the abyss of divine enjoyment thus suddenly revealed. . . . Here was the secret of happiness, about which philosophers had disputed for so many ages, at once discovered; happiness might now be bought for a penny, and carried in the waistcoat-pocket; portable ecstasies might be had corked up in a pint-bottle and peace of mind might be sent down by the mail. (De Quincey, 1901, pp. 169–170)

De Quincey reported that there was an increased sensitivity in both hearing and vision. The increase was not so much of loudness of noises and lights as in the ability of the mind "to construct out of raw organic sound an elaborate intellectual pleasure" (De Quincey, 1901, p. 179).

And finally, the dreams. Opiates at higher doses induce a sleepy, trancelike state called a *nod* during which the user sees visions or dreams (hence the expression "pipe dreams"). These are not like the hallucinations from drugs such as LSD but more like vivid daydreams.

Whatsoever things capable of being visually represented I did but think of in the darkness . . . which once traced in faint and visionary colour. . . . They were drawn out by the fierce chemistry of my dreams into insufferable splendor that fretted my heart. (De Quincey, 1901, p. 224)

Nor are the dreams always visual. Coleridge always claimed that the words to the famous *Kubla Khan* came to him in a trance after he had taken opium. Users of opium are firmly convinced that the creative processes are helped by the drug. As Cocteau (1968), the French poet, playwright, and artist, said:

All children possess the magic power of being able to change themselves into what they wish. Poets, in whom childhood is prolonged, suffer a great deal when they lose this power. This is undoubtedly one of the reasons which drives the poet to use opium. (p. 71)

De Quincey took opium orally, and though he enjoyed the experience well enough, he missed a subjective effect that is usually experienced only by people who inject morphine or heroin or who smoke opium: the rush. The rush is an intense momentary feeling of pleasure experienced after injecting the drug and is a result of the high concentrations delivered suddenly to the brain. Rushes are usually described as sexual, rather like an orgasm in the stomach or in the entire body. As one 17-year-old addict described it, "It's just the most intense wonderful feeling. . . . I worry that I will always be tempted to feel the heroin rush again, because nothing else I've tried comes close to it" (Weil & Rosen, 1983, p. 87).

Systematic Studies of Mood. Many authors who write about the subjective effects of opiates stress the euphoric effects and the "divine enjoyment" that the drug offers. Such writings and other accounts have frequently led theorists to speculate that the origin of the attraction of opiates is the relief of anxiety and depression, but most of the experiments in which mood and emotional behavior are measured objectively find that positive feelings do not last and are replaced with changes in mood and emotion that are mostly negative. In one study conducted at the McLean Hospital in Belmont, Massachusetts, by Roger Meyer, Steven Mirin, and their associates (Meyer & Mirin, 1979), male adult heroin addict volunteers were admitted to the hospital and kept in a ward for 42 days. During that time, for a period of 10 days they were allowed to earn heroin injections. During their stay, the ward staff kept track of their aggressive and social behaviors, and they were administered standardized psychological tests and asked to complete mood scales. This study found that during the first few days of heroin administration, before significant tolerance developed, heroin relieved tensions and produced euphoria. However, as use continued, there was a shift to unpleasant mood states and increased psychiatric symptoms. These unpleasant feelings were relieved for only a brief period of 30 to 60 minutes after each injection. In addition to this deterioration in mood, there was also a decrease in physical activity and social interaction and an increase in aggressive behavior and social isolation. These effects diminished when the subjects were maintained on methadone and when the self-administered heroin was blocked by an opiate antagonist.

The effects on mood also differ with whether the drug is given to experienced users or naive subjects. In a classic study, Lasagana and his colleagues at Harvard (Lasagana, Felsinger, & Beecher, 1955) investigated the changes in mood and subjective effects in different populations and found that former addicts were more likely to experience positive feelings after opiates while nonusers reported sedation, mental clouding, and feelings of sickness. In this experiment, 17 out of 30 former users said that they would like to repeat the experience of morphine a second time, whereas only 2 of 20 nonusers wanted to repeat.

Performance. At low and moderate doses, opiates do not appear to interfere with human performance. Most of these studies have been on patients being maintained on methadone, so the doses are generally high enough to prevent withdrawal but low enough so that nodding does not occur. It has been shown that at these dosages, addicted individuals can maintain good health and productive work for extended periods. There are numerous cases of individuals who administered opiates in one form or another for years but were still able to pursue successful and even brilliant careers. One such individual was Dr. William Stewart Halstead, one of the founders of Johns Hopkins Medical School and one of the most brilliant surgeons of his day. He pioneered in the development of aseptic surgical techniques and the use of cocaine as a local anesthetic and was known as the "father of modern surgery." Yet during his career he was addicted to morphine, a fact that he was able to keep secret from all but his closest friends. In fact, the only time his habit caused him any trouble was when he was attempting to reduce his dosage and started to show withdrawal symptoms (Brecher, 1972, p. 35). This is similar to the finding by Thompson and Schuster (1964) that food-seeking and shock-avoidance behavior of monkeys was not disrupted while monkeys self-administered morphine but was disrupted when they were not allowed access to morphine and started to experience withdrawal. (This research will be discussed at greater length later in this chapter.)

At higher doses, opiates interfere with performance by decreasing the motivation to engage in any activity. This lethargy was remarked on by De

Quincey, who, during a period of excessive opium use, desired to do much writing but could not because of his "powerless and infantile feebleness."

Effects on the Behavior of Nonhumans

Unconditioned Behavior. Morphine has a biphasic effect on spontaneous motor activity (SMA). At low doses, there is an increase in movement, but at higher doses, there is a decrease. In mice, this low-dose stimulation causes "running fits," where the mice run blindly and continuously. This effect can be blocked by nalorphine. In rats, low doses cause an increase in SMA. At higher doses, this behavior takes the form of stereotyped responses that differ from the stereotyped behavior caused by amphetamine (see Chapter 10). Morphine-produced stereotyped behavior covers a wide range of behaviors including social behavior, whereas amphetamine-produced stereotyped behavior involves only short duration, nonsocial behaviors (Schörring & Hecht, 1979). Still higher doses produce a type of catalepsy; the animal's body becomes rigid, and the rat can be molded into almost any position, which it will maintain for extended periods. In primates there does not seem to be an excitatory phase. The main effect is a depression of behavior.

Positively Motivated Behavior. At low doses, opiates tend to increase response rates of most species of animals responding on an FI schedule, whereas higher doses slow FI rates. However, FR rates are not altered at low doses, but high doses diminish responding (Thompson et al., 1970). Unlike amphetamines, the decreases in rate on FI and FR both take place at the same doses. The rate-decreasing effects of opiate agonists can be blocked by low doses of antagonists, but these antagonists at higher doses have effects very similar to agonists.

Aversively Motivated Behavior. As with FI response rates, there are reports of opiates increasing both discrete trials and continuous avoidance of electric shocks at low doses, which is not what you might expect from an analgesic, but at higher doses, opiates slow avoidance behavior without disrupting escape responding (Heise & Boff, 1962).

It might be expected that a drug with noted analgesic properties would increase behavior suppressed by punishment, but this is not the case. Opiates usually only decrease response rates already diminished by response-contingent shock (Geller, Bachman, & Seifter, 1963). It is not clear what effect opiates have on behavior suppressed by noncontingent shock. Both increases and no effect have been reported. It would appear that the ability of opiates to diminish pain is not one of the mechanisms by which the drugs change avoidance behavior.

Effects of Self-Administered Opiates. Travis Thompson and Charles Schuster (1964) conducted one of the earliest experiments in which monkeys were maintained on a schedule of self-administered morphine. Monkeys could give themselves intravenous morphine for a brief period every six hours. After the self-administration behavior was acquired, Thompson and Schuster placed the monkeys on an FR 20 for food and a discrete-trials shock-avoidance schedule between periods of morphine availability. They found that the behavior of the monkeys on these schedules was not impaired by the self-administered drug even though the doses reached rather high levels. The only time they noticed a deterioration in the avoidance or the FR was when the morphine was no longer available and the monkeys were going through withdrawal. This is similar to the experience of Dr. Halstead, the addicted surgeon described earlier.

DRUG STATE DISCRIMINATION

Opiates are readily discriminated from saline by both rats and monkeys. Morphine is not as discriminable as the barbiturates or marijuana, but it is more easily discriminable than the hallucinogens and the stimulants (Overton, 1973). Animals trained to discriminate morphine will generalize to all other opiate agonists such as methadone and codeine, but only partly to mixed opiate agonist/antagonists such as cyclazocine. In addition, rats can be trained to discriminate between morphine and cyclazocine. Discriminative stimulus control of morphine and cyclazocine can be blocked by opiate antagonists, but cyclazocine requires a dose of antagonist 10 to 30 times higher than morphine. This evidence suggests that these drugs have effects on different populations of opiate receptors. Morphine works at the mu receptor, which can be blocked easily by opiate antagonists, but cyclazocine works at both the mu and sigma receptors, with the result that its effects can only be partly blocked by the antagonist. Another reason to believe that the sigma receptor is involved is that PCP is generalized to cyclazocine but not to morphine, and PCP acts on the sigma receptors (Holtzman, 1982).

TOLERANCE

One of the most remarkable features of opiates is the rapidity and extent of the development of tolerance to most of their effects. Figure 11–1

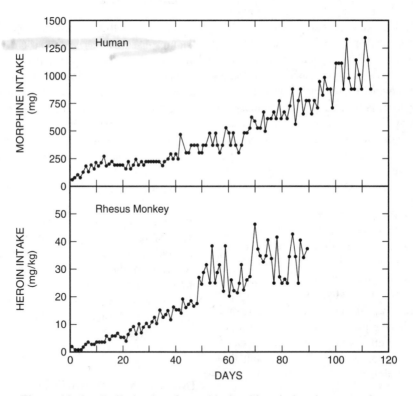

Figure 11–1 Daily intake of morphine and heroin in a human and a rhesus monkey when allowed free access to the drug. In both species intake slowly increases over time and there are no periods of abstinence or voluntary withdrawal. (Adapted from Griffiths, Bigelow, & Henningfield, 1980.)

shows the increasing dose self-administered by two species. Within three or four months of regular use, consumption will increase tenfold or more. In fact, doses taken by a regular user may be sufficiently high to kill a nontolerant individual several times over.

Tolerance develops to different effects at different rates and disappears at different rates. For example, while complete tolerance may develop to the analgesic and positively reinforcing effects, constriction of the pupil recovers only partially with continued opiate use, and the constipating effects never go away.

It is clear that some tolerance is due to changes in opiate metabolism and some is the result of changes in the properties of the opiate receptors. Another likely mechanism of tolerance is learning, since tolerance seems to some extent to be dependent on the environment in which the drug is given (S. Siegel, 1983). (See the discussion of tolerance in Chapter 3.) One interesting theory suggests that tolerance may also result from the development of an immune response to opiates that can be induced by a single administration of the drug (Cochin, 1974).

Cross-Tolerance

Generally, when tolerance has developed to any opiate drug, there will be tolerance to all others. This cross-tolerance does not extend to the depressants, stimulants, or hallucinogens, but there is some degree of cross-tolerance between opiates and alcohol.

WITHDRAWAL

Opiate withdrawal is probably one of the most misunderstood aspects of drug use, largely because of the image of withdrawal that has been portrayed in the movies and popular literature for many years. This popular notion of the severity of heroin withdrawal probably came about in the 1920s and 1930s when heroin addicts had easier

access to cheaper sources of the drug and took it in much greater quantities than are common now. Few addicts these days are able to take enough drug to cause the severe withdrawal symptoms that are shown in the movies. Even in its most severe form, however, opiate withdrawal is not as dangerous or terrifying as withdrawal from barbiturates or alcohol. In fact, withdrawal from alcohol can be fatal, but withdrawal from heroin or any other opiate is never fatal.

Classic heroin withdrawal proceeds in predictable stages. It starts 6 to 12 hours after the last administration of drug, peaks at 26 to 72 hours, and, for the most part, is over within a week. The first sign is restlessness and agitation. Yawning soon appears and may become quite violent. The person is able to stay still only briefly, and paces about with head and shoulders stooped over. The user experiences chills with an occasional hot flash and breathes with short jerky breaths. During this time goose bumps appear on the skin, which takes on the appearance of the skin of a plucked turkey (this is the origin of the expression "going cold turkey"). At this point the addict becomes drowsy and will often fall into a deep sleep known as the *yen* sleep, which may last 8 to 12 hours. After awakening, there are cramps in the stomach, back, and legs; vomiting; and diarrhea. There may also be twitching of the extremities, which causes the hands to shake, and a kicking of the legs (this is the origin of the expression "kicking the habit"). There is also profuse sweating, and the clothes and the bed may become saturated with sweat. These symptoms become progressively less severe and soon disappear altogether.

The severity of the withdrawal depends on the daily dose of the addict and is seldom as severe as this description. For most individuals, withdrawal resembles a bad case of the flu. Even though heroin withdrawal is not life-threatening, it is extremely uncomfortable and is not undertaken lightly.

Withdrawal is similar for all opiates, although it is usually less severe with the less potent opiates such as codeine or propoxyphine. These withdrawal symptoms can be stopped almost instantly at any stage by the administration of any of the opiate drugs. Opiate withdrawal symptoms can also be reduced by alcohol (Ho & Allen, 1981). Withdrawal in a physically dependent individual can be generated almost instantly by the administration of an opiate antagonist.

SELF-ADMINISTRATION IN HUMANS

We tend to think of all heroin users as addicts, but this assumption is certainly not true. Many people appear to be able to maintain what is called an "ice-cream habit" or "chipping," in which heroin is taken occasionally when the drug and opportunities to take it are available. Although chipping is a reality, its extent is unknown because chippers are difficult to detect. They appear to be able to maintain a normal lifestyle and seldom require treatment.

We know a great deal more about the *addicted pattern* of heroin use, which has been extensively studied. In this pattern, the user is often (though not always) physically dependent and attempts to consume sufficient heroin to experience the rush and to avoid withdrawal, usually at least one injection a day. The addict is preoccupied with "taking care of business" or "scoring"—obtaining and taking the drug. This usually occupies most of the addict's attention and money, leaving little time and resources for anything else. The heroin addict typically chooses friends and associates who are also heroin users.

The first exposure to heroin is usually motivated by curiosity and is approached with caution. Frequently, the new user is introduced to the drug by someone he or she trusts. Surveys show that by far the majority of addicts were first given the drug by a friend. Very few were given the drug by a "pusher" or someone unknown to them. It is extremely unlikely that someone could be made into an addict against his or her will by an unscrupulous pusher trying to develop new markets. Figure 11–2 shows the result of a study of the spread of heroin use in a community in England (Alarcon, 1969). Such diagrams make it clear that the spread of the drug can be treated as though it were a communicable disease like the measles.

It is not known how many people exposed to opiates do not become addicts and avoid the ad-

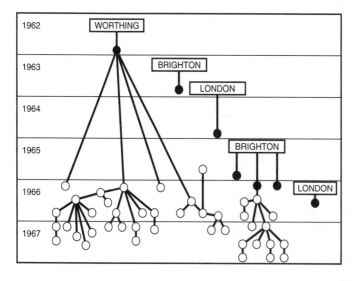

Figure 11–2 How heroin use spread in Crawley, England, from 1962 to 1967. Crawley is a small town of about 62,000 near London. The pattern is that a young person would leave the town and be introduced to heroin use in another community. Such people are indicated by solid circles. On their return some of these would introduce others to the drug as indicated by the lines. There are two main chains started by users from Worthing and Brighton. Altogether, 53 new heroin users were initiated in Crawley. (Alacron, 1969, p. 18.)

dicted lifestyle. We have already seen that the initial experience with heroin is considered unpleasant by the majority of first-time users, and it probably requires considerable persistence to acquire a physical dependence.

At the other end of addiction, there appears to be a *maturing out* of heroin use. Studies have indicated that many addicts spontaneously discontinue use of the drug (Winick, 1962). These addicts usually reach this point in their 30s or 40s after some 5 to 10 years of heroin use. The longer a person has used heroin, the less the chance of maturing out. It is difficult to estimate the number of addicts who eventually mature out; estimates range from more than two-thirds (Winick, 1962) to less than a quarter (Ball & Snarr, 1969).

Patterns of Use

Studies on nonhumans and humans have shown very similar patterns. In both cases, when the drug is freely available, the amount of self-administered drug is carefully regulated. As tolerance develops, the daily dose increases gradually and regularly until it reaches a peak and then remains steady. There are no intake-abstinence cycles as with alcohol and stimulants, and withdrawal symptoms are not seen. Figure 11–1 shows data from similar studies. In one, a human heroin addict self-administered morphine intravenously, and in the other, a rhesus monkey gave himself heroin via the same route (Griffiths, Bigelow, & Henningfield, 1980). For the most part, this pattern is similar to that of the opiate addict who attempts to maintain a fairly constant blood level and avoids withdrawal when it is at all possible to do so.

Trends in Use

While the reported use of heroin in most segments of the population has remained fairly stable since the late 1970s, the Drug Abuse Warning Network (DAWN) reports that heroin-related emergency room admissions have been steadily increasing since 1978 when they accounted for 4 percent of drug-related episodes. In 1993 they accounted for 13 percent. This appears to be a continuing trend. Since 1988 there has been a very large increase in episodes where the reported route of administration was "sniffed," or "snorted." There was a much smaller increase in reports involving heroin "injection." This change reflects a dramatic increase in the purity of heroin in recent years. In 1985, the purity of heroin on the street was usually less than 10 percent—probably why the drug was referred to as "shit." In 1992 the purity of street-level heroin was 73.7 percent. This increase in purity has contributed to a change in the way heroin is administered. One reason why heroin was preferred over morphine in the years after morphine was banned by the Harrison Act of 1914 was because its high lipid solubility meant that it could be taken intranasally (sniffed). The reason why it had to be injected until recently has been the very poor quality of the drug on the street. The recent increase in sniffing arises from the recent improvements in the quality of street drug. It is also motivated by an avoidance of the risks of infections such as AIDS that have been associated with needles (Sabbag, 1994). This recent trend toward a grade of heroin that can be sniffed may herald a surge in use as middle- and upper-class drug users, familiar with snorting cocaine but unhappy about injecting themselves, discover this new heroin.

SELF-ADMINISTRATION IN NONHUMANS

Morphine was the first drug for which intravenous self-administration was demonstrated in nonhumans. We have already discussed one of the first experiments of this type, conducted by Travis Thompson and Charles Schuster and published in 1964. At the time this research was done, it was assumed that physical dependence was an essential aspect of addiction, so Thompson and Schuster used squirrel monkeys that had been made dependent on morphine by injections four times a day for 30 days. The monkeys were then given the opportunity to bar-press for morphine four times a day. The monkeys were placed on an FI-FR chain schedule; to receive the drug, the monkeys were on an FI 2-minute schedule while a tone was turned on. The first response made after two minutes turned off the tone and turned on a white light. While the white light was on, the animals were required to make 25 responses. When this requirement was completed, a red light came on, and an infusion of morphine was given through an intravenous catheter.

The monkeys readily learned this response, and they performed on these schedules in the same manner as they would for any other reinforcer. Thompson and Schuster (1964) also demonstrated that both deprivation from morphine and injections of nalorphine would increase the amount of morphine the monkeys would administer. In later research they demonstrated that nondependent monkeys would also self-administer morphine (R. M. Schuster & Thompson, 1969).

As shown in Figure 11–1, when morphine is freely available, it is self-administered by laboratory animals with great regularity on a daily basis, and the dose slowly increases.

HARMFUL EFFECTS OF OPIATES

Acute Effects

At very high doses, opiates produce a comatose state with pinpoint pupils and severe depression of breathing, which eventually causes death. Unlike barbiturates, opiates lower the seizure threshold and may also cause convulsions at high doses. Opium has been used historically as a poison, so it is not surprising that people die from time to time from accidental overdose (OD) of opiates.

In fact, heroin overdose was the leading cause of death in all males aged 15 to 35 in New York City in 1969 and 1970, and the number of heroin overdose deaths in New York and other large American cities has increased drastically since the 1950s. However, it has been suggested that many of these deaths may not be due to heroin overdose at all. One reason for this suspicion is that analysis of the heroin in the bodies of overdose victims frequently does not show a lethal level of the drug. In addition, others using the same amount of heroin from the same "bag" as the victim have not reported any ill effects. Why, then, are there so many ODs? It is likely that they are not ODs at all. The reason for the high overdose death statistics is the coroners' practice of putting "heroin overdose" on death certificates if no other cause of death is apparent and the individuals were known addicts who had recently shot up heroin (Brecher, 1972).

Even if these deaths were not ODs, what could be killing so many addicts? There are several explanations. One possibility is *quinine,* a drug used to cut or dilute the heroin before it is sold on the streets. Quinine can be lethal when given intravenously, and frequently these OD victims show signs of quinine poisoning such as froth oozing from the nose and mouth. Another explanation is the mixing of heroin with other respiratory depressants such as barbiturates and alcohol. These drugs potentiate the effects of heroin and may make an otherwise normal dose of heroin lethal. The rock singer Janis Joplin died of a heroin overdose after some hard drinking with her friends at a nearby bar.

Another possible cause of an unexplained overdose is a sudden loss of tolerance to the drug. As described in Box 3–1, some tolerance may depend on the specific environment in which the drug is normally given. If the drug is used in a new environment, tolerance is diminished, and what is a normal dose for an addict may suddenly be transformed into a lethal dose.

Chronic Effects

Surprisingly few medical problems arise as a direct result of chronic heroin use. One of these is constipation. Somewhat more serious is a direct link between opiates and cancer. Opiates interfere with the body's ability to repair damaged DNA molecules, and this effect makes them cancer promoters, enhancing the cancer-causing effects of other substances that damage DNA. Like alcohol use, heroin use greatly increases the chance of bladder cancer caused by smoking (Falek et al., 1982).

Though there are some direct health problems caused by opiates, most of the harm done by opiates is indirect and arises from the addicted lifestyles most addicts are forced to adopt. Heroin is expensive, and it may take several hundred dollars a day to support the habit. Because getting the drug takes such priority, housing and nutrition suffer, and so does health. Added to these difficulties is the greatly increased exposure to disease caused by the practice of "shooting up" the drug. These injections are seldom done with clean needles and syringes, and often many people use the same equipment, providing direct access for diseases into the body, including hepatitis and AIDS. Being a heroin addict is not healthy. Between 1972 and 1973 the death rate for addicts was 13.2 per 1,000 population, while the death rate of the general population was 9.3 per 1,000. These figures are even more startling when specific age groups are compared. The death rates in the 16 to 32 age range was 13 times higher for addicts than for the general population (Watterson, Sells, & Simpson, 1976). It is estimated that 21 percent of intravenous drug users in the United States are carriers of the AIDS virus. In certain areas of New York this figure is as high as 60 percent (C. R. Schuster & Pickens, 1988). Apart from disease and overdose problems, heroin addicts are more likely to die from violent death and suicide (Wikler, 1980, p. 4).

Reproduction

In males, chronic opiate use reduces levels of the male sex hormone testosterone. This effect leads to a decrease in sex drive and fertility and may also cause changes in secondary sex characteristics. In women, alteration in hormone levels causes menstrual irregularities, amenorrhea, and a consequent decrease in fertility.

Pregnancies are also complicated by direct and indirect effects of opiates and opiate withdrawal. During pregnancy, the ability of the body to eliminate opiates is increased. The subsequent reduction in circulating levels of opiates leads to increased demand for the drug and increases the probability of withdrawal if the drug supply is irregular or uncertain. It is believed that opiate withdrawal during pregnancy can harm the fetus because it causes a decrease in blood oxygen levels. Numerous other medical complications in the pregnancies of addicted women may arise from the problems of the addicted lifestyle. These complications, which occur in 40 to 50 percent of pregnant addicts, include anemia, cardiac disease, swelling, liver disease, hypertension, pneumonia, tuberculosis, and infections of the urogenital system, such as bladder infections and venereal disease (Kreek, 1982).

Babies born to addicted mothers have low birthweights and are more likely to be premature and to experience illness and complications after birth. In general, these problems are less likely in methadone-maintained mothers than in those using street heroin.

One big problem for babies born to dependent mothers is that right after birth, they have to go through withdrawal because they are no longer exposed to the opiate in the mother's blood. Withdrawal in neonates is similar to adult withdrawal. The symptoms include irritability, respiratory distress, yawning, sneezing, tremors, difficulty in sucking and swallowing, and a peculiar high-pitched cry. Some may even experience seizures. These symptoms start within 72 hours of birth and may last six to eight weeks (Finnegan, 1982).

TREATMENT

History

Ever since opiate addiction was defined in the nineteenth century as a medical problem, there has been pressure on the medical profession to provide some sort of "cure." Prior to that time, alcoholism and opiate use were not considered medical problems but moral problems, indications of a weakness of character or a flaw in personality. They were treated as any other immoral behavior, with punishment and censure. In this context, drug use was only a concern of the medical profession when it led to ill health. For many years after the medical profession undertook to provide treatment for opiate addiction, these ideas of morality continued to influence medical thinking. At first, notions of character weakness were simply transferred to medical jargon; addiction was thought of as a "disease of the will" or "moral insanity." The sorts of treatments generated by these ideas involved in "cultivation of self-control" and the "reeducation of the will." Self-control was equated with health, and so physical exercise and clean living were emphasized, along with the moral leadership of the physician specialist.

By the beginning of the twentieth century, the idea of treating the will had disappeared. Drug-seeking behavior and compulsions were thought to result from organic causes, and the addict was no longer held responsible for the condition. The difficulty with this view was that no organic cause could be identified. One solution was to turn to the drug itself for a cause. It was believed that one effect of opium was the compulsion to use more opium. It therefore followed that the craving would disappear from the mind when the drug was purged from the body, so many treatments of addiction were very similar to the treatments of opiate overdose. In following this line of reasoning, many physicians felt that the best thing to do with an addict was to precipitate sudden withdrawal. The suffering of the patients was not taken into account, and patients were not given any treatment to relieve the withdrawal. It is likely that the old moralistic ideas of punishment contributed to the acceptability of such treatments.

Many other drugs were used at various times to treat opiate addiction. These included atropine, bromides, caffeine, chloral hydrate, cannabis, cocaine, and even the newly discovered heroin.

Therapeutic Communities

A more recent approach to treatment is the therapeutic community such as Daytop, Phoenix House, or Odyssey House. The best example of a therapeutic community is the earliest and the prototype of most others: Synanon, founded in 1958 in California by Charles E. Dederich, a recovered alcoholic. It is staffed by former heroin addicts and operates as a commune. Addicts seeking help are admitted to the community, where they are isolated from the outside world. As in Alcoholics Anonymous, the philosophy of Synanon is that there is no "cure," just control. Users are kept inside and isolated from the neighborhood, friends, and situations that had formerly been part of their addiction and are given social support until they are believed to be in control of the habit. Only then are they permitted to work outside, returning to Synanon every night. Eventually, when they and others are confident that they can control the habit, they are permitted to leave if they want to. Many do not.

Synanon was not started by professionals or governments with any basis in a scientific theory of addiction. It arose spontaneously in response to a social problem. Its aim sounds surprisingly similar to the early moralistic treatments: to restructure an immature, addiction-prone individual into a strong, self-reliant person who no longer needs a drug (Yablonsky & Dederich, 1965).

After years of operation, Synanon claims an abstinence rate of only around 10 percent. Ninety percent of all "graduates" relapse, and this figure probably does not give a true picture of its real effectiveness, since Synanon accepts only the most likely candidates in the first place, those who appeared highly motivated to quit (Brecher, 1972). Therapeutic communities are also only appropriate for younger, unattached addicts, and they are not suitable for those with family and employment responsibilities.

Maintenance Therapies

The British System. Maintenance therapies are based on the philosophy that the real harm done by opiates arises from the fact that they are expensive and illegal. It follows that if addicts have a cheap, reliable source of the drug, they will remain healthy, be free to pursue careers and normal lives, and not be forced into a criminal way of life. In England this approach has been followed for years. An addict can obtain a prescription from a special clinic and have it filled at public expense at any druggist's shop. This approach is known as the *British system,* and it appears to be modestly effective in preventing new cases of heroin addiction, decreasing the death rate in addicts, reducing criminal behavior, and improving the functioning of addicts. It has the added advantage of bringing addicts into regular contact with health professionals and is effective in stopping the spread of AIDS (Bewley, 1974; O'Mara, 1993).

One British writer has suggested that treating addiction as a medical problem in a clinic reduces the glamour of drugs; after all, "sickness is generally less attractive than sin" (Bewley, 1974, p. 160).

Methadone Maintenance. In the United States, various laws made it impossible for doctors to prescribe heroin to addicts, so methadone has been used to prevent withdrawal (Nyswander, 1967). Methadone has several advantages over heroin as a maintenance drug. First, it can be taken orally. Second, it prevents withdrawal symptoms for 24 hours. Third, it acts as an antagonist to heroin. Because it can be taken orally, it is easy to administer and does not have all the associations of shooting up. The fact that it lasts for 24 hours means that it can be administered once a day in a clinic and the user does not need to take it home. And the fact that it blocks the effects of heroin means that addicts on methadone will experience few euphoric effects or rushes if they decide to try heroin. It is not entirely clear why methadone blocks the effect of heroin. We know that methadone competes with morphine for the mu receptors, but it is also possible that the lack of sensitivity to heroin arises from cross-tolerance between methadone and heroin.

Substitution of methadone for heroin is not considered a therapeutic end in itself. Methadone is always used in conjunction with psychological or social treatments. In fact, the success of methadone treatments depends heavily on the addict's having a good, trusting relationship with well-trained staff (Weddington, 1995).

In a typical methadone maintenance clinic, patients are screened to ensure that they really are physiologically dependent on heroin, and then, over the period of several weeks, a dosage of methadone is worked out that will maintain that person free from withdrawal symptoms. Typically, the patient must return to the clinic every day for a drink of methadone. In some programs, addicts who demonstrate that they have been free of heroin and other problems are permitted to take the drug home and are only required to attend two or three times a week.

Over the years that methadone has been used as a maintenance drug in the United States, it has been demonstrated that it reduces sickness and death associated with illicit drug use, normalizes disruptions of immune and endocrine functions, reduces the transfer of HIV, and reduces criminal activity (Ling, Rawson, & Compton, 1994).

Many addicts choose to stay maintained on methadone indefinitely, but as normal lifestyles develop, there are pressures to detoxify altogether. Methadone patients are discriminated against in insurance, licensing, employment, and housing, and the pressures to attend clinics regularly interfere with travel and vacations. Then, too, methadone has uncomfortable side effects such as sweating, sexual dysfunction, and constipation. With patients who appear ready and motivated to discontinue the drug, doses of methadone are slowly decreased over a period of no less than six months so that withdrawal is minimized. This process is best accomplished at a rate that is decided on by the user and that should be very gradual. Even when the methadone reduction is gradual, detoxification becomes difficult when the doses get low.

In general, relapse rates in addicts weaned from methadone are similar to those with other methods—80 to 90 percent—but some reports have been quite impressive (Meritz et al., 1978; Simpson, Joe, & Bracy, 1982; Weddington, 1995). It is estimated that of the half million to one million people in the United States that are addicted to heroin, 100,000 receive methadone maintenance therapy in the 750 to 800 clinics across the country (Ling, Rawson, & Compton, 1994).

LAAM. One new maintenance drug is LAAM. Like methadone, this drug can also be taken orally and blocks the effects of heroin, but its effects last longer than methadone—up to 72 hours—and it needs to be taken only three times a week. The addict need not come to the clinic as often, and the clinic need not send any of the drug home with the addict. After many years of extensive testing, LAAM was formally approved in the United States in 1993 as a maintenance drug for heroin addicts.

LAAM appears to work better than methadone in cases where the addict is unable to get to a clinic on a daily basis because of difficulties with employment, child care, or transportation. There are also some addicts who have problems stabilizing on a dose of methadone, and some who for one reason or another refuse to enter methadone treatment. Many of these people report that LAAM "holds" better than methadone (Ling, Rawson, & Compton, 1994).

Some people believe that LAAM has the capacity to change the face of heroin maintenance therapy. Methadone may still continue to be used for primary treatment in specialized clinics in inner city areas where heroin use flourishes and users require the intensive support of daily clinic visits, but as addicts establish more stable lifestyles, employment, and family lives, it would be more appropriate to switch to LAAM and make it available in a general health care setting (Ling, Rawson, & Compton, 1994).

Buprenorphine. Buprenorphine has been used as an analgesic and is still used experimentally for heroin dependence. It can be taken orally and has a long half-life, although its effects do not last as long as those of LAAM. It binds to mu receptors where it is a partial agonist; that is, it blocks the effects of heroin but has only mild opiate effects itself. Thus it will block heroin withdrawal and only cause mild physical dependence. It therefore is much easier to stop taking buprenorphine than methadone or LAAM, and it is easier to switch to antagonist therapies without experiencing withdrawal (Ling, Rawson, & Compton, 1994).

Antagonist Therapies

As mentioned, one of the advantages of methadone over heroin for maintenance is that methadone works as an antagonist to the effects of heroin. In the presence of methadone, the effect of heroin is greatly diminished. This aspect of methadone is considered beneficial, but it is not the main reason why methadone is used. Methadone is used primarily to prevent withdrawal. An implicit assumption of maintenance therapies is that the primary motivation for taking heroin is the fear of withdrawing. Addicts are therefore maintained on the drug so that they will not be compelled to use heroin from the streets to prevent withdrawal. This assumption may not be correct. We know from studies of self-administration with laboratory animals that physical dependence is not necessary to maintain opiate self-administration. Nondependent monkeys will self-administer opiates at a high rate even though they have never experienced withdrawal. This type of research has shown that drug taking is motivated by the positively reinforcing effects of drugs, not the fear of withdrawal. It is little wonder, then, that drug-seeking behavior persists during and after maintenance and why the heroin-blocking effect of methadone is important.

If the reinforcing effect of the heroin is responsible for its use, there is no need to maintain a person in a physiologically dependent state, but it is important to keep the reinforcing effect of heroin blocked. This is where the antagonists come in. They are very effective heroin blockers and have only minimal agonist properties.

Patients are first withdrawn from heroin and kept abstinent for seven to ten days; otherwise, the antagonist would precipitate withdrawal symptoms. This stage can be difficult, and the dropout rate is very high at this time. There has been considerable benefit using clonidine to relieve the withdrawal, an approach which permits the early use of the antagonist (Gold, 1995). As early as possible, addicts are given daily doses of an antagonist—naloxone, naltrexone, or cyclazocine—when they come for therapy, which is usually at an outpatient day program where they also have educational seminars, recreational activities, and group therapy. The best way to get rid of positively reinforced responses is to extinguish them by allowing the responses to occur but removing the reinforcement. The antagonist accomplishes this purpose by blocking the rewarding effects of heroin when it is used, so that the heroin is no longer a reinforcer. Since the patients in the antagonist therapy treatment are outpatients who are free to spend their evenings and weekends with their friends, they inevitably attempt to use heroin, but this behavior quickly extinguishes and soon disappears.

Early experimental antagonist programs report success in keeping addicts in treatment. At the end of one year, 70 percent were still in the day program, and fewer than half of these were still taking the antagonist. Urine tests for heroin showed that fewer than 2 percent of the patients used heroin (Kleber, 1974). The results of programs such as these suggest that maintenance on antagonists may be more beneficial than maintenance on agonists.

Even though results have been encouraging (Kleber, 1974), an unexpected difficulty has arisen. When drug users know that they are getting an antagonist, they seldom try to shoot up heroin because they "know" that it will not have an effect. When they start taking the antagonist, they usually stop using heroin so suddenly that the positive reinforcing effects of the heroin on heroin-seeking behavior never get a chance to extinguish. Consequently, once the antagonist is discontinued, relapse rates will be high (Martin et al., 1976). In spite of this problem, research has shown that if a person stays in antagonist therapy for two to three months or longer, chances of staying heroin-free after treatment are considerably increased. Success rates with antagonist therapies are much better with people who were highly motivated to quit, have strong family support, and have legitimate professional careers (Jaffe, 1987). Antagonist therapy is beneficial probably because it gives users a chance to decide to remove themselves from the temptation to relapse and permits them to develop other, more socially acceptable sources of reinforcement (Wikler, 1980).

CHAPTER SUMMARY

- The *opiates* are a class of natural and synthetic drugs. *Opium*, derived from the opium poppy, is the source of *morphine* and *codeine*. Heroin is made by slightly altering the morphine molecule to make it more lipid-soluble and consequently more potent. Synthetic opiates such as *methadone* and *LAAM* have a different chemical structure but have the same site of action and similar physiological effects.

- Opium has been used for centuries in the Middle East. It was spread by Arab traders from there to Africa, China, and Europe, where in the sixteenth and seventeenth centuries it was widely used as a medicine. Its popularity grew until the middle of the 1800s, when legal restrictions were placed on its use in England. In the United States all opiates except heroin were banned by the Harrison Act of 1912. Later, in 1924, it too was banned.

- Most opiates are not well absorbed from the digestive system and need to be inhaled or injected for full effect. The opiates are metabolized primarily in the liver and have a half-life of two to four hours except for some synthetics such as methadone or LAAM.

- The body seems to have its own systems that use endogenous opiate-like chemicals called *endorphins* or *enkephalins* both as neurotransmitters and neuromodulators. There are several opiate receptors, but the one that is responsible for reinforcing and analgesic effects is the *mu* receptor.

- One opiate system involves the spinal cord and a part of the brain known as the *central gray*. It is thought that the analgesic properties of the opiates are mediated by this mechanism.

- Opiates cause a sleepy, dreamy state and when taken intravenously cause *rushes,* or feelings of intense pleasure resembling orgasm.

- Chronic opiate use causes constipation and diminished sex drive and sexual performance, but if doses are not too high, chronic use does not interfere with intellectual or physical abilities.

- The opiates slow the behavior of nonhumans responding on both positively and negatively reinforced schedules. There is no indication that these changes are due to analgesia or a decrease in sensitivity to pain or to the fear of painful stimuli.

- Tolerance develops at different rates to the different effects of opiates. Withdrawal symptoms occur after chronic opiate use, and the severity of withdrawal increases with higher chronic doses. These symptoms may last for about three days, and although very unpleasant, they are not life-threatening.

- Humans and nonhumans will readily self-administer opiates whether they are physically dependent or not. The typical pattern is to start at low doses and increase dosage as tolerance develops. Once a stable pattern has been achieved, daily doses seldom change, and there is little variability from day to day. Intake is not cyclic, and voluntary withdrawal symptoms are seldom seen.

- Although chronic opiate use has few serious direct physical effects, the indirect effects of using the drug and the addicted lifestyle can be serious.

- Most attempts to treat chronic heroin use have a very high relapse rate, about 90 percent. The most popular current treatment is maintenance on a long-acting opiate such as methadone or LAAM.

12

Antipsychotic Drugs

Canst thou not minister to a mind diseased;
pluck from the memory a rooted sorrow;
raze out the written troubles of the brain;
and with some sweet oblivious antidote cleanse
the stuff'd bosom of that perilous stuff which
weighs upon the heart?

—Macbeth

Macbeth asked this question of the doctor treating Lady Macbeth. The doctor's answer was no. Modern physicians are a bit better off when it comes to ministering to a mind diseased. In fact, modern psychiatry has been revolutionized by many "antidotes" in the form of anxiolytics, antipsychotics, antidepressants, and antimanics. They are not as wonderful as Macbeth described; they have troublesome side effects, and they do not always work well, but they are probably a good deal better than the treatment that Lady Macbeth was offered.

The drugs that are useful in treating the symptoms of schizophrenic psychoses are called by several names. In North America they are often referred to as *antipsychotics*, while in Europe the term *neuroleptic* is preferred. They are also re-

ferred to as *major tranquilizers*. These three names are derived from three major effects of this class of drugs on behavior.

These drugs are called antipsychotic because their most useful effect is to diminish the symptoms of psychosis. There are two basic types of psychosis, *schizophrenia* and *bipolar disorder* (also called *manic-depressive psychosis*). The drugs referred to as antipsychotic are useful in the treatment of schizophrenic psychosis (described in this chapter) and in the treatment of symptoms of the manic phase of bipolar disorder (described in Chapter 13).

The term *neuroleptic* means "clasping the neuron." It refers to a capacity of these drugs to cause rigidity in the limbs and difficulty of movement similar to that seen in people suffering from Parkinson's disease. This property of these drugs is a persistent and bothersome side effect, and it is indeed strange that a family of drugs should be named after a side effect rather than its most useful therapeutic effect. This name may have been chosen because at one time it was believed that both effects were related; that is, people believed that these drugs would not relieve psychosis unless they were causing neuroleptic effects as well. It is now known that the two types of effects are independent (Creese, 1983). In fact, we now have drugs that seem to be effective antipsychotics but have few, if any, neuroleptic effects.

The term *neuroleptic* is probably more common than *antipsychotic,* but we will use the latter term here because it seems more appropriate to think of drugs in terms of their useful effects rather than their side effects.

The term *major tranquilizer* is also sometimes used to refer to the antipsychotics because they have a sedating effect not only on agitated psychotic patients but also on normal people. This name is inappropriate because it suggests that these drugs are useful only because they "tranquilize" agitated patients. Even though there is a tranquilizing effect, these drugs seem to produce their antipsychotic effect of directly blocking the symptoms of psychosis. Rather than create psychotics who are simply more tranquil or sedated, they cause psychotics to be less psychotic and in many cases less agitated. Another problem is that "major tranquilizer" implies that they are just a stronger version of the "minor tranquilizers," a term sometimes applied to drugs such as the benzodiazepines or barbiturates (see Chapter 7). This terminology is misleading because there is very little similarity in chemistry or effect between the barbiturates and benzodiazepines on the one hand and the antipsychotics on the other.

TYPES OF ANTIPSYCHOTICS

In recent years, a distinction has often been drawn between typical and atypical antipsychotics drugs. The older group, the *typical antipsychotics,* cause neuroleptic or parkinsonian symptoms in addition to their antipsychotic effects, and their therapeutic effect seems to be mostly in treating the positive symptoms of psychosis, the hallucinations and delusional thinking, rather than the negative effects like flattened

affect and alogia. (More on this later.) A number of newer drugs have been developed and introduced in the 1980s and early 1990s that have minimal parkinsonian effects and seem more effective in treating the negative symptoms; these are termed *atypical antipsychotics.* Many atypical antipsychotics are still in the developmental stage and have not been licensed for use.

Typical Antipsychotics

Table 12–1 shows some commonly used antipsychotics with some of their more common trade names. Perhaps the best-known antipsychotic is *chlorpromazine* (Thorazine or Largactil). Others include *promazine* (Sparine), *trifluoperazine* (Stelazine), *fluphenazine* (Prolixin), and *haloperidol* (Haldol).

TABLE 12–1 Typical and Atypical Antipsychotic Drugs

Generic Name	Trade Name
Typical antipsychotics	
Chlorpromazine	Thorazine, Largactil
Promazine	Sparine
Triflupromazine	Vesprin
Thioridizine	Mellaril
Mesoridizine	Serentil
Trifluoperazine	Stelazine
Fluphenazine	Prolixin
Perphenazine	Trilafon
Acetophenazine	Tindal
Prochlorperazine	Stemetil, Compazine
Carphenazine	Proketazine
Thiothixene	Navane
Chlorprothixene	Taractan, Tarasan
Loxapine	Loxitane, Loxapac
Haloperidol	Haldol
Molindone	Lindone, Moban
Atypical antipsychotics	
Clozapine	Clozaril
Respiridone	Resperdal
Raclopride	
Remoxipride	

Sources: J. Davis et al. (1983), p. 25; Churness (1988), pp. 529–530; Jarvik (1970), p. 157.

Atypical Antipsychotics

Thioridazine (Mellaril) has been used for many years and was recognized as causing few parkinsonian symptoms. It is now often classified as an atypical antipsychotic. The next such drug to be developed was *clozapine* (Clozaril). Since the introduction of this drug, several more have been introduced, and many more are being developed. These include *respiridone* (Resperdal), *sulpride* (Sulmatil and Dolmatil), *raclopride, remoxipride, amperozide, zotepidinen,* and *melperone.* Often, these drugs are used in the United Kingdom or other European countries and are slow to be approved for use in the United States.

THE NATURE OF PSYCHOSIS AND SCHIZOPHRENIA

It is probably a good idea at this point to take a brief look at psychosis, the disorder that these drugs are used to treat. Psychotic disorders are characterized by a loss of touch with reality; psychotics reach a state where they completely misunderstand and misinterpret the events going on around them and respond inappropriately in both an intellectual and an emotional sense. They often experience bizarre hallucinations, and their behavior is guided by delusions, beliefs that have no basis in reality.

Psychoses may be brief and temporary, brought on by drugs or some toxin, and psychotic behavior may arise from diseases such as Alzheimer's, but the two major types of psychosis are *bipolar disorder* (which used to be known as *manic depressive psychosis,* discussed in Chapter 13) and *schizophrenia.*

The term *schizophrenia* itself is often misunderstood. The word is derived from the Greek *schizein,* "to split," and *phrēn,* "mind." The splitting referred to, however, is not into two different personalities in the same individual. It is a separation between thought and emotion, different aspects of one personality.

The diagnostic criteria for schizophrenia have been established by the American Psychiatric

---

BOX 12–1   DSM-IV Diagnostic Criteria for Schizophrenia

A. Characteristic Symptoms: Two (or more) of the following, each present for a significant proportion of time during a 1-month period (or less if successfully treated):

(1) delusions
(2) hallucinations
(3) disorganized speech (e.g., frequent derailment or incoherence)
(4) grossly disorganized or catatonic behavior
(5) negative symptoms, i.e., affective flattening, alogia (poverty of speech or thought), or avolition (inability to initiate and persist in goal directed activities)

Note: Only one Criterion A symptom is required if delusions are bizarre or hallucinations consist of a voice keeping up a running commentary on the person's behavior or thoughts, or two or more voices conversing with each other.

Source: American Psychiatric Association (1994), p. 285

BOX 12–2   Schizophrenia: A Case Study

This account of a schizophrenic episode was published in the Journal of Abnormal and Social Psychology *in 1955 ("An Autobiography," 1955). The author is not identified by name, but we are told that she is a college-educated social caseworker and was a 36-year-old mother of three children when she experienced her first schizophrenic episode. Her experience with schizophrenia was at a time before antipsychotic drugs were available, and common treatments were barbiturates (amobarbital) and shock treatment. Compare the symptoms this woman describes with the description of schizophrenia provided in Box 12–1 to see if you feel that she fits the criteria for schizophrenia.*

Most of what follows is based on an unpublished autobiography written in the spring of 1951 shortly after I returned home from the second of the three episodes of my schizophrenic experiences . . .

Shortly after I was taken to hospital for the first time in a rigid catatonic condition,[1] I was plunged into the horror of a world catastrophe. I was being caught up in a cataclysm and totally dislocated. I myself had been responsible for setting the destructive force into motion, although I had acted with no intent to harm, and defended myself with healthy indignation against the accusations of others. If I had done anything wrong I was suffering the consequences along with everyone else. Part of the time I was exploring a new planet (a marvelous and breath-taking adventure) but it was too lonely. I could persuade no one to settle there and I had to get back to earth somehow. The earth, however, had been devastated by atomic bombs and most of its inhabitants killed. Only a few people—myself and the dimly perceived nursing staff—had escaped. At other times I felt totally alone on the new planet.

Association and are published in the *Diagnostic and Statistical Manual of Mental Disorders,* fourth edition (1994), which is more commonly referred to as the *DSM-IV.* Box 12–1 presents the characteristic symptoms for schizophrenia laid out in the DSM-IV.

The symptoms of schizophrenia are often classified into two types, positive and negative. *Positive symptoms* are such things as hallucinations and delusions or irrational beliefs that can be very complex and highly organized. These hallucinations and delusions often involve feelings of grandeur ("I am being spoken to by God") or paranoia ("The CIA is plotting to kill me because I know too much"). The disorder in thinking and speech involves a loosening of associations between ideas; thoughts skip from one subject to another completely unrelated subject without the speaker being aware that the topics are unconnected. The speech of such people has been described as "word salad."

Negative symptoms include *affective flattening* where the person's face is immobile and unresponsive and he or she shows a diminished range of emotional expressiveness. Another negative symptom is *alogia,* or impoverished speech where replies are brief and uncommunicative and seem to reflect diminished thinking. *Avolition* is an inability to initiate or engage in goal-directed activities. The person sits for long periods of time and shows no interest in participating in work or social activities.

After the first few weeks of extreme disorganisation, I began to acquire some relatively stable paranoid delusions. . . .

During the paranoid period I thought I was being persecuted for my beliefs, that my enemies were actively trying to interfere with my activities, were trying to harm me, and at times even trying to kill me. I was primarily a citizen of the larger community. I was trying to persuade people who did not agree with me, but whom I felt could be won over, of the correctness of my belief. . . .

In order to carry through the task which had been imposed upon me, and to defend myself against the terrifying and bewildering dangers of my external situation, I was endowed in my imagination with truly cosmic powers. The sense of power was not always truly defensive but was also connected with a strong sense of valid inspiration. I felt that I had power to determine the weather, which responded to my inner moods, and even to control the movement of the sun in relation to other astronomical bodies. . . . I was also afraid that other people had power to read my mind, and thought I must develop ways of blocking my thoughts from other people. . . .

A mixture of sexual and ethical motivation became apparent during phases when I felt myself to be carrying through a predominantly maternal role and to be symbolically identified with Mary, the Mother of Christ. This identification was poetic; that is, I knew that I was myself and was Mary only in the figurative sense. The "Christ-Child" was apparently the human baby in general, the infant as the symbol of humanity, but I doubt that I would have made this identification if all my children had been girls.

[1]Catatonic schizophrenia is characterized by a state of immobility in which the individual assumes a position without moving for extended periods of time.

Box 12–2 presents a case study of a patient suffering from catatonic schizophrenia, one form of the disease.

HISTORY

Like most drugs in this book that are therapeutically useful, drugs that treat the symptoms of schizophrenia were discovered by accident. In the 1950s a French military surgeon, Henri Laborit, was looking for a preoperative medicine that would relieve patients' anxiety and reduce the high death rate that was associated with surgical shock, an acute and sometimes fatal state of weakness and reduction in vital functions that occurs during surgery. Laborit theorized that shock was caused by excessive release of transmitters such as epinephrine, acetylcholine, and histamine; therefore, he tried out drugs known to block these substances to see if they reduce the incidence of surgical shock. The drugs he tried included atropine, curare, and antihistamines. The first antihistamine Laborit tested was *promethazine*, which was supplied by the Rhône-Poulenc company. Like most antihistamines, it has both antihistamine and sedating properties. Laborit was encouraged by the results he got with promethazine. In 1951, Rhône-Poulenc asked Laborit to try another antihistamine that they had synthesized several years earlier but had rejected because its sedating properties had been too strong. This was *chlorpromazine.*

The results were impressive. Laborit's patients did not lose consciousness but became sleepy and lost interest in everything going on around them (the sedating or tranquilizing effect) and could be anesthetized with a reduced dose of anesthetic. Laborit described the state induced by chlorpromazine as "artificial hibernation." He recognized the significance of this effect and immediately suggested to some psychiatrist friends that the drug might be useful in treating agitated mental patients. Two Parisian psychiatrists named Delay and Deniker learned about these trials and requested samples from Rhône-Poulenc. They administered the drug in higher doses and did not mix it with other drugs as other psychiatrists had been doing. In 1952 they reported some amazing successes, and in 1953 the drug was marketed in Europe as Largactil (Snyder, 1986, p. 71; Sneader, 1985, p. 177; Spiegel & Aebi, 1981, p. 33).

Chlorpromazine was marketed in the United States in 1955 as Thorazine and was very successful. At that time the number of patients in mental hospitals had been climbing steadily, but with the introduction of chlorpromazine, it started to decline dramatically. In the next three decades the resident population of mental institutions in the United States dropped by 80 percent (Hollister, 1983, p. 3), largely as a result of the use of antipsychotics.

ROUTES OF ADMINISTRATION

The antipsychotics are usually taken orally, but preparations are available to be given in i.m. or i.v. injections. They are seldom injected when given as antipsychotics, but they are injected when used as a presurgical or preanesthetic medication because the sedating effects appear more quickly when given parenterally. Intravenous injection also avoids any irregularities or delays in effect arising from erratic absorption from the digestive system. It is doubtful, however, that antipsychotic effects can be significantly speeded by giving the drug parenterally because its antipsychotic effects take several days to develop. The antipsychotics may be injected in circumstances where it may be difficult to induce agitated schizophrenic patients to take the drugs orally.

Because antipsychotic drugs are often taken chronically and patients do not always take them reliably, they are sometimes given in the form of a slowly dissolving depot injection as described in Chapter 1. Depot injections release the drug into the system slowly, and a single injection may be effective for as long as four weeks (Lemberger, Schildkraut, & Cuff, 1987, p. 1288).

ABSORPTION AND DISTRIBUTION

Most antipsychotics are readily absorbed from the digestive system, and once absorbed, they are distributed throughout the body and easily cross the placental and blood-brain barriers. Blood protein binding is considerable, and the drugs tend to be absorbed into body fat and released very slowly.

EXCRETION

The drugs are destroyed entirely by metabolism, and almost no drug is excreted in the urine. It is interesting to note that one of the metabolites of chlorpromazine has antidepressant properties similar to those of imipramine (Creasey, 1979, p. 189). Because of their strong protein binding and their tendency to stay in body fat, antipsychotics have very long half-lives of 11 to 58 hours, and metabolites can be found in the urine months after treatment.

Because of their pharmacokinetics, it is usually appropriate to take them once a day, usually at bedtime so that the sedating effects will be maximal when the patient is sleeping.

NEUROPHYSIOLOGY

Both the antipsychotic properties and the parkinsonian symptoms caused by these drugs are a result of the fact that they block a specific type of dopamine (DA) receptors known as D_2 receptors, and consequently block transmission at DA synapses where the postsynaptic cell uses D_2 receptors. Figure 12–1 shows the relationship between the relative potency of various antipsychotics to block D_2 receptors and their potency as antipsychotic drugs. As you can see, there is an almost perfect correlation between these two effects. This is strong evidence that the two effects are related.

Although the principal therapeutic effect of the antipsychotics is based on their ability to block DA receptors, these drugs can also have effects on many other transmitter systems in the brain. They block the effects of acetylcholine, serotonin, and histamine; they alter the effects of GABA and peptide transmitters; and they block NE receptors and increase NE synthesis and release (Roth, 1983, p. 127). In some cases, these

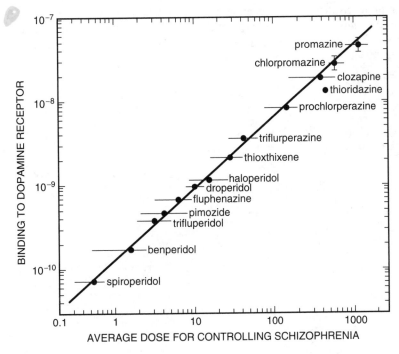

Figure 12–1 The relationship between dopamine binding and the therapeutic effectiveness of various antipsychotic drugs. The vertical axis is an index of the drug's ability to bind to D_2 receptors, and the horizontal axis shows the average dose that is effective in controlling schizophrenia. The relationship is nearly perfect. (Seeman et al., 1976, p. 718.)

effects on other receptor sites appear to be responsible for differences in the effect of different antipsychotic drugs on positive and negative symptoms and in the side effects they cause. More on this later.

DA Brain Systems

Two major brain systems depend on DA as their transmitter; both serve completely different functions but are together responsible for both the antipsychotic effect of these drugs and their main side effects. One system appears to be the *mesolimbic system* discussed in Chapter 5, and the other is the *nigrastriatal system* which is responsible for the smooth movements of the muscles.

The Mesolimbic System. The location of the DA neurons that are blocked by antipsychotic drugs is not known for certain, but it is likely that they are closely associated with the same system that mediates reinforcement. This system has its cell bodies in the *ventral tegmental area (VTA)* of the lower brain and synapses in the *nucleus accumbens (ACC)* in the limbic system. It is sometimes called the *mesolimbic system* (see Figure 12–2). The cell bodies in the VTA also synapse on cells in other parts of the brain, including the frontal cortex and other parts of the limbic system.

It is thought that schizophrenic symptoms are a result of some malfunction in this DA system, probably an excess of DA activity, but the situation is much more complicated. We know that other neurotransmitters are involved in psychosis, including serotonin, and other brain systems also play an important role. Attention has been focused on the role of DA because of the great success that D_2-blocking drugs have had

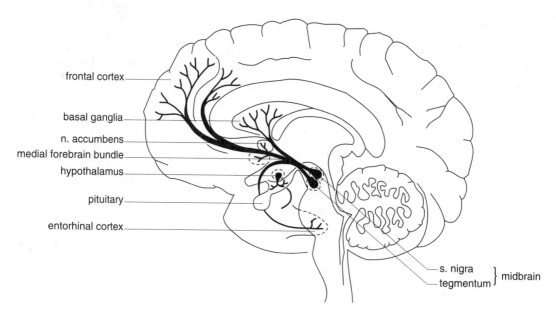

Figure 12–2 Dopamine systems in the human brain. The mesolimbic system originates in the midbrain in the ventral tegmentum and runs to the nucleus accumbens and forward to the forebrain. The nigrastriatal system originates in the midbrain in the substantia nigra and runs forward to the basal ganglia in the striatum.

treating schizophrenia, but the success of the more recent atypical antipsychotics that work at other types of receptors for DA and other transmitters has focused attention elsewhere. In addition, the DA-blocking effect of these drugs occurs as soon as the drug is taken, but the therapeutic effect may be delayed for days or weeks. This delayed effect also suggests that more is involved than just the blocking of excessive DA activity (Carlsson, 1994).

The Nigrastriatal System. The integration of smooth movements is thought to be the function of a part of the brain known as the *basal ganglia,* part of the *striatum.* The basal ganglia are two centers called the *caudate nucleus* and the *putamen* and form part of what is known as the *extrapyramidal motor system* (see Chapter 4). Cell bodies located in the *substantia nigra* in the lower part of the brain (close to the VTA) send axons to synapse in the basal ganglia (close to the ACC; see Figure 12–2). These synapses use DA as the transmitter, and it is known that the functioning of the extrapyramidal motor system depends on normal levels of DA being released at these synapses. When there is a deficiency of dopamine at these synapses, people show symptoms of the movement disorder known as Parkinson's disease. When antipsychotic drugs are given, they block the activity of dopamine in the basal ganglia and can cause parkinsonian movement disorders (sometimes called *extrapyramidal symptoms*).

When typical antipsychotic drugs are taken, they block the excessive activity in the mesolimbic system and relieve the schizophrenic symptoms. Unfortunately, they also block the activity in the nigrastriatal system that cause parkinsonian symptoms and possibly the movement disorder known as *tardive dyskinesia* (discussed later). The newer atypical antipsychotics are an exciting breakthrough. They appear to be able to block dopamine in the mesolimbic system without altering the functioning of the nigrastriatal system and therefore have minimal extrapyramidal movement side effects.

Differences Between Typical and Atypical Antipsychotics

It is still not entirely clear exactly what physiological property or properties of the atypical antipsychotics are responsible for their different effects. It is likely that different atypical antipsychotics are able to spare extrapyramidal functioning by different means (Kane, 1994; Carlsson, 1994). They all are D_2 blockers, and this action still seems to be responsible for their basic antipsychotic effects (Seeman, 1990), but many atypical antipsychotic drugs like raclopride and remoxipride have less affinity (ability to bind and block) for D_2 receptors than the typical antipsychotics. As a result, endogenous dopamine can successfully compete with the drug for the receptors if it is present in sufficient quantities. Since there is considerably more dopamine in the basal ganglia than in the limbic system, low-affinity drugs would have a greater effect in the limbic system than the basal ganglia. This could explain why these drugs are effective against psychotic symptoms but have little effect on movement.

The difference between typical and atypical antipsychotics might also be explained by differences in the other receptor sites that they affect. It is known that drugs that block the cholinergic muscarinic receptors are effective treatments against parkinsonian symptoms. Drugs that block both D_2 receptors and cholinergic muscarinic receptors would be expected to have diminished parkinsonian effects (Creese, 1983, p. 201). Clozapine and thirodizine are both effective ACh blockers.

Another hypothesis that has not been fully tested is that atypical antipsychotics block other types of dopamine receptors that are distributed differently between the mesolimbic and the nigrastriatal systems. It seems clear that D_1 receptors are not involved in the actions of antipsychotics, but a D_3 receptor has recently been identified. It has also been shown that the D_3 receptors occur in much higher concentrations in the mesolimbic system than in the nigrastriatal system. Although it is not true in every case, the atypical antipsychotics are much more effective D_3 blockers than the typical antipsychotic drugs (Schwartz et al., 1990). Unfortunately, drugs that can block D_3 receptors without blocking D_2 receptors have not been developed. The same speculations have been made regarding D_4 receptors, although the distribution of these receptors in the brain is not as well understood.

It is often noted that atypical antipsychotics are more effective in treating the negative symptoms of schizophrenia (flattened affect, alogia, etc.). This effect might be achieved because these drugs alter some other neurotransmitter such as serotonin. Respiridone, for example, is a very potent serotonin blocker as well as being a D_2 blocker.

EFFECTS ON THE BODY

The effects of the different antipsychotics show considerable variation, but not as much variability as can be seen among different individuals taking the same drug. Each drug's effectiveness as an antipsychotic and the sort and intensity of side effects will vary considerably from person to person. This is one reason why there are so many of these drugs on the market. Psychiatrists may try a given individual on a number of different drugs at different doses until one is found that produces the most favorable therapeutic effect and has the fewest side effects.

As we have already seen, the most pronounced side effect is alterations in movement that resemble the symptoms of Parkinson's disease. This effect is reported in about 40 percent of patients on typical antipsychotics. It includes a dulled expression on the face, rigidity and tremor in the limbs, weakness in the extremities, and very slow movements. In addition, about 20 percent of patients show *akathesia,* a condition characterized by uncontrolled restlessness, constant compulsive movement, and sometimes a protruding tongue and facial grimacing.

After taking the typical antipsychotics for a period of time, about 30 percent of patients show a condition called *tardive dyskinesia,* characterized by involuntary repetitive movements of the face such as smacking of the lips and twitching. Unfortunately, with some individuals, the symptoms of tardive dyskinesia are permanent and do not go away after the drug is stopped (Enna & Coyle, 1983, p. 10). It is still too early to say whether the newer atypical antipsychotics eventually cause tardive dyskinesia.

Antipsychotics also seem to cause the body to have trouble regulating temperature, which becomes easily influenced by changes in the environment. In hot environments patients are more susceptible to heat stroke, and in cold climates they are more vulnerable to hypothermia.

In certain susceptible individuals, epileptic seizures may increase. Other side effects include reduced food intake, altered pigmentation of the skin, changes in heart rate and blood pressure (due to the effect of these drugs on NE receptors), dry mouth, impaired vision, constipation (due to anticholinergic effects), and jaundice.

The major problem with clozapine is that it is known to cause a disorder called *agranulocytosis,* a potentially fatal suppression of bone marrow activity. It occurs in 1–2 percent of all patients receiving clozapine and can happen at any time. For this reason, clozapine is only administered to patients who have not responded to any other antipsychotic drug, and patients on this drug must be carefully and continuously monitored.

Lethal Effects

The antipsychotics produce many side effects, but these drugs are not lethal. In fact, they are extremely safe and have a high therapeutic index (see Chapter 1), about 100. For some antipsychotics the therapeutic index is as high as 1,000 (Baldessarini, 1985, pp. 35, 38, 81). It is practically impossible to use antipsychotics to commit suicide.

Effects on Sleep

Antipsychotics at therapeutic doses have very little effect on sleep, but some antipsychotics such as chlorpromazine that have sedating effects will increase sleep time when given at high doses or when first administered. The antipsychotics do not alter sleep cycles or REM sleep (Spiegel & Aebi, 1981, p. 116).

EFFECTS ON THE BEHAVIOR AND PERFORMANCE OF HUMANS

Subjective Effects

Chlorpromazine, when given to healthy subjects, causes a very pronounced feeling of tiredness. Subjects report slower and confused thinking, difficulty in concentrating, and feelings of clumsiness. They also report a need for sleep, dejection, anxiety, and irritability. Simple tasks such as walking seem to take great effort.

Haloperidol is not as sedating as chlorpromazine, but it makes subjects feel internally aroused and externally sedated at the same time; that is, they feel restless and want to do something but also feel restrained and have difficulty moving (Spiegel & Aebi, 1981, p. 62).

The subjective experience of antipsychotics is never described as pleasant. This fact is probably responsible for the poor compliance rates with these drugs; patients often do not take them. This does not appear to be true, however, of at least one atypical antipsychotic, clozapine (Meltzer, 1990a).

Effects on Performance

Surprisingly, few studies of the effects of antipsychotics on cognitive functioning have been conducted. Those that were done have been inconclusive, reporting either no effect, deficits, or improvements (Judd et al., 1987, p. 1469).

EFFECTS ON THE BEHAVIOR OF NONHUMANS

Effects on Unconditioned Behavior

Unlike the antianxiety drugs such as the benzodiazepines, the most remarkable effect of the antipsychotic drugs is that they suppress spontaneous movement in an open field, and higher doses render most laboratory animals immobile. In fact, these animals take on a sort of plastic immobility whereby their limbs will remain in any position in which they are placed as though the animals were made out of modeling clay. It was this immobility that gave rise to the name *neuroleptic*.

At doses that do not seem to have these neuroleptic effects, antipsychotics diminish the frequently and intensity of attack behaviors in most species. This decrease in aggression coincides with an overall decrease in activity, so it is possible that it is a result of an overall debilitation in motor abilities (Miczek & Barry, 1976).

Effects on Positively Reinforced Behavior

In general, the antipsychotic drugs cause a decrease in responding on both the FI and FR schedules, although the effect on FR responding occurs at a much lower dose than the effect on FI. Within the FI, the high rates at the end of the interval are slowed, but the low rates at the beginning of each FI are increased, so there is little change in overall rate. This sort of rate-dependent effect is similar to that seen with many other drugs, including amphetamine.

Effects on Negatively Reinforced Behavior

As far back as 1953, when chlorpromazine was first being tested on humans by Laborit, Simone Courvousier and her associates at the Rhône-Poulenc company (1953) discovered that the drug would decrease avoidance at doses that would have no effect on escape from a shock, an effect now known to be shared by antianxiety drugs such as barbiturates and benzodiazepines. In fact, this was the first time that this technique had been adopted for use in testing drugs, and it has since become one of the most widely used screening device for new psychotherapeutics (Laties, 1986, p. 27).

Chlorpromazine also increases the number of shocks received on a nonsignaled avoidance task. Strangely, the antipsychotics do not seem to have a consistent effect on behaviors suppressed by punishment. Thus they are very different from the barbiturates and benzodiazepines, which greatly increase the rates of punished responding (McMillan & Leander, 1976).

Drug State Discrimination and Dissociation

It has been demonstrated that chlorpromazine will cause dissociation. In one study, rats trained on an avoidance task under the influence of chlorpromazine were unable to remember what they had learned when tested under saline but could recall the task when returned to the drug state again (Otis, 1964). This finding has caused some concern among psychotherapists because psychotherapy involves learning, and often patients receive psychotherapy while they are being treated with these drugs. Consequently, they may not recall what they learned in psychotherapy when they are taken off the drugs.

In drug state discrimination studies, the antipsychotics are not well discriminated. For an antipsychotic to act as a discriminative stimulus, large doses are required, and many more training trials are needed compared with most other behaviorally active drugs (Overton & Batta, 1977; Overton, 1987).

Once an animal has been trained to discriminate an antipsychotic, the response will generalize to most other antipsychotics at sufficiently high doses. There are some exceptions. For example, a rat trained to discriminate clozapine will not generalize to haloperidol or chlorpromazine (Goas & Boston, 1978). There is no generalization be-

tween the antipsychotics and the antidepressants or any other class of drugs (Stewart, 1962).

TOLERANCE

There is no evidence that tolerance develops to the antipsychotic effects of these drugs. Once a patient has been established on a therapeutically effective dose, it is often maintained for years without any decrease in effectiveness. Tolerance seems to develop to the sedating effects of the drugs seen when it is first given, and tolerance also seems to develop to the parkinsonian effects.

WITHDRAWAL

Physical dependence, if it occurs at all, is rare. There are reports of muscular discomfort, exaggeration of psychotic symptoms and movement disorders, and difficulty in sleeping when some antipsychotics are suddenly withdrawn, but such effects are not normally seen even after years of use at normal doses. It is possible that the failure to notice withdrawal symptoms is due to the extremely slow excretion of the drug from the body (Baldessarini, 1985, p. 38).

SELF-ADMINISTRATION

As we have seen in Chapter 5 (see Table 5–1), chlorpromazine is not self-administered by laboratory animals. In fact, these drugs appear to be aversive. In one experiment, monkeys learned to bar-press to avoid infusions. At first the monkeys did not respond to avoid chlorpromazine, but after a week, they were successfully avoiding 90 percent of programmed infusions. It appears that the aversive properties of chlorpromazine develop slowly with repeated doses (Hoffmeister & Wuttke, 1975, p. 424).

Experience with humans is similar. The antipsychotics are never abused; in fact, they are a class of drugs that have considerable compliance problems. *Compliance* refers to the extent to which a patient adheres to a regime of medical treatment. In the case of typical antipsychotics, most schizophrenic patients show poor compliance—they often stop taking their medication, with the usual result that their symptoms reappear. For this reason, various administration techniques have been developed that do not depend on the patient's compliance. Such techniques include administration of depot injections, which slowly release the drug and maintain the appropriate blood levels.

HARMFUL EFFECTS

Reproduction

Apart from the movement disorders already described, the antipsychotic drugs can have serious effects on reproductive functions.

In males, the antipsychotics reduce sexual interest, an effect that may arise from their sedative properties. Sexual performance may also be impaired, the primary difficulty being a failure to ejaculate, with erection and orgasm unaffected. These problems arise from both anticholinergic properties of the antipsychotics and their effect on hormone levels (N. F. Woods, 1984, p. 440). If you look closely at Figure 12–2, you can see that there is a short dopamine pathway running from the hypothalamus to the pituitary. When this system is activated, it suppresses the release of prolactin, a hormone that suppresses male sexual activity. Drugs like cocaine that activate this system can stimulate male sexual performance by suppressing prolactin release, but drugs like antipsychotics that block dopamine have the opposite effect. Atypical antipsychotics do not seem to alter prolactin release.

In females there may be abnormal menstrual cycles and infertility, and in both males and females there is sometimes an enlargement of the breasts, and fluid will sometimes ooze from the nipples (N. F. Woods, 1984, p. 441).

OTHER THERAPEUTIC EFFECTS OF ANTIPSYCHOTIC DRUGS

Antipsychotic drugs are useful in the treatment of other medical problems. They are effective antiemetics; that is, they prevent nausea and vomiting and are useful in the treatment of motion sickness. In addition, they were originally developed by Laborit as presurgical and preanesthetic medications and are still used for that purpose.

A number of movement disorders thought to be a result of excessive dopamine activity in the brain can, not surprisingly, be treated effectively with antipsychotics. These disorders include Huntington's chorea, an inherited degenerative disease. Huntington's is fatal, but antipsychotics help control some of the symptoms. Antipsychotics are also useful in treating Tourette syndrome; Tourette patients show involuntary muscle ticks, twitches, and vocalizations (often swearing). Surprisingly, antipsychotics are also used to treat tardive dyskinesia.

Antipsychotics have also been used to treat hiccups, stuttering, and delirium tremens caused by alcohol withdrawal (Van Woert, 1983) and psychotic behaviors induced by LSD and other hallucinogens.

CHAPTER SUMMARY

- Antipsychotic drugs are also referred to as *neuroleptic* drugs or *major tranquilizers*. They are used in the treatment of schizophrenia.

- *Extrapyramidal motor effects* are common side effects of antipsychotic drugs. These effects constitute a movement disorder similar to *Parkinson's disease*.

- People suffering from schizophrenia lose touch with reality. They misunderstand events going on around them and make inappropriate intellectual and emotional responses to those events. *Positive symptoms* include hallucinations and delusions. *Negative symptoms* include a loss of initiative, flattening of affect, and *alogia*, impoverished speech and thought.
- *Typical antipsychotic drugs* are only effective against positive symptoms, but the newer *atypical antipsychotic drugs* are effective on both positive and negative symptoms and have fewer movement side effects.
- Chlorpromazine was marketed in 1955, and it and other similar antipsychotics have dramatically reduced the number of patients in mental hospitals throughout the world.
- Antipsychotics are administered orally and are distributed throughout the body. They easily cross the placental and blood-brain barriers. Because they are highly lipid-soluble, they have very long half-lives.
- Antipsychotics work by blocking the dopamine D_2 receptors in the *mesolimbic system*. They cause parkinsonian movement disorders and *tardive dyskinesia* by blocking D_2 receptors in the *nigrastriatal system*.
- When given to normal people, antipsychotics cause a feeling of tiredness, and the effects are never described as pleasant.
- Antipsychotics decrease general activity levels of nonhumans, and have a *rate-dependent effect* on operant behavior; that is, low response rates are speeded and high rates are diminished. They decrease avoidance behavior in doses that have no effect on escape behavior.
- *Tolerance* does not appear to develop to the antipsychotic effect of these drugs, and withdrawal symptoms are rare. They are never self-administered by nonhumans and are not abused by humans.
- Antipsychotics can depress sexual interest and performance in males and interfere with menstruation in females.

13

Antidepressants and Mood Stabilizers

There are several types of antidepressants. The first drugs that were successfully used to treat depression were the *monoamine oxidase inhibitors* (*MAOIs*) and the *tricyclic antidepressants* (*TCAs*). Consequently, they are sometimes referred to as *first-generation antidepressants.* Newer drugs have been developed that do not belong to either of these categories, and they are often called *second-generation antidepressants.* This is a diverse group of chemicals that includes the *selective serotonin reuptake inhibitors* (*SSRIs*).

The first MAOI to be used was *iproniazid*, but it is no longer in use. Others include *phenelzine* (Nardil), *tranylcypromine* (Parnate), and *moclobemide* (Ludiomil, available in the United Kingdom and Canada, but not in the United States).

The tricyclic antidepressants (TCAs) are so called because their molecular structure contains three rings. Common TCAs are *imipramine* (Tofranil), *amitriptyline* (Elavil), *desipramine* (Norpramin), *nortriptyline* (Aventyl), and *doxepin* (Adapin).

Some second-generation antidepressants are *maprotiline* (Manerex), *amoxapine* (Asendin),

trazodone (Desyrel), *mianserin* (Tolvon, not used in the United States), *bupropion* (Wellbutrin), and *nomifensine* (Merital, withdrawn). Although many second-generation antidepressants have been used in Europe, strict drug development laws have delayed or prevented the use of many of them in the United States.

The SSRIs include *fluoxetine* (Prozac), *sertraline* (Zoloft), and *paroxetine* (Paxil).

In addition to these drugs, the element *lithium* is also successfully used to treat and prevent the manic-depressive (bipolar) disorder. It is usually sold as the salt lithium carbonate under many different trade names, including Carbolith, Eskalith, Lithonate, and Lithotabs.

THE NATURE OF DEPRESSION AND MANIA

From time to time we all feel sad or "depressed" as a result of things that happen to us, but this condition is not usually accompanied by physical symptoms, and it does not last. There are some people for whom depression is much more serious. For them, there may be no cause in their environment, the depression is deep, and it does not go away or keeps returning for no apparent reason. These people also show a loss of appetite, loss of interest in normally pleasurable activities, loss of energy, problems sleeping, exaggerated feelings of worthlessness and guilt, and haunting thoughts of death and suicide. Box 13–1 presents a summary of the DSM-IV criteria for a major depressive episode. Box 13–2 gives a personal account of depression.

What is interesting is that depression can occur without actually feeling depressed. Often, older people show many of the physical symptoms of depression—insomnia, weight loss, and so on—but do not seem to feel sad. They may, however, show *anhedonia*, a loss of interest in activities that are normally pleasurable. This is nevertheless "clinical depression" or "depressive illness" and can be treated with antidepressants.

Depression is classified as an *affective disorder* or *mood disorder*. Traditionally, mild depression would be "neurotic depression" but serious

BOX 13–1 Criteria for a Major Depressive Episode from the DSM-IV

A. Five (or more) of the following symptoms have been present during the same two-week period and represent a change from previous functioning; at least one of the symptoms is either (1) depressed mood or (2) loss of interest in pleasure.
   (1) depressed mood most of the day, nearly every day, as indicated by either subjective report (e.g., feels sad or empty) or observation made by others (e.g., appears tearful)
   (2) markedly diminished interest in pleasure in all, or almost all, activities most of the day, nearly every day
   (3) significant weight loss when not dieting or weight gain (e.g., a change of more than 5% body weight in a month) or decrease or increase in appetite nearly every day
   (4) insomnia or hypersomnia nearly every day
   (5) psychomotor agitation or retardation nearly every day
   (6) fatigue or loss of energy nearly every day
   (7) feelings of worthlessness or excessive or inappropriate guilt nearly every day
   (8) diminished ability to think or concentrate, or indecisiveness, nearly every day
   (9) recurrent thoughts of death (not just fear of dying), recurrent suicidal ideation without a specific plan, or a suicide attempt or a specific plan for committing suicide
B. The symptoms do not meet the criteria for a Mixed Episode.
C. Symptoms cause clinically significant distress or impairment in social, occupational, or other important areas of functioning.
D. Symptoms are not due to direct physiological effects of a substance (e.g., a drug of abuse or medication) or a general medical condition.
E. Symptoms are not better accounted for by bereavement, i.e., after the loss of a loved one, the symptoms persist for longer than 2 months or are characterized by marked functional impairment, morbid preoccupation with worthlessness, suicidal ideation, psychotic symptoms, or psychomotor retardation.

Source: American Psychiatric Association (1994, p. 327)

BOX 13–2   Depression: A Case Study

This is an extract of a subjective account of depression written by E. George Gray, a British neuroscientist in his fifties who recovered from depression after several years.

I write about severe (not manic) depression. My breakdown started when I began to feel irreversibly ill, and during the following six years I spent two months in one hospital, returned to work prematurely for a year and then finally disintegrated mentally into deeper depression and entered another hospital for five months. . . .

In retrospect I see that since the age of 14, or before, I have suffered bouts of depression of greater or less severity, with one minor breakdown in 1948 after returning from war service. Since I was not aware that I was suffering from depression, I suffered literally in silence, often for months on end. I suspect that many people have similar experiences, and I wonder whether studies have been made on populations to detect them.

I went to my general practitioner some years ago. He rightly diagnosed depression, and prescribed a tricyclic antidepressant. The side effects turned out to be so disturbing that I never returned to him. The point is that "depression" was then just a word to me, when I should have been warned that untreated depression could lead to an extremely serious breakdown (as in fact it did). . . . I remember, just before the crisis, bouncing on to the psychiatrist's couch and putting on a brave front. A few probing questions, and I found myself reduced to tears and wanting to die. Only then did I realize how seriously ill I was. My major breakdown had been coming on for the previous three years.

The tricyclic amitriptyline produced, in me, intolerable side effects. I was for a long time on 60 [mg] daily of the tricyclic antidepressant mianserin,[1] but am now stabilised on 40 [mg]. I have also, during and since my breakdown, been taking 750 [mg] of lithium carbonate daily. My weight is [172 pounds].

Recovering and back to work, on lithium and mianserin, but still with bouts of headache, nausea, insomnia, hand trembling, stuttering and so on. I found diazepam [Valium] of inestimable value during this phase. Particularly traumatic were times when I had to chair a staff meeting or conduct a seminar; on such occasions 2 mg diazepam (chewed and swallowed for rapid absorption) 20 minutes beforehand usually saved the situation.

[1]Mianserin is actually a second-generation antidepressant, Tolvon.
Source: Gray (1983)

---

depression accompanied by physical symptoms was considered a psychosis. The DSM-IV no longer makes this distinction, but it does recognize that schizophrenia (see Chapter 12) may be associated with depression. In such cases the depressed person will also exhibit some of the symptoms of psychosis such as hallucinations and delusions. This is called a *mixed episode*, and the treatment is somewhat different.

Depression has been called the common cold of mental illness because large segments of the population experience it at some time in their lives. Modest estimates suggest that within any six-month period 3 percent of the population of the United States experience a mood disorder, and about 6 percent have one at some point during their lives (some estimates range as high as 26 percent). Women are twice as likely to suffer from depression as men, but there are no gender differences in bipolar disorder. Only about 20 percent of those with depressive illness receive help from a mental health professional (Lickey & Gordon, 1991, p. 149). The resulting disability—in the form of health care utilization, absenteeism (172 million working days annually), injuries at work, and the like—costs an estimated $26 billion annually in the United States (Janicak et al., 1993, p. 207). There are other costs too. The overall mortality rate for depressed people is higher than in normals, and the probability of suicide is twenty times greater in depressed people.

Accounts of depressive illness were recorded by the ancient Greeks, and depression is also common in other cultures and societies. In other cultures, similar symptoms are reported except that in non-Western societies depressed people are more likely to report physical symptoms and less likely to express feelings of guilt and self-reproach (Lickey & Gordon, 1991, p. 175).

Depression is a chronic illness. Eighty-eight percent of those suffering from depression who receive drug therapy improve within 6 months, but less than one-third of these remain well.

For most individuals, depression comes in cycles that may alternate with normal periods, but it may also alternate with *mania*. Mania is the exact opposite of depression. The person becomes excessively elated and hyperactive and takes on many ambitious and grandiose projects. The need

BOX 13–3 DSM-IV Criteria for a Manic Episode

A. A distinct period of abnormally and persistently elevated, expansive, or irritable mood, lasting at least one week (or any duration if hospitalization is necessary).
B. During the period of mood disturbance, three of the following symptoms have persisted (four if the mood is only irritable) and have been present to a significant degree:
   (1) inflated self-esteem or grandiosity
   (2) decreased need for sleep
   (3) more talkative than usual or pressure to keep talking
   (4) flight of ideas or subjective experience that thoughts are racing
   (5) distractibility (attention easily drawn to unimportant or irrelevant external stimuli)
   (6) increase in goal-directed activity or psychomotor agitation
   (7) excessive involvement in pleasurable activities that have a high potential for painful consequences (e.g., engaging in unrestrained buying sprees, sexual indiscretions, or foolish bushiness investments)
C. The symptoms do not meet the criteria for Mixed Episode.
D. The mood disturbance is sufficiently severe to cause a marked impairment in occupational functioning or in usual social activities or relationships with others, or to necessitate hospitalization to prevent harm to self or others, or there are psychotic features.
E. The symptoms are not due to the direct physiological effects of a substance (e.g., a drug of abuse or medication, or other treatment) or a general medical condition.

Source: American Psychiatric Association (1994, p. 332)

for sleep is decreased, the sense of self-esteem is inflated, and behavior is often reckless. Manic individuals become very talkative, and ideas race through their heads. They are easily distractible, and conversation will switch from topic to topic. Manic people often become reckless and foolhardy, engaging in foolish investments or sexual indiscretions. Box 13–3 gives the DSM-IV criteria for a manic episode. The condition in which depression alternates with mania was called *manic-depressive psychosis*, but the DSM-IV now prefers the term *bipolar disorder*.

It has been known for some time that mood is related to the functioning of the monoamines (MAs), in particular, serotonin (5-HT) and norepinephrine (NE), although dopamine (DA) may also play a role. Drugs like cocaine and amphetamine make people feel good because they enhance transmission at these synapses, and drugs like reserpine that deplete the brain of MAs often cause severe depression. The *monoamine theory of depression* in its original form suggested that depression was a result of reduced levels of activity in these monoamine systems. As we shall see, this theory is no longer tenable in its simple form (Siever, 1987; Jimerson, 1987; Meltzer & Lowy, 1987). All of the three MAs are probably involved in some aspect of mood, and they interact with each other in complex ways, but it is now fairly clear that decreased activity in the 5-HT system is a crucial element in depression. All treatments that have been shown to be effective in relieving depression have one thing in common, they ultimately change (almost always increase) transmission at 5-HT synapses (Blier & de Montigny, 1994). It is clear, however, that these increases in 5-HT transmission may be caused by, and may in turn cause changes in, activity of other transmitter systems (even some that do not use MAs)(Charney et al., 1990; Janicak et al., 1993). An increase in 5-HT transmission appears to be a necessary but not sufficient condition for effectiveness against depression (Leonard, 1993). Activity at specific 5-HT synapses may in fact be only one link in a long and complex chain of neurological deficiencies that cause depression and mania.

Three brain systems that use MA transmitters have been implicated in some aspect of mood. All have centers in the midbrain or upper brain stem and send projections forward to the various parts of the limbic system and the forebrain through the medial forebrain bundle: (1) NE fibers that arise in the *locus coeruleus* in the midbrain, (2) serotonergic fibers that originate in areas of the Raphé system, and (3) dopaminergic fibers of the mesolimbic system that originate in the ventral tegmentum.

HISTORY

The antidepressant properties of the MAO inhibitor iproniazid were discovered accidentally. The drug was developed as a treatment for tuberculosis, but it was soon discovered that it had a significant effect on the mood of patients to whom it was given. It relieved depression and made them feel better. Later research soon found that this effect was not a result of the fact that it relieved the symptoms of tuberculosis. When MAO inhibitors were first introduced in the 1950s, they became widely used, but in a few years the initial enthusiasm waned because of several factors. To begin with, iproniazid was taken off the market soon after it was released because of reports that it caused liver damage. It turned out that the liver damage only occurred because the doses used were too high. In addition, some clinical studies concluded that MAOIs were ineffective. Once again, these reports were unfounded. The studies used inadequate research design, and we now know that the doses used were too low. In addition, MAOIs were also known to interact with many other drugs and some foods. It is now known that MAOIs are just as effective as any other treatment for depression (more effective in some types of patients) and that they do not cause liver damage at therapeutic doses. New MAOIs have also been developed that are more specific in their actions, are reversible, and much less likely to interact with diet. This class of drugs is regaining its place as an effective and relatively safe agent in the treatment of depression (Kurtz, 1990).

The tricyclic antidepressants were also discovered by accident. They were discovered as a result of research on antipsychotic drugs (see Chapter 12). In the hope of finding better antipsychotics, many new drugs based on the antipsychotic drug molecule were synthesized, one of which was imipramine. In the late 1950s imipramine was tested on psychiatric patients, and although it did not improve schizophrenic patients, it did elevate the mood of depressed patients. Because the tricyclics are safer than the early MAO inhibitors, many more have been developed, and their use has become common in the treatment of depression.

The popularity of the tricyclics is now being threatened by the newer second-generation antidepressants, which are safer and have fewer of the bothersome side effects of the tricyclic and MAO inhibitor drugs (Shopsin, Cassano, & Conti, 1981; Enna & Eilson, 1987; Leonard, 1993; Feighner & Boyer, 1991), although they do not seem to be more effective or work faster in the treatment of depression. Like the TCAs and MAOIs, many second-generation antidepressants were developed for other purposes, and their antidepressant properties were discovered later.

The first SSRI, fluoxetine (more widely discussed by its trade name Prozac) was introduced in the United States in 1987 and soon received considerable attention in the popular media because it was being used, not to treat depression, but as a means of altering personality (more on this later). The media also carried reports that the drug could precipitate violent aggressive acts and suicide. If such adverse effects occur, however, they are extremely rare, and the use of fluoxetine and other SSRIs continues to increase both in the treatment of depression and as a personality "cosmetic."

Lithium, when given in the form of one of its salts, also works well in preventing both mania and depression that come in cycles in bipolar disorder. This too was discovered accidentally. In the 1940s the Australian psychiatrist John Cade was testing a theory he had that there was a toxin in the blood of manic patients that caused the disease. He proposed that uric acid might protect experimental rats from the effects of this toxin, so he tried to inject rats with uric acid to see if it protected them from the lethal effects of being injected with the urine from manic patients. Unfortunately (or fortunately), he found that the uric acid did not readily dissolve, so he mixed it with lithium to make a soluble salt. He noticed that this mixture calmed the rats and did seem to offer them some protection. Later he found that any salt of lithium would do the same thing, and he concluded that it was the lithium, not the uric acid, that was effective (Snyder, 1986; Sneader, 1985, p. 185). When he tried out the lithium with his manic patients, he achieved amazing successes. Not only did lithium decrease symptoms, but it prevented the recurrence of both mania and depression if taken regularly.

In spite of clear demonstrations of its effectiveness, lithium was slow to be used and was not available commercially in the United States until 1970.

Lithium is particularly effective in the treatment of bipolar disorder because it relieves mania and blocks the recurrence of depression. It is, however, not effective in treating depression once it occurs. For this reason lithium is not classed as an antidepressant. It may be referred to as an "antimanic" drug or a "mood stabilizer." Antidepressants alone are not often used to treat bipolar disorder. While they may relieve depression, they sometimes can induce a manic episode. Lithium is often used in conjunction with an antidepressant in patients with the bipolar disorder, and may also be used with an antidepressant in cases where antidepressants are not effective by themselves.

ABSORPTION

The MAO inhibitors, the tricyclic antidepressants, and many second-generation antidepressants all have similar absorption pharmacokinetics. The TCAs reach maximal blood concentrations in 1–3 hours (although some TCAs may take as long as 8 hours). The absorption of SSRIs is slower, taking 4–8 hrs to reach maximum concentrations. All antidepressants show high levels of protein binding (Preskorn, 1993).

A significant proportion of a dose of most antidepressants is destroyed by the digestive system and liver before it reaches the bloodstream. This *first pass metabolism* is inhibited by alcohol, and as a result, alcohol will greatly increase the amount of drug absorbed from a specific dose. As a result, overdoses of TCAs are much more serious when taken in conjunction with alcohol.

Orally administered lithium is rapidly absorbed, and peak levels in the blood occur between one-half hour and two hours after consumption. However, lithium is much slower in getting inside cells, and this fact probably accounts for the delayed therapeutic effect of the drug (L. E. Hollister, 1983, p. 181).

Lithium has a low therapeutic index of about 3 (Baldessarini, 1985, p. 35), so it is important to keep blood levels from becoming too high at any one time. Because lithium is absorbed rapidly, it peaks in the blood at high levels, and these peaks often exceed the therapeutic window (see Chapter 1). It is also excreted rapidly; therefore, several daily doses are needed to keep the levels from falling below the therapeutic level. This problem is often handled by using slow-release capsules in which the lithium is embedded in a material that dissolves slowly. This technique prevents the rapid rise and high peak blood levels

and also makes it possible to cut back administrations to two per day (Cooper, 1987, p. 1366).

DISTRIBUTION

Antidepressants readily cross the blood-brain and placental barriers. They tend to be concentrated in the lungs, kidneys, liver, and brain. Some antidepressants can be found in significant quantities in breast milk.

Lithium enters and leaves the brain relatively slowly, reaching a peak after more than 24 hours. It seems to be concentrated in some parts of the brain. There is no protein binding. Lithium readily crosses the placental barrier and also finds its way into breast milk easily and should not be used by breast-feeding mothers.

EXCRETION

The MAOIs have a short half-life of 2–4 hours (Preskorn, 1993). Some MAOIs may be taken once a day because they have an irreversible effect on MAO and their effects persist long after they are eliminated from the body. Newer MAOIs like moclobemide have a reversible effect, and two or three daily doses are required. The TCAs have a half-life of about 24 hours and reach a steady-state level in the body after about five days in most people. In most cases, only a single daily dose is needed.

Most second-generation antidepressants have shorter half-lives than the tricyclics and often require more frequent dosing (Rudorfer & Potter, 1987). Some SSRIs have a relatively short half-life and do not have active metabolites. With these drugs a steady-state blood level can be achieved a few days with single daily dosing. However, some of the SSRIs have extremely long half-lives and an active metabolite that has the ability to block the enzyme responsible for its destruction. Fluoxetine, for example, has a half-life of 2–4 days, and its active metabolite, *norfluoxetine*, has a half-life of 7–15 days. It may take as long as 75 days for the drug and its metabolite to reach a steady-state level in the body. It can also take this long for the drug and its metabolite to be completely eliminated from the body after the drug is discontinued.

There is considerable variability between individuals in the pharmacokinetics of the antidepressants. After a fixed daily dose of a tricyclic, individual steady-state blood levels may be as much as 36 times higher in some individuals than others, because some people have a genetic deficiency in one of the enzymes the body uses to destroy these drugs. In such people antidepressants can have extremely long half-lives (Preskorn, 1993; Rudorfer & Potter, 1987). Thus it is necessary to adjust doses for individuals and in many cases monitor blood levels (Simpson & Singh, 1990).

Lithium is excreted unchanged in the urine and has a half-life of between 12 and 21 hours (Hollister, 1983, p. 181). The excretion rate varies considerably among individuals and increases with age to as long as 36 hours (Baldessarini, 1985, p. 96). For this reason the blood levels must be carefully monitored when a patient is started on lithium therapy.

NEUROPHYSIOLOGY

The monoamine oxidase inhibitors (MAOIs) do exactly what their name implies—they block the activity of monoamine oxidase, the enzyme that destroys the monoamines dopamine (DA), norepinephrine (NE), and serotonin (5-HT). With this enzyme blocked, MA transmitters released into the synaptic cleft will not be metabolized, and the level of transmitter can rise as the transmitter accumulates. Activity at the synapse will increase unless the synapse has some other means of adjusting its activity. The effect of the older MAOIs is not selective, and the level of all MAs is affected. Some newer MAOIs, however, selectively affect NE and 5-HT and have little effect on DA.

The tricyclics work in the same way as cocaine (see Chapter 10)—they prevent the reabsorption of monoamines after they have been released into the cleft. The tricyclics affect all the MAs, but they are more selective than the MAOIs; some are more effective in potentiating NE, and others stimulate 5-HT selectively. Another effect of the tricyclics is that they act as anticholinergics, blocking transmission at cholinergic synapses. The effect on 5-HT and NE is believed to be responsible for their therapeutic action, and the anticholinergic effect is responsible for many of the side effects of antidepressants.

As their name suggests, the selective 5-HT reuptake inhibitors (SSRIs) block the ability of presynaptic cells to reabsorb and recycle 5-HT and have the effect of causing a buildup of 5-HT at synapses. This action is specific to 5-HT, and the SSRIs have minimal effect on other MAs.

The second-generation antidepressants also alter activity at MA synapses, although their actions may rely on completely different mechanisms than the tricyclics and may be highly specific to particular MAs. Some of these newer antidepressants, however, seem to have no obvious direct effect on MA transmission (Shopsin, Cassano, & Conti, 1981).

We know that antidepressants have an immediate effect of increasing transmitter levels in MA synapses. In the context of the monoamine theory that states that depression is a result of diminished MA activity this makes sense, but there is a big problem. The effect on transmitters is immediate, taking place as soon as the drug gets to the synapse, but the antidepressants need to be taken continuously for two to three weeks before there is any relief from depression.

This delay must mean one of two things. Either increased activity at MA synapses does not relieve depression and the MA theory of depression is wrong, or antidepressants do not immediately increase activity at the MA synapses because something delays the effect for about two weeks.

When a synapse is overstimulated for a period of time, the postsynaptic cell may reduce the number of receptor sites or reduce the sensitivity of receptor sites. This is called *down-regulation of receptors*. It has been pointed out that down-regulation of some receptors has a time lag of about two weeks, the same delay as the therapeutic effect of antidepressants. This similarity has led to speculation that depression might be caused by supersensitivity of MA systems rather than low levels of transmitter and that the antidepressants work by reducing this supersensitivity by causing the receptors to down-regulate (Sulser, Vetulani, & Mobley, 1978; Lickey & Gordon, 1991, p. 226; Mobley & Sulser, 1981).

Another possibility, and one for which there is even better evidence, is that in 5-HT synapses at least, increased levels of transmitter do not result in an immediate increase in firing because the presynaptic cell is equipped with an autoreceptor, a receptor that detects excessive amounts of 5-HT in the cleft. When it does, it inhibits the release of more 5-HT. Thus reuptake inhibitors like the SSRIs do not cause an immediate increase in conduction at 5-HT synapses. It takes about two weeks for the autoreceptors to habituate to the presence of excess 5-HT. It is only then that conduction at the synapse actually increases (Blier & de Montigny, 1994). Studies of the electrical activity at 5-HT synapses have shown that acute administration of SSRIs does not increase activity; it is only after two weeks of chronic treatment that electrical activity increases greatly. The delay experienced with other types of antidepressants may be a result of similar adjustment mechanisms.

The bulk of evidence supports the theory that depression is a result of diminished activity in the 5-HT system in the brain running from the Raphé nuclei through the medial forebrain bundle to the forebrain, and that mania is a result of the excessive activity in this system. The situation is very complicated, however, and many other explanations of depression and mania exist. These theories involve other neurotransmitters such as GABA, ACh, and DA, the balance between levels of neurotransmitters, second messengers, biological rhythms, hormone levels, and the immune system (Leonard, 1993; Janicak et al., 1993, pp. 211–219).

No one knows how lithium works, but it appears that it stabilizes the neurochemical mechanisms that control mood and keeps them from swinging so radically between extremes. Lithium is known to do a number of things in the brain, including (1) altering the balance of ions such as Cl^- and K^+, which are important in the formation of resting and action potentials; (2) altering the functioning of many transmitters such as 5-HT, NE, DA, ACh, and GABA; and (3) inhibiting the second messenger cyclic AMP. It has also been shown that lithium causes a down-regulation of some NE receptors (Bunney & Garland-Bunney, 1987). It is still not known which of these effects, if any, is responsible for the therapeutic effect of lithium, but the augmentation of 5-HT and its effect on second-messenger activity are the most promising candidates.

EFFECTS OF ANTIDEPRESSANTS AND ANTIMANICS

Effects on the Body

Unlike the psychomotor stimulants, the tricyclics do not stimulate the sympathetic nervous system. Instead, their anticholinergic effects block the parasympathetic nervous system, which uses ACh as a transmitter. These effects are characterized by symptoms that include dry mouth, constipation, dizziness, irregular heartbeat, blurred vision, ringing in the ears, and retention of urine. Excessive sweating is also common. Tremors are seen in about 10 percent of patients receiving the tricyclics. These side effects are usually worse during the first two weeks of treatment or when the dose is increased suddenly. Older patients are also more likely to show confusion and delirium, with incidence as high as

50 percent in patients over 70 (Baldessarini, 1985, p. 191).

The SSRIs may cause symptoms such as nausea, headache, nervousness, and insomnia, all of which, apart from the insomnia, tend to disappear with time.

Patients taking the tricyclics often report an increase in appetite and an increased preference for sweets accompanied by an increase in body weight. One study reported an increase of 1.3 to 2.9 pounds per month. In fact, excessive weight gain has been reported to be the major reason why patients stop taking these drugs. The MAOIs and lithium also cause weight gain, but the opposite effect has been reported with the SSRIs, which are sometimes used to treat obesity and help with weight loss (Boyer and Feighner, 1991, p. 142).

MAOIs alone do not have very marked effects apart from a lowering of blood pressure and postural hypotension (fainting or dizziness after moving to a standing position after sitting or lying down). Unfortunately, MAOIs interact with many other drugs. Drugs like amphetamine, decongestants, and nose drops that cause the release of NE (see Chapter 10) are potentiated by MAOIs because they block the metabolism of NE, which then accumulates. In some cases they block the metabolism of the other drugs or may interact with them in unexplained ways. Drugs potentiated by MAOIs include alcohol and some narcotics.

Another problem with MAOIs is that MAO not only destroys the MAs, but also is responsible for the digestion of some substances in food. One of these substances is *tyramine,* which is found in aged cheese, pickled herring, beer, wine, and chocolate. After eating such foods when MAO is inhibited, tyramine accumulates in the body and causes high blood pressure, which in turn can cause headaches, internal bleeding, and even stroke or death. As a consequence, people on MAOIs have always had to watch their diet closely and were at some risk.

There are actually two types of MAO, MAO-A which is primarily responsible for the breakdown of the 5-HT and NE, and MAO-B which is most active in metabolizing DA. The first type, MAO-A, is located in the intestine and normally metabolizes the tyramine just after it is consumed. Any tyrosine missed by the intestinal MAO-A is destroyed by MAO-B in the liver and the lungs before it gets into general circulation throughout the body. Normally less than 1 percent of tyramine gets past this MAO and into the system (Fitton, Faulds, & Goa, 1992). The older MAOIs blocked both forms of MAO, but new MAOIs like moclobemide selectively block MAO-A and have a minimal effect on MAO-B. As a result, tyrosine that gets past the inhibited MAO-A in the intestine can still be metabolized by the MAO-B in the liver and lungs. Selective MAO-A inhibitors are therefore much safer, and patients do not have to be as careful with their diet (Fitton, Faulds, & Goa, 1992). It also helps if the pill is taken after eating, allowing any dietary tyrosine to be metabolized before the maximum effect of the MAOI takes place.

As many as 90 percent of patients on lithium have complaints about unwanted physical effects. The most common are hand tremors, increased thirst, nausea and vomiting, diarrhea, swelling, and weight gain. After extended treatment, patients may experience fatigue and muscle weakness. Another problem associated with long-term use is kidney damage.

Effects on Sleep

Strangely, the tricyclics cause sleepiness, although this may have more to do with their anticholinergic properties than their MA-stimulating effects. Unlike the antidepressant effect, which takes days to develop, a single dose of a tricyclic can cause drowsiness and is sometimes prescribed to treat insomnia. The drug does not, however, increase total sleeping time. High doses of tricyclics at bedtime can cause nightmares.

Many antidepressants reduce REM time significantly, although some do not seem to have any effect on REM (Spiegel & Aebi, 1981,

p. 116). Reduction in REM sleep may be associated with the drug's antidepressant effects because it has been shown that sleep deprivation, particularly REM deprivation, can actually decrease symptoms of depression temporarily, and sleep can make depression worse (Janicak, et al., 1993, p. 322).

Fluoxetine is reported by some to increase the vividness of their dreams. While some enjoy this side effect, others find it disturbing.

Effects on Personality

In 1990 fluoxetine (Prozac) attracted national attention by appearing on the cover of *Newsweek*. Quoted in that issue was a psychiatrist, Peter Kramer, who had written about giving fluoxetine to people, not to treat depression, but to modify their personalities. Prozac "seemed to give social confidence to the habitually timid, to make the sensitive brash, and to lend the introvert the social skills of a salesman" (Kramer, 1993, p. xv). Kramer quoted one of his patients as saying that the drug had made him feel "better than well." He also coined the term "cosmetic psychopharmacology," suggesting that people could take drugs such as fluoxetine to cover, by neurochemical means, some aspect of their personality that they were not satisfied with in the same way that facial blemishes could be hidden by makeup, or the shape of a nose can be made more attractive by cosmetic surgery.

It has been established that fluoxetine and other SSRIs are useful in treating people with diagnosed personality disorders such as obsessive-compulsive personality, and in the treatment of compulsive behaviors (Gitlin, 1993). However, the use of fluoxetine and SSRIs as a personality cosmetic for people who do not have a diagnosed "disorder" but are not happy with their personality is a matter of some debate. It raises a number of interesting issues, not the least of which concerns the origins of personality. If a drug can cause such immediate and profound changes in personality, this fact has far-reaching implications for the way we view personality. Is our personality determined by our past, our childhood experiences, and the like, as many theorists have believed for years, or is personality determined by 5-HT levels in the Raphé nuclei (Kramer, 1993)?

Some patients who have used fluoxetine as a personality cosmetic have become disenchanted with the changes in themselves over a period of time and discontinued the drug because they felt that it had taken some of the edge or tension out of their lives and made them too bland.

EFFECTS ON THE BEHAVIOR AND PERFORMANCE OF HUMANS

Subjective Effects

The antidepressants do not produce euphoric or even pleasant effects. At low doses, imipramine's effects are similar to those of the antipsychotics. It causes feelings of tiredness, apathy, and weakness. Higher doses produce impaired comprehension and a confusion that is described as unpleasant. Amitriptyline causes feelings of calmness and relaxation (Spiegel & Aebi, 1981, p. 64).

Lithium has few, if any, subjective effects apart from those associated with side effects such as nausea. Subjects sometimes report a feeling of mental slowing and difficulty in concentration (Judd et al., 1987, p. 1467).

Effects on Performance

Acute doses of the tricyclic antidepressants imipramine and amitriptyline can have detrimental effects on vigilance tasks and cause cognitive, memory, and psychomotor impairment that seems to be related to sedation. These drugs should not be used by people who must drive, use heavy equipment, or do intellectual work. Some studies have shown improvement in cognitive functioning after chronic drug treatment, suggesting that these impairments show tolerance. Other studies, however, have not (Lickey & Gordon, 1991, p. 230).

There is no evidence that the nontricyclics have any effect on performance or cognitive functioning (Judd et al., 1987, p. 1468; Spiegel & Aebi, 1981, p. 64), although there are reports that SSRIs cause memory problems.

Extensive systematic studies of mental abilities after acute and chronic lithium administration indicate a small but significant slowing of mental processes. There appear to be few effects on performance of tasks and reaction time. The difficulty appears to be in a slowing of information processing and memory (Judd et al., 1987, p. 1468; Kocsis et al., 1993).

EFFECTS ON THE BEHAVIOR OF NONHUMANS

Positively Reinforced Behavior

Tricyclic antidepressants are more effective in increasing response rates than methamphetamine. They even appear to increase high rates where amphetamine tends to decrease them (Dews, 1962).

There have been few studies of the effects of MAO inhibitors on positively reinforced behavior, largely because of the very long delay in effect with these drugs. Most of these studies have not shown any great effect (McMillan & Leander, 1976).

Negatively Reinforced Behavior

The tricyclic antidepressants tend to decrease avoidance behavior in a discrete-trials situation at doses that have no effect on escape behavior (McMillan & Leander, 1976), thus making them similar to the antianxiety drugs and the antipsychotics.

The tricyclics also do not increase punishment-suppressed behavior. If anything, they tend to decrease it. The tricyclics are similar to amphetamine and the psychomotor stimulants in

this regard. The effects of MAO inhibitors on punished behavior have not been determined.

DISCRIMINATIVE STIMULUS PROPERTIES

Neither the MAO inhibitors nor the tricyclics are discriminable at doses that produce most of their behavioral effects. However, at very high but sublethal doses, they can be discriminated. Lithium does not appear to have any discriminative stimulus properties (Overton, 1982, 1987). There does not appear to be any generalization between the antidepressants and the antipsychotics or any other drug class (J. Stewart, 1962).

TOLERANCE

Tolerance to the side effects of the antidepressants usually occurs within several weeks. There are reports that the therapeutic effectiveness of these drugs may also show some tolerance, but this hypothesis has not been confirmed (Baldessarini, 1985, p. 143).

WITHDRAWAL

Sudden discontinuation of high doses of the tricyclics can cause withdrawal symptoms, which include restlessness, anxiety, chills, muscle aches, and akathesia, a feeling of a compulsion to move (Baldessarini, 1985, pp. 143, 192). For this reason, these drugs should not be discontinued abruptly.

SELF-ADMINISTRATION IN HUMANS AND NONHUMANS

Neither the tricyclic antidepressants nor the MAO inhibitors are self-administered unless prescribed by a physician for the treatment of depression. They are seldom sold illicitly on the street and do not appear to be used nonmedically. Apart from their medical application, it does not appear as though either the tricyclic antidepressants or the MAO inhibitors are reinforcing to either humans or nonhumans (Griffiths, Bigelow, & Henningfield, 1980).

To determine whether imipramine has aversive effects, an experiment was conducted in which monkeys were able to avoid infusions of various doses of imipramine by pressing a lever. Imipramine was avoided only at very high doses. It appears to be one of the few drugs tested that has neither positive nor negative reinforcing properties (Hoffmeister & Wuttke, 1975, p. 425).

Compliance. Because depression is a chronic disorder it is important to find effective ways of preventing relapses. Lithium is effective in preventing relapse if taken chronically. It has also been shown that chronic administration of therapeutic doses of most antidepressants is an effective way of preventing relapse. Patients, however, must be willing to tolerate the side effects of the drug over an extended period of time. Comparative trials have shown that the SSRIs are far superior to any other antidepressant in terms of patients remaining compliant to chronic drug regimens. This success was due to the comparatively low rate of unwanted side effects of the SSRIs (Tollefson, 1993).

HARMFUL EFFECTS

Reproduction

Early studies have found that the tricyclic antidepressants can interfere with male sexual functioning but suggest that the problems are not extensive (Harrison et al., 1986). A more recent study, however, has found evidence that the problem may be more serious than first thought (Monteiro et al., 1987). This study compared a group of patients of both sexes receiving the tricyclic clomiprimine for the obsessive-compulsive disorder with a placebo control group. In response to general questions about sexual functioning, there did not appear to be any difference between the drug group and the controls, but when questioned more closely in a structured interview about changes in sexuality, nearly all (96 percent) of the drug group reported severe difficulties in achieving orgasm. No difficulties were reported in the control group. This effect did not seem to be a result of sedation or fatigue and did not show any tolerance. Delayed or impaired ejaculation has also been reported with the MAO inhibitors (Woods, 1984, p. 439). Also, patients on SSRIs frequently report delayed ejaculation and loss of interest in sex.

There is little evidence that the antidepressants cause any adverse effects to the fetus during pregnancy in humans, but a teratogenic effect has been noted in laboratory animals. As a general rule, they should be discontinued during pregnancy. In one study pregnancy outcomes of women on fluoxetine and tricyclic antidepressants were compared with a matched control group. There were no differences in fetal malformations between the groups, but the women in the fluoxetine and tricyclic antidepressant groups were nearly twice as likely as controls to miscarry (Pastuszak et al., 1993).

Some antidepressants have been detected in breast milk of nursing mothers, but usually there is no evidence of the drug in the blood of the baby. It appears that the first pass metabolism of the baby is able to get rid of the drug before it gets into its system.

Lithium is known to cause cardiac malformations in the developing fetus if taken early in pregnancy (Hollister, 1983, p. 195), so its use should be avoided if pregnancy is possible. Since it readily passes into breast milk, it should not be taken by nursing mothers.

Violence and Suicide

Soon after fluoxetine was introduced to the U.S. market there were reports that it induced intense violent suicidal preoccupations in some patients (Teicher, Glod, & Cole, 1990). In fact, Prozac-induced violence became a defense in some courtrooms and was the subject of extensive coverage by television talk shows. The evidence was largely in the form of case studies. On the other hand, large-scale studies have actually shown that fluoxetine reduces the incidence of suicide and violence, not increases it. The issue has not been clearly settled because it is difficult to research. Such drugs are often prescribed for people who are very agitated, depressed, and suicidal anyway. Suicide after taking an antidepressant drug may represent only a lack of effect, an inability to prevent a suicide, not a drug-induced effect. In addition, if this is a drug that only causes suicide and violence in a small number of people, but reduces it in most others, large-scale studies that average across everyone would not detect it.

Fluoxetine induces an activating effect with racing thoughts, nervousness, and tremor in a number of individuals after being taken for three to four weeks (Boyer & Feighner, 1991). Sometimes this develops to the point where it is called *akathesia*, a movement disorder characterized by restlessness, agitation, an inability to sit still, and a compulsion to be continuously active. Akathesia is also one of the movement disorders seen after the administration of antipsychotics (see Chapter 12). Reports of violence and suicide seem to be associated with this effect of the drug in certain individuals (Rothschild & Locke, 1991). For most, fluoxetine is relatively safe and effective, but like any drug, it has the capacity to cause serious problems for some, and its use and dosage should be monitored closely, especially for the first few weeks.

SSRIs can cause several adverse effects collectively known as the *serotonin syndrome*, especially when taken in combination with other drugs like MAO inhibitors that elevate serotonin. Symptoms of the serotonin syndrome are lethargy, restlessness, confusion, flushing, and tremors. If this syndrome is unrecognized and untreated, hyperthermia, increased muscle tone, and jerky movements may develop. The condition can ultimately cause respiratory, circulatory, and kidney failure if untreated.

Overdose

The tricyclics are the third most common cause of drug-related deaths, exceeded only by alcohol-drug combinations and heroin. The toxicity of the tricyclics is due primarily to their effect on the contractility of the heart muscle. They have a therapeutic index of around 10 to 15. This is a serious concern, especially when these drugs are prescribed to people who are seriously depressed and contemplating suicide. There is considerable variability in the death rates attributed to drugs within the same class. Among the tricyclics, clomiprimine is relatively safe, but many deaths have been attributed to amitriptyline. Tranylcypromine is an MAOI responsible for a high rate of deaths, while the rate of isocarboxazide fatalities is low (Leonard, 1993).

The SSRIs are considerably safer with no overdose deaths attributed to fluoxetine (Boyer & Feighner, 1991; Leonard, 1993).

CHAPTER SUMMARY

- There are three classes of antidepressants: *inhibitors of monoamine oxidase* (*MAO inhibitors*), *tricyclic antidepressants*, and the newer second-generation antidepressants, which include the *selective serotonin reuptake inhibitors* (*SSRIs*). In addition, the element *lithium* is used in the treatment of *bipolar disorder* (formerly called *manic-depressive psychosis*).

- *Depression* has symptoms such as loss of appetite, loss of energy, sleeping problems, intense feelings of guilt or worthlessness, and thoughts of suicide. For some, depression comes in cycles and alternates with *mania*, a state of elated hyperactivity. This condition is called *manic-depressive psychosis* or, more recently, *bipolar disorder*.

- The antidepressants are absorbed orally and reach peak blood levels in about four hours.

- Most tricyclics have very long half-lives; the half-lives of the second-generation antidepressants are usually shorter.

- All agents that act as antidepressants have the effect of increasing transmission at serotonergic synapses. There is a delay of about two weeks in the start of the therapeutic effect of the antidepressants.

- The MAO inhibitors also block the destruction of some toxic substances found in some foods. People taking MAO inhibitors should not eat foods like pickled herring and some types of cheese. Lithium also causes unwanted effects like thirst, tremor, and nausea.

- Tolerance develops to many of the effects of antidepressants. Withdrawal symptoms are sometimes seen when the drug is discontinued abruptly.

- Antidepressants do not appear to be reinforcing in nonhumans and are never abused or taken for recreational purposes.

- The tricyclics and SSRIs have been shown to cause problems in sexual functioning with both sexes reporting difficulty in achieving orgasm. Lithium has been shown to cause cardiac malformations in the fetus when taken by the mother early in pregnancy.

14

Cannabis

... these are exciting times in cannabinoid neurobiology.

—E. L. Gardner (1992, p. 322)

SOURCES

The Cannabis Plant

The *hemp* plant, or *Cannabis sativa*, was given its name and classification by Linnaeus in 1753. It is not known where the plant originated, but it was probably somewhere in central Asia. There are a great many varieties of cannabis, which can vary from small shrubs to bushy 20-foot-high plants. Commonly, the plants can be identified by their distinctive leaves, which are frequently long and slender with serrated edges and grow in groups of five, resembling the fingers of a hand. There are male and female plants. The female plants are bushy and may grow quite tall. The male plants are smaller and not as bushy or vigorous. The female plant must be fertilized by pollen from the male flower to produce seeds. To help collect the wind-borne pollen, the female exudes a sticky resin from its flowering top. The resin also protects the seeds from heat and insects.

Since Linnaeus first classified *C. sativa*, there has been speculation about whether there was more than one species. Based on differences in form and potency, some botanists have identified three species, including *C. sativa*, *C. indica*, and *C. ruderalis* (Grinspoon & Bakalar, 1993). Otherwise it is speculated that there is only one species *C. sativa* of which there are two phenotypes (subspecies or varieties). One is traditionally cultivated in northerly areas for its fiber. It matures rapidly and has a low content of active ingredients and is often called *hemp*. The other type is slow maturing, is traditionally cultivated in more southerly and tropical regions for its intoxicating properties, and has a relatively high content of psychoactive ingredients (Small, 1979).

Active Ingredients

The active ingredient in cannabis is usually reported as something called *delta-9-tetrahydro-*

cannabinol (delta-9-THC), but the chemistry of cannabis is much more complex than that. In fact, there is an entire family of drugs, called the *cannabinoids*, that are found exclusively in cannabis, and each may contribute, either directly or indirectly, to the behavioral effects of the cannabis plant. Over 80 cannabinoids have been identified. The most common is delta-9-THC. Another cannabinoid is *delta-8-THC*, but there is relatively little delta-8-THC in cannabis compared to the delta-9-THC content. (The numbers in these names refer to the places where different parts of the molecule are attached. Because there are two different conventions for numbering the parts of the molecules, the same chemical can have two names. For this reason, you will sometimes see the active ingredients in cannabis called delta-1-THC and delta-6-THC. These are exactly the same as delta-9 and delta-8, respectively). Other cannabinoids are drugs such as *cannabinol (CBN)* and *cannabidiol (CBD)*, but by themselves these are not believed to have any important behavioral effects. The story, however, is not quite this simple, because the amount of active ingredients appears to depend on preparation and route of administration, and these inactive ingredients may alter the potency or metabolism of more active ingredients.

Cannabis is sometimes taken orally, but usually it is burned and the smoke is inhaled. It has been shown that burning changes many of the cannabinoids and appears to create new ones with increased potencies and effects. It is known, for example, that people can get high from smoking marijuana that contains virtually no delta-9-THC but is rich in CBD. Studies have shown that the inactive CBD is converted into delta-9-THC when the plant is burned, and new cannabinoids of unknown potency are also created (Salimenk, 1976; Kephalis et al., 1976).

Not only are the new cannabinoids created during burning, but more are created during digestion when the drug is taken orally, and still more during metabolism. It is still not clear what

effects each of these drugs has, how much each contributes to the effect that cannabis has on behavior, or how each of the cannabinoids interacts with the effects of other cannabinoids. Consequently, the effect of a particular cannabis plant cannot be predicted simply on the basis of the results of an analysis of its ingredients. As if things were not complicated enough, the content of marijuana changes over time, especially if exposed to light and air. With time, THC is apparently converted into CBN (Mechoulam et al., 1976).

Cannabis Preparations

All parts of the cannabis plant contain THC, and the plant is prepared for consumption in various ways. The most familiar to North Americans is *marijuana*. The term *marijuana* is a Mexican-Spanish word that originally referred to a cheap tobacco but later came to refer to the dried leaves and flowers of the cannabis plant. Marijuana is usually smoked in a cigarette, cigar, or pipe but is sometimes baked into cookies or brownies.

In India a distinction is made between *bhang* and *ganja*. Bhang is similar to marijuana. It is the dried leaves of uncultivated cannabis plants, or female plants from which the resin has been removed. Generally, bhang is not very potent. Ganja is made from the tops of female plants from which the resin has not been removed. It is three to four times more potent than bhang. In the West Indies cannabis was imported directly from India, and the Indian term *ganja* rather than the North American *marijuana* is used. In Jamaica the term *ganja* refers to the entire cannabis plant, and the distinction between ganja and bhang is not made.

Hashish, also known as *charas* in India, refers to the dried resin from the top of the female plant. It is originally a pale yellow sap when harvested but turns almost black when dried. It may be consumed in a number of ways. Frequently, it is smoked, either alone or in a mixture with tobacco, or it may be baked in candies or cookies.

There are some delightful stories concerning the way in which hashish was traditionally harvested in Nepal. To maximize the yield, the resin is removed several times before the plant is harvested. Legend has it that in ancient times naked workers were made to run through the fields thrashing their arms about and getting covered with the sap. It was then scraped off their bodies. Newer methods are much less romantic but more sanitary. The resin is squeezed off the plant onto cheesecloth, from which it is later scraped.

A purified variation of hashish is *hash oil* or *red oil*. Hash oil is prepared by boiling the hashish in alcohol (or some other solvent), filtering out the residue, and then permitting the alcohol to evaporate. The cannabinoids are highly soluble in alcohol, which extracts them from the hashish and concentrates them. Depending on the degree of purity, hash oil may range from black or red to light amber. Hash oil is much more concentrated than hashish. It may contain up to 60 percent cannabinoids, and because it is easier to smuggle, it is becoming more popular. Hash oil may be consumed in several ways. It is common to place a drop on the paper of a regular tobacco cigarette, which may then be smoked inconspicuously. Other ways involve placing a drop on hot tinfoil and inhaling the smoke.

Synthetic Cannabinoids

Several synthetic drugs similar to the cannabinoids have been developed, and some are licensed for commercial use. The first was Synhexyl (called Parahexyl in Great Britain). Nabilone is now used clinically to alleviate nausea and distress in patients receiving chemotherapy for cancer, and a synthetic delta 9-THC (Dronabinol) is used for the same purpose. Other substances such as levonantradol and (−)-HU-210 have been developed but not marketed. Win 55212–2 is a synthetic thought to have antagonistic properties (Consroe & Sandyk, 1992).

HISTORY

It is believed that cannabis originated in central Asia, but its early history is difficult to trace because it was cultivated and widely dispersed long before recorded history. The spread of cannabis appears to have occurred in the middle of the second century B.C. The people responsible were the Scythians, a warlike and mobile Middle Eastern tribe related to the Semites. The word *cannabis* is a Scythian word, and the Greek historian Herodotus described the Scythians as having used cannabis. He explained how the Scythians would enter their tents, throw hemp seeds on heated stones, inhale the vapors, and "howl with joy." This procedure was used as a cleansing ceremony after funerals (Benet, 1975).

The Scythians spread cannabis into Egypt by way of Palestine and northward into Russia and Europe, where the Scythian custom of burning cannabis seeds after funerals still remains (Benet, 1975).

In China cannabis has been known since Neolithic times, about 6,000 years ago. The Chinese word *ma* for hemp has been in use for at least 3,000 years. The plant was cultivated for its fiber; for its seed, which was a staple grain; for its intoxicating effects; and for its medicinal effects (Li, 1975, p. 56).

Cannabis has been used for centuries in India. Its use spread there directly from China rather than the Middle East. From India the drug was introduced to Africa by Arab traders who sailed along the east coast of Africa in the twelfth century. It spread across Africa along with the cultural influence of Islam. In Africa it is known as *bangi* or *dagga* (Toit, 1975).

Hemp was introduced into Russia and Eastern Europe by the Scythians, and from there it spread into Western Europe, where it was grown for centuries without its intoxicating properties being widely recognized. It was grown chiefly for its fiber, from which rope was made. It was also commonly used as a medicine.

Despite the fact that cannabis has been used as a folk remedy wherever it has been grown, scientific medical attention was not directed toward the drug until 1839 when W. B. O'Shaughnessy, a young chemistry professor at the University of Calcutta, tried it out on various ailments. He reported that hemp was an effective anticonvulsant and an appetite stimulant. There followed a series of papers that expounded the usefulness of hemp in the treatment of a number of disorders, including tetanus, neuralgia, dysmenorrhea, asthma, gonorrhea, and migraine. It was also reported to be useful in treating addiction to alcohol, opium, and chloral hydrate. There were also claims that hemp might be useful in the treatment of mental illness. One of the earliest of these claims was made in 1845 by the French physician J. J. Moreau de Tors, who used it to treat melancholia, hypomania, and other forms of mental illness (Moreau, 1845/1973). In England, Sir John Russell Reynolds, president of the Royal College of Physicians and physician to Queen Victoria, used marijuana extensively in the treatment of neurological disorders (Consroe & Sandyk, 1992).

In general, the intoxicating effects of the drug remained unnoticed by Europeans until the publication of *Le Club des Hachichins* by the French writer Théophile Gautier in 1846. Gautier was a romantic and flamboyant writer who once offered a reward to anyone who could invent a new pleasure. The reward was earned (but we do not know whether he ever collected) by J. J. Moreau de Tours, the physician just mentioned. Dr. Moreau introduced Gautier to the Club des Hachichins and gave him his first hashish with the words, "This will be subtracted from your share in Paradise." Gautier's account of the effects, quoted later in this chapter, are now a classic description of the drug experience.

The drug that Gautier used was imported from the Middle East and North Africa. No one made the association between hashish and the quantities of hemp that were being grown at that time all over Europe to make rope. Even though he recognized that the two plants were related, Moreau believed that hemp and hashish were different. (What the members of the club received was not what is currently called hashish. Moreau used the term *hashish* to refer to a product made by boiling the plant in butter rather than the cannabis resin.)

In the days of European imperialism, rope was a very important item because empires were built on naval strength and ships could not sail without rope. Hemp did not grow well in England, so its production was encouraged in the American Colonies. Sir Walter Raleigh was ordered to grow hemp in his Virginia colony, and consequently a crop was planted alongside tobacco in 1611, the colony's first season. American hemp proved to be of good quality, and hemp became a staple crop of the American colonies for more than 200 years. One of the better-known hemp growers was George Washington.

It is believed that the use of the cannabis plant for smoking and the word *marijuana* were introduced into the United States by Mexican laborers in the early twentieth century. Marijuana smoking slowly spread through the United Sates, but it was restricted to racial minorities and jazz musicians. This association did much to shape the perceptions of white legislators and to motivate opponents. In the 1920s marijuana started to attract the attention of the authorities and the public, which almost universally condemned it. Alarmist stories appeared in newspapers attributing criminal activity to the drug, especially crimes of violence.

Because there was a shortage of reliable scientific data to the contrary, these accusations went unchallenged. By 1937 most states had laws against marijuana, and the U.S. federal government had passed the *Marijuana Tax Act*, which imposed prohibitive taxes on possession and use, effectively eliminating the legitimate medical use of marijuana, and driving recreational users underground. Soon most other Western countries had antimarijuana laws. In Canada, marijuana is classed as a "narcotic" and included in the *Narcotic Control Act* with the opiate drugs (and cocaine).

The medical profession represented by the American Medical Association has always supported the position of the U.S. federal government, and in 1970 the result was the *Controlled Substances Act*. This act ignored the previous century of accumulating medical evidence and declared that marijuana had no potential medical use and had a high potential for abuse.

In spite of these laws (or perhaps because of them), the popularity of marijuana continued to grow until it reached its peak in the 1970s and started to level off. Throughout the 1980s and early 1990s use in the United States declined considerably, but that decline may be coming to an end (see "Self-Administration": "Patterns of Use.")

ABSORPTION

The cannabinoids are extremely lipid-soluble, so lipid-soluble, in fact, that they will hardly dissolve in water. When taken orally, the cannabinoids are absorbed from the digestive system rather slowly because they do not dissolve and become dispersed throughout the digestive fluid. Oral absorption may be aided by adding oil to the plant material before consumption. This is often done by baking it in some food like cookies or brownies.

Absorption by the oral route is slow and incomplete, so when taken orally, the dose must be doubled or tripled to have the same effect as when inhaled (Institute of Medicine, 1982, p. 21). The peak effects after oral administration usually occur after one to three hours and may last five hours or longer (Paton & Pertwee, 1973b; Agurell et al., 1984). Oral administration is also more likely to cause nausea or vomiting (Grinspoon, 1969).

Smoking cannabis plant material is an efficient route of administration. Normal smoking causes about 50 percent of the cannabinoids in a marijuana cigarette to enter the lungs, and of that, virtually all enters the body (Manno et al., 1974). Effects may begin to be felt within a few minutes and reach a peak after 30 to 60 minutes. Because of a widespread belief that absorption increases with the duration of each puff, experienced marijuana smokers will take a deep draw on the marijuana cigarette and then hold the smoke in the lungs for 10 to 20 seconds. In fact, holding the smoke in the lungs may not contribute much to absorption of THC. It appears that the depth of an inhalation is much more important than duration in determining THC absorption (Azorlosa, Greenwald, & Stitzer, 1995).

DISTRIBUTION

Because of their high lipid solubility, the cannabinoids are distributed to all areas of the body according to blood flow, but after a while they tend to become concentrated in the lungs, the kidneys, and the bile of the liver. Very little remains in the brain.

METABOLISM

Metabolism starts as soon as the cannabinoids enter the body. There is some metabolism in the lungs if the drug is inhaled and some in the intestine if the drug is taken orally, but most of the metabolism takes place in the liver. Delta-9-THC is primarily converted into a substance known as 11-hydroxy-delta-9-THC. This is believed to be more active than delta-9 but does not penetrate the brain as easily and so has an equivalent effect. These substances are then rapidly converted into numerous other metabolites, some of which have effects on their own. These effects may be similar to those of THC, but some may be different. Most of these metabolites are less lipid-soluble and are more easily excreted (Mechoulam et al., 1976).

While CBD is thought to have only a slight effect of its own, it appears to have a direct effect on the metabolism of THC. It blocks the enzyme that converts delta-9-THC, slows its metabolism, and prolongs its duration of action. By contrast, CBN may speed the metabolism of THC (Mechoulam et al., 1976). It is also possible that CBD and CBN interact with THC in other ways. For example, these substances may alter the distribution of THC by displacing it from binding sites in the blood and increasing the amount of THC available for distribution to the brain (Siemens, Kalant, & Nie, 1976).

Blood levels of delta-9-THC and its main metabolites fall rather rapidly at first. This initial decline is due to redistribution and has a half-life of about 30 minutes in humans, but this is followed by a phase with a much slower rate of decline and a half-life of 50 to 60 hours. During this phase, the rate of metabolism is limited by the rate at which the THC is released from body fat into the blood, which is quite slow. After about one week, 20 to 30 percent of administered THC and its metabolites remain in the body. Traces may be detected in the body as long as 30 days later (Institute of Medicine, 1982, p. 20).

Figure 14–1 shows the rated "high" produced by different doses of THC administered by different routes.

There is evidence that cannabis users can metabolize and excrete the cannabinoids faster than nonusers, although this effect is not big and probably does not account for the development of any tolerance (Agurell et al., 1984). Research with laboratory animals has not shown that the development of tolerance is related to any change in cannabinoid absorption, distribution, or metabolism (Dewey, Martin, & Harris, 1976).

The subjective high does not parallel the blood levels of THC. The maximum subjective effect is usually reported while the THC blood levels are falling. This delayed effect may be due to the finding that THC levels in the brain continue to increase for several hours after the drug has been consumed. The drug never reaches very high lev-

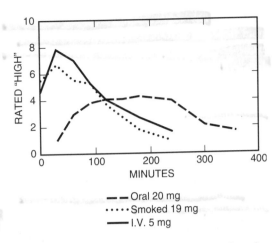

Figure 14–1 The time course for intensity of subjective "high" after consuming various doses of THC via different routes of administration. (Adapted from Agurell et al., 1984.)

els in the brain. In fact, the amount of THC in the brain probably is no more than 1/6,000 the administered dose (Bronson, Latour, & Nahas, 1984).

NEUROPHARMACOLOGY

Up until the late 1980s the mechanism by which cannabinoids alter neural functioning was a mystery. There was plenty of evidence that they work at a receptor site, but receptor sites for cannabinoids had never been identified. In addition, cannabinoids have many effects in common with general anesthetics; for example, they are highly lipid-soluble and alter the fluidity of membranes. In 1990 an announcement was made that a receptor for cannabinoids had been identified by two scientists at the National Institute of Mental Health in Bethesda, Maryland. Both scientists had been working on different problems independently in adjacent labs in the same building.

Researchers in the laboratory of Miles Herkinham had been working with radioactive levonantradol. Levonantradol is a synthetic cannabinoid that had been developed as a medicine but had psychological effects too similar to THC to be useful. By making it radioactive, it is possible to see where it goes in the brain of laboratory animals. Using this technique, the scientists in Herkenham's lab were creating a map of where levonantradol ended up in the brain and presumed that it was binding to a cannabinoid receptor at these sites.

In the neighboring laboratory of Tom I. Bonner, Linda Matsuda had discovered a gene that would make a receptor site. They were trying to find a receptor for substances that modulate pain, but the receptor they found did not bind any known pain neurotransmitter; in fact, it did not seem to bind any known neurotransmitter. Matsuda did know, however, exactly where in the brain these receptors were found—she had made a map. When Matsuda heard of Herkinham's map, she went down the hall and they compared maps. It was apparent in an instant that the two maps were similar—the mystery receptors were in exactly the same place in the brain where the radiolabeled levonantradol ended up. It did not take long for the two researchers to confirm that Matsuda's receptor was in fact a cannabinoid receptor (Restak, 1993).

The maps of Herkinham and Matsuda showed that cannabinoid receptors are concentrated primarily in the cortex, hippocampus, cerebellum, and basal ganglia, but occur also in the hypothalamus, brain stem, and spinal cord (Howlett, Evans, & Houston, 1992). Interestingly, we now know that cannabinoid receptors are not confined to the nervous system; they have been found in areas such as the spleen (Mechoulam, Hanus, & Martin, 1994). These receptors are structurally different from the ones found in the brain and seem to be associated with the effects of cannabinoids on immune functions. The peripheral receptor also appears to be affected by CBN. These discoveries raise the possibility that there may be numerous subtypes of cannabinoid receptors, as there are with the receptors for other neurotransmitters and neuromodulators. If there are different subtypes of cannabinoid receptors and they mediate different cannabinoid effects, it may be possible to develop medicines that can selectively produce medically useful cannabinoid effects with a minimum of side effects.

Like the discovery of the opioid receptor, the discovery of the cannabinoid receptor has stimulated research into the nature of the endogenous ligand—the substance or substances that occur naturally in the body and act at the receptor. Such a substance has been identified by William Devane and Raphael Mechoulam at the Hebrew University of Jerusalem who call it *anandamide* after the Sanskrit word *ananda*, meaning "internal bliss" (Restak, 1993; Mechoulam, Hanus, & Martin, 1994). These researchers have also found two more anandamides, and it is likely that there are more yet to be discovered.

These discoveries stimulated an explosion of research, the full impact of which has yet to be felt, and will likely lead to new drugs and medicines as well as a better understanding of where and how THC and the cannabinoids alter the functioning of the brain and change behavior.

Cannabinoid receptors and their endogenous ligand appear to function more as neuromodulators than as neurotransmitters. There are numerous demonstrations that cannabinoids most likely produce their effects by altering the functioning of many other neurochemicals. They have been shown to alter functioning of NE, DA, 5-HT, ACh, histamine, opioid peptides, and prostaglandins. Cannabinoids are known to increase synthesis of NE, DA, 5-HT, and GABA. They can potentiate the actions of NE, ACh, GABA, and opiate peptides, and they can alter the functioning of receptors for NE, DA, and ACh. Not all of these effects, however, are likely to be mediated via the cannabinoid receptor; some may be achieved directly by other means (Pertwee, 1992).

Cannabinoid receptors are found in the nucleus accumbens and it is clear that they function to increase activity in the mesolimbic dopamine reward system. They perform this function by potentiating the effects of endogenous opioid peptides, which in turn act as neuromodulators of dopamine transmission. This effect appears to be responsible for the reinforcing effects of cannabinoids (Gardner, 1992).

EFFECTS OF CANNABIS

Effects on the Body

Low and moderate doses of marijuana have predictable physiological effects on most people. The commonest effect is bloodshot eyes caused by a dilation of the small blood vessels in the whites of the eyes. This effect reaches a peak about an hour after smoking. It causes no discomfort to the user. Once it was also thought that marijuana caused dilation of the pupils, but systematic research has not demonstrated this as a reliable effect. In fact, accurate measurements of pupil diameter have shown a very slight decrease in pupil size, but this cannot be detected without instruments (Domino, Rennick, & Pearl, 1974). It seems that any dilation seen after marijuana use is a result of the darkened conditions where the drug is usually consumed and not the drug itself. Heavy marijuana use can sometimes be detected because the user looks "stoned." It has been shown that this stoned look arises from a slight droop in the eyelids (Domino, Rennick, & Pearl, 1974).

Another effect is the sensation of having a dry mouth and compulsion to drink. This frequently induces some users to drink alcoholic beverages while smoking marijuana. There is also an intense feeling of hunger known as the *munchies* that is strongest about three hours after smoking, when other effects have declined. This increase in appetite appears to show tolerance after a few weeks of continuous marijuana use, and appetite is actually depressed.

Smoking marijuana also causes a reliable increase in heart rate, which can go as high as 160 beats per minute in some individuals. There are also unpredictable fluctuations in blood pressure and body temperature. Nausea and vomiting sometimes result, especially after the user has been moving around. At higher doses, headaches are sometimes reported (Paton & Pertwee 1973b).

Medically Useful Effects

Some effects on the body that are not normally noticed have some medical usefulness. For example, THC reduces the pressure of the fluid in the eyeball. Glaucoma, a condition in which pressure in the eyes is too high, has been successfully treated with marijuana. In a rather famous case in the United States, a young man with glaucoma was prosecuted for growing marijuana but won his case by arguing that it was necessary to break the law in order to treat his glaucoma (Grinspoon, 1971, p. 397; Grinspoon & Bakalar, 1993).

THC can act as an antiemetic, a drug that stops nausea and vomiting. Nabilone, a synthetic cannabinoid, is now frequently used to treat the nausea and sickness of people receiving chemotherapy for cancer.

THC has been shown effective as an anticonvulsant. It also has properties as an antibiotic and can reduce some types of tumors. THC is also a bronchodilator that could be useful in the treatment of asthma, and it has analgesic properties. It also shows some promise in treating movement disorders and spasticity (Braude & Szara, 1976, vol. 2; S. Cohen & Stillman, 1976; Institute of Medicine, 1982).

Marijuana has a long history of being used as a medicine in many cultures. Unfortunately, few systematic controlled studies exist that properly evaluate marijuana or any cannabinoids in the treatment of disease. In addition, no cannabinoid has yet been found that does not cause the subjective high and other effects like memory distortion. As a result, only a few synthetic cannabinoids, like nabilone, are licensed and currently in use. However, now that the cannabinoid receptor has been identified, an increased understanding of how the cannabinoids produce their various effects may soon make it possible to isolate specific medically useful effects and design cannabinoids that will produce them (Consroe & Sandyk, 1992).

Effects on Sleep

Marijuana causes drowsiness and increases sleeping time in humans, but higher doses interfere with sleep, causing restlessness and insomnia (Tart & Crawford, 1970). Habitual users may have difficulty getting to sleep (Paton & Pertwee, 1973b).

Low doses of marijuana cause slight changes in sleep stage patterns, and many studies have found no effect on sleep. At higher doses, the effects are clear-cut: Marijuana has a unique effect on sleep stages. In addition to depressing total REM sleep, it also depresses the total eye movement activity during REM. Unlike the barbiturates, however, there is a large increase in stage 4 slow-wave sleep. When the drug is withdrawn, there is a mild rebound of REM sleep time on the first night but a very large and persistent rebound of eye movement activity. Stage 4 drops to normal and then increases again after the first night. This large increase in eye movement during withdrawal is not accompanied by the poor quality of sleep, frequent wakening, or nightmares seen with barbiturates (Feinberg et al., 1975).

EFFECTS ON THE BEHAVIOR AND PERFORMANCE OF HUMANS

Subjective Effects

The first European writer to describe the effects of cannabis was Théophile Gautier, who was a member of the Club des Hachichins of Paris in the middle of the nineteenth century. Gautier's accounts must be considered with some skepticism because they were written primarily to entertain rather than inform. Gautier was an artist, not a scientist, and a rather creative and romantic artist at that. And again, the drug that Gautier and the other club members took was not what we know as hashish but the very potent dawamesc, made by boiling the cannabis plant in oil or butter. In addition, dawamesc contains cantharis (a supposed aphrodisiac also known as Spanish fly), which has unpredictable toxic effects (Grinspoon, 1971, p. 58). Gautier's experiences are therefore not typical of contemporary North American use, but much of what he reports is characteristic of the hallucinogenic effects of cannabis intoxication at high doses. Gautier's account is classical, and in spite of its embellishments and inaccuracies, it has shaped the expectancies and prejudices of users and opponents through the years.

After a vivid description of the setting, an old house on an island in the Seine, and of being given his portion of the drug, Gautier relates how he and the other club members dined in ornate and exotic surroundings. By the end of the meal, Gautier began to feel the effect of the drug in the form of an enhancement of both sensitivity and enjoyment of the senses.

All of a sudden, a red flash passed beneath my eyelids, innumerable candles burst into light and I felt bathed in a warm clear glow. I was indeed in the same place, but it was different as a sketch is from a painting: everything was larger, brighter, more gorgeous. (Gautier, 1966, p. 169)

As a result of the large dose he had taken, Gautier soon started to hallucinate. Initially, all his companions disappeared, leaving only their shadows on the wall, and he was visited by a personification of hashish, a character called Ducas-Carota of the Golden Pot. Ducas-Carota was followed by a succession of distorted figures, and Gautier experienced another common effect: everything seemed extremely funny.

As though I were the lord of the feast, each shape came in turn into the luminous circle whereof I occupied the center, with an air of grotesque deference to mutter in my ear, banter, none of which I now remember, but which at the time I found prodigiously witty, and which excited me to the maddest gaiety. (p. 170)

Gautier laughed until he thought he would burst.

Later, Charles Baudelaire, another member of the club, was to publish his accounts of the hashish experience. Other classical descriptions were written by Fitzhugh Ludlow, the American son of an abolitionist minister and friend of Mark Twain, and the American traveler and diplomat Baynard Taylor (Solomon, 1966; Ebin, 1961).

Mood Changes and Getting High. A more typical experience with marijuana is characterized by swings of mood from euphoric gaiety with hilarious laughter to placid dreaminess. The experience is nearly always pleasant, with a feeling of well-being and joyfulness usually referred to as *being high*, but occasionally there are feelings of anxiety and foreboding even at low doses in hospitable surroundings.

When cannabis is consumed socially, as it most often is, there is frequent laughing and singing. Almost anything seems funny, and the most innocent event or statement may ignite gales of contagious laughter. If the drug is taken alone or in a quiet setting, the user may spend time predominantly in a dreamy state *getting off* on, or concentrating on, the subjective experience. It is frequently felt that perceptions are keener and that sensory effects are felt more intensely and enjoyed more. Just as slightly funny things seem hilarious, mundane thoughts and insights may take on the greatest significance and importance. Artists and musicians frequently feel that creativity is enhanced.

Although physical activity sometimes increases and people feel that their actions are effortless, they generally avoid tasks requiring effort and prefer instead to remain passive.

In spite of consistent reports from users that marijuana elevates mood, when subjective changes in feelings are measured systematically by a test like the POMS, findings are not at all clear-cut. Both positive and negative changes in mood have been reported (R. T. Jones & Benowitz, 1976; Rossi et al., 1974), and the pattern of responding to mood scales appears to be unique. For example, in one study, smoking marijuana caused an increase in scales indicating stimulation and at the same time increased scores on scales associated with sedation. There were no changes in scales indicating euphoria or positive mood states (Chait et al., 1988).

Many researchers believe that the reason for variability in subjective ratings between studies is that environment can have a considerable influence on how the drug changes mood. The effects of surroundings on mood have been investigated, but it has been found that differences such as smoking in a neutral as opposed to a psychedelic environment or watching television, listening to rock music, or carrying on a conversation have no effect on subjective self-ratings. One factor that does seem to be important, however, is the mood of others. In an experiment in 1978, it was shown that mood self-ratings are not correlated with ratings of intoxication, but after subjects took marijuana, mood ratings were highly correlated with the mood of the other subjects in the experiment, whether they were high or not. Thus it would seem that after smoking marijuana, a person becomes more susceptible to being influenced by the mood of others (Rossi, Kuehnle, & Mendelson, 1978).

But whatever the reason for the variability, one's first experience with the drug seems to be an important determinant of later use. One study of college students showed that those who reported positive effects at first experience were also more likely to use the drug sooner the second time and use it regularly later (Davidson & Schenk, 1994).

Perception

Though one of the subjective effects of the cannabinoids is an increased sensory sensitivity, subjective testing of sensory thresholds has found only decreases in sensitivity or no change in auditory, visual, and tactile thresholds (R. T. Jones, 1978). The cannabinoids also cause a loss of sensitivity to pain, which indicates that the drug has analgesic properties.

The time-distorting effect of cannabis has been demonstrated experimentally (Domino, Rennick, & Pearl, 1976), although not to the extent described by Gautier. Weil, Zinberg, and Nelson (1968) found that three subjects out of nine judged a five-minute speech to be 10 minutes long. Increases in subjective time rate (people experience time passing more quickly) is one of the most reliable behavioral effects of cannabis (Chait & Pierri, 1992).

Memory

It does not appear that marijuana has an effect on the ability to recall material already well learned or recognition memory (the ability to recognize words or figures), but it does disrupt the ability to recall words or narrative material (Chait & Pierri, 1992). The problems occur primarily in short-term memory in which information is held actively in the brain for short periods. While intoxicated with cannabis, people frequently show what has been called *temporal disintegration*—they lose the ability to retain and coordinate information for a purpose. If they are required to hold information in the brain for any length of time, it frequently gets lost before it can be used. It is not unusual, for example, for people under the influence of cannabis to start a sentence and then stop halfway through because they forgot what they started to say. When such things happen, others who have been using the drug are not likely to remember either. The result is some very disjointed conversations (Weil & Zinberg, 1969). Some users have described this

inability to hold things in short-term storage by saying that thoughts come so quickly that it is difficult to keep from being distracted by them. It is quite likely that the deficits in short-term memory and the distorted time sense are related, since we depend on our memories to help us judge the passage of time.

It has been pointed out that there is a similarity between the effects of cannabis on memory and the symptoms of Korsakoff's psychosis, a neurological disorder seen in long-term alcoholics (see Chapter 6). One symptom of Korsakoff's psychosis is a memory disorder and a disorientation in time that is caused by damage to the limbic system and hippocampus. This similarity has led to speculation that cannabis affects memory by blocking the functions of the hippocampus (Miller & Drew, 1974). This is a likely hypothesis in light of the fact that cannabinoid receptors are found in high concentrations in the hippocampus.

Attention

There also appears to be a deficit on tasks requiring vigilance or sustained attention, particularly if the task is of long duration (over 50 min) (Chait & Pierri, 1992). Just as cannabis creates an inability to retain thoughts, it also appears to make attention more distractible. Many researchers report that subjects are not able to concentrate on the tasks they are doing after being given marijuana. They are easily distracted, usually by events in their own minds. Being easily distracted can interfere with many different types of tasks (De Long & Levy, 1974).

Creativity

One of the subjective effects of cannabis is that it helps to improve appreciation of art, even art produced by the user. There is a widespread belief that the drug increases the creativity of artists. This belief may have arisen largely because the drug was widely used by musicians and artists. Nevertheless, there is no consistent evidence from objective research showing that creativity is enhanced (Chait & Pierri, 1992) or that artists who use marijuana are more successful than artists who are not users (Grinspoon, 1971, p. 157).

Performance

Trying to summarize the effects of cannabis on the various measures of performance is nearly impossible. There is no doubt that certain tasks are impaired by the drug at high doses, but results are so variable that it is difficult to be specific. As we have seen, variability between experimental findings can arise from differences such as experience of subjects, instructions, motivation, setting, and dosage. These are only a few of the factors that can contribute to the confusion—and no doubt have done so (Chait & Pierri, 1992).

An example of this confusion can be found in experiments on hand-eye coordination using a pursuit rotor wherein subjects are required to track a moving target manually. One experiment found that marijuana impaired this ability in novice subjects, but the performance of experienced subjects actually improved with marijuana (Weil, Zinberg, & Nelson, 1968). This sort of finding is not unusual.

Another factor that complicates the findings in performance tasks is that deficits in performance may not indicate a loss of the specific ability being measured. Many experiments show an increase in mean reaction time (although some do not). A careful analysis of the data, however, shows that the slowing is a result of a few rather long reaction times in an otherwise normal performance. These occasional long latencies appear to be due to lapses in attention and an inability to concentrate on the task rather than an inability to move the hand. In another experiment, subjects were required to pursue a moving dot on an oscilloscope screen with another dot that they could control by hand. Marijuana interfered with performance, but the interference was not a result of

lack of coordination. It was the result of a lack of motivation and interest in the task. One subject stopped following the moving dot and drew patterns on the screen with the dot that he controlled (Manno et al., 1974).

In general, however, simple reaction time appears to be unaffected by marijuana, but in complex and choice-reaction-time tests, accuracy but not speed is likely to be affected. Marijuana is often reported to impair hand-eye coordination tasks such as the digit symbol substitution and the pursuit rotor.

Driving

Numerous studies have been conducted on the effects of marijuana on driving and flying, and most have reported impaired performance, although such effects are not reported for all individuals (Klonoff, 1974; Chait & Pierri, 1992).

Studies in a driving simulator have shown that marijuana has little effect on the ability to control a car but impairs the subject's ability to attend to peripheral stimuli. Thus marijuana-intoxicated drivers might be able to stop a car as fast as they normally could, but they may not be as quick to notice things that they should stop for, probably because they are attending to internal events rather than to what is happening on the road (Moskowitz, Hulbert, & McGlothlin, 1976).

EFFECTS ON THE BEHAVIOR OF NONHUMANS

Unconditioned Behavior

THC has a biphasic effect on SMA; in many species there is an increase in activity followed by a depression. The depressant effect is more powerful and appears in more species, lasts longer, and is more resistant to tolerance. At high doses, the decrease in motion is called *ataxia* and is accompanied by a loss of motor control and by fine tremors. Laboratory animals assume one posture without moving for long periods. Monkeys stare into space or look at their hands and occasionally appear as though they were hallucinating (Paton & Pertwee, 1973a).

One effect that was noticed early in animal experimentation was a taming effect, or a reduction in aggression. Animals that are normally aggressive and hard to handle became tame and placid after receiving THC. TCH will reduce the attack behavior of the dominant member of a pair of rats and will also diminish the ability of a submissive rat to defend itself in a fight. Predatory attack behavior of several species is also reduced.

In rats, THC causes a decrease in food intake and a subsequent weight loss. THC is about half as potent as amphetamine in suppressing food intake, but unlike amphetamine, THC causes an increased preference for sweet sugar solutions. This may be related to the munchies effect in humans (Sofia, 1978).

THC is as potent as morphine in reducing the response of laboratory rats to painful stimuli as measured by a number of tests. CBN also has analgesic effects but is only as potent as aspirin. No analgesic effects were found for CBD (Sofia, 1978). The metabolites of THC are probably more potent than the parent compound. These analgesic effects can be blocked by naloxone, the opiate antagonist, suggesting that the analgesic effects of the cannabinoids are mediated by the opiate system.

Positively Reinforced Behavior

In general, the effect of THC on FR responding is to depress most responding. After a period of time, responding suddenly returns to its normal rate and pattern. Responding on an FI schedule is depressed, but there does not appear to be a change in the typical patterning of the FI. Also, VI rates are decreased, but some researchers have reported an increase at low doses of THC in some species. Unlike many drugs, THC does not appear to affect different schedules differently (McMillan & Leander, 1976).

Negatively Reinforced Behavior

Like the barbiturates and the benzodiazepines, THC decreases avoidance responding at doses that do not alter escape responding in a discriminated avoidance task, which means that it has antianxiety effects. But the effects of THC on a continuous avoidance task are variable; both increases and decreases have been reported. You might expect that a drug that has both antianxiety and analgesic effects would increase punished behavior, but neither delta-9-TCH nor delta-8-THC appears to increase behavior suppressed by punishment with electric shock (McMillan & Leander, 1976). In this regard, THC is very unlike the barbiturates and other antianxiety drugs.

In general, the effects of the cannabinoids on operant behavior are probably more similar to the effects of opiates than to those of any other drug class.

DISSOCIATION AND DRUG STATE DISCRIMINATION

Dissociation

Both delta-9-TCH and delta-8-THC cause dissociation of an avoidance task in rats. Rats were unable to transfer what they learned in the drug state to the nondrug state. There was a symmetrical inability to transfer what they learned in the nondrug state to the drug state (Henricksson & Järbe, 1971). Dissociation has also been demonstrated in humans using marijuana. In one study, subjects were asked to learn a list of words after taking a placebo and then to recall the list after smoking marijuana, and vice versa. Subjects had difficulty transferring the information acquired in one state to the other state. This effect was not very powerful because the loss of recall could be overcome by prompting and cuing the subjects by reminding them of word categories (Stillman et al., 1976). In another study, only *asymmetrical dissociation* was found: Information acquired while the subjects were not intoxicated was remembered after smoking marijuana, but information acquired during marijuana intoxication was not remembered when sober (Darley & Tinklenberg, 1974).

Dissociation has not been demonstrated for motor skill and perceptual tasks such as card sorting or on the pursuit rotor task or signaled avoidance even though marijuana did impair performance on these tasks (Järbe & Mathis, 1992).

Drug State Discrimination

Rats are easily able to discriminate THC from placebo when it is administered i.v., i.p., or orally. The stimulus properties are evident as early as 7½ minutes after injection and peak at 30 minutes but are still reliable at 60 minutes. A training dose of delta-9-THC would generalize to delta-8-THC and the 11-hydroxy metabolite but would not generalize to CBD (Balster & Ford, 1978), although some generalization occurs to CBN (Järbe & Mathis, 1992). Interesting interactions do occur with these other naturally occurring cannabinoids because in some experiments CBD has been shown to enhance and prolong the stimulus effects of THC (Järbe and Mathis, 1992).

Many other drugs have been tested to learn whether the THC response generalizes to them, but so far no such generalization has been discovered. It would seem that THC has unique stimulus properties and will not generalize to any other substance (Krimmer & Barry, 1977; Ford et al., 1984).

Experienced marijuana smokers can easily learn to distinguish marijuana cigarettes containing 0 percent from marijuana cigarettes containing 2.7 percent THC. They were able to make the discrimination within 90 seconds of taking the first puff. They were successfully able to identify marijuana containing 1.7 percent, but they identified 0.09 percent marijuana as a placebo (Chait et al., 1988).

TOLERANCE

In laboratory animals, tolerance develops rapidly to the effects of THC on operant behavior. Depending on the dose and the route of administration, complete tolerance may develop after five or six days of repeated injections of THC (Abel, McMillan, & Harris, 1974). This tolerance lasts for more than a month, and there is cross-tolerance between delta-9-THC and its 11-hydroxy metabolite (Kosersky, McMillan, & Harris, 1974). Tolerance also develops within a few days to increases in motor activity but much more slowly to the depression activity. There is no tolerance at all to the anorexia effects or the discriminative stimulus effects. Tolerance does not appear to be due to alterations in absorption, metabolism, or distribution of the drug (Dewey, Martin, & Harris, 1976).

There is some disagreement about the development of tolerance in humans. Many marijuana users have reported that there is a sensitization or *reverse tolerance* to the drug—they become more sensitive to the effects rather than less sensitive with repeated use. Reverse tolerance has never been shown in laboratory studies with nonhumans or humans. There are several reasons why reverse tolerance is observed only outside the laboratory. One is likely a matter of dosage. In laboratory studies, dosage is carefully measured in terms of the amount of drug consumed, but outside the laboratory, users calculate their consumption in terms of the number of joints (marijuana cigarettes) they smoke. With experience, people learn to inhale more efficiently so that they are able to get more drug into their bodies from a given amount of marijuana. Therefore, they will require fewer joints to get high. In addition, experience may be required for a person not only to learn how to get high but also to learn the sorts of activities, situations, and company that contribute to the high. All these factors could contribute to the observation that over time, fewer joints are needed to get high.

In one study, subjects were given rather high doses of THC orally every four hours for 12 days, and a number of measures were taken. Subjective assessments of the intensity of the high decreased considerably over the course of the experiment. Tolerance also developed to the effect on heart rate. This tolerance was still evident one week after the drug was discontinued. The disruptive effects of high doses of marijuana on cognitive and motor performance also disappeared (Jones & Benowitz, 1976). It is unlikely, however, that tolerance to THC occurs unless high blood levels are maintained for an extended period. In another study, subjects were required to smoke one marijuana cigarette per day for 28 consecutive days, and measures of subjective intoxication level, performance on a learning task, and heart rate were taken. On this drug regime, which is more similar to normal patterns of use, there was no evidence of any sensitization or tolerance (Frank et al., 1976).

WITHDRAWAL

Withdrawal symptoms have been seen after prolonged administration of high doses in nonhumans. These symptoms are not severe and frequently appear as an increase in motor behavior.

Withdrawal symptoms have been reported with humans. In the high-dose study mentioned earlier, human volunteers took high doses of oral THC every four hours. When the drug was stopped, the subjects reported a sense of "inner unrest" after six hours. By 12 hours after the last dose of THC, subjects reported a variety of symptoms including hot flashes, sweating, runny nose, loose stools, hiccups, and loss of appetite. Other symptoms that were noticed by the experimenters were irritability, restlessness, and insomnia (Jones & Benowitz, 1976). Like tolerance, withdrawal is only likely after high continuous levels of cannabis in the blood. In the study where subjects were required to smoke only one marijuana cigarette a day for 28 days, no with-

drawal symptoms were reported (Frank et al., 1976).

SELF-ADMINISTRATION

THC is one of those drugs that is self-administered by humans but not by nonhumans (Griffiths, Bigelow, & Henningfield, 1980). Though several attempts have been made, there are few accounts of any species other than humans voluntarily consuming cannabis or cannabinoids.

Yet it is seldom difficult to get humans to take cannabis. In a hospital ward setting, Mendelson and his associates (1976) conducted an experiment in which subjects were required to press a button to gain points with which they could buy marijuana cigarettes. A joint could be earned for about 30 minutes work. Extra points could be saved for money at the end of the experiment. In this experiment were two groups of subjects, casual and heavy users of marijuana. The number of joints smoked by each group was far less than the number available but showed a slight increase over the 26 days of the experiment. Casual users smoked about two joints per day at the beginning and increased to three by the end of the experiment. The heavy users started at four a day and ended at about seven. Apart from this slight increase, the amount consumed was fairly stable from day to day without any cyclic patterns or periods of abstinence, although there was a big increase on the last day marijuana was available. No evidence of withdrawal was seen when use was stopped. In this study, it seemed that there was a level of high that most users tried to achieve, and they stopped when they achieved this effect. In other words, they titrated the dose.

Marijuana self-administration in humans in experimental settings has been demonstrated a number of times since then, but curiously, it has not yet been shown that THC content is important. In one recent experiment (Kelly et al., 1994) marijuana cigarettes with 0 and 2.3 percent THC were smoked with equal frequency even though self-reports of "high," "potency," and "liking" were higher for the THC-containing marijuana.

Titration

The ability of users to titrate the dose was studied in another experiment in which experienced marijuana users were given joints of different potencies and asked to smoke until they achieved a "nice high." To some extent these experienced users did smoke fewer high-potency joints than low-potency joints before they stopped, but the compensation was far from perfect. The subjects smoked 60 percent more of the weak marijuana than the strong marijuana, but even after this compensation, they administered a 250 percent higher dose to themselves when the strong joints were available (Cappell & Pliner, 1974). On the basis of this experiment, it seems that even experienced users are not able to adjust their intake accurately in the face of variations in potency of the marijuana they are smoking. It also casts doubt on the notion that there is such a thing as a "social high" that can be determined on the basis of an administered dose. Factors other than dosage must control marijuana intake.

Even though people in experiments will smoke as many marijuana cigarettes with 0 percent THC as they do with 2.4 percent THC (Kelly et al., 1994), choice experiments have shown that the reinforcing effect of marijuana increases with increased THC content. In a preference study, experienced users sampled marijuana of two different potencies (0.63 and 1.95 percent THC). During the choice phase of the experiment, subjects chose the high-potency marijuana much more often than the low-potency marijuana (Chait & Burke, 1994).

Effect of Tolerance

In the Mendelson experiment, in which moderate and heavy marijuana users are allowed unrestricted access to marijuana, both groups increased their intake over the course of the experiment. Such increases over time are usually thought of as a compensation for the development of tolerance to the subjective effect of the drug, but we have already seen that rather large doses are needed before tolerance develops. The relationship between tolerance and consumption was investigated in a similar study in the same laboratory. This experiment (Babor et al., 1975) measured the development of tolerance to the effects on heart rate, the subjective high, and total consumption. It was found that tolerance developed only in a group of heavy users and not in the moderate user groups. Figure 14–2 shows the development of tolerance to the subjective high feeling and the actual consumption of marijuana in both groups. Though both groups increased consumption, only one showed tolerance. It is therefore likely that the increase in use is not a result of decreased high due to tolerance. The researchers suggested that the increase is due to social factors instead.

Patterns of Use

In North America cannabis is a social drug. In the 1970s most marijuana was smoked in groups. On some occasions it may have been consumed in large public gatherings like rock concerts or large parties, but most of the time the groups were gatherings of close friends and acquaintances. The drug was consumed in an almost ritualistic manner. A pipe or joint was passed from one person to another in a circle, each person taking a drag or passing it if feeling sufficiently high. More recently, solitary use of the drug has become more common, and the ritualism has declined.

The social nature of marijuana may also be responsible for the initiation of marijuana use. Only a very small percentage of users first smoke marijuana alone. There can be no doubt that the strong social reinforcement and the feelings of shared pleasure and intimacy contribute considerably not only to the start of drug use but to the drug's continued use as well.

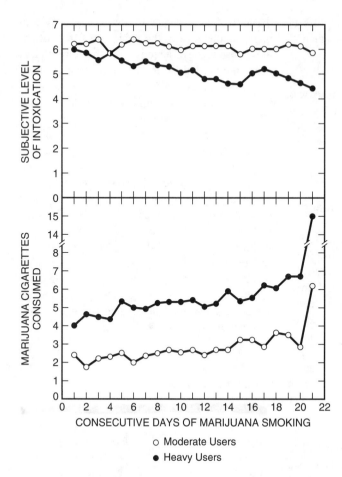

Figure 14–2 The development of tolerance to the subjective high feeling and the actual consumption of marijuana in subjects permitted to smoke as much marijuana as they want for 21 days in a laboratory study. Even though all subjects increased consumption, only subjects classified as heavy users before the experiment showed tolerance to the subjective effect of the drug. The vertical axis of the top panel gives the level of subjective intoxication, from 1—straight, to 7—stoned. (Babor et al., 1975.)

In some countries where cannabis is a traditional drug with a long history, the pattern and extent of use are quite different from that of Europe and North America, where cannabis use is recent. In countries such as India, Egypt, Greece, Morocco, and Jamaica, the majority of cannabis users take it extensively every day, and there is little casual use. But in the United States, the vast majority of users are casual, and only a small percentage use it daily. Compared with other countries, relatively small amounts are consumed in North America. It has been estimated that a casual cannabis user can get "stoned" on 5 to 6 mg of THC, and the average daily user in the United States consumes about 50 mg THC per day.

Compare this level to that of the average daily user in Eastern countries, who consumes 200 mg per day. In addition, marijuana use is not as persistent in the United States as in other countries. Most Westerners who start using cannabis eventually decrease use and stop, but in countries where use is more extensive, it may persist for 20 to 40 years.

According to the National Household Survey on Drug Abuse, between 1985 and 1992 the number of marijuana users in the United States declined from 9.3 percent of the population to 4.3 percent, and the number of frequent marijuana users (once a week or more) dropped from 4.6 to 2.4 percent (U.S. DHHS, 1994). This decline may have bottomed out, because there was little difference between 1992 and 1994 (U.S. DHHS, 1995). At the same time, however, the potency of the marijuana smoked has increased considerably. In the 1960s, 2.0 percent THC content in marijuana was considered above-average potency. In 1990 the average THC content was 3.6 percent, and in 1993 it was 5.4 percent.

Even though there are fewer smokers than there used to be, marijuana is increasingly involved in hospital emergency room incidents. The Drug Abuse Warning Network (DAWN) reports that there was an 86 percent increase in marijuana-related incidents between 1990 and 1993 (22 percent from 1992 to 1993). It appears that the increased potency is causing problems for those who continue to use the drug.

We may well be seeing a slow transformation of cannabis use from the casual, social use of the 1960s and 1970s to the more serious high-dose pattern typical of cultures where cannabis products have been available for a much longer time.

HARMFUL EFFECTS

Cannabis is a drug of great controversy. Probably no other drug in recent times has generated more public concern and debate and stimulated more research into its safety or lack of it. This body of scientific literature is highly specialized, confusing, and often contradictory, and it is often misrepresented in the popular media, which have tended to publicize only certain research findings and to ignore others. It has been difficult for the nonexpert to keep track of it all. There can be little wonder that people generally are confused and that those with particular biases have no trouble supporting their position.

Marijuana has been accused of having many harmful effects, some of which we shall discuss. It will be obvious to anyone after reading this section that cannabis, like any other drug, has a great number of effects on many systems of the body, some of which have the potential for great

harm. It should also be obvious that even though the potential for harm exists, especially at high doses, there are very few hard data to show that the drug really does any harm. The cause of this lack of data may be that there is no harm, but it may also be that reliable data are difficult to collect.

Violence and Aggression

One of the oldest beliefs about cannabis is that it causes violence and aggression and is associated with crime, but there are absolutely no systematic data to support the myth. In long-term studies where marijuana was given to individuals in controlled hospital ward settings, increases in violence were never reported. In addition, mood rating scales generally showed decreases in feelings of hostility and increases in friendliness.

Numerous surveys and field studies, using a variety of techniques, have compared criminal behavior and crimes of violence in groups of marijuana users and nonusers, and in the vast majority of these studies no connection has been found. In fact, if there was a correlation, it was with a decrease in violence. For example, one study showed that among a certain population of young criminal males, marijuana is used specifically to reduce aggression rather than to increase it (Tinklenberg, 1974). Though there may be isolated cases of idiosyncratic or unusual violent reactions of some individuals after taking marijuana, these ordinarily occur in people with a prior psychiatric disturbance or when other drugs are used at the same time.

Mental Disturbance

Many early studies, particularly from Eastern countries like India, claimed that a substantial proportion of inmates of mental institutions were there because of cannabis-related disorders. But studies in the United States have not found any evidence that marijuana can cause psychoses in normal people. However, it does appear to be able to precipitate full-blown psychoses in those with psychotic tendencies, and it will intensify schizophrenic and paranoid symptoms that already exist (Choptra & Smith, 1974).

Sometimes when the drug is taken in larger doses than usual, and the user is overcome with overwhelming anxiety and paranoid feelings. Such states often lead to a trip to a hospital emergency department. At higher doses another reaction to cannabis is the *adverse psychotic reaction,* a panic that arises from the hallucinations and perceptual distortions. This effect is commonly referred to as a *freak-out.* Users lose touch with reality and feel that they may be going insane, and they panic. Freak-outs usually occur when the drug is taken in unusual and stressful circumstances, if more drug is consumed than the user is accustomed to, or if the cannabis is mixed with other drugs. Freak-outs are much more common with hallucinogens such as LSD than with cannabis. They usually can be effectively treated by being quietly "talked down," but in severe cases, a benzodiazepine tranquilizer can be effective (Dinwiddie & Farber, 1995).

Permanent Intellectual Impairment and Brain Damage

It is known that long-term heavy use of alcohol results in brain damage and a loss of mental functions, and recently there have been reports that the same sort of thing might occur with marijuana. In North Africa and other places where cannabis is used for long periods at high doses, there are reports of *cannabis dementia*. One British study has even reported evidence of a shrinking of the brain, along with the same sort of loss of functions seen in alcoholics. As usual, it is difficult to be sure that the deficits in these studies are really due to the marijuana and not to some other drug the individual might have taken or something else in the environment. To help answer this question, Kevin Fehr and her colleagues at the Addiction Research Foundation of Ontario (1976) administered THC to rats in large daily doses for six months. The THC caused an impairment of maze learning that still existed two months after the drug was discontinued. The researchers concluded that it was likely that the drug had caused some sort of permanent brain damage. In fact, other studies have shown that there are alterations in rat brain structure and function, especially in the hippocampus, after chronic exposure to THC (Seallet, 1991).

In a study with rhesus monkeys, William Silkker and his colleagues at the National Center for Toxicological Research in Jefferson, Arkansas, trained monkeys to perform certain behavioral tasks including a progressive ratio schedule of lever pressing for banana-flavored food pellets and a delayed conditioned discrimination task. One group of monkeys was exposed to the human equivalent of smoking four to five low- to medium-potency marijuana cigarettes through a mask that covered the nose and mouth every day for a year. A second group was exposed to the same only on weekends, and there were appropriate control animals that received the smoke, but without the THC. During the exposure, there were effects on behavior and some hormone levels, probably resulting from stress, but seven months after the exposure there were no detectable differences in behavior, hippocampal volume, neuron size, or synaptic and dendritic anatomy (Silkker et al., 1992).

It has been pointed out that comparisons between rats, monkeys, and humans should take into account the duration of exposure relative to the organism's life span. Three months' exposure is normally required to cause neurotoxic effects in rats. This is about 8 to 10 percent of a rat's life span. The monkey equivalent would be three years, and the equivalent exposure in humans would be seven to ten years (Seallet, 1991).

Amotivational Syndrome

It has sometimes been observed that when a young person starts smoking marijuana, systematic changes occur in that person's lifestyle, ambitions, motivation, and possibly personality.

These changes have been collectively referred to as the *amotivational syndrome*, whose symptoms are

apathy, loss of effectiveness, and diminished capacity or willingness to carry out complex, long-term plans, endure frustration, concentrate for long periods, follow routines, or successfully master new material. Verbal facility is often impaired both in speaking and writing.

Such individuals exhibit greater introversion, become totally involved with the present at the expense of future goals and demonstrate a strong tendency toward regressive, childlike, magical thinking. (McGlothlin & West, 1968, p. 372)

There is no doubt that many young individuals have changed from clean, aggressive, upwardly mobile achievers into the sort of person just described at about the same time as they started smoking marijuana. What is not clear, however, is a causal relationship between the loss of middle-class motivations and cannabis.

Evidence for the existence of an amotivational syndrome, however, has been found in the experiment described earlier in which rhesus monkeys were exposed to the smoke from a marijuana cigarette every day for a year (Silkker et al., 1992). These monkeys pressed a lever for banana-flavored food pellets on a progressive ratio schedule. Each time the pellet was received, the ratio requirement increased and more presses were required (see Chapter 2). Silkker and associates found that during exposure to marijuana smoke, breaking points were considerably lower than they were for controls and that they returned to normal when exposure to the smoke was discontinued. Thus the monkeys exposed to marijuana smoke were not as willing to work hard for an attractive food as nonexposed monkeys. Since their animals responded normally on other tasks for the same food pellets, the researchers argued that this result was analogous to the amotivational syndrome seen in humans and was not a result of either a loss of the ability to respond or loss of appetite.

Laboratory studies with humans have found no evidence of amotivational syndrome. The Mendelson experiment, in which hospitalized volunteers worked on an operant task to earn money and marijuana for 26 days, showed that the marijuana smoked did not influence the amount of work done by either the casual-user group or the heavy-user group; all remained motivated to earn and take home a significant amount of money in addition to the work they did for the marijuana.

The issue is not clearly settled, but it is curious that the only clear experimental evidence demonstrating a motivation loss is from research with nonhumans. Even if there is no specific motivational effect, it is clear that cannabis affects attention and memory, and these are intellectual capacities usually considered necessary for success in educational institutions. Achievement motivation must be high indeed in any individual who combines high levels of cannabis use with a successful academic career. It is quite likely that the task requirements in an educational institution are more similar to the progressive ratio schedule in the monkey experiment than they are to button pressing of research subjects on a hospital research ward.

Progression to Other Drugs

There are claims that marijuana is a "gateway" drug; that is, it is a stepping-stone on the road to the use of more dangerous drugs. In support of this stepping-stone theory are studies that show that virtually all heroin users had used marijuana before they adopted heroin (Golub & Johnson, 1994). In addition, studies have shown that the more a person uses marijuana, the greater is the probability that the person will use other drugs as well (Mullins, Vitola, & Michelson, 1975).

These data suffer from the same difficulty as the research on the amotivational syndrome: No causal relationship can be established. The fact that marijuana is used before heroin does not mean that marijuana use *caused* heroin use. Likewise, most people drink soda pop before they drink alcohol, but this fact does not mean that soda pop causes alcohol drinking.

At the heart of the progression hypothesis is the idea that users develop tolerance to "mild" drugs, become bored with their effects, and escalate to more powerful drugs. If this were true, we might expect that users would abandon marijuana when they progress to other drugs, but this does not appear to be the case. Marijuana is seldom abandoned in favor of other drugs. Instead, the usual pattern is to adopt the use of other drugs along with marijuana. The stepping-stone hypothesis has no pharmacological support. There is no pharmacological reason why the use of one drug should lead to the use of a totally different drug.

Even though a causal relationship cannot be proved, we cannot dismiss the correlation between the use of marijuana and other drugs; there must be an explanation, and, like the amotivational syndrome, it probably has more to do with sociology than with pharmacology. Heavy marijuana use does not predispose a person pharmacologically to use other drugs, but it provides the social settings, motivation, and opportunity to use other drugs. In addition, the personality traits of curiosity and risk taking that might motivate a person to use marijuana are also likely to motivate the use of other drugs as well.

Reproduction

Though not all researchers have been able to replicate the finding, marijuana seems to lower the levels of the male sex hormone testosterone in both human and nonhuman males. However, it is not yet apparent whether this finding has any biological significance. The levels of testosterone vary greatly from one individual to another and within the same individual throughout the course of a day. We do not know as yet whether a marijuana-induced suppression of testosterone will make any difference in the face of this great natural variability.

There has been some speculation on problems that might be caused by low testosterone levels, although no reliable data have been collected to show that these effects occur more frequently among marijuana users. One might suspect that low sex hormone levels would reduce sex drive and fertility in men. It has been shown that cannabis does reduce sperm production and alters sex drive in rats. In human males, extensive marijuana smoking reduces sperm production and sperm mobility, and there may be a consequent loss in fertility (Hembree, Zeidenberg, & Nahas, 1976).

Testosterone is also important at an earlier stage of development. At 8 to 10 weeks of development in the uterus, the male fetus starts to secrete testosterone, which is important in the differentiation and development of the brain and the male urogenital system, including the sex organs. Suppression of testosterone caused by the mother's cannabis use at this time could disrupt this phase of development (Kolodny, 1975). Also serious is the reduction of testosterone at specific stages of development. Testosterone levels are vitally important in the growth spurt and the physiological changes that take place at puberty in males. Lowered testosterone levels might be expected to alter or delay these changes. Because it is not uncommon for marijuana to be used at or before puberty, its effect on testosterone levels could be a problem.

In a large-scale study between 1984 and 1989, more than 7,000 pregnant women in the United States were studied and their drug use histories were recorded. Eleven percent of these women reported using marijuana during pregnancy. Marijuana use was not associated with low birthweight or prematurity. By comparison, 35 percent of the women smoked tobacco, and this history was associated with low birthweight (Shiono et al., 1995).

Some functional differences have been detected in children exposed prenatally to cannabinoids through maternal marijuana smoking. One study showed abnormal sleep patterns in newborns that persisted at least till the age of three in cannabis-exposed children (Dahl et al., 1995).

Immunity

It has been clearly established that marijuana reduces activity in the body's immune system, which fights invading microorganisms and disease. This reduction has even caused speculation that THC might be effective in stopping the body's rejection of tissue after transplant operations. Again, the clinical significance of this effect has not been determined. We might suspect that marijuana users would be more susceptible to disease than nonusers, but adequate statistical data on this issue are difficult to obtain and have not been collected (Munson, 1975).

Respiration

Marijuana has both a positive and a negative effect on breathing. To begin with, THC appears to act as a bronchodilator; it increases the diameter of the bronchi, the small airways in the lungs, and for this reason it alleviates the symptoms of asthma. However, marijuana smoke inhaled for long periods of time causes a decrease in the size of the lung passages, causing asthma. These effects create a most unusual situation. A chronic marijuana smoker may suffer from asthma caused by the marijuana smoke, but the asthmatic symptoms can be relieved for a short while by smoking marijuana (Tashkin et al., 1976).

In addition to the effect on air passages in the lungs, marijuana smoke is like tobacco smoke in that it decreases the activity of macrophages in the lungs. The macrophages attack foreign substances and bacteria in the lungs and help to protect lung tissue from infection. We do not yet know whether marijuana smokers have an increased incidence of lung diseases and infections (McCarthy et al., 1976), but on the basis of what

we know about tobacco smoke, it is likely that a relationship will be found.

Cancer

Evidence is clear that tobacco smoke is associated with cancer. What about marijuana smoke? Even though marijuana users typically inhale much less smoke than tobacco users, the smoke from marijuana contains 50 to 70 percent more carcinogenic material than tobacco smoke, and marijuana smokers typically inhale more deeply and hold the smoke in the lungs longer than tobacco smokers. Surprisingly little research has been done in this area, and results are frequently confounded by the fact that most marijuana smokers also smoke tobacco. It seems likely that marijuana accelerates the carcinogenic effects of tobacco smoke. Even though the median age for developing cancer is between 55 and 65, one study of people less than 45 with lung cancer found that almost all smoked both tobacco and marijuana (Sridhar et al., 1994). Clearly a lot more work needs to be done in this area.

EPILOGUE

Psychopharmacological McCarthyism?

When Lester Grinspoon began studying marijuana in 1967 he claimed that he had no doubt that he would find it was a harmful drug used by more and more foolish people. He took as his job the task of revealing the dangers of marijuana. Instead, after three years of study, he concluded that he had been wrong and that his belief that the substance was dangerous was unfounded. In 1971 he wrote a book titled *Marihuana Reconsidered* (Grinspoon, 1971) in which he said so. He naively believed that people would come to understand that marijuana was much less harmful than legal drugs such as alcohol and tobacco and, consequently, that marijuana would be legal within ten years.

Not only was he wrong, but in another book published in 1993, he comments that there is something special about illicit drugs, "If they don't always make the user behave irrationally, they certainly cause many nonusers to behave that way" (Grinspoon & Bakalar, 1993, p. ix). Grinspoon points out that instead of legalization, the climate has deteriorated so seriously that we are now in a period of what he calls "psychopharmacological McCarthyism" where it is not even acceptable to state in public that a drug like marijuana might have beneficial effects. He points to the widespread public condemnation of published research that found that adolescents who had engaged in some drug experimentation with marijuana were better adjusted than those who had not.

As another example of psychopharmacological McCarthyism, Grinspoon points to mandatory drug testing. In the McCarthy era, people were forced to take loyalty oaths or risk losing their jobs or reputations. Grinspoon calls drug testing a "chemical loyalty oath." Just as loyalty oaths did little to enhance national security of the United States, mandatory drug testing is of little use in preventing or treating drug abuse; instead, Grinspoon claims that it is little more than shotgun harassment designed to enhance outward conformity.

CHAPTER SUMMARY

- There may be three species of cannabis plant, although many believe that there is only one species, *Cannabis sativa*, with two distinct phenotypes. One, widely called *hemp*, has low levels of active ingredient. The other phenotype grows in warmer climates, has a high content of active ingredient, and is used primarily as an intoxicant.

- The primary active ingredient in cannabis is *delta-9-tetrahydrocannabinol (THC)*.

- *Marijuana* is made from the dried leaves and flowers of the cannabis plant and is not very potent. *Hashish* is the resin from the flowering tops of the female plant and is 10 times more potent than marijuana. Hashish can be refined and concentrated into a liquid called *hash oil* or *red oil*.

- THC is absorbed very poorly from the digestive system and is usually inhaled in the form of smoke, which is a much more efficient system of administration. After inhalation, effects may begin in 30 to 60 minutes. The effects disappear within an hour or so.

- In the late 1980s a receptor for THC was isolated and located in many parts of the brain. Later, at least one endogenous cannabinoid was discovered.

- THC has several physiological effects: It causes bloodshot eyes, decreases the pressure in the eyeball, increases appetite and heart rate, and can act as an antiemetic and an anticonvulsant.

- At high doses, cannabis acts like a hallucinogen, but at the low doses common in North American use, the drug is reported to cause a pleasurable high. Cannabis causes *temporal disintegration;* that is, the user loses the ability to store information in the short term and is easily distracted.

- Cannabis can interfere with driving performance.

- THC has distinctive stimulus properties and will cause dissociation in both humans and nonhumans. The stimulus properties will generalize to other cannabinoids but not to any other drug.

- Tolerance develops to most of the effects of the cannabinoids.

- Withdrawal symptoms have been reported in humans and nonhumans but are usual only after continuous administration of fairly high doses. Some of the withdrawal symptoms reported are hot flashes, runny nose, loose stools, and sweating.

- Cannabinoids are not self-administered by nonhumans. Humans will work to earn marijuana and will titrate dosage, though not very accurately.
- The belief that cannabis causes violence and aggression has no support in research. It is known to interfere with immune processes and to lower the levels of testosterone in males, but the exact clinical significance of these findings for reproduction and susceptibility to disease in marijuana users is not known.

15

Hallucinogens

Many names have been suggested for drugs in this class. These include *phantasticant, psychotomimetrics* (psychosis mimics), and *psychedelics* (mind-manifesters). The most common name in use these days is *hallucinogens*, which covers all drugs that cause the user to have hallucinations. There are several problems with this definition, however. One is that almost any drug will cause hallucinations if taken in sufficient quantities. High doses of many substances will cause a *toxic psychosis* during which hallucinations are likely, just as we can experience hallucinations during a high fever or at times of great thirst or hunger. To get around this difficulty, we might say that drugs classed as hallucinogens may be distinguished from all other drugs because they cause hallucinations at doses that have few toxic effects; the hallucinations are a direct result of the drug and not an indirect effect of drug poisoning. As we proceed through this chapter, however, it will become apparent that this distinction is not easy to make. Some drugs, such as LSD, cause vivid hallucinations at doses

many thousands of times lower than their toxic doses, but others, such as scopolamine, are potent poisons that also cause a trancelike state. It is difficult to determine whether hallucinations experienced in this state are a direct result of the drug or a result of the fact that the body has been poisoned.

Yet another difficulty is that it is not clear exactly what constitutes a hallucination. A hallucination is usually thought of as an altered or distorted perception of reality, but the more we try to pin the concept down, the harder the task. We all are able to make ourselves experience distorted realities. We can push in on our closed eyelids and see colored lights. We can make ourselves dizzy and the world will appear to spin around. But are these hallucinations? If they are not, what distinguishes them from the drug-induced experience? If we drink too much alcohol, and have double vision, we can see two of everything. Is this drug-induced hallucination the same as a mescaline-induced vision? Clearly, it is not easy to define a hallucination exactly, and as a result, the working classification *hallucinogen* must remain imprecise. This lack of precision should cause us little difficulty as long as we remain aware of the difficulties with the term.

In addition, we will see that there are many drugs that are hallucinogens at higher doses but are not commonly taken in hallucinogenic doses. We must be careful, then, not to use the term *hallucinogen* as though it could explain the reason why the drug is used. It may be that the hallucinations are only a coincidental similarity among drugs that are otherwise unrelated. It is conventional, however, to class these drugs together, as we shall do in this chapter.

TYPES OF HALLUCINOGENS

Because there are so many hallucinogens, it is necessary to subdivide the category into classes. Many categories have been suggested based on the structure of the molecule of the drug or the perceived differences in effect, but the simplest way to divide the hallucinogens is to separate them according to the neurotransmitter that they resemble. It is probably no accident that most of the hallucinogens bear a chemical resemblance to neurotransmitters. We will consider the hallucinogens that are similar to serotonin, norepinephrine, and acetylcholine. Because there are a number that are not similar to any transmitter yet discovered, we will also have a miscellaneous category. Note that cannabis is included as a hallucinogen in many discussions, but in this book it has been given a chapter of its own. This special status does not reflect any special property of cannabis, which might well have been included in the miscellaneous section of this chapter. Cannabis was given a chapter of its own because of its widespread use and because of the abundance of information on it.

HALLUCINOGENS SIMILAR TO SEROTONIN

LSD

In recent times, perhaps the best-known hallucinogen has been LSD, a synthetic drug. However, a number of similar chemicals occur naturally in the ergot fungus that infects grains, especially rye. During the Middle Ages in Europe there were outbreaks of what is now called *ergotism*, caused by eating the fungus-infected grain. There were two kinds of effects, caused by different fungi. One kind severely constricted blood flow to the limbs and made them feel excessively warm. Eventually this condition would lead to gangrene, and the limb would just fall off. In 1039 a religious order was formed in France to treat people afflicted with this kind of ergotism. The patron saint of this order was St. Anthony, and the disease became known as *St. Anthony's fire* because of the sensation of heat. The other type of ergotism was characterized by convulsions, delirium, and hallucinations. That these afflictions were caused by the fungus was not discovered until more than 700 years later, in 1777. St. Anthony's fire was caused by derivatives of lysergic acid in the ergot fungus.

The story of LSD begins in the twentieth century. One of the effects of the lysergic acid derivatives in ergot was contractions of the uterus, a fact that was known to midwives, who used it to aid in childbirth. This prompted Albert Hoffman of the Sandoz drug company in Basel, Switzerland, to experiment with the derivatives of lysergic acid in the hopes of finding a new medicine. He had no inkling that he was dealing with a hallucinogen. In 1938 he synthesized a series of lysergic acid compounds but found none of them particularly interesting and went on to other things. Five years later, in 1943, Hoffman made a new batch of the twenty-fifth derivative (which he called LSD-25) and tried some new experiments, but he began to feel very peculiar and had to go home. He suspected that the reason for his strange sensations was that he had accidentally taken some of the LSD-25. To test this theory, a few days later he deliberately ingested 0.25 mg (250 micrograms), which he thought was an extremely small dose. His plan was to start with a dose that was so small that it would have no effect and slowly work up, but he had not reckoned on the extreme potency of LSD. A quarter of a milligram is a rather large dose, several times what is required to cause a powerful hallucinatory effect. Hoffman experienced the first LSD trip.

The drug was then distributed for testing to laboratories in Europe and the United States, where it was thought that it might be a useful drug in the treatment of mental disorders and alcoholism or at least a means of studying psychotic behavior. Some researchers, like Humphry Osmond at the University of Saskatchewan, believed that LSD offered the power to provide great personal insights and possessed considerable psychotherapeutic potential. LSD was used in experiments in mental hospitals and laboratories until the mid-1960s, when it broke out of the laboratory and into the street. Several factors were responsible for this escape. One was that the government of the United States passed new regulations against LSD use, and another was Dr. Timothy Leary.

How can passing a law against a drug increase its use? In this case the answer is simple. Prior to the restrictions on LSD in the early 1960s, the drug was only available for experimentation from Sandoz Laboratories, and the supply was generally enough to satisfy the small number of users. When Sandoz started to limit the availability of LSD in response to the new laws, illegal laboratories started to manufacture it. Because the drug was easy to make and only small quantities were needed, the market was soon flooded, and the drug became cheap and widely available. The clandestine labs in the United States even started to export LSD to other countries (Brecher, 1972).

The reason the U.S. government restricted LSD was not that the drug was believed to have popular appeal. LSD was restricted because of the large number of babies born deformed after their mothers had used the drug *thalidomide*, which was also being distributed as a new drug for testing at that time (see Chapter 4). The thalidomide tragedy led to a general tightening of all drug regulations.

Timothy Leary was a research professor in the department of Social and Human Relations at Harvard University who was always considered by his colleagues to be a bit unconventional and radical in his views. The psychedelic revolution began for Leary in 1960 when he was in Mexico and he ate some mushrooms containing *psilocybin* that caused him to have a "full-blown conversion experience." He returned to Harvard where he and his colleague, Richard Alpert, distributed psilocybin to as many people as they could get to take it. In 1961 they tried LSD, started a new religion, and adopted LSD as a sacrament. In 1963, Leary and Alpert were dismissed from Harvard, a move that generated considerable publicity for both them and the drug. They coined the phrase that was to become the philosophy of the hippie movement of the 1960s: "Turn on, tune in, drop out."

LSD had its heyday during the 1960s and early 1970s, the years of the hippie movement, which reached its peak at the Woodstock Music Festival in 1969. LSD has not vanished since then, but the pattern of its use is now somewhat different. In the 1960s, LSD was used as a true psychedelic: High doses were consumed in order to achieve personal or cosmic insights. Using these high doses was not always a pleasurable experience. Gordon Wasson, who explored the religious use of many hallucinogenic plants, was asked once why he did not take hallucinogens all the time. He replied, "Ecstasy is hard work." It has been suggested that drug users in more recent years are not as interested in insight as they are in pleasure (Baumeister & Placidi, 1983).

LSD is now taken in smaller doses so that the effect is a euphoric high similar to that of marijuana, and powerful mind-altering states are neither desired nor achieved. For enlightened discussion of the career of both LSD and Leary, see Grinspoon and Bakalar (1979b), Baumeister and Placidi (1983), and Lee and Shlain (1985).

LSD is sold on the street as "hits." A hit is a dose of LSD absorbed in a blotter, capsule, or sugar cube. In the 1970s a hit contained about 100 micrograms of LSD with a range of 0 to 300 micrograms (James & Bhatt, 1972). Other estimates suggest that a typical hit is 40 to 70 micrograms in spite of the fact that sellers usually claim a hit is about 300 micrograms (Barron, Lowinger, & Ebner, 1970).

LSD is effective orally and is usually taken by this route. Effects usually begin between 30 and 90 minutes after ingestion. Only 1 percent of the drug ever reaches the brain. There are few physical side effects, the most consistent being a dilation of the pupils. The half-life of LSD is about 110 minutes in humans. It is extensively metabolized in the liver, and the metabolites are secreted into the digestive system in the bile and excreted in the feces (Brown, 1972).

Psilocybin

Psilocybin is found in several species of mushrooms that are native to North America. These are popularly known as *magic mushrooms* or *Mexican mushrooms*. Most varieties are found only in the southern United States and Mexico, but some species grow all over the continent. One of the more widespread varieties is in the genus *Psilocybe*. Figure 15–1 shows a drawing of an example of a *Psilocybe*. Other genera of mushrooms that contain psilocybin are *Conobybe*, *Paneolis*, and *Stropharia*.

These mushrooms have been considered sacred in Mexico and Central America for thousands of years. Early clay figurines with mushroomlike horns dating back 1,800 years have been discovered, and mushroom-shaped stones from about 500 B.C. have been excavated at Mayan sites in Guatemala. At the time of their

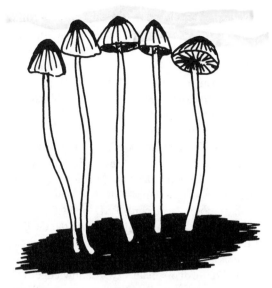

Figure 15–1 A common species of *Psilocybe* mushroom (magic mushroom).

conquest of the Aztecs, the Spanish found an important religious cult that used these mushrooms as a sacrament. The mushrooms were called *teonanácatl*, which means "God's flesh." This cult was suppressed by the Spanish, and use of the mushroom was forced underground. There is also evidence that these mushrooms were used by native people of South America. Mushroom statues have been found in Colombia, and records of the Jesuit missionaries report that the native peoples of the western Amazon in Peru consumed a "tree fungus." However, there is no known contemporary use of these mushrooms in South America.

Only recently have the mushrooms used by the Aztecs been identified. Gordon Wasson, a retired banker, made the discovery in 1952 when he ate 12 of the mushrooms as part of an Indian ceremony in the remote mountains of Mexico. His accounts of his experiences were published in *Life* magazine. In 1958, Albert Hoffman, who discovered LSD, isolated two substances from the *Psilocybe* mushroom. He called them *psilocybin* and *psilocin* (De Ropp, 1961, p. 153).

Psilocybe mushrooms played a role in the story of Timothy Leary. Seven magic mushrooms caused his conversion to the psychedelic philosophy, although his name later became associated primarily with LSD. Like LSD, psilocybin was used extensively by the hippie subculture but was never as popular as LSD, largely because it was more difficult to manufacture and less potent than LSD, so much more needed to be made. It was cheaper to make and sell LSD, and the effects were similar. "Magic mushrooms" were sold, but these were almost always common edible mushrooms laced with LSD or PCP. *Psilocybe* use decreased in the 1970s with the decline of LSD and hippiedom, although there has been a resurgence in the popularity of psilocybin. This is largely due to the spread of the knowledge that psilocybin-containing mushrooms grow well not just in Mexico but all over North America.

Orally, 4 to 8 mg of psilocybin is required to produce a hallucinogenic effect in humans. Thus LSD is about 100 times more potent, but the effects of both drugs are qualitatively the same if dosage adjustments are made. Psilocybin is also more potent and less toxic than mescaline (Schultes & Hoffman, 1979, p. 77). When taken orally, its effects may be experienced within 30 minutes. Some 25 percent is excreted unchanged, mostly in the urine; 5 percent is metabolized; and we do not know what happens to the other 70 percent. Psilocybin is converted into psilocin in the body; behavioral effects in nonhumans are closely related to the levels of psilocin, so it appears that psilocin is the active agent rather than psilocybin (Brown, 1972).

Lysergic Acid Amide

Another drug that we owe to the Aztecs is *lysergic acid amide* (also called *engine*), an ingredient of the seeds of the plant we call the *morning glory*. The Aztecs called it *ololiuqui*, "the flower of the virgin." The structure of the molecule of lysergic acid amide is very similar to that of LSD, but the effects are somewhat different.

The Spanish recorded the use of ololiuqui by the Mexican Indians in the early seventeenth century, and they identified the drug as coming from the morning glory. In modern times some doubt arose as to whether that plant was actually a hallucinogen because there was no recent evidence of any use of morning glory in Mexico, and no other member of the family of plants to which morning glory belonged was then known to contain a drug. It was even suggested that ololiuqui was really derived from another plant (*Datura*) and that the Aztecs deliberately identified the morning glory to the Spanish ecclesiastical authorities to misdirect their persecution of hallucinogen use. We know now that ololiuqui is presently used by the Indians of Oaxaca in Mexico to aid prophecy and the divination of disease (Schultes, 1978).

When swallowed whole, the seeds have no effect. The drug is prepared by grinding the seeds, soaking them in water, and then straining the water through a cloth. Some varieties of morning glory seeds sold by garden seed companies are effective hallucinogens, but care should be used because these seeds are frequently treated with fungicides and preservatives that contain mercury and can be highly toxic. The major active ingredient in the morning glory seeds, lysergic acid amine, was discovered and identified first by Albert Hoffman in 1960. (You should be getting familiar with that name by now.) Its discovery was surprising because this was the first time that a lysergic acid derivative had been found in a plant higher than a fungus (Schultes & Hoffman, 1980). It turned out that many members of the family of plants that the morning glory belongs to, the Convolvulaceae, also contain LSD-like drugs.

Lysergic acid amide is about a tenth as potent as LSD. It is readily absorbed when taken orally. In small doses, the drug causes a dreamy state after about 20 minutes, but the thought processes remain alert. These effects are short-lived and leave no hangover. In higher doses, the same sort of state is intensified, and the user falls into a sleep after about an hour. The drug does not cause the intense visual hallucinations characterized by LSD unless taken in extremely high doses (Brown, 1972).

Dimethyltryptamine (DMT)

Dimethyltryptamine (DMT) can be found in several plants. Most of the 45 to 60 species of the genus *Virola* contain it in their bark. These trees are found in the jungles of South and Central America, and the drug is used by the native peoples of the Amazon and Orinoco rivers.

Just after the turn of the twentieth century, a German anthropologist named Koch-Grunberg recorded how the bark of the virola was prepared by a witch doctor of the Yekwana Indians. The witch doctor stripped the bark off the tree, pounded it, and then boiled the bark until all the water had boiled off. The remaining sediment was toasted over a fire and then powdered with a knife. The powder was then sniffed into the nostrils. This snuff is known by many names, the most common being *yankee* in Colombia and *parica* in Brazil. It is used by witch doctors and shamans for the diagnosis and treatment of disease and for divination, prophecy, and magic.

DMT is easily synthesized and was first produced in 1931. It is much less potent than LSD (the effective dose is 1 mg/kg). The effects start soon after administration and are usually gone within an hour.

Synthetic DMT was used as a hallucinogen along with LSD by the hippie subculture. It was also known by the name *businessman's lunch* because its effects were so brief that it could be used to produce a hallucinatory experience during a lunch hour.

Bufotenine

There are a number of derivatives of DMT. One of them, *5-hydroxy-DMT*, is also known as *bufotenine*, and it is spread widely throughout several plant and animal species. There are traces of bufotenine in virola snuffs, but bufotenine is the principal ingredient in another South American jungle snuff known as *yopo* or *cohoba*, which is made from the beans of several species of trees of the genus *Anadenanthera*. When Columbus arrived in the New World, he recorded the use of a strong hallucinogenic snuff by the native Indians, and every other explorer of Central and South America recorded similar activities over a wide area.

Bufotenine was first isolated in the United States in 1954 by V. L. Stromberg of the National Heart Institute from the seeds of the *Anadenanthera peregrina*, which also contain some other DMT variants. Over 120 years after being collected, bufotenine was identified in seeds of this tree that were gathered by the British explorer and botanist Richard Spruce, who studied and recorded the use of many hallucinogenic plants in South America in the nineteenth century. Bufotenine is also found in the flesh of a fish called the *dream fish*, which is caught in the Norfolk Islands. It was originally discovered in the skin of a species of toad from which it derives its name; toads belong to the family *bufonidae*. Bufotenine is one of only a few hallucinogens found in both animal and plant tissues. Remember that toads were a principal ingredient in witches' brews. Because toads are easy prey to many predators, they secrete vile-tasting and sometimes poisonous substances from glands in their skin as a form of protection. These substances include several neurotransmitters, toxins, and bufotenine-like chemicals that vary from species to species (Lyttle, 1993).

Bufotenine does not appear to have hallucinogenic effects when administered orally; it must be injected or inhaled to have this effect. It is also common for the South American snuff user to mix the snuff with ashes or lime from ground seashells. This mixture aids in absorption throughout the nasal membranes because these drugs are bases and the lime reduces ionization and speeds absorption.

In 1989 and 1990, reports started circulating in the popular media that a new craze, "toad licking," was sweeping the world of illicit drug users. It was attributed to "hippies" in Australia who would reportedly boil toads to extract "toad venom" which they would then consume in some undescribed manner to get "high." The press interviewed various experts, but very few cases of "toad licking" were ever actually found, although it seems that two men ended up in a hospital after intense bouts of vomiting caused by eating secretions from the backs of toads that they had spread on crackers. Nevertheless, there were attempts in Canada and the United States to pass specific anti-toad-licking legislation (Lyttle, 1993). The toad-licking "problem" appears to have been entirely created by overeager media, since it is clear that bufotenine is not active when consumed orally.

Harmine and Harmaline

Harmine and *harmaline* are found in several plants; perhaps the best known are the members of the genus *Bainsteriopsis*, a vine that grows in the tropical jungles of South America. The active ingredient was identified in 1928 as harmine. Some tribes of South American native peoples prepare from the bark of the vine a drink that has many names including *ayahuasca, coapi, pinde,* and *yage* (one of the first people to record the use of ayahuasca was Richard Spruce in 1851), but in some locales the Indians just chew the dried stem. They use it for magic, prophecy, and divination and claim that the drug makes the user telepathic.

Harmine does not appear to cause hallucinations in the manner of LSD. Instead, it induces a trancelike state during which bright-colored images appear when the eyes are closed. There is no feeling of ecstasy or euphoria. The effective dose given s.c. is between 25 and 75 mg in man (Schultes & Hoffman, 1980, p. 178). This makes it considerably less potent than DMT or LSD.

The drink is usually prepared from the bark of the plant, but in some places the Indians also use additives, often from other plants, that increase greatly the potency and duration of the experience. One of these additives is the leaf of the same *Bainsteriopsis* vine, which contains a drug related to DMT. It is believed that harmine acts as an MAO inhibitor, so it would also block the metabolism of drugs like DMT, and this action would greatly enhance their effect. It is for this reason that the mixture of ayahuasca and the *Bainsteriopsis* leaves is so potent.

Ibogaine

Closely related to harmaline is a family of chemicals known as the *iboga derivatives*, which include *ibogaine* and *ibogamine*. They are ingredients in the root of the shrub *Tabernanthe iboga*, which is native to Central and West Africa. The root is chewed by the residents of this region in a manner similar to the chewing of coca leaves by the Indians of the Andes. It is said to reduce hunger, allay fatigue, and act as an aphrodisiac. In larger doses, it causes confusion and drunkenness and can induce visions, but it is not commonly used for its hallucinatory properties.

The iboga root has great significance in the history and culture of Gabon in West Africa. It is used in an initiation rite in several secret societies and is also eaten by sorcerers before they communicate with the spirit world or before they ask for advice from their ancestors. The use of iboga is still growing in Gabon. The custom has served to unify warring tribes in their resistance to the spread of Christianity, Islam, and other European and foreign influences (Schultes & Hoffman, 1980, p. 236).

Ibogaine has attracted considerable attention recently because of claims that it can cure addictions. Some people who have taken ibogaine to experience its hallucinogenic effects immediately stopped taking other drugs without any withdrawal and completely lost any desire or craving for drugs. In rats, ibogaine has been shown to reduce self-administration of both cocaine and morphine (Glick et al., 1994) immediately after administration. This finding can be explained by the fact that the drug induces tremors that could interfere with lever pressing. Interestingly, however, the reduced self-administration persisted in some rats for several days, long after the tremors were gone. The effect on cocaine intake seems to be stronger when the ibogaine is repeatedly administered once a week for three weeks (Cappendijk & Dzoljic, 1993). A similar effect of ibogaine has been observed with morphine self-administration (Glick et al., 1991).

There is a lack of properly controlled trials of ibogaine on human addicts, but there are individual cases where the drug did appear to cause astonishing results, not only blocking withdrawal effects of heroin, but completely eliminating any craving or any desire to use heroin, alcohol, or tobacco in some long-time heroin addicts. Cases are also reported where the drug has had no lasting effect at all (Sheppard, 1994).

Studies on the discriminative stimulus properties of ibogaine have shown that the drug effect is discriminable and will generalize only partially to MDA and LSD and a variety of other active substances that alter dopamine and serotonin brain systems, indicating that its subjective effects are unique (Schechter & Gordon, 1993).

In rats it has been observed that ibogaine kills a specific type of brain cell in a part of the cerebellum. It is not known whether this effect is likely to occur in humans, but such concerns have hampered testing of the drugs on human addicts. Deaths have also been reported in association with ibogaine use, but it is not clear that ibogaine was the cause (Sheppard, 1994).

HALLUCINOGENS THAT RESEMBLE NOREPINEPHRINE

Mescaline

Mescaline is the active ingredient in a cactus known as the *peyote (Lephophora williamsii)*, which is native to the deserts of Mexico and the southwestern United States. The peyote is a small, spineless cactus that barely sticks out of the ground and has a thick, tuberous root. It has been used for centuries in Mexico and, like *Psilocybe* mushrooms and morning glory seeds, was a sacred plant of the Aztecs.

Numerous Indian legends concern the origins of peyote, most involving a similar theme. An Indian is lost alone in the desert and is about to give up and die when he eats peyote and discovers its effects.

The first European account of peyote use in Mexico was a description by the Spanish in the seventeenth century of Aztec use, but there is archaeological evidence that peyote has been used for at least 8,000 years. The Spanish noted that peyote was used as a medicine, to foresee and predict the future, and to "discern who has stolen from them some utensil." The Spanish felt that the peyote visions were "satanic trickery" and made vigorous efforts to stamp it out. They only succeeded in driving it into the hills and remote areas, where it survived. The Mexican Indians use peyote primarily in a long ceremony during which there is much dancing.

Although the Indians of the southwestern United States had known about peyote for many years, not until the end of the nineteenth century did they begin to use it extensively. They built a new ceremony around its use, incorporated elements of both their own traditional religious beliefs and Christianity, and formed a new religion now called the *Native American Church*. It has spread from Mexico to Canada and has some 250,000 members. By a special act of the United States Congress, the use of peyote was made legal as a sacrament of this church in 1970 (Schultes & Hoffman, 1980, p. 199), although individual states may still pass laws against it.

Only the top part of the cactus is used. It is cut into thick slices and set in the sun to dry. The slices shrivel into wrinkled brown disks called *mescal buttons*, from which the term *mescaline* is derived. These buttons are placed in the mouth and sucked and chewed until they disintegrate and are swallowed. During a peyote ceremony, an Indian may consume as many as 12 of these buttons. They have a particularly disagreeable and nauseating odor and a bitter taste (De Ropp, 1961).

There is some confusion about the use of the term *mescal*. Mescal is also the name of an alcoholic drink made from fermentation of the agave cactus. This mescal does not contain mescaline. The situation is further confused by the presence of yet another mescal, a bean called the *mescal bean* (also known as *red* or *coral bean*), which is the seed of a tree (*Saphora secundaflora*) that grows in northern Mexico and Texas. This bean does not contain mescaline either, but it does contain a drug called *cytisine* that resembles nicotine and is quite toxic. It is believed that the mescal bean was worshipped and used ceremonially in the so-called *red bean dance* before the evolution of the peyote cult. In modern times, use of the mescal bean as a drug has died out apart from its use as a necklace by the *roadmen*, the leaders of the peyote ceremony. In fact, the red bean dance ceremony probably developed into the peyote ceremony when the much less toxic cactus was substituted for the mescal bean and the term *mescal* was switched from the bean to the cactus. There are reports that when this transition was taking place, the mescal bean and the mescal button were used together. This would have been a particularly potent combination (Schultes & Hoffman, 1980, p. 159).

Mescaline was one of the earliest hallucinogens isolated from plant material and identified. It was isolated from peyote at the end of the nineteenth century by the German chemist Arthur Heffter. Heffter isolated several substances from peyote and tried them all himself until he found the one that caused pronounced visual hallucinations, and he called that *mescaline*. In 1919 the structure of mescaline was determined and the drug was first synthesized. Mescaline was used as a hallucinogen by Timothy Leary and the hippies of the 1960s, but, like psilocybin, it was not as easy to manufacture as LSD and was less po-

tent. Consequently, most of what was sold on the street as mescaline was really something else, usually LSD. A hallucinogenic dose of mescaline is about 200 mg, making it about 1/4,000 as potent as LSD.

Mescaline is absorbed readily from the digestive system. After oral consumption, the first symptoms are nausea, vomiting, tremor, and incoordination. After about an hour or so follows a period of LSD-like psychological effects that may last for several hours. The half-life of mescaline is 1½ to 2 hours. The drug is excreted in the urine, about half of it metabolized (Brown, 1972).

STP and Synthetic Mescaline-Like Drugs

The structure of the mescaline molecule has been altered to form a family of drugs that is actually closer to amphetamine. These drugs may be thought of as a cross between amphetamine and mescaline, and many such drugs have been discovered. Much of this research was done in the hope of finding a drug with a medically useful property. Unfortunately, the only use for these new substances has been in the drug subculture, where they are used as hallucinogens. Table 15–1 lists several of the better-known

TABLE 15–1 Some Synthetic Mescaline Drugs and Their Potency Relative to Mescaline

Drug	Potency Relative to Mescaline*
DMA	8.0
MDA	3.0
MMDA	3.0
DOM	80.0
DOET	100.0
DOAM	10.0
TMA	0.5

Sources: Grinspoon & Bakalar (1979b), p. 23; Shulgin (1978).
*The potency number represents the number of times the dose of the drug must be divided to produce an effect equivalent to a given dose of mescaline.

mescaline derivatives and their potency relative to mescaline. For the most part, these substances are more potent than mescaline, considerably more toxic, and cause more unpleasant side effects such as headaches and nausea. During the heyday of hallucinogens in the 1960s, many synthetics were invented and manufactured in clandestine labs in an attempt to circumvent the law, which only identified specific chemicals as illegal. They have become known as "designer drugs" and appeared on the street with a bewildering variety of names. Because many were not screened for adverse effects as commercially developed drugs must be, some had extremely toxic effects. One drug specifically destroyed neurons in the basal ganglia and created severe Parkinson's disease. Some of these substances were so toxic that they caused a number of deaths. These drugs are much less common now, but some, like MDMA, are still around and still a source of concern.

Perhaps the best known of these synthetics is *DOM*, which is *2,5-dimethoxy-4-methylamphetamine*. It was synthesized in 1963 and appeared on the street in San Francisco in 1967. DOM was also known on the street as *STP*, after the engine oil additive. STP was also supposed to stand for "super terrific psychedelic." Another name for STP was *LBJ* (Lyndon Baines Johnson).

MDMA is *3,4-methylenedioxymethamphetamine*. Unlike many of the designer drugs, it was not invented in an attempt to circumvent the law. It was originally synthesized by the Merck drug company and was patented in 1914. It was never developed or used for any purpose until the late 1960s, when it first appeared on the drug scene (R. K. Siegel, 1986). It is also commonly known as *ecstasy* (other names include *X, Adam, MDM, M&M*, and the *yuppie drug*) and achieved considerable popularity in the mid-1980s.

It has about the same potency as MDA. A dose of 75 to 100 mg induces a state similar to that caused by marijuana or low doses of phencyclidine with no hallucinations and an enhanced awareness of emotions and sensations (Lamb &

Griffiths, 1987; R. K. Siegel, 1986). Prior to July 1985, when it was reclassified by the U.S. government, some psychiatrists gave MDMA to their patients because it seemed to enhance intimacy and communication between the patient and the therapist (Verebey, Alrazi, & Jaffe, 1988; Adler et al., 1985).

The drug can be taken orally and reaches a peak blood level in about two hours. The majority of the drug is either excreted unchanged or metabolized to MDA.

MDMA appears to be relatively free of acute adverse effects with only about 20 mentions in hospital emergency room admissions in 1986, a number that has not increased even in the face of increasing illicit use. MDMA is not a drug of the streets; users of MDMA appear to be more highly educated middle-class intellectuals (Newmeyer, 1993).

MDMA was reclassified and its use was banned, even for psychotherapeutic purposes, because it was discovered that the drug has neurotoxic effects. It has been shown that a dose of about four times the normal effective dose causes a depletion of serotonin in the brain of rats one week after a single administration. This is similar to the effects of PMA (described later), which has caused a number of deaths (Schmidt, 1987).

Two other drugs in this group are of interest. *TMA* is about twice as potent as mescaline and causes many of the usual synthetic mescaline-like effects, but it also causes intense anger and hostility, so much so that in one experiment the researchers feared that some subjects, if provoked, might have shown "homicidal violence" (Shulgin, 1978). Another drug, *PMA*, was developed in a clandestine lab in Canada in the early 1970s and was distributed in the illicit drug market in the United States and Canada. This drug is extremely potent, second only to LSD, but it is also very toxic and has a therapeutic index of 2.5, making it very dangerous to use. A number of deaths were attributed to PMA before warnings could be spread about it.

Myristicin and Elemicin

Myristicin and *elemicin* are drugs that are found in the fruit of members of the genus of tree *Myristica*. The best known is *Myristica fragrans*, or *nutmeg*. The nutmeg tree is native to tropical Asia and became known in Europe through the trade of two spices derived from it. *Nutmeg* is made from the seeds of the tree, and *mace* is derived from the fruit. Nutmeg and mace are very similar chemically, but they differ in the amounts of essential oils they contain and so have a different taste and fragrance. Both contain myristicin and elemicin and, to a lesser extent, a large number of related compounds. Despite a few reports of nutmeg being consumed in India mixed with tobacco or *betel*, or in Egypt as a hashish substitute, nutmeg has not been widely used as a hallucinogen, probably because of the variability of its hallucinogenic effect and the toxic effects that follow its use. These include headache, nausea, and dizziness. The drug is not very potent in its psychological effects, and large quantities, at least a teaspoonful, must be taken. The effects include visual hallucinations, but not with the frequency of LSD; auditory hallucinations, distortions of time and space, and a feeling of floating.

While there are few reported uses of nutmeg as a hallucinogen, it has been used since ancient times in India and Malaya as a medicine in the treatment of a variety of disorders, including digestive disorders and kidney troubles, fever, tuberculosis, asthma, and heart disease (Weil, 1979).

Myristicin closely resembles the synthetic MMDA, and the elemicin molecule is closely related to TMA.

HALLUCINOGENS SIMILAR TO ACETYLCHOLINE

Anticholinergics

A large number of plants from all over the world contain drugs that block the muscarinic receptor sites for acetylcholine. The three major natural *anticholinergics* are *atropine, hyoscyamine,* and *scopolamine (hyoscine)*. There are also a number of synthetic anticholinergics that are used to treat the symptoms of Parkinson's disease and the parkinsonian symptoms sometimes resulting from the use of antipsychotics (see Chapter 12). Two of these are *benzotropine* and *trihexyphenidyl*.

The plants that contain anticholinergic drugs belong to the family Solanaceae and have been used throughout recorded history and probably much earlier. Their use is particularly widespread because they are found in so many species of plants with wide distribution. Wherever they are used, by whatever society or culture, their use has two common elements: They have been associated with sorcery, magic, and witchcraft, and they are reputed to be aphrodisiacs. Another interesting effect reported by all of the users of anticholinergics is that they give the sensation of flying.

Other members of the Solanaceae are also well known. They include the potato, tomato, eggplant, and pepper. Many of these plants, especially the potato and the tomato, though perfectly safe, were believed to be poisonous, and few people would dare to eat them. Only in recent times have tomatoes become a popular food. When the potato was first imported to Europe from Peru, it was not accepted because of its resemblance to the *mandrake*.

An ancient source of anticholinergics is the root of the mandrake (*Mandragora officinarum*). This plant grows on dry, stony ground and is native from the Mediterranean to the Himalayas. The mandrake has a large taproot that is usually divided and resembles the human body, a fact that was given great significance by magicians and sorcerers. It was believed that care should be taken when the root was removed from the ground. If the root was pulled out roughly, the mandrake would shriek, with dire results for anyone hearing it, as described in this passage from *Romeo and Juliet*: "And shrieks like the Mandrakes torn out of the earth, / That living mortals hearing them run mad."

The Greeks believed that the witch Circe used the mandrake, and this association with witches and magic persisted into the Middle Ages. Many unfortunate women of the time were put to death as witches merely for possessing a mandrake root. Mandrake was one of the secret ingredients witches were reputed to have used in their brews, along with monkshood, deadly nightshade, hemlock, fat from a stillborn baby, toads, and soot. This concoction was supposed to make them fly (Ricciuti, 1978).

Another plant used by witches for the same purpose was the *deadly nightshade (Atropa belladonna)*, which is native to central and southern Europe, northern Africa, and the Middle East, but it has been spread to North America and around the world. The berries of the plant have traditionally been used as a poison; hence the ominous-sounding name. The genus and species names also refer to two ancient uses of the plant. One ancient use, as a poison, is indicated in the name *Atropa*, after Atropos, one of the Greek Fates, who cut the thread of life and was responsible for death. The species name *belladonna*, literally "beautiful woman," refers to the practice of putting a drop of the juice of this plant into the eyes to dilate the pupils so as to make the user more attractive.

Deadly nightshade was also used by witches in the Middle Ages, which gave rise to other names such as *devil's herb, sorcerer's herb, enchanter's nightshade*, and *apples of Sodom* (Le Strange, 1977).

Henbane (Hyoscyamus niger) also contains anticholinergics. It is native to Europe, Asia, and India but has now spread around the world. The plant was known to the ancient Egyptians, and an account of it appears in the *Ebers Papyrus*, written in 1500 B.C. It was known to the Greeks, who called it *hyoskyamos*, which means "hog bean," because hogs would eat the plant without ill effects. Like mandrake, it was used by the Greeks as a painkiller and anesthetic. It was also used in Europe by witches, who would roast the seeds and leaves and inhale the smoke. The henbane plant is also used extensively in Europe and

North America in folk medicine (Schultes & Hoffman, 1979).

Another anticholinergic-containing plant is *Datura (Datura stramonium)*, also known as *jimson* or *Jamestown weed* or *thornapple*. The origins of the plant are not known, but it has grown in North America and India for centuries. It too was extensively used as a poison and by witches, even in North America, where the Aztecs, quite independently from the European witchcraft tradition, used datura for magical purposes.

Datura has a long history of association with crime, not that it induced criminal behavior, but it was used by criminals to kill or sedate their victims. In India it was supposed to have been used by the followers of a cult who robbed and killed in the service of Kali, the god of destruction. It was used by professional poisoners in Europe in the Middle Ages, but worst of all, it was supposed to have been used by white slavers who mixed it with an aphrodisiac and gave it to unwilling girls.

In addition to these nefarious uses, datura also had a place in traditional medicines. It was used in India as a sedative and for treating diseases of the feet. In Europe and North America it was used to treat asthma, epilepsy, delirium tremens, rheumatism, and menstrual pains.

Synthetic Anticholinergics. Interestingly, a number of cases of abuse of the synthetic anticholinergics have been reported. Usually these drugs were prescribed for medical reasons, and the patients used them to produce euphoria. They have been used both to improve mood and to produce a hallucinogenic experience (Dilsaver, 1988).

MISCELLANEOUS HALLUCINOGENS

Ibotinic Acid

Ibotinic acid is the active ingredient in the *Amanita muscaria* mushroom, which grows on all continents except South America and Australia. It is usually found in forests of pine, spruce, or birch. It is a large, toadstoollike mushroom with a scabby top and may range in color from creamy white to pinkish orange to scarlet. It is also known as *fly agaric* because of its ability to intoxicate and sedate flies. Figure 15–2 shows a drawing of an *Amanita muscaria*. There are many species of amanita, some edible and some highly poisonous. The *Amanita muscaria* is one of the toxic varieties, but if taken in a subtoxic dose, it has remarkable effects.

The tribes of Siberia had no intoxicant other than aminita mushrooms until they were introduced to alcohol by the Russians. They harvested the mushrooms and ate them raw, dried them over a slow fire, or consumed them in an extract in water or reindeer milk. Consumed orally, the drug is readily absorbed, and intoxication starts within an hour. It is marked by twitching and trembling of the limbs and numbing of the feet. There is a euphoric feeling and a sense of lightness of the feet that often leads to dancing. There then follows a period of vivid-colored hallucinations. Occasionally there is vigorous, sometimes violent activity. The episode ends in a deep sleep (Schultes & Hoffman, 1979).

In addition to being used in India, Siberia, Russia, and other northern European countries, amanita also appears to have been used by the native peoples in North America, specifically the Ojibwas of Michigan (Schultes & Hoffman, 1979).

For many years the active ingredient in amanita was believed to be *muscarine*, a drug that stimulates muscarinic cholinergic receptor sites (see Chapter 4), but the effects of muscarine could not account for all the observed effects of the mushroom. Subsequent research in Switzerland and Japan has shown that the principal ingredient in the amanita is a substance called ibotinic acid. Also present are *muscamole* and *muscazone*. It is also likely that ibotinic acid is metabolized to muscamole, which is the real active ingredient.

Figure 15–2 The *Aminita muscaria* mushroom.

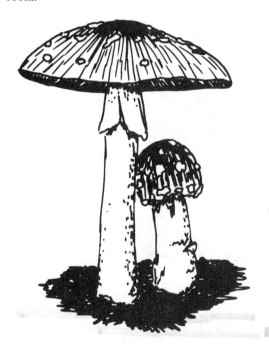

Phencyclidine and Ketamine

Phencyclidine, also known as *PCP*, is a synthetic drug developed by the Parke-Davis Company as an analgesic and anesthetic in 1963 and marketed as Sernyl. For this purpose it proved very effective and safe because it did not depress the heart, blood pressure, or respiration. It caused a trancelike state rather than a loss of consciousness. It has been classified as a *dissociative anesthetic* because it seemed to separate people from sensory experience. In 1965 it was withdrawn from the market because patients reported that while they were recovering from the drug, they experienced delirium, disorientation, and agitation. It was then marketed as Sernylan, and its use was restricted to nonhumans. It started to be sold on the street in 1965 under the names *crystal, angel dust, hob,* and *horse tanks.* However, it did not become popular during the 1960s. Not until the decline of LSD in the 1970s did PCP use start to increase. Before PCP became popular in its own right, it was more widely used than most people suspected because it was often mixed with other drugs or sold as something else like THC, mescaline, or psilocybin.

When PCP was introduced on the street in the 1960s, it was sold in the form of tablets or capsules for oral administration. It is seldom sold in that form now because of its unpredictable delay in action and difficulty in controlling the dose. Currently, it is sold as saltlike crystals that can be sprinkled on mint leaves, parsley, tobacco, or even marijuana and smoked. PCP can also be snorted into the nostrils or dissolved in water and injected. This latter route provides a rush and is more efficient, since no drug is wasted as with snorting or smoking. PCP is readily absorbed through most moist tissues and so can be administered through the eyes, rectum, or vagina.

PCP is not really a hallucinogen in the sense that LSD is. Taken at doses of 5 to 10 mg, the drug causes relaxation, warmth, a tingling feeling, and a sense of numbness. There are euphoric feelings, distortions in body image, and a feeling of floating in space. These effects wear off after four to six hours and are sometimes followed by a mild depression that may last for 24 hours to a week. At higher doses, the user may become stuporous or even comatose. Psychotic behavior occurs frequently and may include anything from manic excitation to catatonia, in which the user assumes one position and does not move for a prolonged period of time. There may be sudden mood changes accompanied by laughing and crying; disoriented, confused, and delusional thought; drooling; and repetitive actions. This psychotic state may slowly disappear as the drug level declines, but sometimes the psychosis requires hospitalization and lasts for weeks.

PCP has the reputation of causing people to be violent and to commit violent uncontrolled acts toward other people. In fact, people have used PCP as a defense in criminal cases by claiming that they had smoked a marijuana cigarette that, unknown to them, had been laced with PCP, and this caused them to be violent. A recent, careful examination of the literature on the drug has not found any systematic evidence that PCP specifically causes violent or criminal behavior. It is true that the psychotic state induced by large doses of PCP causes disorientation, agitation, and hyperactivity that are difficult to manage and have the potential for injury to the individual and others nearby. However, PCP does not seem to turn normal, innocent people into dangerous and violent criminals (Brecher et al., 1988). Research and experience with laboratory animals even suggest that PCP has a taming effect on normally aggressive animals (Balster, 1987).

Traditionally, PCP is used sporadically like LSD, but continuous use is becoming more common. When the drug is used every day, tolerance develops, and there is some evidence of dependence and withdrawal symptoms (Grinspoon & Bakalar, 1979b).

The drug is entirely metabolized and excreted in the urine. Its metabolism is slow, and traces may be found in the urine for a week.

Since PCP has become popular, a number of variants have been invented and sold; these include TCP, PCE, PCPY, and PCC. For more information, see Linder, Lerner, and Burns (1981).

Ketamine is a drug with effects similar to those of PCP. It was marketed as Ketalar in 1969. It is a more potent anesthetic and has a shorter duration of action than PCP. Ketamine is used as an anesthetic for children (Brown, 1972).

NEUROPHYSIOLOGY

The neurophysiology of hallucinogens is complex and not well understood. One difficulty is that the hallucinogens are not a homogeneous group. There are many types of drugs called hallucinogens that have very different neurophysiological effects. Since all the serotonin-like and the norepinephrine-like hallucinogens have in common the fact that they alter serotonergic transmission, it would be reasonable to suspect that the hallucinogenic effect of these drugs results from their action on serotonergic synapses. For example, the prototype hallucinogen LSD is a potent serotonin antagonist; it blocks the serotonin receptors. But this property by itself cannot be the only explanation for the hallucinogens because there are other serotonin-blocking drugs that do not cause hallucinations at all. Because many other drugs that are hallucinogenic also affect serotonergic transmission, it is apparent that serotonin blocking is necessary for the hallucinations to happen, but there must be some other effect as well. No one knows what this other effect might be.

It is quite clear that the hallucinations caused by the anticholinergics such as scopolamine are a result of the blocking of transmission at cholinergic synapses.

The dissociative anesthetics such as PCP are a mystery. They are known to alter the levels of some transmitters and appear to have their own receptor sites in the brain, which may indicate that there is likely a naturally occurring substance in the brain that also uses these sites. One receptor site that is sensitive to PCP is similar but not identical to the sigma receptor described in Chapter 11 on opiate drugs, and is also receptive to the mixed opiate agonist-antagonists such as cyclazocine (Johnson, 1987). The location and function of sigma receptors are not known, but they have been the subject of considerable investigation because they may play a role in understanding schizophrenia. Both PCP and cyclazocine cause symptoms similar to psychotic behavior. It is believed that a more complete understanding of the PCP receptor and the substance that activates it naturally may provide insights into the nature of mental illness.

In addition to altering the functioning of norepinephrine, dopamine, acetylcholine, and serotonin and being active at the sigma receptor, PCP blocks the activity of receptors for excitatory amino acids such as glutamate and aspartate which are transmitters in many parts of the brain, including the cortex (Johnson, 1987). PCP has a receptor site located in the ion channel normally controlled by a NMDA receptor for glutamate or glycine. When occupied by PCP, this receptor blocks the ion channel making these transmitters ineffective (Dinwiddie & Farber, 1995).

EFFECTS ON THE BEHAVIOR AND PERFORMANCE OF HUMANS

Subjective Effects

How does a scientist go about studying hallucinations? Hallucinations are, by definition, in the realm of subjective experience, and one of the first principles of scientific inquiry is that all scientific data must be public and observable to anyone. It is, however, possible to study the verbal reports of people who are experiencing or have experienced hallucinations, but then arises the problem of how to organize such a mass of words into something meaningful. Heinrich Kluver (1966), who started his work in the 1920s, combined reports of subjects in his own experiments on mescaline and those of other researchers and noticed that there were consistencies. Most of what these people described consisted of vivid visual images, and the researchers were aware all the time that the images were not real. If they closed their eyes, they would see these images against a black background; if they opened their eyes, the images would be projected on whatever they were looking at. Kluver noticed that the images were frequently geometric patterns, and he identified four types of patterns. The first he described as being like a grating or lattice; the second, like a cobweb; the third, like a tunnel, funnel, or cone; and the fourth, like a spiral. Kluver remarked that images of these types also appear in fever deliriums, insulin hypoglycemia, and states that occur just before drifting off to sleep (*hypnogogic states*). Unfortunately, what Kluver described was only the first of two stages of imagery; the second stage described by others is more complex and involves meaningful images, images of people, animals, and places. Even during this phase there are some common elements among individuals. For example, 60 to 70 percent of all subjects report seeing small animal or human figures that are friendly and caricature-like, and 72 percent of all subjects report religious imagery.

Despite the great interest of these observations, no comprehensive systematic or scientific work was attempted until the 1970s. The problem was tackled with surprising ingenuity and success by Ronald K. Siegel of the University of California at Los Angeles. Siegel adopted a variation of the technique of trained introspection, which had been used by the early German schools of psychology. Siegel trained his observers to use a code to describe their experiences. They were able to code the type of image, color, and movement using a series of letters and numbers that they could express as fast as the images appeared. When they demonstrated that they were well trained, Siegel then gave them a series of blind tests in which they were given placebos or any of a number of drugs in random order and left in a darkened room to report their experiences. Neither the subjects nor the researchers scoring the imagery codes knew what drug had been given.

Whereas the subjects given placebos saw a predominance of random forms, those getting the hallucinogenic drugs saw far more lattice and tunnel forms, confirming the observations of Kluver. During control sessions, subjects primarily saw black and violet forms, but in hallucinogenic sessions, they saw more colors, ranging into the yellow, orange, and red end of the spectrum. Finally, in all conditions aimless and pulsating movement was reported, but in hallucinogenic sessions there was an increase in "explosive" movement.

After demonstrating that all of these drugs appeared to create similar types of images, Siegel was also able to demonstrate that at higher doses people sometimes go through a phase where they see themselves being swept up into their own hallucination. This is followed by a stage where the images lose their geometric quality and become meaningful pictures of real objects. These images can change rapidly, as fast as 10 times a second. The change is not without a pattern, as each image appears to be related to the one before it. Figure 15–3 illustrates this point. Siegel also noted that the images during this stage were related to the subject's surroundings. For example, sounds such as footsteps induced an image of someone walking. Another interesting finding is that the colors appeared to shift from the blue end of the spectrum to the red end as the effect of the drug increased in intensity.

Because all these drugs have such similar effects, Siegel wondered whether the similarities were not due to cultural factors, since all his subjects came from a similar culture (UCLA). To answer this question, he went to visit a remote tribe of Huichol Indians in the Sierra Madre range of Mexico. These Indians make brightly colored pictures of their peyote visions from colored yarn. What he found was that the experiences pictured by the Huichols in their yarn paintings were identical to those reported by the subjects in his laboratory.

Siegel postulated that the nature and structure of hallucinations must be determined by the nature of and structure of the visual system and the brain, not by the drug, because (1) these hallucinatory experiences are similar among vastly different drugs; (2) this experience is similar to the effects produced by other nondrug hallucinations, such as those from fever, hypoglycemia, and migraine headaches; and (3) the experiences are similar between cultures. In other words, the hallucinations are a result of nonspecific interference in brain functioning; the drug intensifies what might be considered normal background noise in the perceptual systems, and this noise is then organized by the normal processes of perception and cognition into images and patterns (Siegel & Jarvik, 1975; Siegel, 1977).

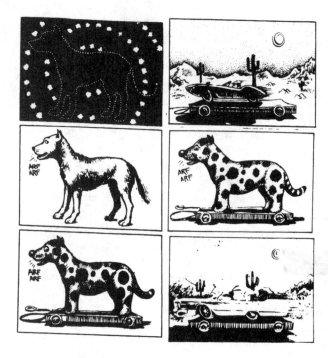

Figure 15–3 This series of drawings (read from top to bottom, column by column) illustrates the systematic changes in complex meaningful imagery reported after mescaline. Note that each scene contains an element of the previous one. Drawings by David Sheridan, pen and ink. (From Siegel & Jarvik, 1975.)

This study addresses only one property of the hallucinogenic experience, the visual, but there is a great deal more to the effect of hallucinogens than images. The experience often has a profound effect on emotions, insights, and feelings, which are not as easily studied and can only be conveyed by less scientific modes of expression, as we shall see.

Subjective Accounts

So many people have taken hallucinogenic drugs and then written about the experience that it is difficult to know where to begin. As with those who wrote about hashish, many of these people are more interested in producing literature than science, but then again, the subjective experience of taking a hallucinogen cannot survive translation into strictly scientific terms.

Perhaps the best scientific account of a hallucinogenic effect was of Albert Hoffman, the discoverer of LSD, who first took the drug acciden-

tally. His account is valuable because it is totally unaffected by expectancy. Hoffman had no idea what a hallucinogenic experience should be like. He was not even aware that he would have one, so his observations are free from influences of culture and expectation. This account is from his laboratory notebook.

Last Friday . . . in the midst of my afternoon work in the laboratory I had to give up working. I had to go home because I experienced a very peculiar attack of dizziness. At home I went to bed and got into a not unpleasant state of drunkenness which was characterized by an extremely stimulating fantasy. When I closed my eyes (the daylight was most unpleasant to me) I experienced fantastic images of an extraordinary plasticity. They were associated with an intense kaleidoscopic play of colors. After about two hours this condition disappeared. (Stoll, 1949)

Hoffman's account of an LSD trip seems flat and uninspired, but it does convey in straightforward language that there were spectacular visual effects and that he actually liked it, but its sterility missed the emotional impact that many people experience after taking hallucinogens. In general, many people find that these drugs induce feelings with great religious significance. It is perhaps for this reason that we find hallucinogens throughout the world associated with worship and religion, such as the peyote of the Native American Church. The religious nature of the hallucinogenic experience is described here by R. Gordon Wasson (1972) in this account of his participation in a Mazatec Indian *Psilocybe* mushroom rite:

It permits you to see more clearly than our perishing mortal eyes can see, vistas beyond the horizons of this life, to travel backwards and forwards in time, to enter other planes of existence, even (as the Indians say) to know God. It is hardly surprising that your emotions are profoundly affected and you feel that an indissoluble bond unites you and the others who have shared in this sacred agape. All that you see during this night has a pristine quality; the landscape, the edifices, the carvings, the animals—they look as though they had come straight from the Maker's workshop. (p. 197)

Another commonly reported effect of the hallucinogens is that they seem to provide insight into one's past and into one's own mind, revealing repressed thoughts and unrecognized feelings. Such insights are similar to those that psychoanalysis attempts to achieve through psychotherapy. It was this sort of effect that inspired Humphry Osmond to suggest that hallucinogens might be useful tools in psychotherapy and prompted him, along with Aldous Huxley, to suggest the term *psychedelic*, which means "mind-manifesting" or "mind-expanding" (Osmond, 1957). Here is an example from the experiences of psychologist Bernard Aaronson, who took LSD as part of an experiment:

We sat on the bench under the trees and talked about the loneliness of being, and talked about how people are forever needing things they expect you to provide.

For what seemed a long time, I cried as I have not cried since I was a baby, for all the people in the world who need things and whose needs cannot be met. I cried too for all the people around me that I botched in the giving or to whom I cannot give because I am depleted. . . . I expressed great hostility toward both my parents and with H.'s help analyzed my feelings as they derived from my relationship with each of them. I analyzed my relationship with my next older brother, and examined the meaning in my life of my relationship with that friend whom I love the most. (Aaronson & Osmond, 1970, pp. 47–48)

Another commonly reported experience is the greatly enhanced pleasure derived from viewing art and, especially, listening to music.

Ordinarily I am not particularly susceptible to music. This time, lying on the cot, I became acutely aware of the Montoya record playing. This was more than music: the entire room was saturated with sounds that were also feeling—sweet, delicious, sensual—that seemed to be coming from somewhere deep down inside me. I became mingled with the music, gliding along with the chords. Everything I saw and felt was somehow inextricably interrelated. This was pure synesthesia, and I was part of the synthesis. I suddenly "knew" what it was to be simultaneously a guitar, the sounds, the ear that received them, and the organism that responded, in what was the most profoundly consuming aesthetic experience I have ever had. (Jerry Richardson in Aaronson & Osmond, 1970, p. 53)

A more complete account of the subjective experiences of hallucinogens is beyond the scope of this book. A good selection of accounts of drug experiences may be found in Grinspoon and Bakalar (1979b).

Perception

As we have seen, people who use LSD frequently report that their perceptions are much keener and that sight and hearing become more acute. There have been a few studies of the effects of LSD on visual sensory thresholds, but their results are not consistent. In general, however, impairments of sensory functions attributable to LSD are reported more often than improvements (Hollister, 1978).

While it is clear that LSD increases the enjoyment of music, it has not yet been established whether there are any changes in auditory thresholds. The perception of the passage of time is distorted in most individuals; however, the direction of distortion is not consistent. In most cases, time is perceived as slowing down (10 seconds seems more like 20), but in some experiments the reverse has been reported (Hollister, 1978).

It is known that PCP has analgesic effects (it was developed as an analgesic), but it is surprising that LSD also seems to provide some relief from pain (Leavitt, 1974, p. 326).

Performance

One of the difficulties with measuring human performance under the influence of hallucinogens is maintaining the motivation of the subject to cooperate. Like marijuana, hallucinogens frequently cause subjects to become inattentive to the task and so caught up in internal experiences that they lose their motivation to perform as well as they are capable on tasks that they may feel are irrelevant at the time. It has been suggested that Carlos Castaneda (1973), an anthropology student who wrote extensively about his experiences after taking several different types of hallucinogens, could not have had the experiences he describes because he claims to have been able to continue to take notes while under the influence of the drugs (R. K. Siegel, 1981).

The available data mostly show that LSD and PCP both impair reaction time. Oddly enough, performance on a pursuit rotor task may be improved by LSD but impaired by PCP (Rosenbaum et al., 1959).

Functioning on intellectual tasks is also impaired. Like THC, LSD causes a deficit in immediate memory. Other impairments are seen in problem solving and cognitive functions such as mental addition and subtraction, color naming, concentration, and recognition (Hollister, 1978, p. 397). Although no studies of the effects of PCP on memory in humans have been conducted, PCP does seem to be more disruptive of memory in nonhumans than LSD, THC, opiates, and other psychoactive drugs (Balster, 1987).

Claims have been made that LSD-like hallucinogens improve creativity, but again as with THC, these are difficult to substantiate experimentally. There is little doubt that LSD changes the sort of work done by artists, but it is doubtful whether these changes are improvements.

EFFECTS ON THE BEHAVIOR OF NONHUMANS

Unconditioned Behavior

The effects of LSD-like hallucinogens on the behavior of nonhumans are variable. Large doses of LSD and mescaline appear to increase spontaneous motor activity of mice in an open field (Brimblecombe & Pinder, 1975). Increases in activity have also been reported for scopolamine and other anticholinergics (Baez, 1976).

At low doses, LSD appears to enhance the sexual activity of male rats, but at high doses sexual activity is inhibited. Aggressive behavior and attack behavior in rats may be either enhanced or inhibited by LSD and other hallucinogens, depending on the situation. Some aggressive animals may be tamed by the drug, but others that are normally tame may attack their handlers after ingesting LSD. It appears that these changes reflect a general enhancement of reactivity or responsiveness rather than a specific increase in aggression (Miczek & Barry, 1976).

In spite of the claims that they are aphrodisiacs, anticholinergics inhibit sexual behavior in both male and female rats, and the anticholinergics also inhibit both aggressive and defensive behavior (Miczek & Barry, 1976).

Effects on Positively Reinforced Behavior

The LSD-like hallucinogens slow or block responding on an FR schedule. This effect remains fairly constant throughout the session, but responding returns suddenly as the drug wears off. Both LSD and mescaline increase responding during the early part of an FI when it is normally low. In the latter part of the interval, LSD causes increases in the high rates, but mescaline decreases this responding just as amphetamines do. The effects of these drugs on responding on a VI schedule are variable. Some researchers report increases, and some report decreases (McMillan & Leander, 1976).

Effects on Negatively Reinforced Behavior

LSD has a rather specific effect on shock avoidance. Like many antianxiety drugs, it blocks signaled shock avoidance at doses well below those that interfere with escape responding. Mescaline also blocks avoidance, but there are no data on whether this effect occurs at doses that also interfere with escape. Unlike LSD, the anticholinergics depress avoidance behavior only at doses that also depress escape responding (Seiden & Dykstra, 1977).

Not much is known about the effect of hallucinogens on shock-suppressed behavior, but LSD does not seem to increase it (McMillan & Leander, 1976). This effect is quite different from that of the antianxiety drugs, which increase both avoidance and shock-suppressed behavior.

DRUG STATE DISCRIMINATION

Nonhumans readily learn to discriminate hallucinogenic drugs from saline in either a T-maze or a Skinner box. In general, responses controlled by one hallucinogen generalize to most other hallucinogens but not to drugs that are not usually classed as hallucinogens. Table 15–2 shows which drugs generalize to various hallucinogens and which do not.

The stimulus cue of LSD is not blocked by cholinergic blockers such as atropine, opiate antagonists such as naloxone, or dopamine blockers such as chlorpromazine. Although there is some variability between drugs and laboratories, it appears that the stimulus properties of LSD can be blocked by central-acting serotonin agonists but not by peripheral serotonin agonists; these findings indicate that serotonin receptors in the CNS must somehow be involved in the subjective effects of LSD. Serotonin is further implicated in studies where rats were trained to perform a response when given electrical stimulation of the Raphé nuclei, a serotonin-containing system implicated in sleep (see Chapter 4). Later this response was performed by rats given LSD, indicating that the Raphé stimulation was felt as being similar to LSD. In addition, LSD injected

TABLE 15–2 Drugs That Generalize to Hallucinogens and Those That Do Not

Drug	Will Generalize to	Will Not Generalize to
LSD	Mescaline, psilocybin, scopolamine, cyclazocine, THC	Barbital, amphetamine, morphine, methadone, chlorpromazine
Mescaline	DOM, DOET	Amphetamine, cocaine
Ditran	Atropine	PCP
Atropine	Scopolamine	Pentobarbital
PCP	Ketamine, SKF 10,047	Ditran, THC, pentobarbital, morphine, chlorpromazine

Source: Kuhn, White, & Appel (1977), pp. 142–143.

directly into the Raphé system produces the same stimulus effects as when given i.p. All these data support the notion that the subjective effects of LSD depend on serotonin receptors in the Raphé system (Hirschorn, Hayes, & Rosecrans, 1975).

While not as much is known about psilocybin, mescaline, and the synthetic mescaline-like drugs, it appears that serotonin is important in their stimulus effects as well.

At this point it may be reasonable to ask whether the stimulus effect of these hallucinogens in rats and monkeys has anything to do with the hallucinogenic effect in humans. Of course, it is impossible to say for sure one way or the other because we have no way of knowing whether a rat or a monkey experiences what we call a hallucination, but we do have evidence that suggests that the two effects are the same. There is a very high correlation between potency of a number of hallucinogenic drugs in humans and their potency in producing discriminable stimuli in nonhumans ($r = .964$) (Glennon, Rosecrans, & Young, 1982).

Two types of hallucinogens differ from the others in that they do not appear to use serotonin for their stimulus effects. They are the anticholinergics and the dissociative anesthetics PCP and ketamine. The stimulus properties of atropine and the anticholinergics can be blocked by central-acting cholinergic stimulants but not by those that act on the periphery; this fact indicates that the central cholinergic synapses mediate the effect of the anticholinergic hallucinogens.

It is interesting that the mixed opiate agonist/antagonist cyclazocine will generalize to PCP. It has also been demonstrated that there is generalization between cyclazocine, PCP, and a new drug called *SKF 10,047*, a powerful agonist at the sigma receptor. The stimulus effects of PCP are not affected by manipulations of serotonin level or by anticholinergics. The discriminable effects of PCP apparently arise from its effect at a specific receptor, probably the sigma receptor, and this effect is probably not mediated by any well-understood transmitter (Browne, 1982).

TOLERANCE

Tolerance develops rapidly to the effect of LSD, psilocybin, and mescaline on humans. If LSD is taken repeatedly, its effects disappear within two or three days; no amount of drug will be effective. This tolerance dissipates quickly, and sensitivity returns within a week. This is one reason why these drugs are seldom taken continually. The ability of LSD to disrupt the operant behavior of nonhumans also shows rapid tolerance. There is cross-tolerance between LSD and psilocybin and mescaline but no cross-tolerance between LSD and *d*-amphetamine or THC (Brown, 1972, p. 50).

Tolerance also develops to the effects of PCP. Users frequently only need a few puffs of a PCP-laced cigarette to get high when they first try the drug, but within two to six weeks, they are smoking one or two joints at a time to accomplish the same effect. Tolerance has also been demonstrated in nonhumans and appears to take place at physiological, pharmacokinetic, and behavioral levels (Balster, 1987).

WITHDRAWAL

No withdrawal symptoms to the serotonin or norepinephrine hallucinogens have been found, but research with nonhumans has shown that there may be some withdrawal after continual use of PCP. The symptoms include vocalizations, grinding of the teeth, diarrhea, difficulty staying awake, and tremors. No systematic studies of PCP withdrawal in humans have been done.

Withdrawal symptoms have been reported for people who abuse the synthetic anticholinergics. They include depression, and they can last for two weeks (Dilsaver, 1988).

SELF-ADMINISTRATION

In laboratory studies, nonhumans do not self-administer most hallucinogens. Mescaline, LSD,

DOM, and the anticholinergics are not self-administered, but there are exceptions. One is MDA, a synthetic mescaline-like drug that is chemically similar to amphetamine and shares some of its effects. It is likely that it is the amphetamine-like effects of MDA rather than its hallucinogenic properties that support self-administration. The other hallucinogen that is self-administered by nonhumans is PCP (Griffiths, Bigelow, & Henningfield, 1980). PCP is self-administered by monkeys, dogs, baboons, and rats either by intravenous infusion or orally (Balster, 1987; Carroll, 1993).

Not only do most hallucinogens lack reinforcing effects in nonhumans, but many also appear to have aversive effects. It has been demonstrated that laboratory animals work to avoid being given drugs like LSD and DOM. In one experiment, rhesus monkeys learned to press a lever to turn off a stimulus that normally preceded an infusion of LSD or DOM and thus prevented the infusion (Hoffmeister & Wuttke, 1975).

Outside the laboratory, however, there are reports that nonhumans will, from time to time, consume plants that contain hallucinogenic drugs. In fact, the hallucinogenic properties of some plants were supposed to have been discovered by observing the behavior of animals that had eaten the plants. For example, the hallucinogenic properties of the iboga root were supposedly first discovered when the natives of Gabon and the northern Congo observed that boars and gorillas ate the roots and went into a wild frenzy (Siegel & Jarvik, 1975). There are also reports that dogs in Hawaii enjoy eating *Psilocybe* mushrooms and that mongooses prefer to eat the species of toad that contains bufotenine.

The self-administration of hallucinogens in human cultures is almost universal and very ancient, but hallucinogen use is different from the use of most other drugs. First, with the possible exception of PCP, it is never continual. It is indulged in sporadically and on special occasions. The use of hallucinogens in most cultures is usually associated with religious ceremonies, and frequently the drugs are taken only by priests and shamans for the purpose of divination, talking to the dead, or seeking direction from a deity. Even in modern Western culture, hallucinogens are usually taken episodically. They may be used regularly by some people, but the rapid development of tolerance bars a continuous trip. At the height of its popularity in the 1960s, some people used LSD as often as possible and organized their lives around its use. These "acid heads" have become much less common in recent times and were likely a phenomenon of the hippie lifestyle. Unlike other heavily used drugs such as alcohol, hallucinogen use does not increase over time with most people. Initially, there may be a period during which a user will start taking the drug more frequently, but after a few years most hallucinogen users mature out; that is, they get tired of the experience, and their use decreases or stops altogether.

Patterns of PCP use are similar. Most users are experimental or occasional, but some become heavy chronic users. Unfortunately, in the case of PCP, there is no rapid development of tolerance to discourage continuous intoxication. Like that of the acid heads, a lifestyle goes along with heavy PCP use. Chronic PCP use begins as a social phenomenon and usually continues within a close-knit social group. The members of such groups develop family-like caring relationships and a loyalty that seldom develops in groups of users of any other drug. However, as PCP use intensifies, PCPers become more solitary and dissociate themselves from their group. At this point other social relationships also deteriorate (Linder, Lerner, & Burns, 1981).

HARMFUL EFFECTS

Acute Toxicity

Psilocybin, LSD, and mescaline are not very toxic. There are no recorded cases of anyone dying from an overdose of any of these drugs, but other hallucinogens have a lower safety margin. The synthetic analogues of mescaline, such as MDA and DOM, are more toxic, but there is still a fairly wide margin of safety with most of these drugs.

The anticholinergic hallucinogens are considerably more dangerous. These are traditional poisons and have been responsible for many deaths throughout history. They must be taken with great care. Fortunately, anticholinergics are not popular in modern Western culture and will probably remain unpopular because of their unpleasant side effects.

Of real concern is PCP. A lethal dose of PCP is 10 to 15 times the effective dose. Though toxic effects may vary, high doses cause coma, convulsions, and respiratory arrest. Brain hemorrhage and kidney failure have also been reported. The lethal effects of PCP are potentiated by the presence of depressant drugs such as alcohol or barbiturates in the body.

Psychotic Behavior

Again, the hallucinogens are sometimes also called *psychotomimetic* drugs (drugs that mimic psychosis), and indeed, there are many similarities between psychoses and the effects of the hallucinogens. However, the psychotic behavior seen under the influence of hallucinogens such as LSD, mescaline, and psilocybin apparently does not persist after the drug has worn off unless the person has psychotic tendencies already, in which case any powerful emotional experience would be sufficient to precipitate psychosis.

A great deal has been made in the media of the sort of behavior that may be provoked by the acute effects of such drugs. For example, stories appear occasionally about young LSD users jumping out of windows because they believed that they could fly. There are also reports of murders being committed under the influence of the drug. There can be no doubt that events such as these occur, but they are extremely rare and probably occur with no greater frequency under

the influence of LSD than under the influence of alcohol or any other drug.

Much more common, but of less concern, is the *acute psychotic reaction* or *freak-out*. This occurs when the user is having a "bad trip," an unpleasant experience. Freak-outs happen when the experience is unpleasant and the user forgets that the experience is caused by a drug. The user fears going permanently insane. The reaction is panic. Such panic reactions are not normally seen in experienced users and are frequently a result of an unusually high dose or a mixture of drugs. Panic reactions do not constitute a serious medical emergency. Panicky trippers can usually be *talked down*—put in close contact with someone who talks to them constantly, reassuring them that the state is drug induced and that it will get better. If their attention can be concentrated on this fact, the effects of the drug can be decreased and the panic dispelled. For example, in one case a young man reported after he was talked down from a freak-out that the drug was causing every object in his entire world to melt and change shape, but if he concentrated on the person talking to him, that person was the only object that remained constant.

One disturbing effect of many hallucinogens is that some of the effects may be experienced briefly at various times long after the drug has worn off. These episodes are called *flashbacks*. There is a similar effect called *trailing phenomena* in which objects seem to move in a jerky, discontinuous fashion as though being illuminated by stroboscopic light. No one understands flashbacks or trailing phenomena. They may occur unpredictably for years after even a single use of LSD. They normally last only a few seconds or minutes and are frequently associated with the use of other drugs such as marijuana or with times of emotional stress. One theory of flashbacks is that they are manifestations of a temporal lobe seizure, but there is little evidence to support this view (Hollister, 1978).

Acute behavioral effects of PCP can sometimes be responsible for injury and death. For example, users have drowned in pools or hot tubs while trying to swim to increase a sensation of floating. In addition, because the drug is an anesthetic, rather severe injuries have been tolerated or self-inflicted without pain or any effort at avoidance. Though the exact frequency of this sort of event has not been documented, it is probably more likely to happen with PCP than with LSD and the other serotonin-like and norepinephrine-like hallucinogens.

Long-lasting psychotic behavior has been reported after PCP use, even in individuals without any psychotic tendencies. This PCP psychosis may last several months.

Genetic Damage

In 1967, near the height of psychedelic revolution, when hallucinogens were being used widely by many young people, a paper was published in the journal *Science* by Maimon Cohen and his colleagues (Cohen, Marinello, & Back, 1967). The article was a report of an experiment in which LSD was added to a culture of blood cells. The cells were allowed to divide, and it was found that there was damage to the chromosomes of the white blood cells. This fact was widely reported in the popular press as evidence that LSD caused birth defects and cancer, and it served as the basis for a propaganda campaign against LSD. Since that first study there has been a torrent of research on the topic, but we do not seem to be much further ahead than in 1967. There is little doubt that LSD does break chromosomes in cultured cells in the laboratory, but other drugs, even aspirin, do this to the same extent. Studies with LSD users are confusing. Some have shown that there is more chromosome damage in their blood cells than in matched nonusers, but this finding has not always been replicated. It has also not yet been established whether this breakage, if it really does happen, has any significance for human health and reproduction. Studies are contradictory. Some show that LSD users have no greater incidence of babies with birth defects

than matched controls have, while other studies claim to have found that the rate of abortions, premature deliveries, and birth defects is slightly higher among LSD users than nonusers. Clearly, the burden of proof still rests with those who accuse LSD of genetic damage, but we should not forget that even though the LSD-caused genetic harm has not been proved, it cannot be assumed that there is no harm either (Grinspoon & Bakalar, 1979b). Remember, it took many years before the harmful effects of both tobacco and alcohol during pregnancy were documented.

Drugs can cause birth defects by means other than damaging genes. If the drug is present while the embryo is developing in the uterus, it is possible for a drug to interfere with certain stages of development and cause abnormalities without altering genes. Experimental testing of this sort, where LSD is given to pregnant females, cannot ethically be done on humans. In nonhumans, damage is only seen when very high doses of LSD, doses many hundred times higher than a normal human dose, are given to pregnant females. Though this sort of finding is unconvincing, it should not be ignored. It is always safer to avoid any sort of drug during pregnancy and not take chances.

CHAPTER SUMMARY

- *Hallucinogens* are a class of drugs that cause hallucinations. There are many kinds of hallucinogens that cause hallucinations by different physiological processes. Some resemble the neurotransmitter *serotonin*, some resemble *norepinephrine*, some are similar to *acetylcholine*, and others, like the *dissociative anesthetics*, are not similar to any neurotransmitter.

- LSD is an extremely potent hallucinogen that resembles serotonin. It is probably the best-known hallucinogen. It was synthesized in 1943 but did not become popular until the 1960s, when it was extensively used.

- *Psilocybin* and *psilocin* are found in the mushroom of the genus *Psilocybe*. Psilocybin is less potent than LSD but has similar effects. *Lysergic acid amide,* which is found in the seeds of the morning glory, is about a tenth as potent. *Dimethyltryptamine (DMT)* has effects very similar to those of LSD but is much shorter-acting. It is found in trees of the genus *Virola* in South America.

- *Bufotenine,* similar to DMT, is found in many species of plants and several animal species including toads and fish.

- *Harmine* and *harmaline* are found in the *Bainsteriopsis* vine of South America. They are less potent than LSD or DMT.

- *Ibogaine* is a drug from the root of the *iboga* plant of Central and West Africa. There are recent reports that ibogaine will eliminate opiate withdrawal and decrease motivation to use a wide variety of drugs.

- *Mescaline* is the prototype drug that resembles norepinephrine. It is found in the *peyote cactus* of the deserts of Mexico and the southwestern United States. Mescaline is about 1/400 as potent as LSD but has many LSD-like effects.

- Many synthetic mescaline-like drugs have been developed and were used widely during the 1960s. These include *MDA* and *DMA*. They are generally more potent and more toxic than mescaline.

- *Myristicin* and *elemicin* are found in nutmeg. Widely used as a spice, nutmeg is seldom used as a hallucinogen, probably because of its toxic side effects.

- A number of drugs resemble acetylcholine and act as *anticholinergics* because they block cholinergic transmission. Two are *atropine* and *scopolamine,* found in a wide variety of plants including *mandrake root, deadly nightshade* or *belladonna, henbane,* and *jimson weed* or *datura.*

- *Phencyclidine* (PCP) and *ketamine* are classed as dissociative anesthetics. They induce a trancelike state with feelings of euphoria, warmth, numbness, and body distortions.

- The subjective effects of hallucinogens are difficult to study. In general, the hallucinatory experience starts out with colored visions of tunnel, spiral, and lattice shapes that move. Meaningful images start to become incorporated into these images, and finally there is a rapid succession of meaningful scenes.

- Performance is usually impaired by hallucinogens because the user has difficulty remaining motivated and attending to the task.

- *Tolerance* develops rapidly to LSD. When it is taken repeatedly, its effects disappear in two or three days, but the tolerance disappears within a week. Tolerance also develops to PCP, but it is much less extensive and develops more slowly.

- With the exception of PCP and MDA, hallucinogens are not self-administered by nonhumans. In humans, hallucinogens are taken in an occasional or sporadic fashion, although PCP is sometimes used chronically. Most people mature out after a few years.

- Most hallucinogens are not toxic and have a high therapeutic index; however, PCP and the anticholinergics are much more dangerous, and overdoses are more likely. Some synthetic mescaline-like drugs are also very toxic.

Glossary

Acetaldehyde: a metabolite of ethanol. The body converts ethanol to acetaldehyde by the enzyme alcohol dehydrogenase.

Acetylcholinesterase: AChE; an enzyme that destroys acetylcholine.

Action potential: the momentary breakdown of the resting potential of a neuron.

Acute tolerance: the very rapid development of tolerance within a single drug administration, so that at the same blood level, the drug has less effect when blood level is falling than when it is rising.

Additive effects: occur when the presence of one drug shifts the dose response curve of another drug to the left. In other words, the drugs have similar effects that add together.

Adverse psychotic reaction: also known as a freak-out; after large doses of a hallucinogen, persons may lose touch with the fact that their condition is a result of taking a drug, and they panic. They may feel that they are going insane.

Agonist: a substance that causes the normal physiological change that occurs in response to the occupation of a receptor site.

Akathesia: a movement disorder sometimes seen in psychiatric patients using antipsychotic drugs.

Alcohol dehydrogenase: the enzyme that converts ethanol to acetaldehyde. The higher the level of alcohol dehydrogenase in the body, the faster ethanol is metabolized. This enzyme is also responsible for the conversion of methanol to formaldehyde.

All-or-none law: if a stimulus is sufficient to depolarize a neuron past its threshold, it will produce an action potential. All action potentials are the same no matter how strong the stimulus that produced them.

Amethystic: a drug believed to have the ability to antagonize the effect of alcohol.

Analgesic: a drug such as morphine or aspirin that relieves pain.

Anandamide: The name given to the endogenous substance that binds to the THC receptor.

Antagonism: drugs are said to be antagonistic if one drug shifts the dose response curve of the other to the right. In other words, one drug diminishes the effectiveness of the other. Also, a substance that will block the natural function of a transmitter is said to be an *antagonist* of that transmitter.

Anticholinergic: a drug that blocks cholinergic synapses. Such drugs stop the functioning of the parasympathetic nervous system and cause dilated pupils, blurred vision, and dry mouth.

Antiemetic: a drug that prevents nausea and vomiting.

Anxiolytics: this term refers to a class of drugs that includes the barbiturates and the benzodiazepines that relieve anxiety.

ARCI: Addiction Research Center Inventory; a paper-and-pencil test developed specifically to assess the abuse potential of drugs. The complete questionnaire consists of 550 true/false items covering a broad range of physical and subjective effects.

Artery: a blood vessel that carries blood away from the heart.

Ataxia: a decrease in movement or a loss of the ability to move.

Atypical antipsychotic drug: an antipsychotic drug that is effective against negative symptoms of schizophrenia and has minimal parkinsonian side effects.

Avoidance task: in a typical avoidance task an animal is given a signal that precedes an electric shock. The animal can avoid the shock if it responds during the warning signal. This task is often used to determine the effects of a drug on anxiety and fear, since it is presumed that it is the fear of the shock that motivates responding.

Axon: a projection from the cell body of a neuron that carries action potentials to synapses on other neurons.

Axon hillock: a place where an axon attaches to the cell body of a neuron.

BAL: blood alcohol level; the BAL is usually measured by the Breathalyzer and may be expressed either as a percent or in mg per 100 ml of blood.

Basal ganglia: two ganglia, the caudate nucleus and the putamen, that control movement.

Behavior therapy: a therapeutic approach based on operant and respondent conditioning. It seeks to change a person's behavior without being concerned with personality or motivation.

Behavioral teratology: also known as functional teratology. This is a malfunction in the brain that is expressed as a behavioral deficit and that has been caused by a teratogen during the development of the nervous system.

Behavioral tolerance: the development of tolerance as a result of either operant or respondent conditioning.

Behaviorism: a school of psychology founded by John B. Watson which maintains that the only thing that psychologists should study is behavior because behavior is public and observable and can be studied scientifically.

Between-subjects design: an experimental design where the control and experimental conditions are given to different groups of subjects.

Biogenic amines: see monoamines.

Bipolar disorder: a psychiatric condition where mood swings cyclically between mania and depression. It used to be called manic-depressive psychosis.

Blood-brain barrier: a covering on the capillaries in the brain and spinal cord that blocks many drugs that are not lipid-soluble from getting into the brain.

Bolus: an area of high concentration of a drug in the body just after it has been administered before it has had time to diffuse throughout the body.

Breaking point: the ratio of a progressive ratio schedule where an organism stops responding.

Cacao: this term refers to the cacao tree (*Theobroma cacao*) and its seeds.

Caffeinism: a disorder with symptoms of anxiety, insomnia, irregular heartbeat, and irritability caused by consuming too much caffeine.

Cannabinoids: drugs found in the cannabis plant. These include various form of THC, cannabinol, and cannabidiol.

Cannabis: a generic name given to plants of the species *Cannabis sativa*.

Capillary: the tiniest blood vessel, only big enough for a single red blood cell to pass through, that carries nutrients and removes wastes from body tissues.

Catecholamines: CA; a family of substances used as transmitters in the nervous system. They include epinephrine, norepinephrine, and dopamine.

Center: the name given to a grouping of cell bodies in the central nervous system; also called a nucleus.

Central gray: a system in the brain that mediates pain perception. It is also known as the periaqueductal gray.

CER: conditioned emotional response. A stimulus that reliably precedes a shock will cause an animal to suppress responding for food when it is presented, even though this suppression does nothing to diminish or avoid the shock.

Cerebellum: a large area at the back of the brain that controls the initiation and integration of movement.

CFF: critical frequency at fusion; the frequency at which a flickering light appears steady. It is a measure of visual sensitivity.

Chemical name: the name of a drug that indicates its chemical makeup and its structure. This name is usually long and has many letters and numbers.

Cirrhosis: scarring. Cirrhosis of the liver is the development of scar tissue in the liver. It can result from long-term, high-dose consumption of alcohol.

Clonidine: a drug that suppresses withdrawal symptoms from opiate drugs. It has been used to detoxify addicts maintained with methadone.

Coca: the bush from which cocaine is derived.

Cocaine freebase: the free radical of cocaine, usually made by separating the cocaine molecule from the hydrochloride molecule of cocaine HCl, the form in which cocaine is usually sold in the United States.

Cocoa: this term is used to refer to the processed products of the cacao bean.

Compliance: the extent to which a patient adheres to a regime of medical treatment.

Control group: the group or condition in an experiment to which the effect of an experimental manipulation is compared. In behavioral pharmacology, control subjects are usually given a placebo.

Cortex: the name given to the outer covering of an organ. In the brain the "cortex" is the cerebral cortex.

Crack: a crystalline form of cocaine made by mixing cocaine HCl with baking soda and water and then boiling away the water. Crack is consumed by inhaling the vapor when the crystals are burned. The presence of the base, the baking soda, speeds up the absorption and intensifies the effect.

Cross-dependence: occurs where one drug will relieve withdrawal symptoms of another drug.

Cyclic AMP: cyclic adenosine monophosphate; this substance serves several functions in the body. It is a second messenger in neural transmission, and it increases glucose production in cells.

Dale's principle: an early principle of neurophysiology formulated by Sir Henry Dale, which stated that each neuron normally makes, stores, and releases only one type of transmitter. A number of exceptions to this principle have been found.

Delirium tremens: the "DTs"; a stage of alcohol withdrawal characterized by profound disorientation, disorders of perception, tremors, restlessness, and hallucinations. It is normally seen only in a small percentage of alcoholics.

Dendrites: projections from the cell body of a neuron that receive information from other neurons.

Dependence: a state where withdrawal symptoms are seen when a repeatedly administered drug is discontinued or the dose is lowered.

Dependent variable: the variable in an experiment that is measured by the experimenter.

Depolarization: a reduction in the resting potential of a neuron. If the resting potential is reduced to the threshold, an action potential is generated.

Diffusion: the process by which substances move from an area of high concentration to an area of low concentration.

Disinhibition: an alcohol-produced effect where behavior normally suppressed by fear of adverse consequences is released.

Dissociation: the inability to transfer information acquired while under the influence of a drug to the nondrug state and vice versa. It is also known as state dependent learning.

Dissociative anesthetic: a category of hallucinogens developed as anesthetics that would not cause significant respiratory depression. The two that were developed were PCP and ketamine. PCP is still used as a veterinary anesthetic.

Distillation: a process where a fluid containing alcohol (usually a fermented beverage) is heated and the vapors are condensed. The condensed vapors have a higher alcoholic content than the original fluid.

Dopamine: DA; a catecholaminergic transmitter.

Dose response curve: DRC; a graph showing the effect of different doses of a drug. The horizontal axis shows the dose, and the vertical axis represents the effect.

Double-blind experiment: an experiment where neither the researchers nor the subjects know which subjects are in the experimental condition and which are in the control condition. This procedure controls for the influence of the placebo effect and experimenter bias.

DRL: differential reinforcement of low rates; a schedule where reinforcement is given for a response only if a fixed period of time has elapsed without any responding.

DSM-IV: the revised fourth edition of the *Diagnostic and Statistical Manual of Mental Disorders.* This manual is put out by the American Psychiatric Association (1994). It establishes the criteria for diagnosing mental disorders, and it is constantly undergoing revisions.

ED_{50}: the dose of a drug that has an effect on half of tested subjects, or the dose that produces half the maximum effect of the drug.

Elasticity: a measure of the nature of changes in demand for a product in response to changes in its price. Elastic demand means that as the price increases, demand declines at a faster rate, i.e., less is spent for the product (it has a coefficient greater than -1.0). If the same or more is spent on the product, demand is inelastic (it has a coefficient less than -1.0).

Endorphin: a combination of the words "endogenous" and "morphine," it refers to a string of amino acids (polypeptides) that is formed in the body and works at opiate receptors.

Enkephalin: a short string of amino acids (polypeptides) produced in the body, which acts at opiate receptors.

Enzyme induction: levels of enzyme can be increased by repeated administration of a drug that requires that enzyme for its metabolism.

Enzyme: a chemical in the body that speeds a chemical reaction. Enzymes in the body control metabolism.

EPSP: excitatory postsynaptic potential; depolarization of the postsynaptic membrane.

Escape: a task where an animal is required to make a response to escape from a noxious stimulus, usually an electric shock.

Experimenter bias: if an experimenter knows which subjects in an experiment belong to which group, this knowledge may influence the outcome of the research.

FDA: Food and Drug Administration. A branch of the United States government responsible for the classification and regulation of drugs.

Fermentation: the process by which yeasts convert sugar and water into ethanol and carbon dioxide. The term is also used to describe part of the curing process of tobacco and tea, but in these cases, true fermentation is not involved.

Fetal alcohol syndrome: FAS; a deformity in infants caused by the mother's alcohol consumption during pregnancy. Some symptoms include small eyes, drooping eyelids, and a misshapen mouth. Mental retardation may also be a component of the FAS.

Fixed interval (FI) schedule: on this schedule reinforcement is contingent on the first response to occur after a fixed period of time since the previous reinforcement or some other event. For example, on an FI 5 min, the first response after five minutes have elapsed is reinforced.

FI: see fixed interval schedule.

Fight/flight response: activation of the sympathetic nervous system that prepares the body for the sudden expenditure or energy at times of fear and anger.

First pass metabolism: any metabolism that takes place in the body (often in the stomach or liver) before the drug reaches general circulation.

Fixed ratio (FR) schedule: on this schedule reinforcement is given for the first response made after a certain fixed number of responses have been made. On an FR10, a reinforcement would be given for every tenth response.

Flavor toxicosis learning: a rapid, one-trial form of learning that occurs when an organism becomes sick after eating something new. In the future the organism will not like the taste of the new food and will resist eating it even though it may not have been the food that made it sick.

Fluidity: a change in the physical characteristics of membrane similar to swelling. It is a result of having molecules of alcohol or an anesthetic dissolved in the lipid layer of the membrane. This change may be responsible for the effects of these drugs on nervous tissue.

Formication: a sensation of having insects crawling just under the surface of the skin, also known as crank bugs or cocaine bugs. It is experienced after chronic high doses of an adrenergic stimulant like cocaine or amphetamine.

FR: see fixed ratio schedule.

GABA: gamma-aminobutyric acid, an inhibitory transmitter in the central nervous system.

Ganglion (plural, ganglia): the name given to a grouping of cell bodies of neurons in the peripheral nervous system.

Generic name: the shortened form of the chemical name of a drug that is generally used in research reports and textbooks.

Glial cells: cells in the nervous system that provide structural and metabolic support for the neurons. They have no excitable properties of their own.

Grand mal seizure: the most severe type of epileptic seizure.

Grayout: a period of time for which a person has no memory because of alcohol consumption. Memories can usually be restored by reminding the person of what happened. Grayout appears to be a result of an inability to recall while sober memories stored while intoxicated—in other words, dissociation.

Half-life: the length of time required for the body to get rid of half of the circulating drug.

Harrison Narcotic Act: an act passed in 1914 by the United States Congress that made it illegal to use opium and morphine and made it illegal for physicians to prescribe opiates to those addicted.

Hash oil: also known as red oil; it is made by extracting the cannabinoids from hashish in a solvent and then evaporating the solvent. It has a high drug content and is very potent.

Hashish: the resin that is extruded from the flowering top of the female cannabis plant.

Hemp: the common name for *Cannabis sativa;* it is more usually applied to the type of plant used primarily for fiber rather than the plant grown for consumption.

Hyperpolarization: increasing the resting potential of a nerve cell. This inhibits the cell by making it harder to fire.

Hypothalamus: a motivation control center in the brain. It is part of the limbic system and contains pleasure centers.

Iatrogenic: physician-caused. An iatrogenic disease or disorder is one that results from a medical treatment.

Independent variable: the variable in an experiment that is manipulated by the experimenter.

Indoleamine: a class of monoamine to which serotonin (5-HT) belongs.

Intramuscular: i.m.; an injection into a muscle.

Intraperitoneal: i.p.; an injection through the stomach muscle that leaves the drug in the peritoneal cavity.

Intravenous: i.v.; an injection directly into a vein.

Introspection: internal observation of what is going on in one's own mind, a method used by early psychologists.

Ion: a molecule or atom that carries an electric charge.

Ion channel: an opening or pore in the membrane of a nerve cell that allows specific ions to pass through. Some ion channels are open all the time (nongated channels), and others are opened by specific stimuli such as changes in membrane potential or the occupation of an associated receptor site (gated channels).

Ion trapping: the tendency for acids to ionize when dissolved in basic solutions means that they tend to get trapped on the basic side of a membrane. Similarly, bases get trapped on the acidic side of a membrane.

Ionophore: see ion channel.

IPSP: inhibitory postsynaptic potential; increase in the resting period of the postsynaptic membrane.

Korsakoff's psychosis: a disorder characterized by confusion and memory loss as a result of brain damage caused by heavy drinking.

L-DOPA: a metabolic precursor of the catecholamines.

LAAM: l-alpha-acetylmethadol; a synthetic opiate drug that can be taken orally and will prevent withdrawal symptoms in a heroin addict for three days. It has been used as a maintenance drug for heroin addicts.

Laudanum: a mixture of opium and alcohol that was a popular patent medicine in the nineteenth century.

LD$_{50}$: the dose of a drug that has a lethal effect in half of tested subjects.

Limbic system: an interconnected group of brain structures that controls motivation and emotion. Some of the centers that make up the limbic system are the hypothalamus, the amygdala, and the septum.

Lipid: another name for fat.

Locus coeruleus: a noradrenergic center in the lower brain that sends projections forward to the cortex and limbic system. Its functions include responding to stress, panic, anxiety, and modulation of mood and reinforcement.

Major tranquilizer: this term is sometimes used to describe a drug used to treat psychotic symptoms.

The term *antipsychotic* is more frequently used and is more accurate.

Mania: a highly aroused, excited state during which an individual may be delirious or agitated.

Manic-depressive psychosis: a condition where there are repetitive cycles in mood between mania and severe depression. The term *bipolar disorder* is now preferred.

MAO: monoamine oxidase; one of the enzymes used by the body to metabolize catecholamines.

MAO inhibitor: a type of antidepressant that increases levels of catecholamines by inhibiting the action of MAO.

Matching: a process where alcoholics are matched with particular treatments that will be maximally effective for their particular needs.

Matching law: law states that the relative rate of responding on an alternative will match the relative rate of reinforcement on that alternative.

Maturing out: as some drug users get older, they sometimes spontaneously discontinue or decrease their drug use.

Medial forebrain bundle: a bundle of axons running through the hypothalamus that is associated with pleasure centers.

Medulla: a section of the lower part of the brain that controls autonomic functioning.

Mescal: an alcoholic drink made by fermenting the agave cactus. It does not contain mescaline.

Mescal bean: also known as the red or coral bean. It contains cytisine and has in the past been used in ceremonies of the Indians of the southwest United States. The beans do not contain mescaline, but the ceremonies that used the mescal bean now use peyote, and this is probably the origin of the use of the word *mescaline* to refer to the active ingredient of peyote and of the term *mescal button*.

Mescal button: a dried slice of a peyote cactus.

Mescaline: a hallucinogen that resembles norepinephrine. It is the active ingredient of the peyote cactus.

Mesolimbic system: a dopamine brain system running between the ventral tegmental area and the nucleus accumbens that is responsible for reward. It is also thought to be the main site of action for antipsychotic drugs.

Metabolic tolerance: tolerance that is a result of increases in the metabolism of a drug.

Metabolite: a substance created by the metabolic processes of the body.

Methadone maintenance: a system of treating heroin addicts that is used widely in the United States; heroin withdrawal symptoms are blocked by daily administration of oral methadone.

Minor tranquilizer: this term is used to describe drugs such as the barbiturates and the benzodiazepines that are used to treat anxiety. The term *minor* distinguishes these drugs from the *major tranquilizers,* which are not really related and are used to treat psychosis.

Monoamines: MA; a class of chemicals that contains epinephrine, norepinephrine, dopamine, and serotonin. They are also referred to as biogenic amines.

Mucous membrane: a membrane that is normally kept moist, such as those in the mouth or eyes.

Muscarinic receptor: a cholinergic receptor that can be stimulated by muscarine and blocked by scopolamine or atropine.

Myelin: a fatty covering on axons that speeds transmission of action potentials along the axon.

Nabilone: a synthetic cannabinoid drug used to treat the nausea and sickness of people undergoing chemotherapy for cancer.

Naloxone: a pure opiate antagonist that blocks opiate receptors.

Narcotic: the term is short for "narcotic analgesic" and originally referred to the opiate drugs that made people sleepy (narcotic) and also relieved pain (analgesic). The term is now widely used to refer to many habit-forming drugs.

Native American Church: a religion started by the Indians of the southwestern United States. It is a combination of Christianity and their own traditional religious beliefs. They use peyote as part of their religious ceremony.

Negative symptoms: symptoms of schizophrenia referring to the absence of normal aspects of personality. These include alogia, impoverished speech, and affective flattening—diminished emotional expressiveness.

Nephron: a functional unit of the kidney.

Nerve: a bundle of axons in the peripheral nervous system.

Nesbitt's paradox: the paradoxical observation that smoking tobacco causes arousal, but most smokers report that they smoke to calm themselves.

Neuroleptic: a term that literally means "clasping the neuron." It refers to antipsychotic drugs.

Neuromodulator: a substance released in a synapse that causes a slow, long-acting effect on the reactivity of the postsynaptic cell, modifying its responsiveness to neurotransmitters. It may either increase or decrease the action of neurotransmitter, or it may shorten or prolong their activity.

Neuron: a nerve cell.

Nicotine bolus: when tobacco smoke is rapidly inhaled into the lungs, the blood in the lungs at that time receives a high nicotine content; this nicotine-charged blood is called a nicotine bolus, and the nicotine concentration may last for several seconds, long enough to reach the brain, before the nicotine is dispersed.

Nicotine bolus theory: a theory proposed by M. A. H. Russell that proposes that the nicotine bolus is the source of the reinforcing property of nicotine.

Nigrastriatal system: a dopamine brain system that runs between the striatum and the basal ganglia. It is responsible for smooth movement of muscles. It can be damaged by continued use of antipsychotics, resulting in a movement disorder resembling Parkinson's disease.

Operant conditioning: an operant is a type of behavior that is voluntary and is not elicited by a discrete, identifiable stimulus. The conditioning of an operant by the presentation of a reinforcer is called operant conditioning.

Opiates: a family of drugs that have properties similar to opium.

Opium: the sap derived from the ripened seedpod of the opium poppy. It contains morphine and codeine.

Optical isomer: when two drugs are identical except that one is the mirror image of the other, they are said to be optical isomers of each other. The two forms designated "l" and "d," are abbreviations of "levo" and "dextro."

Parasympathetic nervous system: the part of the autonomic nervous system that controls the normal vegetative functioning of the body such as digestion of food and regulation of heart rate and blood pressure.

Parenteral: a route of administration that involves injection.

Parkinson's disease: a movement disorder that is a result of a deficiency of dopamine in the basal ganglia of the brain.

Patch: the transdermal nicotine patch used to treat symptoms of nicotine withdrawal in smoking cessation programs.

Paw lick test: a test of analgesia where a rat is placed on a hot plate and the time before the animal licks its paw is measured. The longer the latency, the greater the analgesia.

Peptide: also polypeptide; a chain of amino acids linked in a specific order. Some peptides act as neurotransmitters and seem to work at opiate receptor sites.

Periaqueductal gray: a system in the brian that mediates pain perception. It is also known as the central gray.

Petit mal seizure: a mild epileptic seizure.

Phantasticant: another name for a hallucinogenic drug.

Phenotype: a group of individuals with similar appearance and characteristics, but not necessarily the same genetic makeup.

Phosphodiesterase: an enzyme that regulates the levels of cyclic AMP in the body.

Physiological tolerance: tolerance that is a result of compensatory changes in the physiology of the body that diminish the effect of a drug.

pKa: the pH at which a drug is 50 percent ionized.

Placebo: a simulated drug administration. A placebo could be a saline injection or a sugar pill. Placebos are frequently used as an experimental control in drug research.

Placebo effect: when a placebo is given to subjects who believe they are getting a drug, frequently they show effects of the drug they think they are getting.

Pleasure center: a center in the brain that causes the experience of pleasure when stimulated. It is also known as a "reward center" because nonhumans learn to work to receive electrical stimulation of this location.

PNS: peripheral nervous system; all the nerves outside the brain and spinal cord.

Positive symptoms: hallucinations, delusions, and thinking disorders indicative of schizophrenia.

Potentiation: see superadditive effect.

Profile of Mood States: POMS; a paper-and-pencil test designed to measure current mood. The subjects are asked to rate an adjective like "happy" or "nervous" on a five-point scale as to whether it applies to them at that moment.

Progressive ratio schedule: a schedule where the subject is required to work for a reinforcement on a fixed ratio that progressively gets greater and greater until the organism no longer responds. This technique is often used to determine the reinforcing power of a reinforcer.

Protein binding: a property of some drugs to attach themselves to protein molecules in the blood. Since the protein molecules cannot leave the blood, neither can a protein-bound drug, and it cannot get to its site of action.

Psychedelic: a term that means "mind-manifesting" that was used to describe hallucinogenic drugs. It refers to the ability of many of these drugs that cause feelings of insight into the psyche or mind.

Psychological tool theory: a theory of nicotine use that claims that people use tobacco in order to alter the level of arousal so that an optimal level will be obtained and the body will operate at peak efficiency.

Psychotomimetic: a drug that produces effects that mimic psychosis. The term was first used to describe hallucinogens, but it is not accurate. The state caused by LSD and many other hallucinogens is similar to, but distinguishable from, true psychotic behavior.

P300: a brain wave that appears in the EEG 300 milliseconds after an anticipated stimulus. Both alcoholics and their sons who have never had a drink show a diminished P300. This fact has been taken as evidence that the brains of alcoholics and those at risk of developing alcoholism are different from normal brains.

Punishment: when responding is suppressed because it is followed by an event such as an electric shock, it is said to be punished.

Raphé system: a system of nuclei in the brain that controls sleep.

Rate dependent effect: the effects of many drugs on a behavior seem to depend on the rate of the behavior that is being performed. Behavior being performed at a low frequency is usually speeded up, and high-frequency behavior is usually slowed.

Reinforcement: an event that will increase the frequency of an operant response upon which it is contingent. In a respondent conditioning task, the reinforcement refers to the presentation of the unconditioned stimulus.

REM rebound: an increase in the percentage of REM sleep when REM has been suppressed for a period of time and the REM suppressing agent is discontinued.

REM sleep: rapid eye movement sleep, also called paradoxical sleep; a period during sleep when the EEG shows rapid, low-voltage activity (beta waves) which is normally only seen during waking. The eyes also move rapidly under closed lids. REM sleep is usually correlated with dreaming.

Respondent conditioning: a respondent is a type of behavior like a reflex that is elicited by a discrete identifiable stimulus. The conditioning of respondents to conditioned stimuli (CS) is called respondent conditioning or classical conditioning.

Resting potential: the potential difference between the inside and the outside of a neuron. The inside is usually –70 millivolts with respects to the outside.

Reticular activating system: a diffuse projection system that activates the entire cortex when aroused by incoming stimuli. It maintains arousal in the cortex.

Reverse tolerance: occurs when the response to a drug increases with repeated administration; also known as sensitization.

Rush: an intense feeling of pleasure experienced after some drugs are injected intravenously or sniffed.

Saline: a weak solution of salt (sodium chloride). Normal or physiological saline is 0.09 percent salt. It resembles the salt concentration of body fluids.

Schedule-induced polydipsia: an organism can be induced to drink enormous quantities of water (or any drug) simply by delivering small quantities of food on a regular basis. The food may be a reinforcement for responding on an FI schedule, or it may not be contingent on any behavior.

Schedule of reinforcement: the pattern on which operant responses are reinforced.

Schizophrenia: a psychotic disorder that can take on various forms. It is generally characterized by a loss of touch with reality, feelings of paranoia, and erratic, confused speech.

Second messenger: a substance released inside a neuron in response to a neurotransmitter interacting with a receptor site on the postsynaptic membrane in a synapse. The second messenger causes a change in the resting potential or the reactivity of the postsynaptic cell.

Second order schedule: a schedule where a reinforcer is paired with a stimulus. The organism responds on a short schedule, e.g., an FR for the stimulus alone. Each of these FRs is considered as a single response on another schedule such as an FI 60 min. Thus the stimulus and the reinforcer are paired after the completion of the first FR after the end of the FI has been completed.

Sensitization: occurs when the response to a drug increases with repeated administration; also known as reverse tolerance.

SI units: Système International d'Unités. Many journals report drug concentrations this way. The SI unit is millimoles per liter (mmol/l).

Sigma receptor: a receptor site in the brain that is stimulated by several mixed agonist/antagonist opiates like cyclazocine. It is also thought to be affected by phencyclidine. Activity at this receptor is believed to be related to psychosis.

Somatic nervous system: the part of the peripheral nervous system made up of the motor nerves that control voluntary muscles, and the sensory nerves carrying information from the conscious senses into the CNS.

Speed ball: a combination of heroin and cocaine (or amphetamine).

Spontaneous motor activity: SMA; the total amount of behavior of an organism in an unstructured environment, usually an open field. Amount of activity may be measured by observation or a number of electronic or other automated means.

SSRI: selective serotonin re-uptake inhibitor. A class of antidepressant drugs, the best known of which is fluoxetine (Prozac).

State dependent learning: the inability to transfer information acquired while under the influence of a drug to the nondrug state and vice versa; also known as dissociation.

Stepping-stone theory: the theory that suggests that people progress from "soft" and relatively mild, harmless drugs to "hard" or powerful and dangerous drugs because they soon tire of the mild drug and crave something stronger.

Stereotyped behavior: the repetitive and compulsive performing of a simple behavior without obvious purpose. It is seen in both humans and nonhumans after high doses of MA stimulants and other drugs.

Subcutaneous: s.c.; an injection where the drug is left just under the skin.

Superadditive effects: potentiation; when the effect of two drugs mixed together is greater than added. This effect is usually apparent when one normally ineffective drug increases the effectiveness of a second drug.

Sympathetic nervous system: the part of the autonomic nervous system that prepares the body for the sudden expenditure of energy in time of crisis, as in the fight/flight response.

Sympathomimetic: a name given to a class of drugs that have effects on the body similar to arousal of the sympathetic nervous system.

Synapse: the place where action potentials from one neuron release chemicals that influence the firing of another neuron.

Synaptic cleft: the tiny gap between neurons at a synapse.

Synesthesia: a hallucinogenic experience where sensory experiences cross sensory modalities (sounds are seen and sights are heard, for example).

Tardive dyskinesia: an irreversible movement disorder often caused by continuous use of antipsychotic drugs.

Temporal disintegration: the loss in the ability to retain information in the short-term memory and to coordinate it for purpose. It is seen after consumption of cannabinoid drugs.

Teratogens: drugs that cause malformations of the fetus.

Terminal bouton: the enlargement at the end of an axon that forms the presynaptic part of a synapse.

THC: tetrahydrocannabinol. This term is used as an abbreviation for the name of one type of active ingredient in marijuana. Two of these ingredients are delta-9-THC and delta-8-THC.

Therapeutic window: the range of blood levels of a therapeutic drug between a level so low that it is not effective and a level so high that there are undesirable toxic effects.

Threshold: the lowest intensity of a stimulus or the smallest change in some property or a stimulus that can be detected by a sense organ.

Time course: a figure plotting the changes in the effects of a drug over time from the time it was administered.

Titration: adjusting a dose of a drug in order to maintain a particular blood level or effect.

Toad licking: the practice of licking, sucking, or otherwise obtaining the secretion or venom from the skin of toads. It is believed to contain bufotenine, a hallucinogen.

Tolerance: the decrease in potency of a drug with repeated administration or, conversely, the necessity to increase the dose of a drug in order to maintain the same effect when the drug is given repeatedly.

Tourette syndrome: a neurological disorder where patients show muscle ticks and involuntary vocalizations.

Tract: a bundle of axons in the central nervous system.

Trade name: the commercial name of a drug. The trade name is made up by a drug company, and the drug is marketed and advertised under this name. The trade name can be distinguished by the fact that it is always capitalized.

Tricyclic: a type of commonly used antidepressant.

Turkey drugs: These are preparations that look in all regards like a controlled psychoactive drug (e.g., amphetamine) but instead contain a drug or a combination of drugs that are not controlled substances such as caffeine.

Typical antipsychotic drug: an older type of antipsychotic drug that is effective against positive symptoms of schizophrenia and will cause parkinsonian symptoms.

Variable interval: VI; a schedule of reinforcement in which the reinforcement is given on the basis of the passage of time, but the length of time is randomly determined. On a VI 10 schedule, a subject would be reinforced on the average every 10 minutes.

Variable ratio: VR; a schedule of reinforcement on which the reinforcement is given on the basis of number of responses, but the number is randomly determined. On a VR 10 schedule, a subject would be reinforced on the average after every ten responses.

Vehicle: a liquid in which a drug is dissolved or suspended so that it becomes a fluid and may be injected.

Vein: a blood vessel that carries blood to the heart.

Vesicles: spherical structures in the terminal bouton that contain the neurotransmitter.

VI: see variable interval schedule.

Vigilance: the ability to detect a specific signal in an array of signals.

VR: see variable ratio schedule.

Wernicke's disease: damage to the brain caused by a deficiency of thiamin. It is common to many alcoholics and causes Korsakoff's psychosis.

Withdrawal symptoms: physiological changes that occur when a continually administered drug is discontinued or the dose is lowered. Usually, the higher the dose of the drug, the more severe the withdrawal. Withdrawal symptoms are different with different drugs.

Within-subjects design: an experiment design where the control and experimental conditions are given to the same subjects at different times.

References

Aaronson, B., & Osmond, H. (1970). *Psychedelics.* Garden City, NY: Anchor/Doubleday.

Abel, E. L. (1989). *Behavioral teratogenesis and behavioral mutagenesis.* New York: Plenum.

Abel, E. L., McMillan, D. E., & Harris, L. S. (1974). Delta-9-tetrahydrocannabinol: Effects of route of administration on onset and duration of activity and tolerance development. *Psychopharmacologia, 35,* 29–38.

Abel, E. L. & Sokol, R. J. (1989). Alcohol consumption during pregnancy: The dangers of moderate drinking. In *Alcoholism: Biomedical and genetic aspects,* ed. H. W. Goode and D. P. Agarwal (pp. 216–227). New York: Pergamon Press.

Adler, J., Abramson, P., Katz, S., & Hager, M. (1985, April 15). Getting high on "Ecstasy." *Newsweek,* p. 96.

Agurell, S., Lindgren, J., Ohlsson, A., Gillispie, H. K., & Hollister, L. (1984). Recent studies on the pharmacokinetics of delta-1-tetrahydrocannabinol in man. In *The cannabinoids: Chemical, pharmacological, and therapeutic aspects,* ed. S. Agurell, W. L., Dewey, & R. E. Willett (pp. 165–184). Orlando, FL: Academic Press.

Alarcon, R. de. (1969). The spread of heroin abuse in a community. *Bulletin on Narcotics, 21*(3), 17–22.

Alcoholics Anonymous. (1980). *Dr. Bob and the good oldtimers.* New York: Alcoholics Anonymous World Services.

Aldrich, A., Aranda, J. V., & Neims, A. H. (1979). Caffeine metabolism in the newborn. *Clinical Pharmacology and Therapeutics, 25,* 447–453.

Aldrich, M. R., & Baker, R. W. (1976). Historical aspects of cocaine use and abuse. In *Cocaine: Chemical, biological, clinical, social and treatment aspects,* ed. S. J. Mule (pp. 1–12). Boca Raton, FL: CRC Press.

Alexander, B. K., Beyerstein, B. L., Hadaway, P. F., & Coambs, R. B. (1981). Effects of early and later colony housing on oral ingestion of morphine in rats. *Pharmacology, Biochemistry and Behavior, 15,* 571–576.

Alexander, B. K., & Schweighofer, A. R. F. (1988). Defining "addiction." *Canadian Psychology, 29,* 151–162.

American Psychiatric Association. (1987). *Diagnostic and statistical manual of mental disorders* (3rd ed., rev.). Washington, DC.

American Psychiatric Association. (1994). *Diagnostic and statistical manual of mental disorders,* 4th ed. (DSM-IV). Washington DC.

American Society of Hospital Pharmacists. (1987). *Drug information '87.* Bethesda, MD: American Society of Hospital Pharmacists.

Anderson, K. (1975). Effects of cigarette smoking on

learning and retention. *Psychopharmacologia, 41,* 1–5.

Angrist, B., & Gershon, S. (1969). Amphetamine-induced schizophreniform psychosis. In *Schizophrenia: Current concepts and research,* ed. D. V. Sira Sinkar (pp. 508–524). Hicksville, NY: P.J.D. Publications.

Angrist, B., & Sudilovsky, A. (1978). Central nervous system stimulants. In *Handbook of psychopharmacology,* vol. 11, ed. L. L. Iverson, S. D. Iverson, & S. H. Snyder (pp. 95–165). New York: Plenum.

Annis, H. (1988). Patient-treatment matching in the management of alcoholism. In *Problems of drug dependence,* ed. L. S. Harris (pp. 152–161). NIDA Research Monograph 90. Washington, DC: U.S. Government Printing Office.

Arber, E. (1895). *English reprints: A counterblaste to tobacco* (by James I of England). Westminster: A. Constable.

Armitage, A. K. (1973). Some recent observations relating to the absorption of nicotine from tobacco smoke. In *Smoking behavior: Motives and incentives,* ed. W. L. Dunn (pp. 83–91). Washington, DC: V. H. Winston and Sons.

Armor, D. J., Polach, J. M., & Stambul, H. B. (1978). *Alcoholism and treatment.* New York: Wiley.

Arnaud, Maurice J. (1993). Metabolism of caffeine and other components of coffee. In *Caffeine, coffee and health,* ed. S. Garattini. New York: Raven Press.

Ashley, M. J. (1982). Alcohol consumption, ischemic heart disease and cerebrovascular disease: An epidemiological perspective. *Journal of Studies on Alcohol, 43,* 869–887.

Ashton, H. (1984). Benzodiazepine withdrawal: An unfinished story. *British Medical Journal, 288,* 1135–1140.

Ashton, H., & Stepney, R. (1982). *Smoking: Psychology and pharmacology.* London: Travistock Publications.

Aston, R. (1972). Barbiturates, alcohol and tranquilizers. In *The chemical and biological aspects of drug dependence,* ed. S. J. Mule & H. Brill (pp. 37–54). Cleveland, OH: CRC Press.

Ator, N., & Griffiths, R. R. (1992). Oral self-administration of triazolam, diazepam and ethanol in the baboon: Drug reinforcement and benzodiazepine physical dependence. *Psychopharmacology, 108*(3), 301–312.

Atweh, S. F., & Kuhar, M. J. (1983). Distribution and physiological significance of opioid receptors in the brain. *British Medical Bulletin, 39,* 47–52.

Austin, G. A. (1985). *Alcohol in Western society from antiquity to 1800.* Santa Barbara, CA: ABC-Clio Information Services.

An Autobiography of a Schizophrenic Experience. (1955). *Journal of Abnormal and Social Psychology, 512,* 677–689.

Axelrod, J., & Reisental, J. (1953). The fate of caffeine in man and a method for its estimation in biological materials. *Journal of Pharmacology and Experimental Therapeutics, 107,* 519–523.

Azorlosa, J. L., Greenwald, M. K., & Stitzer, M. L. (1995). Marijuana smoking, effects of varying puff volume and breathhold duration. *Journal of Pharmacology and Experimental Therapeutics, 272*(2), 560–569.

Babor, T. F. (1985). Alcohol, economics and the ecological fallacy: Toward an integration of experimental and quasi-experimental research. In E. Single & T. Storm, (eds.), *Public drinking and public policy* (pp. 161–190). Toronto: Addiction Research Foundation.

Babor, T. F., Berglas, S., Mendelson, J. H., Ellingboe, J., & Miller, K. (1983). Alcohol: Effect on the disinhibition of behavior. *Psychopharmacology, 80,* 53–60.

Babor, T. F., Mendelson, J. H., Greenberg, I., & Kuehnle, J. C. (1975). Marijuana consumption and tolerance to physiological and subjective effects. *Archives of General Psychiatry, 32,* 1548–1552.

Baekeland, F. (1977). Evaluation of treatment methods in chronic alcoholism. In *The biology of alcoholism,* vol. 5, ed. B. Kissen & H. Begleiter (pp. 385–440). New York: Plenum.

Baez, L. A. (1976). Effects of drugs on arousal and consummatory behavior. In *Behavioral pharmacology,* ed. S. D. Glick & J. Goldfarb (pp. 140–175). St. Louis, MO: Mosby.

Baird, D. D. (1992). Evidence for reduced fecundity in female smokers. In *Effects of smoking on the fetus, neonate and child,* ed. D. Poswillio & E. Alberman (pp. 5–22). Oxford: Oxford University Press.

Baker, R.C., & Jerrells, T. R. (1993). Immunological aspects. In *Recent developments in alcoholism,* vol. 11, ed. M. Galanter (pp. 249–271). New York: Plenum Press.

Baldessarini, R. J. (1985). *Chemotherapy in psychiatry: Principles and practice.* Cambridge, MA: Harvard University Press.

Balfour, D. J. K. (1982). The pharmacology of nicotine dependence: A working hypothesis. *Pharmacology and Therapeutics, 15,* 239–250.

Ball, J. C., & Snarr, R. W. (1969). A test of the maturation hypothesis with respect to opiate addiction. *United Nations Bulletin on Narcotics, 21,* 9–13.

Balster, R. L. (1987). The behavioral pharmacology of phencyclidine. In *Psychopharmacology: The third generation of progress,* ed. H. Y. Meltzer (pp. 1573–1579). New York: Raven Press.

Balster, R. L., & Ford, R. D. (1978). The discriminative stimulus properties of cannabinoids: A review. In *Drug discrimination and state dependent learning,* ed. B. T. Ho, D. W. Richards, & D. L. Chute (pp. 131–147). Orlando, FL: Academic Press.

Barnes, G., & Elthrington, L. G. (1973). *Drug dosage in laboratory animals: A handbook.* Berkeley: University of California Press.

Barone, J. J., & Roberts, H. (1984). Human consumption of caffeine. In *Caffeine: Perspectives from recent research,* ed. P. B. Dews (pp. 59–73). Berlin: Springer-Verlag.

Barrett, J. E., & DiMascio, A. (1966). Comparative effects on anxiety of the "minor tranquilizers" in "high" and "low" anxious student volunteers. *Diseases of the Nervous System, 27,* 483–486.

Barron, S. P., Lowinger, P., & Ebner, E. (1970). A clinical examination of chronic LSD use in the community. *Comprehensive Psychiatry, 11,* 69–79.

Barrows, S., & Room, R. (1991). Social history and alcohol studies. In *Drinking: Behavior and belief in modern history,* ed. S. Barrows & R. Room (pp. 1–25). Berkeley: University of California Press.

Barry, H., III. (1988). Psychoanalytic theory of alcoholism. In *Theories of alcoholism,* ed. C. D. Chaudron & D. A. Wilkinson (pp. 103–141). Toronto: Addiction Research Foundation.

Barry, H., III, & Kubina, R. K. (1972). Discriminative stimulus characteristics of alcohol, marijuana and atropine. In *Drug addiction: Experimental pharmacology,* vol. 1, ed. J. M. Singh, L. Miller, & H. Lal (pp. 3–16). Mt. Kisco, NY: Futura.

Barry, H., III, McGuire, M. S., & Krimmer, E. C. (1982). Alcohol and meprobamate resemble phenobarbital rather than chlordiazepoxide. In *Drug discrimination: Applications in CNS pharmacology,* ed. F. C. Colpaert & J. F. Slangen (pp. 219–233). Amsterdam: Elsevier Biomedical.

Battig, K., & Grandjean, E. (1957). Étude physiologique et pharmacologique d'une réaction de fuite conditionnelle chez le rat. *Journal de Physiologie, 49,* 41–44.

Baumeister, R. F., & Placidi, K. S. (1983). A social history and analysis of the LSD controversy. *Journal of Humanistic Psychology, 23*(4), 25–58.

Beasley, Joseph D. (1987). *Wrong diagnosis–wrong treatment: The plight of the alcoholic in America.* New York: Essential Medical Information Systems, Inc.

Becker, G. S., Grossman, M., & Murphy, K. M. (1988). An empirical analysis of cigarette addiction. *American Economic Review, 84*(3), 396–418.

Becker, H. S. (1963). *Outsiders: Studies in the sociology of deviance.* New York: Free Press.

Beckett, A. H., Gorrod, J. W., & Jenner, P. (1971a). Analysis of nicotine-l'-N-oxide in urine in the presence of nicotine and cotenine, and its application to the study of *in vivo* nicotine metabolism in man. *Journal of Pharmacy and Pharmacology, 23,* 55S–61S.

Beckett, A. H., Gorrod, J. W., & Jenner, P. (1971b). The effects of smoking on nicotine metabolism *in vivo* in man. *Journal of Pharmacy and Pharmacology, 23,* 62S–67S.

Belleville, J. W., Forrest, W. H., Shroff, P., & Brown, B. W. (1971). The hypnotic effects of codeine and secobarbital and their interactions in man. *Clinical Pharmacology and Therapeutics, 2,* 607–612.

Benet, S. (1975). Early diffusion and folk use of hemp. In *Cannabis and culture,* ed. V. Rubin (pp. 31–50). The Hague: Mouton.

Benowitz, N. L., & Henningfield, J. E. (1994). Establishing a nicotine threshold for addiction. *New England Journal of Medicine, 331*(2), 123–125.

Bergman, J., & Johanson, C. E. (1985). The reinforcing properties of diazepam under several conditions in rhesus monkeys. *Psychopharmacology, 86,* 108–113.

Bergsman, A., & Jarpe, G. (1969). Comments on free prescription of central stimulants and narcotic drugs. In *Abuse of central stimulants,* ed. F. Sjoquist & M. Tottie (pp. 275–279). Stockholm: Almqvist & Wiksell.

Berridge, V., & Edwards, G. (1981). *Opium and the people.* London: St. Martin's Press.

Besser, G. (1967). Some physical characteristics of auditory flicker fusion in man. *Nature, 214,* 17–19.

Betts, T. A., Clayton, A. B., & MacKay, G. M. (1972). Effects of four commonly used tranquilizers on low-speed driving performance tests. *British Medical Journal, 4,* 580–584.

Beveridge, G. W. (1971). The skin in acute barbiturate poisoning. In *Acute barbiturate poisoning,* ed. H. Matthews (pp. 129–134). Amsterdam: Excerpta Medica.

Bewley, T. H. (1974). Treatment of opiate addiction in Great Britain. In *Opiate addiction: Origins and treatment,* ed. S. Fisher & A. M. Freeman (pp. 141–161). New York: Wiley.

Bezchilbnyk, K. Z., & Jeffries, J. J. (1981). Should psychiatric patients drink coffee? *Canadian Medical Association Journal, 124*, 357–358.

Bickel, W. K., DeGrandpre, R. J., Higgins, S. T., & Hughes, J. R. (1990). Behavioral economics of drug administration: 1. Functional equivalence of response requirement and drug dose. *Life Sciences, 47*, 1501–1510.

Bickel, W. K., Highs, J. R., DeGrandpre, R. J., Higgins, S. T., & Rozzuto, P. (1992). Behavioral economics of drug self-administration: 4. The effects of response requirement on the consumption of and interaction between concurrently available coffee and cigarette. *Psychopharmacology, 107*, 211–216.

Bickerdyke, J. (1971). *The curiosities of ale and beer.* New York: Blom.

Bigelow, G., & Liebson, I. (1972). Cost factors controlling alcoholic drinking. *Psychological Record, 22*, 305–314.

Bixler, E. O., Scharf, M. B., Leo, L. A., & Kales, A. (1975). Hypnotic drugs and performance: A review of theoretical and methodological considerations. In *Hypnotics: Methods of development and evaluation,* ed. F. Kagan, T. Harwood, K. Rickels, & H. Sorer (pp. 175–195). Jamaica, NY: Spectrum.

Blier, P., & de Montigny, C. (1994). Current advances and trends in the treatment of depression. *Trends in Pharmacological Science, 15*(7), 220–226.

Boer, G. J., Feenstra, M. G. P., Mirmiran, M., Swaab, D. F., & Van Haaren, F. (1988). *The biochemical basis of functional teratology. Progress in brain research,* vol. 73. Amsterdam: Elsevier.

Boland, F., Mellor, C., & Revusky, S. H. (1978). Chemical aversion treatment of alcoholism: Lithium as the aversive agent. *Behavior Research and Therapy, 16*, 401–409.

Bonati, M., & Garattini, S. (1984). Interspecies comparison of caffeine disposition. In *Caffeine: Perspectives from recent research,* ed. P. B. Dews (pp. 48–56) Berlin: Springer-Verlag.

Bond, A. J., & Lader, M. H. (1973). The residual effects of flurazepam. *Psychopharmacologia, 32*, 223–235.

Bonnet, M. H., & Arand, D. L. (1992). Caffeine use as a model of acute and chronic insomnia. *Sleep, 15*, 526–536.

Boston, L. N. (1908). Delirium tremens (*mania e potu*). *Lancet, 1*, 18.

Bowers, M. B., Jr. (1987). The role of drugs in the production of schizophreniform psychosis and related disorders. In *Psychopharmacology: A third generation of progress,* ed. H. Y. Meltzer (pp. 819–823). New York: Raven Press.

Bows, H. A. (1965). The role of diazepam (Valium) in emotional illness. *Psychosomatics, 6*, 336–340.

Boyer, W. F., & Feighner, J. P. (1991). Side effects of the selective serotonin re-uptake inhibitors. In *Selective serotonin re-uptake inhibitors,* ed. J. P. Feighner & W. F. Boyer (pp. 133–152). Chichester, England: John Wiley & Sons.

Bozarth, M. A. (1983). Opiate reward mechanisms mapped by intracranial stimulation. In *The neurobiology of opiate reward processes,* ed. J. E. Smith & J. D. Lane (pp. 313–359). Amsterdam: Elsevier Biomedical.

Bozarth, M. A., & Wise, R. A. (1984). Anatomically distinct opiate receptor fields mediate rewards and physical dependence. *Science: 244*, 516–517.

Bozarth, M. A., & Wise, R. A. (1985). Toxicity associated with long-term intravenous heroin and cocaine self-administration in the rat. *JAMA, 253*, 81–83.

Brady, J. V., Griffiths, R. R., Heinz, R. D., Ator, N. A., Lucas, S. E., & Lamb, R. J. (1987). Assessing drugs for abuse liability and dependence potential in laboratory primates. In *Methods of assessing the reinforcing properties of abused drugs,* ed. M. A. Bozarth (pp. 45–86). New York: Springer-Verlag.

Braude, M. C., & Szara, S. (1976). *Pharmacology of marijuana,* 2 vols. Orlando, FL: Academic Press.

Brecher, E. M. & the editors of Consumer Reports (1972). *Licit and illicit drugs.* Mt. Vernon, NY: Consumers Union.

Brecher, E. M., Wang, B. W., Wong, H., & Morgan, J. P. (1988). Phencyclidine and violence: Clinical and legal issues. *Journal of Clinical Psychopharmacology, 8*, 397–401.

Brenesova, V., Oswald, I., & Loudon, J. (1975). Two types of insomnia: Too much waking or not enough sleep. *British Journal of Psychiatry, 126*, 439–445.

Brimblecombe, R. W., & Pinder, R. M. (1975). *Hallucinogenic agents.* Bristol, England: Wright-Scientechnica.

Britton, D. R., El-Wardnay, Z. S., Brown, C. P., & Bianchine, J. R. (1978). Clinical pharmacokinetics of selected psychotropic drugs. In *Handbook of psychopharmacology,* vol. 13, ed. L. L. Iverson, S. D. Iverson, & S. H. Snyder (pp. 299–344). New York: Plenum.

Bronson, M., Latour, C., & Nahas, G. G. (1984). Distribution and disposition of delta-9-tetrahydrocannabinol (THC) in different tissues in the rat. In *The cannabinoids: Chemical, pharmacologic, and therapeutic aspects*, ed. S. Agurell, W. L. Dewey, & R. E. Willette (pp. 309–317). Orlando, FL: Academic Press.

Brookes, L. G. (1985). Central nervous system stimulants. In *Psychopharmacology: Recent advances and future prospects*, ed. S. D. Iverson (pp. 264–277). Oxford: Oxford University Press.

Brooks, J. E. (1952). *The mighty leaf: Tobacco through the centuries*. Boston: Little Brown.

Brown, F. C. (1972). *Hallucinogenic drugs*. Springfield, IL: Thomas.

Browne, R. G. (1982). Discriminative stimulus properties of phencyclidine. In *Drug discrimination: Applications in CNS pharmacology*, ed. F. C. Colpaert & J. L. Slangen (pp. 109–122). Amsterdam: Elsevier Biomedical.

Bunney, W. E., & Garland-Bunney, B. L. (1987). Mechanism of actions of lithium in affective illness: Basic and clinical implications. In *Psychopharmacology: A third generation of progress*, ed. H. Y. Meltzer (pp. 553–565). New York: Raven Press.

Burg, A. W. (1975). Physiological disposition of caffeine. *Drug Metabolism Reviews, 4*, 199–228.

Busto, U., Issac, P., & Adrian, M. (1986). Changing patterns of benzodiazepine use in Canada. *Clinical Pharmacology and Therapeutics* (Abstr. A23), 184.

Butschky, M. F., Bailey, D., Henningfield, J. E., & Pickworth, W. B. (1994). Smoking without nicotine delivery decreases withdrawal in 12-hour abstinent smokers. *Pharmacology, Biochemistry and Behavior, 50*(1), 91–96.

Caddy, G. R., & Block, T. (1983). Behavioral treatment methods for alcoholism. In *Recent developments in alcoholism*, ed. M. Galanter (pp. 139–165). New York: Plenum.

Caldwell, J. (1976). Physiological aspects of cocaine usage. In *Cocaine: Chemical, biological, clinical, social and treatment aspects*, ed. S. J. Mule (pp. 187–200). Boca Raton, FL: CPR Press.

Callahan, M. M., Robertson, R. S., Branfman, A. R., McCormish, M. F., & Yesair, D. W. (1983). Comparison of caffeine metabolism in three nonsmoking populations after oral administration of radiolabelled caffeine. *Drug Metabolism and Disposition, 11*, 211–217.

Campbell, J. C., & Seiden, L. S. (1973). Performance influence on the development of tolerance to amphetamine. *Pharmacology, Biochemistry and Behavior, 1*, 703–708.

Campbell, J. H. (1971, October). Pleasure-seeking brains: Artificial tickles, natural joys of thought. *Smithsonian*, pp. 14–23.

Cannizzaro, G., Nigito, S., Provenzano, P. M., &

Vitikova, T. (1972). Modification of depressant and disinhibitory action of flurazepam during short-term treatment in the rat. *Psychopharmacologia, 26*, 173–184.

Cappell, H., & Pliner, P. (1974). Cannabis intoxication: The role of pharmacological and psychological variables. In *Marijuana: Effects on human behavior*, ed. L. L. Miller (pp. 233–264). Orlando, FL: Academic Press.

Cappendijk, S. L., & Dzoljic, M. R. (1993). Inhibitory effects of ibogaine on cocaine self-administration in rats. *European Journal of Pharmacology, 241*(2–3), 261–265.

Carlsson, A. (1969). Biochemical pharmacology of amphetamines. In *Abuse of central stimulants*, ed. F. Sjoquist & M. Tottie (pp. 305–310). Stockholm: Almqvist & Wiksell.

Carlsson, A. (1994). The search for the ideal medications: Developing a rational neuropharmacology. In *Schizophrenia: From mind to molecule*, ed. N. C. Andreasen (pp. 161–172). Washington, DC: American Psychiatric Press.

Carney, J. M. (1982). Effects of caffeine, theophylline and theobromine on schedule controlled responding in rats. *British Journal of Pharmacology, 75*, 451–454.

Carroll, M. E. (1993). The economic context of drug and nondrug reinforcers affects acquisition and maintenance of drug reinforced behavior and withdrawal effects. *Alcohol and Drug Dependence, 33*, 201–210.

Carroll, M. E. (1995). Reducing drug abuse by enriching the environment with alternative drug reinforcement. In *Advances in behavioral economics*, vol. 3, ed. L. Green, & J. H. Kagal (Chapter 2). Norwood, NJ: Ablex.

Carroll, M. E., & Meisch, R. A. (1984). Increases in food reinforced behavior due to food deprivation. In *Advances in behavioral pharmacology*, vol. 4, ed. T. Thompson, P. B. Dews, & J. E. Barrett (pp. 47–88). Orlando, FL: Academic Press.

Carroll, M. E., Rodefer, J. S., & Rawleigh, J. M. (1995). Concurrent self-administration of ethanol and an alternative nondrug reinforcer in monkeys: Effects of income (session length) on demand for drug. *Psychopharmacology, 120*, 1–9.

Carvalho, L. P. de, Greckshk, G., Chapouthier, G., & Rossier, J. (1983). Anxiogenic and non-anxiogenic benzodiazepine antagonists. *Nature, 301*, 64–66.

Castaneda, C. (1973). *The teachings of Don Juan*. Los Angeles: Simon & Schuster/University of California Press.

Chait, L. D., & Burke, K. A. (1994). Preference for high- versus low-potency marijuana. *Pharmacology, Biochemistry and Behavior, 49*(3), 643–647.

Chait, L. D., Evans, S. M., Grant, K. A., Kamien, J. B., Johanson, C. E., & Schuster, C. R. (1988). Discriminative stimuli and subjective effects of smoked marijuana in humans. *Psychopharmacology, 94*, 206–212.

Chait, L. D., & Griffiths, R. R. (1982). Differential control of puff duration and interpuff interval in cigarette smokers. *Pharmacology, Biochemistry and Behavior, 17*, 155–158.

Chait, L. D., & Perri, J. (1992). Effects of smoked marijuana on human performance: A critical review. In *Marijuana/Cannabinoids: Neurobiology and neurophysiology*, ed. L. Murphy and A. Bartke (pp. 387–424). Boca Raton, FL: CRC Press.

Chait, L. D., Uhlenhuth, E. H., & Johanson, C. E. (1986). The discriminative stimulus and subjective effects of *d*-amphetamine, phenmetrazine and fenfluramine in humans. *Psychopharmacology, 89*, 301–306.

Charney, D. S., Southwick, S. M., Delgado, P. L. & Krystal, J. H. (1990). Current status of the receptor sensitivity hypothesis of antidepressant action. In *Psychopharmacology of depression*, ed. J. D. Amsterdam. (pp. 13–34). New York: Marcel Dekker.

Chaudron, C. D., & Wilkinson, D. A. (Eds.). (1988). *Theories of alcoholism.* Toronto: Addiction Research Foundation.

Cheney, R. H. (1925). *Coffee.* New York: New York University Press.

Cherry, N., & Kernan, K. (1976). Personality scores and smoking behavior: A longitudinal study. *British Journal of Preventative and Social Medicine, 30*, 123–131.

Choptra, I. C., & Smith, J. W. (1974). Psychotic reaction following cannabis use in East Indians. *Archives of General Psychiatry, 30*, 24–27.

Churness, V. H. (1988). Antipsychotic agents. In *Clinical pharmacology and nursing*, ed. C. L. Bare & B. R. Williams (pp. 522–533). Springhouse, PA: Springhouse Publishing.

Cochin, J. (1974). Factors influencing tolerance to and dependence on narcotic analgesics. In *Opiate addiction: Origins and treatment*, ed. S. Fisher & A. M. Freeman (pp. 23–42). New York: Wiley.

Cocteau, J. (1968). *Opium: The diary of a cure*, trans. M. Crossland & S. Road. London: Peter Owen.

Cohen, M. M., Marinello, M. J., & Back, N. (1967). Chromosomal damage in human leukocytes induced by lysergic acid diethylamide (LSD). *Science, 155*, 1417.

Cohen, S., & Stillman, R. C. (1976). *The therapeutic potential of marijuana.* New York: Plenum.

Colpaert, F. C. (1977). Discriminative stimulus properties of benzodiazepines and barbiturates. In *Discriminative stimulus properties of drugs*, ed. H. Lal (pp. 93–106). New York: Plenum.

Colvin, M. (1983). A counselling approach to outpatient benzodiazepine detoxification. *Journal of Psychoactive Drugs, 15*, 105–108.

Conger, J. (1951). The effect of alcohol on conflict behavior in the albino rat. *Quarterly Journal of Studies on Alcohol, 12*, 1–29.

Consroe, P., & Sandyk, R. (1992). Potential role for cannabinoids for therapy of neurological disorders. In L. Murphy & A. Bartke (Eds.), *Marijuana/cannabinoids neurology and neurophysiology* (pp. 459–524). Boca Raton, FL: CRC Press.

Cooper, T. B. (1987). Pharmacokinetics of lithium. In *Psychopharmacology: A third generation of progress*, ed. H. Y. Meltzer (pp. 1365–1375). New York: Raven Press.

Costa, E. (1985). Preface. In *Chronic treatments in neuropsychiatry: Advances in biochemical pharmacology*, vol. 40, ed. D. Kemali & G. Racagni (pp. 5–6). New York: Raven Press.

Costello, R. M. (1980). Alcoholism treatment effectiveness: Slicing the outcome variance pie. In *Alcoholism treatment in transition*, ed. G. Edwards & M. Grant (pp. 113–127). London: Croom Helm.

Courvousier, S., Fournel, J., Ducrot, R., Kolsky, M., & Koetschet, P. (1953). Propriétés pharmacodynamiques du chlor-hydrate de chloro-3(diméthylamino-3'proply)-10-phenorthiazine (4.560 R.P.) *Archives Internationales de Pharmacodynamie et de Thérapie, 92*, 305–361.

Crawford, R. J. M. (1981). Benzodiazepine dependency and abuse. *New Zealand Medical Journal, 94*, 195.

Creasey, W. A. (1979). *Drug disposition in humans.* New York: Oxford University Press.

Cree, J. E., Meyer, J., & Hailey, D. K. (1973). Diazepam in labor: Its metabolism and effect on clinical condition and thermogenesis of the newborn. *British Medical Journal, 4*, 251–255.

Creese, I. (1983). Receptor interactions of neuroleptics. In *Neuroleptics: Neurochemical, behavioral, and clinical perspectives*, ed. J. T. Coyle & S. J. Enna (pp. 183–222). New York: Raven Press.

Crowley, T. J. (1987). Clinical issues in cocaine abuse. In *Cocaine: Clinical and behavioral aspects*, ed. S. Fisher, A. Raskin, & E. H. Uhlenhuth (pp. 193–211). New York: Oxford University Press.

Curson, D. (1985). Alcohol. In *Psychopharmacology:*

Recent advances and future prospects, ed. S. D. Iverson (pp. 254–263). Oxford: Oxford University Press.

Cushman, P. (1981). Neuro-endocrine effects of opioids. *Advances in Alcohol and Substance Abuse, 1*(1), 77–99.

Dahl, R. E., Scher, M. S., Williamson, D. E., Robles, N., & Day, N. (1995). A longitudinal study of prenatal use: Effects on sleep and arousal at age three years. *Archives of Pediatric and Adolescent Medicine, 149*(2), 145–150.

Daniell, H. W. (1971). Smoker's wrinkles: A study in the epidemiology of "crow's feet." *Annals of Internal Medicine, 75,* 873–880.

Darley, C. F., & Tinklenberg, J. R. (1974). Marijuana and memory. In *Marijuana: Effects on human behavior*, ed. L. L. Miller (pp. 73–102). Orlando, FL: Academic Press.

Darwin, C. (1882). *The descent of man*. New York: Appleton.

Davidson, E. S., & Schenk, S. (1994). Variability in subjective responses to marijuana: Initial experiences of college students. *Addictive Behaviors, 19*(5), 531–538.

Davis, D. L. (1962). Normal drinking in recovered alcohol addicts. *Quarterly Journal of Studies on Alcohol, 23,* 94–104.

Davis, J., Janicak, P., Linder, R., Maloney, J., & Avkovic, I. (1983). In *Neuroleptics: Neurochemical, behavioral and clinical perspectives*, ed. J. T. Coyle & S. J. Enna (pp. 15–64). New York: Raven Press.

Davis, T. R. A., Kensler, C. J., & Dews, P. B. (1973). Comparison of behavioral effects of nicotine, *d*-amphetamine, caffeine and dimethylheptyltetra-hydrocannabinol in squirrel monkeys. *Psychopharmacologia, 32,* 51–65.

De Freitas, B., & Schwartz, G. (1979). Effects of caffeine in chronic psychiatric patients. *American Journal of Psychiatry, 136,* 1337–1338.

DeGrandpre, R. J., Bickel, W. K., Rizvi, S. A. T., & Hughes, J. R. (1993). The behavioral economics of drug self-administration: 7. Effects of income on drug choice in humans. *Journal of the Experimental Analysis of Behavior, 59,* 483–500.

de Lint, J., & Schmidt, W. (1971). The epidemiology of alcoholism. In *Biological basis of alcoholism*, ed. Y. Israel & J. Mardones (pp. 423–442). New York: Wiley/Interscience.

De Long, F., & Levy, B. I. (1974). A model of attention describing the cognitive effects of marijuana. In *Marijuana, effects on human behavior*, ed. L. L. Miller (pp. 103–120). Orlando, FL: Academic Press.

Dement, W., & Kleitman, N. (1957). Cyclic variations in EEG during sleep and their relation to eye movements, body motility and dreaming. *Electroencephalograph and Clinical Neurophysiology, 9,* 673–680.

Deneau, G., Yanagita, T., & Seevers, M. H. (1969). Self-administration of psychoactive substances by the monkey: A measure of psychological dependence. *Psychopharmacologia, 16,* 30–48.

Deneau, G. A., & Inoki, R. (1967). Nicotine self-administration in monkeys. *Annals of the New York Academy of Sciences, 142,* 277–279.

Depoortere, R. Y., Li, D. H., Lane, M. W., & Emmett-Oglesby, M. W. (1993). Parameters of self-administration of cocaine in rats under a progressive-ratio schedule. *Pharmacology, Biochemistry and Behavior, 45,* 539–548.

De Quincey, T. (1901). *The confessions of an English opium-eater*. London: Macmillan.

De Ropp, R. S. (1961). *Drugs and the mind*. New York: Grove Press.

Desmond, P. V., Patwardham, R. V., Schenker, S., & Hoyumpa, A. M. (1980). Short-term ethanol administration impairs the elimination of chlordiazepoxide (Librium) in man. *European Journal of Clinical Pharmacology, 18,* 275–278.

Dewey, W. L., Martin, B. R., & Harris, L. S. (1976). Chronic effects of delta-9-THC in animals: Tolerance and biochemical changes. In *Pharmacology of marijuana*, vol. 2, ed. M. C. Braude & S. Szara (pp. 585–594). Orlando, FL: Academic Press.

de Wit, H. (1989). Ethanol self-administration in males with and without an alcoholic first-degree relative. Unpublished manuscript.

de Wit, H., & Chutuape, M. A. (1993). Increased ethanol choice in social drinkers following ethanol preload. *Behavioral Pharmacology, 4,* 29–36.

de Wit, H., & Griffiths, R. R. (1991). Testing the abuse liability of anxiolytic and hypnotic drugs in humans. *Drug and Alcohol Dependence, 28*(1), 83–111.

de Wit, H., & Johanson, C. E. (1987). A drug preference procedure for use with human volunteers. In *Methods of assessing the reinforcing properties of abused drugs*, ed. M. A. Bozarth (pp. 559–572). New York: Springer-Verlag.

de Wit, H., Johanson, C. E., & Uhlenhuth, E. H. (1984). Reinforcing properties of lorazepam in normal volunteers. *Drug and Alcohol Dependence, 13,* 31–41.

de Wit, H., Perri, J., & Johanson, C. E. (1989). Assessing pentobarbital preference in normal human volunteers using a cumulative dosing procedure. *Psychopharmacology, 99,* 416–421.

de Wit, H., Uhlenhuth, E. H., & Johanson, C. E. (1987). The reinforcing properties of amphetamine in overweight subjects and subjects with depression. *Clinical Pharmacology and Therapeutics, 42,* 127–136.

Dews, P. B. (1955). Studies on behavior: 1. Differential sensitivity to pentobarbital of pecking performance of pigeons depending on the schedule of reward. *Journal of Pharmacology and Experimental Therapeutics, 114,* 393–401.

Dews, P. B. (1958). Studies on behavior: 4. Stimulant actions of methamphetamine. *Journal of Pharmacology and Experimental Therapeutics, 122,* 137–147.

Dews, P. B. (1962). A behavioral output enhancing effect of imipramine in pigeons. *International Journal of Neuropharmacology, 1,* 265–272.

Dews, P. B. (1984). Behavioral effects of caffeine. In *Caffeine: Perspectives from recent research,* ed. P. B. Dews (pp. 86–103). Berlin: Springer-Verlag.

Dews, P. B., & Wenger, G. R. (1977). Rate dependency of the behavioral effects of amphetamine. In *Advances in behavioral pharmacology,* vol. 1, ed. T. Thompson & P. B. Dews (pp. 167–227). Orlando, FL: Academic Press.

Dietch, J. T., & Jennings, R. K. (1988). Aggressive dyscontrol in patients treated with benzodiazepines. *Journal of Clinical Psychiatry, 49,* 184–188.

Dilsaver, S. C. (1988). Antimuscarinic agents as substances of abuse: A review. *Journal of Clinical Psychopharmacology, 8,* 14–22.

DiMascio, A. (1973). The effects of benzodiazepines on aggression: Reduced or increased? In *The Benzodiazepines,* ed. S. Garattini, E. Musi, & L. O. Randall (pp. 433–440). New York: Raven Press.

Dinwiddie, S. H., & Farber, N. B. (1995). Pharmacological therapies of cannabis, hallucinogens, phencyclidine and volatile solvent addiction. In *Pharmacological therapies for alcohol and drug addiction,* ed. N. S. Miller & M. S. Gold, (pp. 213–216). New York: Marcel Dekker.

DiPadova, C., Roine, R., Frezza, M., Gentry, R. T., Baraona, E., & Lieber, C. S. (1992). Effects of ranitidine on blood alcohol levels after ethanol ingestion: Comparison with other H$_2$-receptor antagonists. *JAMA, 267*(1), 83–86.

DiPadova, C., Worner, T. M., Julkunnen, R. J. K., & Lieber, C. S. (1987). Effects of fasting and chronic alcohol consumption on the first-pass metabolism of ethanol. *Gastroenterology, 92,* 1169–73.

Ditmar, E. A., and Dorian, V. (1987). Ethanol absorption after bolus ingestion of an alcoholic beverage: A medico-legal problem, part II. *Canadian Society of Forensic Sciences Journal, 20*(2), 61–69.

Dole, V. P. (1980). Addictive behavior. *Scientific American, 234*(6), 138–154.

Domino, E., Rennick, P., & Pearl, J. H. (1974). Dose-effect relations of marijuana smoking on various physiological parameters in experienced male users: Observations on limits on self-titration intake. *Clinical Pharmacology and Therapeutics, 15,* 514–520.

Domino, E., Rennick, P., & Pearl, J. H. (1976). Short-term neuropsychopharmacological effects of marijuana smoking in experienced male users. In *Pharmacology of Marijuana,* vol. 1, ed. M. C. Braude & S. Szara (pp. 585–594). Orlando, FL: Academic Press.

Domino, E. F. (1967). Electroencephalographic and behavioral arousal effects of small doses of nicotine: A neuropsychopharmacological study. *Annals of the New York Academy of Sciences, 142,* 216–244.

Domino, E. F. (1973). Neuropsychopharmacology of nicotine and tobacco smoking. In *Smoking behavior: Motives and incentives,* ed. W. L. Dunn (pp. 5–32). Washington, DC: V. H. Winston and Sons.

Domino, E. F., & Yamamoto, K. I. (1965). Nicotine: Effect on the sleep cycle of the cat. *Science, 150,* 637–638.

Domjan, M. (1993). *Domjan and Burkhard's principles of learning and behavior.* Pacific Grove, CA: Brooks/Cole Publishing Company.

Dubowski, K. M. (1985). Absorption, distribution and elimination of alcohol: Highway safety aspects. *Journal of Studies on Alcohol* (Suppl.), *10,* 98–108.

Dundee, J. W., & McIlroy, P. D. A. (1982). A history of the barbiturates. *Anesthesia, 37,* 726–734.

Dunhill, A. H. (1954). *The gentle art of smoking.* New York: Putnam.

Dunlop, M., & Court, J. M. (1981). Effects of maternal caffeine ingestion on neonatal growth in rats. *Biology of the Neonate, 39,* 178–184.

Dworkin, S. I., & Smith, J. E. (1987). Neurobiological aspects of drug-seeking behavior. In *Advances in behavioral pharmacology, Vol. 6: Neurobehavioral pharmacology,* ed. T. Thompson, P. B. Dews, & J. E. Barrett (pp. 1–44). Hillsdale, NJ: Erlbaum.

Ebin, D. (1961). *The drug experience.* New York: Orion Press.

Eikelboom, R., & Stewart, J. (1982). Conditioning of drug-induced physiological responses. *Psychological Reviews, 89,* 529–572.

Ellenwood, E. H., Linnoila, M., Angle, H. V., Moore, J. W., Skinner, J. T., III, Easler, M.,

& Molter, D. W. (1981). Use of simple tasks to test for impairment of complex skills by a sedative. *Psychopharmacologia, 73*, 350–354.

Enna, S. J., & Coyle, J. T. (1983). Neuroleptics. In *Neuroleptics: Neurochemical, behavioral, and clinical perspectives*, ed. J. T. Coyle & S. J. Enna (pp. 1–14). New York: Raven Press.

Enna, S. J., & Eilson, M. S. (1987). Second-generation antidepressants. In *Handbook of pharmacology*, vol. 19, ed. L. L. Iverson, S. D. Iverson, & S. H. Snyder (pp. 609–632). New York: Plenum.

Evans, S. M., & Griffiths, R. R. (1992). Caffeine tolerance and choice in humans. *Psychopharmacology, 108*, 51–59.

Eysenck, H. J., & Eaves, L. J. (1980). *The causes and effects of smoking*. London: Maurice Temple Smith.

Fagerström, K. O., Schneider, N. G., & Lunell, E. (1993). Effectiveness of nicotine patch and nicotine gum as individual versus combined treatments for nicotine withdrawal symptoms. *Psychopharmacology, 111*, 271–277.

Falek, A., Madden, J. J., Shafer, D. A., & Donahoe, R. M. (1982). Opiates as modulators of genetic damage and immunocompetence. *Advances in Alcohol and Substance Abuse, 1*(3–4), 5–20.

Falk, J. L., & Feingold, D. A. (1987). Environmental and cultural factors in the behavioral action of drugs. In *Psychopharmacology: The third generation of progress*, ed. H. Y. Meltzer (pp. 1503–1510). New York: Raven Press.

Fehr, K. A., Kalant, H., LeBlanc, A. E., & Knox, G. C. (1976). Permanent learning impairment after chronic heavy exposure to cannabis or ethanol in the rat. In *Marijuana: Chemistry, biochemistry and cellular effects*, ed. G. G. Nahas (pp. 495–506). New York: Springer-Verlag.

Feighner, J. P., & Boyer, W. F. (1991). *Selective serotonin re-uptake inhibitors*. Chichester, England: John Wiley & Sons.

Feinberg, I., Jones, R., Walker, J., Cavness, C., & Floyd, T. (1975). Effects of marijuana extract and tetrahydrocannabinol on electroencephalographic sleep patterns. *Clinical and Pharmacological Therapy, 19*, 782–794.

Feldman, P. E. (1962). An analysis of the efficacy of diazepam. *Journal of Neuropsychiatry, 3*(Suppl. 1), S62–S67.

Ferguson, G. A. (1966). *Statistical analysis in psychology and education*. New York: McGraw-Hill.

Fielding, J. E. (1985a). Smoking: Health effects and control (first of two parts). *New England Journal of Medicine, 313*, 491–498.

Fielding, J. E. (1985b). Smoking: Health effects and control (second of two parts). *New England Journal of Medicine, 313*, 555–561.

Finagrette, H. (1988). *Heavy drinking: The myth of alcoholism as a disease*. Berkeley: University of California Press.

Finnegan, L. P. (1982). Outcome of children born to women dependent on narcotics. *Advances in Alcohol and Substance Abuse, 1*(3–4), 55–101.

Firebaugh, W. C. (1972). *The inns of Greece and Rome*. New York: Blom.

Fischman, M. W., & Schuster, C. R. (1982). Cocaine self-administration in humans. *Federation Proceedings, 41*, 204–209.

Fischman, M. W., Schuster, C. R., Resnekov, L., Shick, J. F. E., Krasnegor, N. A., Fennell, W., & Freeman, D. X. (1976). Cardiovascular and subjective effects of intravenous cocaine administration in humans. *Archives of General Psychiatry, 33*, 983–989.

Fitton, A., Faulds, D., & Goa, K. L. (1992). Moclobemide: A review of its pharmacological properties and therapeutic use in depressive illness. *Drugs, 43*(4), 561–596.

Fletcher, C., & Doll, R. (1969). A survey of doctors' attitudes to smoking. *British Journal of Social and Preventive Medicine, 23*(3), 145–153.

Ford, R. D., & Balster, R. L. (1977). Reinforcing properties of intravenous procaine in monkeys. *Pharmacology, Biochemistry and Behavior, 6*, 289–296.

Ford, R. D., Balster, R. L., Dewey, W. L., Rosecrans, J. A., & Harris, L. S. (1984). The discriminative stimulus properties of delta-9-tetrahydrocannabinol: Generalization to some metabolites and congeners. In *The cannabinoids: Chemical, pharmacologic, and therapeutic aspects*, ed. S. Agurell, W. L. Dewey, & R. E. Willette (pp. 545–561). Orlando, FL: Academic Press.

Forrest, D. (1973). *Tea for the British*. London: Chatto & Windus.

Forrest, W. H., Jr., Bellville, J. W., & Brown, B. W., Jr. (1972). The interaction of caffeine with pentobarbital as a nighttime hypnotic. *Anesthesiology, 36*, 37–41.

Frank, I. M., Lessin, P. J., Tyrrell, E. D., Hahn, P. M., & Szara, S. (1976). Acute and cumulative effects of marijuana smoking on hospitalized subjects: A 36-day study. In *Pharmacology of Marijuana*, vol. 2, ed. M. C. Braude, & S. Szara (pp. 673–680). Orlando, FL: Academic Press.

Fraser, H. F. (1957). Tolerance to and physical dependence on opiates, barbiturates and alcohol. *Annual Review of Medicine, 8*, 427–440.

Freemon, F. R. (1975). A critical review of the all-night polygraphic studies of sleeping medications. In *Hypnotics: Methods of development and evaluation*, ed. F. Kagan, T. Harwood, K. Rickels, A. D. Rudzik, & H. Sorer (pp. 41–57). Jamaica, NY: Spectrum.

French, R. V. (1884). *Nineteen centuries of drink in England*. London: Longman.

Frezza, M., DiPadova, C., Pozzato, G., Terpinm, M., Baraona, E., & Leiber, C. S. (1990). High blood alcohol levels in women: The role of decreased gastric alcohol dehydrogenase activity and first pass metabolism. *New England Journal of Medicine, 322*(2), 95–99.

Froehlich, J. C., & Li, T.-K. (1993). Opioid peptides. In *Recent developments in alcoholism*, vol. 11, ed. M. Galanter (pp. 187–205). New York: Plenum Press.

Garattini, S., Mussini, E., Marcucci, F., & Guaitani, A. (1973). Metabolic studies on benzodiazepines in various animal species. In *The benzodiazepines*, ed. S. Garattini, E. Mussini, & L. O. Randall (pp. 75–97). New York: Raven Press.

Gardner, E. L. (1992). Cannabinoid interactions with brain reward systems—The neurobiological basis of cannabinoid abuse. In L. Murphy & A. Bartke (Eds.), *Marijuana/cannabinoids neurology and neurophysiology* (pp. 275–336). Boca Raton, FL: CRC Press.

Garfield, E. (1983). Current comments. *Current Contents, 18*, 5–14.

Garfinkle, L., & Siverberg, E. (1991). Lung cancer and smoking trends in the United States over the past 25 years. *Cancer, 41*, 137–145.

Gautier, T. (1966). The hashish club. In *The marijuana papers*, ed. D. Solomon (pp. 163–178). Indianapolis: Bobbs-Merrill.

Gauvin, D. V., Cheng, E. Y., & Holloway, F. A. (1993). Behavioral Correlates. In *Recent developments in alcoholism*, vol. 11, ed. M. Galanter (pp. 281–30). New York: Plenum Press.

Gauvin, D. V., Harland, R. D., Michaelis, R. C., & Holloway, F. A. (1989). Caffeine-phenylethylamine combinations mimic the cocaine discriminative cue. *Life Sciences, 44*, 67–73.

Gawin, F. H., & Kleber, H. (1987). Issues in cocaine abuse treatment research. In *Cocaine: Clinical and behavioral aspects*, ed. S. Fisher, A. Raskin, & E. H. Uhlenhuth (pp. 174–192). New York: Oxford University Press.

Gay, G. R., & Inaba, D. S. (1976). Acute and chronic toxicology of cocaine abuse: Current sociology, treatment and rehabilitation. In *Cocaine: Chemical, biological, clinical, social and treatment aspects*, ed. S. J. Mule (pp. 245–252). Boca Raton, FL: CRC Press.

Geller, I., Bachman, E., & Seifter, J. (1963). The effects of reserpine and morphine on behavior suppressed by punishment. *Life Sciences, 4*, 226–231.

George, F. R., & Goldberg, S. R. (1989). Genetic approaches to the analysis of addiction processes. *Trends in Pharmacological Science, 10*, 78–83.

George, F. R., Ritz, M. C., & Elmer, G. I. (1991). The role of genetics in vulnerability to drug dependence. In *The biological basis of drug tolerance and dependence*, ed. J. Pratt (pp. 265–295). London: Academic Press.

George, W. H., & Marlatt, G. A. (1983). Alcoholism: The evolution of a behavioral perspective. In *Recent developments in alcoholism*, vol. 1, ed. M. Galanter (pp. 105–138). New York: Plenum.

Giannini, A. J., Burge, H., Shaheen, J. M., & Price, W. A. (1986). Khat: Another drug of abuse. *Journal of Psychoactive Drugs, 18*, 155–158.

Giannini, A. J., Miller, N. S., & Turner, C. E. (1992). Treatment of khat addiction. *Journal of Substance Abuse Treatment, 9*, 379–382.

Gilbert, R. M. (1976). Caffeine: A drug of abuse. In *Research advances in alcohol and drug problems*, vol. 3, ed. R. J. Gibbins, Y. Israel, H. Kalant, R. E. Popham, W. Schmidt, & R. G. Smart. New York: Wiley/Interscience.

Gilbert, R. M. (1984). Caffeine consumption. In *The methylxanthine beverages and foods: Chemistry, consumption and health effects*, ed. A. Spiller (pp. 185–213). New York: Alan R. Liss.

Gitlin, M. J. (1993). Pharmacotherapy for personality disorders: Conceptual framework and clinical strategies. *Journal of Clinical Psychopharmacology, 13*(5), 343–353.

Glad, W., & Adesso, V. J. (1976). The relative importance of socially induced tension and behavioral contagion for smoking behavior. *Journal of Abnormal Psychology, 85*, 119–121.

Glennon, R. A. (1987). Psychoactive phenylisopropylamines. In *Psychopharmacology: A third generation of progress*, ed. H. Y. Meltzer (pp. 1627–1634). New York: Raven Press.

Glennon, R. A., Rosecrans, J. A., & Young, R. (1982). The use of the drug discrimination paradigm for studying hallucinogenic agents: A review. In *Drug discrimination: Applications in CNS pharmacology*, ed. F. C. Colpaert & J. L. Slangen (pp. 69–98). Amsterdam: Elsevier Biomedical.

Glennon, R. A., Young, R., Martin, B. R., & Dal Cason, T. A. (1994). Methcathinone ("cat"): An enantiometric potency comparison. *Pharmacology, Biochemistry and Behavior, 50*(4), 601–606.

Glick, S. D., Kuehnle, M. E., Raucci, J., Wilson, T. E., Larson, D., Keller, R. W., Jr., & Carlson, J. N., (1994). Effects of iboga alkaloids on morphine and cocaine self-administration in rats: Relationship to tremorigenic effects and to effects on dopamine release in nucleus accumbens and striatum. *Brain Research, 657*(1–2), 14–22.

Glick, S. D., Rossman, K., Steindorf, S., Maisonneuve, I. M., & Carlson, J. N. (1991). Effects and aftereffects of ibogaine on morphine self-administration in rats. *European Journal of Pharmacology, 195*(3), 341–345.

Goas, J. A., & Boston, J. E. (1978). Discriminative stimulus properties of clozapine and chlorpromazine. *Pharmacology, Biochemistry and Behavior, 8*, 235–241.

Gold, M. S. (1995). Pharmacological therapies for opiate addiction. In *Pharmacological therapies for alcohol and drug addiction,* ed. N. S. Miller & M. S. Gold (pp. 159–174). New York: Marcel Dekker.

Gold, M. S., & Miller, N. S. (1995a). Pharmacological therapies for addiction, withdrawal, and relapse. In *Pharmacological therapies for drug and alcohol addictions,* ed. N. S. Miller & M. S. Gold (pp. 11–30). New York: Marcel Dekker.

Gold, M. S., & Miller, N. S. (1995b). The neurobiology of drug and alcohol addictions. In *Pharmacological therapies for alcohol and drug addiction,* ed. N. S. Miller & M. S. Gold (pp. 31–44). New York: Marcel Dekker.

Goldberg, L. (1943). Quantitative studies on alcohol tolerance in man: The influence of ethyl alcohol on sensory, motor, and psychological functions referred to blood alcohol in normal and habituated individuals. *Acta Physiologica Scandanavica* (Suppl.), *16*, 5.

Goldberg, S. R. (1976). The behavioral analysis of drug addiction. In *Behavioral pharmacology,* ed. S. D. Glick & J. Goldfarb (pp. 283–316). St. Louis: Mosby.

Goldberg, S. R., & Schuster, C. R. (1970). Conditioned nalorphine-induced abstinence changes: Persistence in post morphine-dependent monkeys. *Journal of the Experimental Analysis of Behavior, 14*, 33–46.

Goldberg, S. R., & Spealman, R. D. (1983). Suppression of behavior by intravenous injections of nicotine or by electric shocks in the squirrel monkey: Effects of chlordiazepoxide and mecamylamine. *Journal of Pharmacology and Experimental Therapeutics, 244*, 334–340.

Goldberg, S. R., Spealman, R. D., & Goldberg, D. M. (1981). Persistent behavior at high rates maintained by intravenous self-administration of nicotine. *Science, 214*, 573–575.

Goldman, D. (1993). Genetic transmission. In *Recent developments in alcoholism,* vol. 11, ed. M. Galanter (pp. 232–248). New York: Plenum Press.

Goldstein, A. (1964). Wakefulness caused by caffeine. *Naunyn-Schmiedebergs Archiv für Experimentelle Pathologie und Pharmakologie, 284*, 269–278.

Goldstein, A., Kaizer, S., & Warren, R. (1965). Psychotropic effects of caffeine in man: 2. Alertness, psychomotor coordination and mood. *Journal of Pharmacology and Experimental Therapeutics, 150*, 146–151.

Goldstein, A., Kaizer, S., & Whitby, O. (1969). Psychotropic effects of caffeine in man: 4. Quantitative and qualitative differences associated with habituation to coffee. *Clinical Pharmacology and Therapeutics, 10*, 489–497.

Goldstone, S., Boardman, W., & Lhamon, W. (1958). The effects of quintal barbitone, dextroamphetamine, and placebo on apparent time. *British Journal of Psychology, 49*, 324–328.

Golub, A., & Johnson, B. D. (1994). The shifting of importance of alcohol and marijuana as gateway substances among serious drug abusers. *Journal of Studies on Alcohol, 55*(5), 507–514.

Gorelick, D. A. (1993). Pharmacological treatment. In *Recent developments in alcoholism,* vol. 1, ed. M. Galanter (pp. 413–427). New York: Plenum.

Gorelick, D. A. (1995). Pharmacological therapies for cocaine addiction. In *Pharmacological therapies for alcohol and drug addiction,* ed. N. S. Miller & M. S. Gold (pp. 143–158). New York: Marcel Dekker.

Goth, A. (1984). *Medical pharmacology: Principles and concepts.* St. Louis: Mosby.

Graham, H. N. (1984). Tea: The plant and its manufacture; chemistry and consumption of the beverage. In *The methylxanthine beverages and foods: Chemistry, consumption and health effects,* ed. G. A. Spiller (pp. 29–74). New York: Liss.

Grant, K. A., & Barrett, J. E. (1991). Blockade of the discriminative stimulus effects of ethanol with 5-HT$_3$ receptor antagonists. *Psychopharmacology, 104*, 451–456.

Gray, E. G. (1983). Severe depression: A patient's thoughts. *British Journal of Psychiatry, 143*, 319–322.

Greden, J. F. (1974). Anxiety of caffeinism: A diagnostic dilemma. *American Journal of Psychiatry, 131*, 1089–1092.

Greden, J. F., Foutaine, P., Lubetsky, M., & Chamberlin, K. (1978). Anxiety and depression associated with caffeinism among psychiatric inpatients. *American Journal of Psychiatry, 135*, 963–966.

Greden, J. F., Proctor, A., & Victor, B. (1981). Caffeinism associated with greater use of other psychotropic agents. *Comprehensive Psychiatry, 22*, 565–571.

Greenblatt, D. J., & Shader, R. I. (1974). *The benzodiazepines in clinical practice.* New York: Raven Press.

Griffiths, P. (1967). *The history of the Indian tea industry.* London: Weidenfield & Nicholson.

Griffiths, R. R., Bigelow, G. E., & Henningfield, J. E. (1980). Similarities in animal and human drug taking behavior. In *Advances in substance abuse,* vol. 1, ed. N. K. Mello (pp. 1–90). Greenwich, CT: JAI Press.

Griffiths, R. R., Bigelow, G. E., & Lieberson, I. (1979). Human drug self-administration: Double-blind comparison of pentobarbital, diazepam, chlorpromazine and placebo. *Journal of Pharmacology and Experimental Therapeutics, 210*, 301–310.

Griffiths, R. R., Lamb, R. J., Sannerud, C. A., Ator, N., & Brady, J. V. (1991). Self-injection of barbiturates and benzodiazepines. *Psychopharmacology, 103*(2), 154–161.

Griffiths, R. R., Lucas, S. E., Bradford, L. K., Brady, J. V., & Snell, J. D. (1981). Self-injection of barbiturates and benzodiazepines in baboons. *Psychopharmacology, 75*, 101–109.

Griffiths, R. R., & Mumford, G. K. (1995). Caffeine—A drug of abuse? In *Psychopharmacology: The fourth generation of progress,* ed. F. E. Bloom & D. J. Kupfer. New York: Raven Press.

Griffiths, R. R., & Sannerud, C. A. (1987). Abuse and dependence on benzodiazepines and other anxiolytic/sedative drugs. In *Psychopharmacology: The third generation of progress,* ed. H. Y. Meltzer (pp. 1535–1542). New York: Raven Press.

Griffiths, R. R., & Woodson, P. (1988). Caffeine physical dependence: A review of human and laboratory animal studies. *Psychopharmacology, 94*, 437–451.

Grilly, D. M. (1989). *Drugs and human behavior.* Boston: Allyn & Bacon.

Grinspoon, L. (1969). Marijuana. *Scientific American, 221*(6), 17–25.

Grinspoon, L. (1971). *Marihuana reconsidered.* Cambridge, MA: Harvard University Press.

Grinspoon, L., & Bakalar, J. B. (1976). *Cocaine.* New York: Basic Books.

Grinspoon, L., & Bakalar, J. B. (1979a). The amphetamines: Medical uses and health hazards. In *Amphetamine use, misuse and abuse,* ed. D. R. Smith (pp. 260–274). Boca Raton, FL: CRC Press.

Grinspoon, L., & Bakalar, J. B. (1979b). *Psychedelic drugs reconsidered.* New York: Basic Books.

Grinspoon, L., & Bakalar, J. B. (1993). *Marijuana, the forbidden medicine.* New Haven, CT: Yale University Press.

Grinspoon, L., & Hedblom, P. (1975). *The speed culture.* Cambridge, MA: Harvard University Press.

Groppetti, A., & Di Giulio, A. M. (1976). Cocaine and its effect on biogenic amines. In *Cocaine: Chemical, biological, clinical, social and treatment aspects,* ed. S. J. Mule (pp. 93–102). Boca Raton, FL: CRC Press.

Gunne, L. M., & Anggard, E. (1972). *Pharmacokinetic studies with amphetamines: Relationship to neuropsychiatric disorders.* Paper presented at the International Symposium on Pharmacological Kinetics, Washington, DC.

Gupta, R. C., & Koefed, J. (1966). Toxicological statistics for barbiturates, other sedatives, and tranquilizers in Ontario: A ten-year study. *Canadian Medical Association Journal, 94*, 863–865.

Haefely, W. (1983). The biological basis of benzodiazepine actions. *Journal of Psychoactive Drugs, 15*, 19–40.

Haertzen, C. A., & Hickey, J. E. (1987). Addiction Research Center Inventory (ARCI): Measurement of euphoria and other effects. In M. A. Bozarth (Ed.), *Methods of assessing the reinforcing properties of abused drugs,* (pp. 489–524). New York: Springer-Verlag.

Haglund, B., & Cnattingius, L. (1990). Cigarette smoking as a risk factor for sudden infant death syndrome. *American Journal of Public Health, 80*(1), 29–32.

Hallstrom, C., & Lader, M. H. (1981). Benzodiazepine withdrawal phenomenon. *International Pharmacopsychiatry, 16*, 235–244.

Hanson, H. M., Witloslawski, J. J., & Campbell, E. H. (1967). Drug effects in squirrel monkeys trained on a multiple schedule with a punishment contingency. *Journal of the Experimental Analysis of Behavior, 10*, 565–569.

Harris, R. T., Glaghorn, J. L., & Schoolar, J. C. (1968). Self-administration of minor tranquilizers as a function of conditioning. *Psychopharmacologia, 13*, 81–88.

Harrison, W. M., Rabkin, J. G., Erhardt, A. A., Stewart, J. W., McGrath, T. J., Ross, D., & Quitkin, F. M. (1986). Effects of antidepressant medication on sexual function: A controlled study.

Journal of Clinical Psychopharmacology, 6(3), 144–148.

Heimstra, N. W., Bancroft, N. R., & De Kock, A. R. (1967). Effects of smoking on sustained performance on a simulated driving task. *Annals of the New York Academy of Sciences, 142*, 295–307.

Heise, G. A., & Boff, E. (1962). Continuous avoidance as a baseline for measuring the behavioral effects of drugs. *Psychopharmacology, 3*, 264–282.

Hembree, W. C., III, Zeidenberg, P., & Nahas, G. G. (1976). Marijuana's effect on human gonadal functions. In *Marijuana: Chemistry, biochemistry and cellular effects*, ed. G. G. Nahas (pp. 521–532). New York: Springer-Verlag.

Henningfield, J. E., Lucas, S. E., & Bigelow, G. E. (1986). Human studies of drugs as reinforcers. In *Behavioral analysis of drug dependence*, ed. S. R. Goldberg, & I. P. Stollerman (pp. 69–122). Orlando, FL: Academic Press.

Henningfield, J. E., Miyasato, K., & Jasinski, D. R. (1985). Abuse liability and pharmacodynamic characteristics of intravenous and inhaled nicotine. *Journal of Pharmacology and Experimental Therapeutics, 234*, 1–12.

Henningfield, J. E., Miyasato, K., Johnson, R. E., & Jasinski, D. R. (1983). Rapid physiological effects of nicotine in humans and selective blockade of effects by mecamylamine. In *Problems of drug dependence*. National Institute on Drug Abuse Monograph No. 43. Washington, DC: U.S. Government Printing Office.

Henricksson, B. G., & Järbe, T. U. (1971). The effect of two tetrahydrocannabinols (delta-9-THC and delta-8-THC) on conditioned avoidance learning in rats and its transfer to normal state conditions. *Psychopharmacologia, 22*, 23–30.

Herman, C. P. (1974). External and internal cues as determinants of the smoking behavior of light and heavy smokers. *Journal of Personality and Social Psychology, 30*, 664–672.

Heyman, G. M. (In press). Resolving the contradictions of addiction. *Behavioral and Brain Sciences*.

Higgins, S. T., Delaney, D. D., Budney, A. J., et al. (1991). A behavioral approach to achieving initial cocaine abstinence. *American Journal of Psychiatry, 148*(9), 1218–1224.

Higgitt, A. C., Lader, M. H., & Fonagy, P. (1985). Clinical management of benzodiazepine dependence. *British Medical Journal, 291*, 688–690.

Hirschorn, I. D., Hayes, R. L., & Rosecrans, J. A. (1975). Discriminative control of behavior by electrical stimulation of the dorsal Raphé-nucleus: Gen-

eralization to lysergic acid diethylamide (LSD). *Brain Research, 84*, 134–138.

Hirsh, K. (1984). Central nervous system pharmacology of the dietary methylxanthines. In *The methylxanthine beverages and foods: Chemistry, consumption and health effects*, ed. G. A. Spiller (pp. 235–301). New York: Liss.

Ho, A. K. S., & Allen, J. P. (1981). Alcohol and the opiate receptor: Interactions with the endogenous opiates. *Advances in Alcohol and Substance Abuse, 1*(1), 53–75.

Ho, B. T., & Johnson, K. M. (1976). Sites of neurochemical action of delta-9-tetrahydrocannabinol interaction with reserpine. In *Marijuana: Chemistry, biochemistry and cellular effects*, ed. G. G. Nahas (pp. 367–382). New York: Springer-Verlag.

Hoebel, B. G., Hernandez, L., Schwartz, D. H., Mark, G. P., & Hunter, G. A. (1989). Microdialysis studies of brain norepinephrine, serotonin and dopamine release during ingestive behavior. *Annals of the New York Academy of Sciences, 575*, 171–191.

Hoffmeister, F. H., & Wuttke, W. (1969). On the actions of psychotropic drugs on the attack and aggressive-defensive behavior of mice and cats. In *Aggressive behavior*, ed. S. Garattini & E. G. Sigg (pp. 273–280). New York: Wiley/Interscience.

Hoffmeister, F. H., & Wuttke, W. (1973). Self-administration of acetylsalicylic acid and combinations with codeine and caffeine in rhesus monkeys. *Journal of Pharmacology and Experimental Therapeutics, 186*, 266–275.

Hoffmeister, F. H., & Wuttke, W. (1975). Psychotropic drugs as negative reinforcers. *Pharmacological Reviews, 27*, 419–428.

Hollister, L. B., Motzenbecker, F. P., & Degan, R. O. (1961). Withdrawal reactions from chlordiazepoxide ("Librium"). *Psychopharmacologia, 2*, 63–68.

Hollister, L. E. (1978). Psychotomimetic drugs in man. In *Handbook of psychopharmacology*, vol. 11, ed. L. L. Iverson, S. D. Iverson, & S. H. Snyder (pp. 389–425). New York: Plenum.

Hollister, L. E. (1983). *Clinical pharmacology of psychotherapeutic drugs*. New York: Churchill Livingstone.

Holtzman, S. G. (1982). Discriminative stimulus properties of opioids in the rat and squirrel monkey. In *Drug discrimination: Applications in CNS pharmacology*, ed. F. C. Colpaert & J. L. Slangen (pp. 17–36). Amsterdam: Elsevier Biomedical.

Hommer, D. W., Skolnick, P., & Paul, S. M. (1987). The benzodiazepine/GABA receptor complex and anxiety. In *Psychopharmacology: The third genera-*

tion of progress, ed. H. Y. Meltzer (pp. 977–983). New York: Raven Press.

Horger, B. A., Wellman, P. J., Morien, A., Davis, B. T., & Schenk, S. (1994). Caffeine exposure sensitizes to the reinforcing effects of cocaine. *Motivation, Emotion, Feeding, Drinking, Sexual Behavior, 2,* 53–56.

Howlett, A. C., Evans, D. M., & Houston, D. B. (1992). The cannabinoid receptor. In *Marijuana/Cannabinoids: Neurobiology and neurophysiology*, ed. L. Murphy, and A. Bartke (pp. 35–72). Boca Raton, FL: CRC Press.

Huang, J., & Ho, B. T. (1974). Discriminative stimulus properties of *d*-amphetamine and related compounds in rats. *Pharmacology, Biochemistry and Behavior, 2,* 669–673.

Hughes, J. R. (1986). Genetics of smoking: A review. *Behavior Therapy, 17,* 335–345.

Hughes, J. R., Gust, S. W., Skoog, K., Keenan, R. M., & Fenwick, J. W. (1991). Symptoms of tobacco withdrawal: A replication and extension. *Archives of General Psychiatry, 48,* 52–59.

Hughes, J. R., Higgins, S. T., & Bickel, W. K. (1994). Nicotine withdrawal versus other drug withdrawal syndromes: Similarities and differences. *Addiction, 89,* 1461–1470.

Hughes, J. R., Higgins, S. T., Bickel, W. K., & Hunt, W. K. (1989, May). *Caffeine is a reinforcer in humans.* Paper presented to the Behavioral Pharmacology Society, Annapolis, MD.

Hughes, J. R., Higgins, S. T., Gulliver, S., & Mireault, G. (1987, June 6). *Dependence on caffeine in moderate coffee drinkers.* Paper presented to the International Study Group Investigating Drugs as Reinforcers, Philadelphia.

Hughes, J. R., Higgins, S., & Hatsukami, D. (1990). Effects of abstinence from tobacco: A critical review. In *Advances in alcohol and drug problems, Volume 10*, ed. L. T. Kozlowski (pp. 317–398). New York: Plenum.

Hunter, B. E., Walker, D. W., & Riley, J. N. (1974). Dissociation between physical dependence in volitional ethanol consumption: The role of multiple withdrawal episodes. *Pharmacology, Biochemistry and Behavior, 2,* 523–529.

Hutchison, R. R., & Emley, G. S. (1973). Effects of nicotine on avoidance, conditioned suppression and aggression response measures in animals and man. In *Smoking behavior: Motives and incentives*, ed. W. L. Dunn (pp. 171–196). Washington, DC: V. H. Winston and Sons.

Institute of Medicine. (1982). *Marijuana and health.* Washington, DC: National Academy Press.

Inturrisi, C. G., Schultz, M., Shin, S., Umas, J. G., Angel, L., & Simon, E. J. (1983). Evidence from opiate binding studies that heroin acts through its metabolites. *Life Sciences, 33*(Suppl. 1), 773–776.

Issac, P. F., & Rand, M. J. (1972). Cigarette smoking and plasma levels of nicotine. *Nature, 236,* 308–310.

Jaffe, J. H. (1987). Pharmacological agents in the treatment of drug dependence. In *Psychopharmacology: The third generation of progress*, ed. H. Y. Meltzer (pp. 1605–1616). New York: Raven Press.

Jaffe, J. H. (1992). Current concepts of addiction. In *Addictive states*, ed. C. P. O'Brien & J. H. Jaffe (pp. 1–21). New York: Raven Press.

Jaffe, J. H., Cascella, N. G., Kumor, K. M., & Sherer, M. A. (1989). Cocaine-induced cocaine craving. *Psychopharmacology, 97,* 59–64.

James, Jack J. (1991). *Caffeine and health.* London: Academic Press.

James, S. H., & Bhatt, S. (1972). Analysis of street drugs. *Journal of Drug Education, 2,* 197–210.

Janicak, P. G., Davis, J. M., Preskorn, S. H., & Ayd, F. J., Jr. (1993). *Principles and practice of pharmacology.* Baltimore, MD: Williams & Wilkins.

Janke, W., & DeBus, G. (1968). Experimental studies on antianxiety agents with normal subjects: Methodological considerations and a review of the main effects. In *Psychopharmacology: A review of progress, 1957–1967*, ed. H. E. Efron (pp. 205–208). Washington, DC: U.S. Government Printing Office.

Järbe, T. U. C., & Mathis, D. A. (1992). Dissociative and discriminative stimulus functions of cannabinoids/cannabinometics. In *Marijuana/cannabinoids neurology and neurophysiology*, ed. L. Murphy & A. Bartke (pp. 425–458). Boca Raton, FL: CRC Press.

Jarvik, M. E. (1970). Drugs used in the treatment of psychiatric disorders. In *The pharmacological basis of therapeutics*, ed. L. S. Goodman & A. Gillman (pp. 51–203). London: Collier-Macmillan.

Jarvik, M. E. (1973). Further observations on nicotine as the reinforcing agent in smoking. In *Smoking behavior: Motives and incentives*, ed. W. L. Dunn (pp. 33–50). Washington, DC: V. H. Winston and Sons.

Jarvik, M. E. (1979). Biological influences on cigarette smoking (NIDA Research Monograph No. 26). In *The behavioral aspects of smoking*, ed. N. E. Krasnegor (pp. 7–45). Washington, DC: U.S. Government Printing Office.

Jarvis, Martin J. (1994). A profile of tobacco smoking. *Addiction, 89,* 1371–1376.

Jasinski, D. R., Johnson, R. E., & Henningfield, J. E. (1984). Abuse liability assessment in human subjects. *Trends in Pharmacological Sciences, 5,* 196–200.

Javid, J. I., Musa, M. N., Fischman, M., Schuster, C. R., & Davis, J. M. (1983). Kinetics of cocaine in humans after intravenous and intranasal administration. *Biopharmaceutics and Drug Disposition, 4,* 9–18.

Jellinek, E. M. (1960). *The disease concept of alcoholism.* New Haven, CT: Hillhouse Press.

Jick, H. (1988). Early pregnancy and benzodiazepines. *Journal of Clinical Pharmacology, 8,* 159–160.

Jimerson, D. V. (1987). The role of dopamine mechanism in affective disorders. In *Psychopharmacology: A third generation of progress,* ed. H. Y. Meltzer (pp. 505–512). New York: Raven Press.

Johanson, C. E., & Uhlenhuth, E. H. (1980). Drug preference and mood in humans: Diazepam. *Psychopharmacology, 71,* 269–273.

Johnson, H. (1965). A case history: A surgeon's cure of tobacco habituation. *Medical Times, 93,* 437.

Johnson, K. M., Jr. (1987). Neurochemistry and neurophysiology of phencyclidine. In *Psychopharmacology: The third generation of progress,* ed. H. Y. Meltzer (pp. 1581–1588). New York: Raven Press.

Johnston, L. D., O'Malley, P. M., & Bachman, J. G. (1994). National Survey results in drug use. In *Monitoring the future study (Volume 2, 1975–1993)* (pp. 11–25). Washington, DC: National Institute on Drug Abuse, U.S. Department of Health and Human Services.

Jones, E. (1953). *Sigmund Freud: Life and work,* vol. 1. London: Hogarth Press.

Jones, K. L., & Smith, D. W. (1975). The fetal alcohol syndrome. *Teratology, 12,* 1–10.

Jones, R. (1987). Tobacco dependence. In *Psychopharmacology: The third generation of progress,* ed. H. Y. Meltzer (pp. 1589–1595). New York: Raven Press.

Jones, R. T. (1978). Marijuana: Human effects. In *Handbook of psychopharmacology,* vol. 12, ed. L. L. Iverson, S. D. Iverson, & S. H. Snyder (pp. 373–412). New York: Plenum.

Jones, R. T., & Benowitz, N. (1976). The 30-day trip: Clinical studies of cannabis tolerance and dependence. In *Pharmacology of marijuana,* vol. 2, ed. M. C. Braude & S. Szara (pp. 627–642). Orlando, FL: Academic Press.

Jowett, B. (1931). *The dialogues of Plato,* vol. 5 (3rd ed.). London: Oxford University Press.

Judd, L. J., Squire, L. R., Butters, N., Salmon, D. P., & Paller, K. A. (1987). Effects of psychotropic drugs on cognition and memory in normal humans and animals. In *Psychopharmacology: A third generation of progress,* ed. H. Y. Meltzer (pp. 1467–1475). New York: Raven Press.

Juergens, S. M. (1993). Benzodiazepines and addiction. *Psychiatric Clinics of North America, 16*(1), 75–86.

June, H. L., Colker, R. E., Domanagu, K. R., et al. (1992). Ethanol self-administration in deprived rats: Effects of RO-4513 alone and in combination with flumazenil (RO 15–1788). *Alcoholism: Clinical and Experimental Research, 16,* 11–16.

Kalant, H., & Kalant, O. J. (1979). Death in amphetamine users: Causes and rates. In *Amphetamine use, misuse and abuse,* ed. D. R. Smith (pp. 169–188). Boca Raton, FL: CRC Press.

Kalant, H., LeBlanc, E., & Gibbins, R. J. (1971). Tolerance to, and dependence on, ethanol. In *Biological basis of alcoholism,* ed. Y. Israel and J. Mardonez (pp. 235–269). New York: Wiley/Interscience.

Kalant, O. J. (1973). *The amphetamines* (2nd ed.), Toronto: University of Toronto Press and Charles C. Thomas.

Kalix, P. (1994). Khat, an amphetamine-like stimulant. *Journal of Psychoactive Drugs, 26*(1), 69–74.

Kallman, W. M., Kallman, M. J., Harry, G. J., Woodson, P. P., & Rosecrans, J. A. (1982). Nicotine as a discriminative stimulus in human subjects. In *Drug discrimination: Applications in CNS pharmacology,* ed. F. C. Colpaert & J. L. Slangen (pp. 211–218). Amsterdam: Elsevier Biomedical.

Kaminski, B. J., & Griffiths, R. R. (1994). Intravenous self-injection of Methcathinone in the baboon. *Pharmacology, Biochemistry and Behavior, 47,* 981–983.

Kanarek, R. B., & Marks-Kaufman, R. (1988). Dietary modulation of oral amphetamine intake in rats. *Physiology and Behavior, 44,* 501–505.

Kanarek, R. B., & Marks-Kaufman, R. (1989). Environmental modulation of drug self-administration. Paper presented to the Behavior Pharmacology Society, Annapolis, MD.

Kane, J. M. (1994). Efficacy, mechanisms, and side effects of typical and atypical neuroleptics. In N. C. Andreasen (ed.), *Schizophrenia: From mind to molecule* (pp. 173–188). Washington, DC: American Psychiatric Press.

Kay, D. C., Eisenstein, R. B., & Jasinski, D. R. (1969). Morphine effects on human REM state, waking state and NREM sleep. *Psychopharmacologia, 14,* 404–416.

Kaye, S., & Haag, H. B. (1957). Terminal blood alcohol concentration in ninety-four fatal cases of acute alcoholism. *JAMA, 165*, 451–452.

Keenan, R. M., Henningfield, J. E., & Jarvik, M. E. (1995). Pharmacological therapies: Nicotine addiction. In *Pharmacological therapies for alcohol and drug addiction*, ed. N. S. Miller & M. S. Gold (pp. 239–264). New York: Marcel Dekker.

Kelleher, R. T. (1976). Characteristics of behavior controlled by scheduled injections of drugs. *Pharmacological Reviews, 27*, 307–323.

Kelleher, R. T., & Morse, W. H. (1964). Escape behavior and punished behavior. *Federation Proceedings, 22*, 808–817.

Kelleher, R. T., & Morse, W. H. (1968). Schedules using noxious stimuli: 3. Responding maintained with response-produced electric shocks. *Journal of the Experimental Analysis of Behavior, 11*, 819–838.

Keller, M. (1972). The oddities of alcoholics. *Quarterly Journal of Studies on Alcohol, 33*, 1147–1148.

Kellogg, C. K. (1988). Benzodiazepines: Influence on the developing brain. In *Biochemical basis of functioning neuroteratology: Permanent effects of chemicals on the developing brain*, vol. 73, ed. G. R. Boer, M. G. P. Feenstra, M. Mirmiran, D. F. Swaab, & F. Van Haaren (pp. 207–228). Amsterdam: Elsevier Biomedical.

Kellogg, C. K., Tervo, D., Ison, J., Paisi, T., & Miller, R. K. (1980). Prenatal exposure to diazepam alters behavioral development in rats. *Science, 207*, 205–207.

Kelly, T. H., Foltin, R. W., Mayr, M. T. & Fishman, M. W. (1994). Effects of delta-9-tetrahydrocannabinol and social context on marijuana self-administration by humans. *Pharmacology, Biochemistry and Behavior, 49*(3), 763–768.

Kephalis, T. A., Burns, J., Michael, C. M., Miras, C. J., & Papidakis, D. P. (1976). Some aspects of cannabis smoke chemistry. In *Marijuana: Chemistry, biochemistry and cellular effects*, ed. G. G. Nahas (pp. 39–50). New York: Springer-Verlag.

Kihlman, B. A. (1977). *Caffeine and chromosomes*. Amsterdam: Elsevier.

Kissen, B., & Kaley, M. M. (1974). Alcohol and cancer. In *The biology of alcoholism*, vol. 3, ed. B. Kissen & H. Begleiter (pp. 481–511). New York: Plenum.

Kleber, H. D. (1974). Clinical experiences with narcotic antagonists. In *Opiate addiction: Origins and treatment*, ed. S. Fisher & A. M. Freeman (pp. 211–220). New York: Wiley.

Klonoff, H. (1974). Effects of marijuana on driving in a restricted area and on city streets: Driving performance and physiological changes. In *Marijuana, effects on human behavior*, ed. L. L. Miller (pp. 359–397). Orlando, FL: Academic Press.

Kluver, H. (1966). *Mescal and mechanisms of hallucination*. Chicago: University of Chicago Press.

Kobler, J. (1973). *Ardent spirits: The rise and fall of prohibition*. New York: Putnam.

Kocsis, J. H., Shaw, E. D., Wilner, P., et al. (1993). Neuropsychiatric effects of lithium discontinuation. *Journal of Clinical Psychopharmacology, 13*(4), 268–275.

Kolata, G. (1991). Temperance: An old cycle repeats itself. *New York Times, 40*, 35.

Kolodny, R. C. (1975). Research issues in the study of marijuana and male reproductive physiology in humans. In *Marijuana and health hazards*, ed. J. R. Tinklenberg (pp. 71–81). Orlando, FL: Academic Press.

Kosersky, D. S., McMillan, D. E., & Harris, L. S. (1974). Delta-9-tetrahydrocannabinol and 11-hydroxy-delta-9-tetrahydrocannabinol: Behavioral effects and tolerance development. *Journal of Pharmacology and Experimental Therapeutics, 189*, 61–65.

Kozlowski, L. T., & Henningfield, J. E. (1995). Thinking the unthinkable: The prospect of regulation of nicotine in cigarettes by the United States government. *Addiction, 90*, 165–167.

Kramer, M. S. (1987). Determinants of low birthweight: Methodological assessment and meta-analysis. *Bulletin of the World Health Organization, 65*, 663–737.

Kramer, P. D. (1993). *Listening to Prozac*. New York: Viking.

Kreek, M. J. (1982). Opioid disposition and effects during chronic exposure in the perinatal period in man. *Advances in Alcohol and Substance Abuse, 1*(3–4), 21–53.

Krimmer, E. C., & Barry, H., III. (1977). Discriminative stimuli produced by marijuana constituents. In *Discriminative stimulus properties of drugs*, ed. H. Lal (pp. 121–136). New York: Plenum.

Kuhn, D. M., White, F. J., & Appel, J. B. (1977). Discriminative stimulus properties of hallucinogens: Behavioral assay of drug action. In *Discriminative stimulus properties of drugs*, ed. H. Lal (pp. 137–154). New York: Plenum.

Kulhanek, F., Linde, O. K., & Meisenberg, G. (1979). Precipitation of antipsychotic drugs in interaction with coffee or tea. *Lancet, 2*, 1130.

Kumor, K., Sherer, M., Muntander, C., Jaffee, J. H., & Herning, R. (1988). Pharmacological aspects of cocaine rush. In *Problems of drug dependence, 1988*, ed. L. S. Harris (NIDA Research Monograph No. 90). Washington, DC: U.S. Government Printing Office.

Kurtz, N. M. (1990). Monoamine oxidase inhibiting drugs. In *Pharmacotherapy of depression*, ed. J. D. Amsterdam (pp. 93–109). New York: Marcel Dekker.

Laegried, L., Olegard, R., Wahlström, J., & Conradi, N. (1987). Abnormalities in children exposed to benzodiazepines in utero. *Lancet, 8527*(1), 1–109.

Laisi, U., Linnoila, T., Seppala, J. J., & Mattila, M. J. (1979). Pharmacokinetic and pharmacodynamic interactions of diazepam with different alcoholic beverages. *European Journal of Clinical Pharmacology, 16*, 263–270.

Lamb, R. J., & Griffiths, R. R. (1987). Self-injection of d,1-3,4-methylenedioxymethamphetamine (MDMA) in the baboon. *Psychopharmacology, 91*, 268–272.

Landis, C., & Zubin, J. (1951). The effects of thonzyalamine hydrochloride and phenobarbital sodium on certain psychological functions. *Journal of Psychology, 31*, 181–200.

Lankester, E. R. (1889). Mithradatism. *Nature, 40*, 149.

Lasagana, L., Felsinger, J. M., & Beecher, H. K. (1955). Drug-induced mood changes in man. *JAMA, 157*, 1006–1020.

Laties, V. G. (1986). Lessons from the history of behavioral pharmacology. In *Developmental behavioral pharmacology: Advances in behavioral pharmacology*, vol. 5, ed. N. K. Krasenegor, D. B. Gray, & T. Thompson (pp. 21–42). Hillsdale, NJ: Erlbaum.

Latimer, D., & Goldberg, J. (1981). *Flowers in the blood*. New York: Franklin Watts.

Le, A. D., Poulos, C. X., & Cappell, H. (1979). Conditioned tolerance to the hypothermic effect of ethyl alcohol. *Science, 206*, 1109.

Leavitt, F. (1974). *Drugs and behavior*. Philadelphia: Saunders.

Lee, M. A., & Shlain, B. (1985). *Acid dreams: The CIA, LSD and the sixties rebellion*. New York: Grove Press.

Lee, M. T. (1984). *The effects of alcohol on body sway and balance on the ascending and descending limbs of the blood alcohol curve*. Honours thesis, Memorial University of Newfoundland.

Leiber, C. S. (1977). Metabolism of alcohol. In *Metabolic Aspects of Alcoholism*, ed. C. S. Leiber (pp. 1–30). Baltimore, MD: University Park Press.

Leiber, C. S., & De Carli, L. M. (1977). Metabolic effects of alcohol on the liver. In *Metabolic aspects of alcoholism*, ed. C. S. Leiber (pp. 31–80). Baltimore, MD: University Park Press.

Lemberger, L., Schildcrout, S., & Cuff, G. (1987). Drug delivery systems: Applicability to neuropsychopharamcology. In *Psychopharmacology: A third generation of progress*, ed. H. Y. Meltzer (pp. 1285–1295). New York: Raven Press.

Leonard, B. E. (1993). The comparative pharmacology of new antidepressants. *Journal of Clinical Pharmacology, 54* (8, suppl.), 3–15.

Le Strange, R. (1977). *A history of herbal plants*. London: Angue & Robertson.

Levin, Edward D. (1992). Nicotinic systems and cognitive function. *Psychopharmacology, 108*, 417–431.

Levine, H. G. (1981). The vocabulary of drunkenness. *Journal of Studies on Alcohol, 42*, 1038–1051.

Lewitt, E. M. (1989). US tobacco taxes: Behavioral effects and policy implications. *British Journal of Addiction, 84*, 1217–1235.

Li, H. (1975). The origin and use of cannabis in eastern Asia. In *Cannabis and culture*, ed. V. Rubin (pp. 51–62). The Hague: Mouton.

Lickey, M. E., & Gordon, B. (1991). *Medicine and mental illness: The use of drugs in psychiatry*. New York: Freeman and Company.

Linder, R. L., Lerner, S. E., & Burns, R. S. (1981). *PCP: The devil's dust*. Belmont, CA: Wadsworth.

Ling, W., Rawson, R. A., & Compton, M. A. (1994). Substitution pharmacotherapies for opioid addiction: From methadone to LAAM and buprenorphine. *Journal of Psychoactive Drugs, 26*(2), 119–128.

Linnoila, M., & Hakkinen, T. (1974). Effects of diazepam and codeine alone and in combination with alcohol, on simulated driving. *Clinical Pharmacology and Therapeutics, 15*, 368–373.

Lister, R. G., & Nutt, D. J. (1987). Is RO 15–4513 a specific alcohol antagonist? *Trends in Neuroscience, 10*, 223–225.

Litten, R. Z., & Allen, J. P. (1993). Reducing the desire to drink: Pharmacology and neurobiology. In *Recent developments in alcoholism*, vol. 1, ed. M. Galanter (pp. 325–344). New York: Plenum.

Lombardo, J. A. (1986). Stimulants and athletic performance (part 1 of 2): Amphetamines and caffeine. *The Physician and Sportsmedicine, 14*(11), 128–140.

Loomis, T. A., & West, T. C. (1958). Comparative sedative effects of a barbiturate and some tranquilizer drugs on normal subjects. *Journal of Pharma-*

cology and Experimental Therapeutics, 122, 525–531.

Lowe, G. (1982). Alcohol-induced state-dependent learning: Differentiating stimulus and storage hypothesis. *Current Psychological Research, 2,* 215–222.

Lowe, G. (1988). State dependent retrieval effects with social drugs. *British Journal of Addictions, 83,* 99–103.

Lyon, M., & Robbins, T. (1975). The action of central nervous system drugs: A general theory concerning amphetamine effects. *Current Developments in Psychopharmacology, 2,* 80–163.

Lyttle, T. (1993). Misuse and legend in the "toad licking" phenomenon. *International Journal of the Addictions, 28*(6), 521–538.

Macdonald, S. (1986). The impact of increased availability of wine in grocery stores on consumption: Four case histories. *British Journal of Addiction, 81,* 381–387.

MacLeod, C. M., Dekaban, A. S., & Hunt, E. (1978). Memory impairment in epileptic patients: Selective effects of phenobarbital concentrations. *Science, 202,* 1102–1104.

Malcolm, R., Brady, K. T., Johnston, A. L., & Cunningham, M. (1993). Types of benzodiazepines abused by chemically dependent inpatients. *Journal of Psychoactive Drugs, 25*(4), 315–319.

Maltzman, I. (1994). Why alcoholism is a disease. *Journal of Psychoactive Drugs, 26,* 13–31.

Mangan, G. L., & Golding, J. (1978). An "enhancement" model of smoking maintenance? In *Smoking behaviour: physiological and psychological influences,* ed. R. E. Thornton (pp. 87–114). Edinburgh: Churchill Livingstone.

Manno, J. E., Manno, B. R., Kiplings, G. F., & Forney, R. B. (1974). Motor and mental performance with marijuana: Relationship to dose of delta-9-tetrahydrocannabinol and its interaction with alcohol. In *Marijuana: Effects on human behavior,* ed. L. L. Miller (pp. 45–72). Orlando, FL: Academic Press.

Mark, L. C. (1971a). Pharmacokinetics of barbiturates. In *Acute barbiturate poisoning,* ed. H. Matthew (pp. 75–84). Amsterdam: Excerpta Medica.

Marks, V., & Kelly, J. F. (1973). Absorption of caffeine from tea, coffee, and Coca-Cola. *Lancet, 1,* 827.

Marsden, C. D. (1977). Neurological disorders induced by alcohol. In *Alcoholism: New knowledge and new responses,* ed. G. Edwards & M. Grant (pp. 189–198). London: Croom Helm.

Martin, W. R., Eades, C. G., Thompson, J. A., Huppler, R. E., & Gilbert, P. E. (1976). The effects of morphine- and nalorphine-like drugs in the non-dependent and morphine-dependent chronic spinal dog. *Journal of Pharmacology and Experimental Therapeutics, 197,* 517–532.

Masuki, K., & Iwamoto, T. (1966). Development of tolerance to tranquilizers in the rat. *Japanese Journal of Pharmacology, 16,* 191–197.

Maxwell, Milton A. (1984). *The Alcoholics Anonymous experience: A close up view for professionals.* New York: McGraw-Hill.

McCarthy, C. R., Cutting, M. B., Simmons, G. A., Pereira, R., Laguardia, R., & Humber, G. L. (1976). The effects of marijuana on the *in vitro* function of pulmonary alveolar macrophages. In *Pharmacology of marijuana,* vol. 1, ed. M. C. Braude & S. Szara (pp. 211–216). Orlando, FL: Academic Press.

McCarthy, R. G. (1959). *Drinking and intoxication.* New York: Free Press.

McClelland, D. C., Davis, N. W., Kalin, R., & Wanner, E. (1972). *The drinking man.* New York: Free Press.

McCord, J. (1972). Some differences in backgrounds of alcoholics and criminals. *Annals of the New York Academy of Sciences, 197,* 183–187.

McGlothlin, W. H., & West, L. J. (1968). The marijuana problem: An overview. *American Journal of Psychiatry, 125,* 370–378.

McKim, E. M. (1991). Caffeine and its effects on pregnancy and the neonate. *Journal of Nurse-Midwifery, 36*(4), 226–231.

McKim, W. A. (1980). The effects of caffeine, theophylline and amphetamine on the operant responding of the mouse. *Psychopharmacology, 68,* 135–138.

McKim, W. A., & Mishara, B. L. (1987). *Drugs and aging.* Toronto: Butterworths.

McKim, W. A., & Quinlan, L. T. (1991). Changes in alcohol consumption with age. *Canadian Journal of Public Health, 82,* 231–234.

McMammy, M. C., & Schube, P. G. (1936). Caffeine intoxication. *New England Journal of Medicine, 215,* 616–620.

McMillan, D. E., & Leander, J. D. (1976). Effects of drugs on schedule-controlled behavior. In *Behavioral pharmacology,* ed. S. D. Glick & J. Goldfarb (pp. 85–139). St. Louis, MO: Mosby.

Meade, T. W., & Wald, N. J. (1977). Cigarette smoking patterns during the working day. *British Journal of Preventive and Social Medicine, 31*(1), 25–29.

Mechoulam, R., Hanus, L., & Martin, B. (1994).

The search for endogenous ligands of the cannabinoid receptor. *Biochemical Pharmacology, 48*(8), 1537–1544.

Mechoulam, R., McCallum, N. K., Lander, N., Yagen, B., Ben Zvi, Z., & Levy, S. (1976). Aspects of cannabis chemistry and metabolism. In *Pharmacology of marijuana*, vol. 1, ed. M. C. Braude & S. Szara (pp. 39–46). Orlando, FL: Academic Press.

Meisch, R. A. (1975). The function of schedule-induced polydipsia in establishing ethanol as a positive reinforcer. *Pharmacological Review, 27*, 465–473.

Meisch, R. A. (1977). Ethanol self-administration in infrahuman species. In *Advances in behavioral pharmacology*, vol. 1, ed. T. Thompson & P. B. Dews (pp. 35–84). Orlando, FL: Academic Press.

Meisch, R. A., & Carroll, M. E. (1987). Oral drug self-administration: Drugs as reinforcers. In *Methods for assessing the reinforcing properties of abused drugs,* ed. M. A. Bozarth (pp. 143–160). New York: Springer-Verlag.

Meisch, R. A., & Lemaire, G. A. (1993). Drug self-administration. In *Drug Self-Administration,* ed. F. Van Haaren (pp. 257–300). Amsterdam: Elsevier Science Publishers.

Mellinger, G. D., Balter, M. B., & Uhlenhuth, E. H. (1984). Prevalence and correlates of long-term regular use of anxiolytics. *JAMA, 25*, 375–379.

Mello, N. K. (1978). Alcoholism and the behavioral pharmacology of alcohol, 1967–1977. In *Psychopharmacology: A generation of progress*, ed. M. A. Lipton, A. Di Mascio, & K. F. Killam (pp. 1619–1637). New York: Raven Press.

Mello, N. K. (1987). Alcohol abuse and alcoholism. In *Psychopharmacology: The third generation of progress*, ed. H. Y. Meltzer (pp. 1515–1520). New York: Raven Press.

Mello, N. K., & Mendelson, J. H. (1972). Drinking patterns during work-contingent and non-contingent alcohol acquisition. *Psychosomatic Medicine, 34*, 139–164.

Mello, N. K., & Mendelson, J. H. (1987). Operant analysis of human drug self-administration: Marijuana, alcohol, heroin, and polydrug use. In *Methods for assessing the reinforcing properties of abused drugs,* ed. M. A. Bozarth (pp. 525–558). New York: Springer-Verlag.

Meltzer, H. Y. (1990a). Clozapine: Pattern of efficacy in treatment resistant schizophrenia. In *Novel antipsychotic drugs*, ed. H. Y. Meltzer (pp. 33–46). New York: Raven Press.

Meltzer, H. Y. (1990b). The mechanism of action of clozapine in relation to its clinical advantages. In *Novel antipsychotic drugs*, ed. H. Y. Meltzer (pp. 1–14). New York: Raven Press.

Meltzer, H. Y., & Lowy, M. T. (1987). The serotonin hypothesis of depression. In *Psychopharmacology: A third generation of progress*, ed. H. Y. Meltzer (pp. 513–526). New York: Raven Press.

Melzack, R. (1990). The tragedy of needless pain. *Scientific American, 262*, 27–33.

Mendelson, H. H., Kuehnle, J. C., Greenberg, I., & Mello, N. K. (1976). The effects of marijuana use on human operant behavior: Individual data. In *Pharmacology of marijuana*, vol. 2, ed. M. C. Braude & S. Szara (pp. 643–653). Orlando, FL: Academic Press.

Mendelson, W. B. (1979). Pharmacologic and electrophysical effects of ethanol in relation to sleep. In *Biochemistry and pharmacology of ethanol*, vol. 2, ed. E. Majchrowitz & E. P. Noble (pp. 467–484). New York: Plenum.

Meritz, M., Kleber, H. D., Riordan, C. E., & Solbetz, F. W. (1978). A follow-up study of patients successfully detoxified from methadone maintenance: Year two. In *Drug abuse: Modern trends, issues and perspectives*, ed. A. Schecter, H. Alksne, & E. Kaufman (pp. 308–315). New York: Dekker.

Meyer, R. E., & Mirin, S. M. (1979). *The heroin stimulus.* New York: Plenum.

Miczek, K. A., & Barry, H., III. (1976). Pharmacology of sex and aggression. In *Behavioral pharmacology*, ed. S. D. Glick & J. Goldfarb (pp. 176–257). St. Louis, MO: Mosby.

Miller, K. W. (1993). Molecular mechanisms by which general anesthetics act. In *Mechanisms of drugs of anesthesia*, 2nd ed., ed. S. Feldman, C. F. Scurr, & W. Paton (pp. 181–200). London: Edward Arnold.

Miller, L. L., & Drew, W. G. (1974). Cannabis: Neural mechanisms and behavior. In *Marijuana: Effects on human behavior*, ed. L. L. Miller (pp. 158–188). Orlando, FL: Academic Press.

Minifie, B. W. (1970). *Chocolate, cocoa and confectionary science and technology.* Westport, CT: Avi.

Mirsky, I. A., Piker, P., Rosebaum, M., & Lederer, H. (1945). "Adaptation" of the central nervous system to various concentrations of alcohol in the blood. *Quarterly Journal of Studies on Alcohol, 2*, 35.

Mishara, B., & Kastenbaum, R. (1980). *Alcohol and old age.* Orlando, FL: Grune & Stratton.

Mitchell, M. C. (1985). Alcohol-induced impairment of central nervous system function: Behavioral skills involved in driving. *Journal of Studies on Alcohol* (Suppl.), *10*, 109–119.

Mobley, B. L., & Sulser, F. (1981). Down-regulation of the central noradrenergic receptor system by antidepressant therapies: Biochemical and clinical aspects. In *Antidepressants: Neurochemical, behavioral and clinical perspectives*, ed. S. J. Enna, J. B. Malick, & E. Richelson (pp. 31–51). New York: Raven Press.

Modrow, H. E., Holloway, F. A., & Carney, J. M. (1981). Caffeine discrimination in the rat. *Pharmacology, Biochemistry and Behavior, 14*, 683–688.

Moeschlin, S. (1971). Clinical features of acute barbiturate poisoning. In *Acute barbiturate poisoning*, ed. H. Matthew (pp. 117–128). Amsterdam: Excerpta Medica.

Money, K. E., & Miles, W. S. (1974). Heavy water nystagmus and the effects of alcohol. *Nature, 247*, 404–405.

Monteiro, W. O., Noshirvani, I. M., Marks, I. M., & Elliott, P. T. (1987). Anorgasmia from clomipramine in obsessive-compulsive disorder: A controlled trial. *British Journal of Psychiatry, 151*, 107–112.

Moreau, J. J. (1973). *Hashish and mental illness*, ed. H. Peters & G. G. Nahas, trans. G. J. Barnett. New York: Raven Press. (Originally published in 1845.)

Morrison, C. F. (1967). The effects of nicotine on operant behavior of rats. *International Journal of Neuropharmacology, 6*, 229–240.

Morrison, C. F. (1969). The effects of nicotine on punished behavior. *Psychopharmacologia, 14*, 221.

Morrison, C. F. (1974). The effects of nicotine and its withdrawal on the performance of rats on signalled and unsignalled avoidance schedules. *Psychopharmacologia, 38*, 25–35.

Morrison, C. F., & Stephenson, J. A. (1969). Nicotine injections as the conditioned stimulus in discrimination learning. *Psychopharmacologia, 15*, 351–360.

Morrison, C. F., & Stephenson, J. A. (1972a). Effects of stimulants on observed behavior of rats on six operant schedules. *Neuropharmacology, 12*, 297–310.

Morrison, C. F., & Stephenson, J. A. (1972b). The occurrence of tolerance to a central depressant effect of nicotine. *British Journal of Pharmacology, 45*, 151–156.

Moskowitz, J., Hulbert, S., & McGlothlin, W. H. (1976). Marijuana: Effects on simulated driving performance. *Accident Analysis and Prevention, 8*, 45–50.

Mullins, C. J., Vitola, B. M., & Michelson, A. E. (1975). Variables related to cannabis use. *International Journal of Addictions, 10*, 481–502.

Mumford, G. K., Evans, S. M., Kamiski, B. J., et al. (1994). Discriminative stimulus and subjective effects of theobromine and caffeine in humans. *Psychopharmacology, 115*, 1–8.

Munson, S. E. (1975). Marijuana and immunity. In *Marijuana and health hazards*, ed. J. R. Tinklenberg (pp. 39–46). Orlando, FL: Academic Press.

Murphree, N. B., Pfeiffer, C. C., & Price, L. (1967). Electroencephalographic changes in man following smoking. *Annals of the New York Academy of Sciences, 142*, 245.

Myerson, R. M. (1971). Effects of alcohol on cardiac and muscular function. In *Biomedical basis of alcoholism*, ed. Y. Israel & J. Mardones (pp. 183–208). New York: Wiley/Interscience.

Naeye, R. L., & Peters, C. E. (1984). Mental development of children whose mothers smoked during pregnancy. *Obstetrics and Gynecology, 64*, 601–607.

Naranjo, C. A., & Sellers, E. M. (1986). Clinical assessment and pharmacology of the alcohol withdrawal syndrome. In *Recent developments in alcoholism*, vol. 4, ed. M. Galanter (pp. 265–281). New York: Plenum.

National Academy of Sciences. (1979). *Report of a study: Sleeping pills, insomnia, and medical practice* (Publ. No. IOM–79–04). Washington, DC: National Academy of Sciences Institute of Medicine.

Nehlig, A., Daval, J-L., & Debry, G. (1992). Caffeine and the central nervous system: Mechanisms of action, biochemical, metabolic and psychostimulant effects. *Brain Research Reviews, 17*, 139–170.

Nehlig, A., & Debry, G. (1994). Caffeine and sports activity: A review. *International Journal of Sports Medicine, 15*(5), 215–223.

Neims, A. H., Bailey, J., & Aldrich, A. (1979). Disposition of caffeine during and after pregnancy. *Clinical Research, 20*, 236A.

Newmeyer, J. A. (1993). X at the crossroads. *Journal of Psychoactive Drugs, 25*(4), 341–342.

Nicholl, J., & O'Cathain, A. (1992). Antenatal smoking, postnatal passive smoking and sudden infant death syndrome. In *Effects of smoking on the fetus, neonate and child*, ed. D. Poswillio & E. Alberman (pp. 138–170). Oxford: Oxford University Press.

Nriagu, J. O. (1983). Saturnine gout among the Roman aristocrats. *New England Journal of Medicine, 308*, 660–663.

Nyswander, M. (1967). The methadone treatment of heroin addiction. *Hospital Practice, 2*(4), 27–33.

O'Brien, C. P. (1976). Experimental analysis of conditioning factors in human narcotic addiction. *Pharmacological Reviews, 27*, 533–543.

OECD. (1978). *Road research: New research on the*

role of alcohol and drugs in road accidents. A report prepared by an OECD road research group. Organization for Economic Co-operation and Development, September 1978.

Ogbourne, A. C., & Glaser, F. B. (1981). Characteristics of affiliates of Alcoholics Anonymous. *Journal of Studies on Alcohol, 42,* 661–675.

Olds, J., & Milner, P. M. (1954). Positive reinforcement produced by electrical stimulation of the septal area and other regions of the rat brain. *Journal of Comparative and Physiological Psychology, 47,* 419–427.

O'Mara, R. (1993). Maintenence isn't cure, but it is limiting HIV, crime in Britain's drug picture. *The Sun,* September 19, 6A.

O'Neil, S., Tipton, K. F., Prichard, J. S., & Quinlan, A. (1984). Survival after high blood alcohol levels: Association with first order elimination kinetics. *Archives of Internal Medicine, 144,* 641–642.

Osmond, H. (1957). A review of the clinical effects of psychotomimetic agents. *Annals of the New York Academy of Sciences, 66,* 418–434.

Österberg, E. (1992). Effects of alcohol control measures on alcohol consumption. *International Journal of the Addictions, 27*(2), 209–225.

Oswald, I., Lewis, S. A., Tangey, J., Firth, H., & Haider, I. (1973). Benzodiazepines and human sleep. In *The benzodiazepines,* ed. S. Garattini, E. Mussini, & L. O. Randall (pp. 613–625). New York: Raven Press.

Oswald, I., & Thacore, V. R. (1963). Amphetamine and phenmetrazine addiction: Physiological abnormalities in the abstinence syndrome. *British Medical Journal, 2,* 427–434.

Otis, L. S. (1964). Dissociation and recovery of a response learned under the influence of chlorpromazine or saline. *Science, 143,* 1347–1348.

Overall, J. E. (1987). Introduction: Methodology in psychopharmacology. In *Psychopharmacology: A third generation of progress,* ed. H. Y. Meltzer (pp. 995–996). New York: Raven Press.

Overton, D. A. (1964). State dependent or "dissociated" learning produced with pentobarbital. *Journal of Comparative and Physiological Psychology, 57,* 3–12.

Overton, D. A. (1972). State-dependent learning produced by alcohol and its relevance to alcoholism. In *The biology of alcoholism,* vol. 2, ed. B. Kissen & H. Begleiter (pp. 193–217). New York: Plenum.

Overton, D. A. (1973). State-dependent learning produced by addicting drugs. In *Opiate addiction: Origins and treatment,* ed. S. Fisher & A. M. Freeman (pp. 61–67). New York: Wiley.

Overton, D. A. (1977). Comparison of ethanol, pentobarbital and phenobarbital using drug vs. drug discrimination training. *Psychopharmacology, 53,* 195–199.

Overton, D. A. (1982). Comparison of the degree of discriminability of various drugs using the T-maze drug discrimination paradigm. *Psychopharmacology, 76,* 385–395.

Overton, D. A. (1987). Applications and limitations of the drug discrimination method for the study of drug abuse. In *Methods of assessing the reinforcing properties of abused drugs,* ed. M. A. Bozarth (pp. 291–340). New York: Springer-Verlag.

Overton, D. A., & Batta, S. K. (1977). Relationship between abuse liability of drugs and their degree of discriminability in the rat. In *Predicting dependence liability of stimulant and depressant drugs,* ed. T. Thompson & K. R. Unna (pp. 125–135). Baltimore, MD: University Park Press.

Owen, R. T., & Tyrer, P. (1983). Benzodiazepine dependence: A review of the evidence. *Drugs, 25,* 385–398.

Parke, D. V. (1971). Biochemistry of the barbiturates. In *Acute barbiturate poisoning,* ed. H. Matthew (pp. 7–54). Amsterdam: Excerpta Medica.

Parsons, W. D., & Neims, A. H. (1978). Effects of smoking on caffeine clearance. *Clinical Pharmacology and Therapy, 24,* 40–45.

Pastuszak, A., Schick-Boschetto, B., Zuber, C., Feldkamp, M., Pinelli, M., Sihn, S., et al. (1993). Pregnancy outcome following first-trimester exposure to fluoxetine (Prozac). *JAMA, 269*(17), 2246–2248.

Paton, W. D. M., & Pertwee, R. C. (1973a). The actions of cannabis in animals. In *Marijuana,* ed. R. Mechoulam (pp. 192–287). Orlando, FL: Academic Press.

Paton, W. D. M., & Pertwee, R. C. (1973b). The actions of cannabis in man. In *Marijuana,* ed. P. Mechoulam (pp. 288–334). Orlando, FL: Academic Press.

Pattison, E. M., Sobel, M. B., & Sobel, L. C. (1977). *Emerging concepts of alcohol dependence.* New York: Springer.

Paul, S. M., Marangos, P. J., Goodwin, F. K., & Slotnick, P. (1980). Brain-specific benzodiazepine receptors and putative endogenous benzodiazepine-like compounds. *Biological Psychiatry, 15,* 407–428.

Pavlov, I. (1927). *Conditioned reflexes.* New York: Dover.

Pendrey, M. L., Maltzman, I. M., & West, L. J. (1982). Controlled drinking by alcoholics? New findings and a reevaluation of a major affirmative study. *Science, 217,* 169–175.

Perkins, K. A., Grobe, J. E., Epstein, L. H., Caggiula, A. R., & Stiller, R. L. (1992). Effects of nicotine on subjective arousal may be dependent on baseline subjective state. *Journal of Substance Abuse, 4*(2), 131–141.

Pertwee, R. G. (1992). *In Vivo* interactions between psychotropic cannabinoids and other drugs involving central and peripheral neurochemical mediators. In *Marijuana/Cannabinoids: Neurobiology and neurophysiology,* ed. L. Murphy, and A. Bartke (pp. 165–218). Boca Raton, FL: CRC Press.

Peters, J. M. (1967). Caffeine-induced haemorrhagic automutilation. *Archives Internationales de Pharmacodynamie et de Thérapie, 169,* 139–146.

Petursson, H., & Lader, M. H. (1981). Withdrawal from long-term benzodiazepine treatment. *British Medical Journal, 283,* 643–645.

Pfaus, J. G., & Pinel, P. J. (1988). Alcohol inhibits and disinhibits sexual behavior in the male rat. Unpublished manuscript.

Phillis, J.W., & O'Regan, M. H. (1988). The role of adenosine in the central actions of the benzodiazepines. *Progress in Neuro-Psychopharmacology and Biological Psychiatry, 12,* 384–404.

Pickens, R., & Thompson, T. (1968). Cocaine-reinforced behavior in rats: Effects of reinforcement magnitude and fixed-ratio size. *Journal of Pharmacology and Experimental Therapeutics, 161,* 122–129.

Pierce, I. H. (1941). Absorption of nicotine from cigarette smoke. *Journal of Laboratory and Clinical Medicine, 26,* 1322–1325.

Pollin, W. (1977). *Research on smoking behavior* (NIDA Research Monograph No. 17, DHEW Publ. No. ADM 78–581). Washington, DC: U.S. Government Printing Office.

Pomerleau, C. S., & Pomerleau, O. F. (1992). Euphoriant effects of nicotine in smokers. *Psychopharmacology, 108,* 460–465.

Pomerleau, O. F., & Pomerleau, C. S. (1984). Neuroregulators and the reinforcement of smoking: Toward a biobehavioral explanation. *Neuroscience and Biobehavioral Reviews, 8,* 503–513.

Popham, R. E., Schmidt, W., & de Lint, J. (1976). The effects of legal restraint on drinking. In *The biology of alcoholism,* vol. 4, ed. B. Kissen & H. Begleiter (pp. 579–625). New York: Plenum.

Porjesz, B., & Begleiter, H. (1987). Evoked brain potentials and alcoholism. In *Neuropsychology of alcoholism,* ed. O. A. Parsons, N. Butters, & P. E. Nathan (pp. 45–63). New York: Guilford Press.

Porsolt, R. D., Pawelec, C., & Jalfre, M. (1982). Use of a drug discrimination procedure to detect amphetamine-like effects of antidepressants. In *Drug discrimination: Applications in CNS pharmacology,* ed. F. C. Colpaert & J. L. Slangen (pp. 193–210). Amsterdam: Elsevier Biomedical.

Post, R. M., Cutler, N. R., Jimmerson, D. C., & Bunney, W. E., Jr. (1981). Dopaminergic mechanisms in affective illness. In *Recent advances in neuropsychopharmacology,* ed. B. Angrist, G. D. Burows, M. Lader, O. Lingjaerde, G. Sedvall, & D. Wheatly (pp. 55–62). Oxford: Pergamon Press.

Post, R. M., Weiss, S. R. B., Pert, A., & Uhde, T. W. (1987). Chronic cocaine administration: Sensitization and kindling effects. In *Cocaine: Clinical and behavioral aspects,* ed. S. Fisher, A. Raskin, & E. H. Uhlenhuth (pp. 109–173). New York: Oxford University Press.

Preskorn, S. H. (1993). Pharmacokinetics of antidepressants: Why and how they are relevant to treatment. *Journal of Clinical Psychiatry, 54*(9) (Suppl.), 14–33.

Preston, K. L., Griffiths, R. R., Clone, E. J., Darwin, W. D., & Gorodetzky, C. W. (1986). Diazepam and methadone blood levels following concurrent administration of diazepam and methadone. *Alcohol and Drug Dependence, 18,* 195–202.

Pritchard, W. S., Robinson, J. H., & Guy, T. D. (1992). Enhancement of continuous performance task reaction time by smoking in non-deprived smokers. *Psychopharmacology, 108,* 437–442.

Raw, M. (1978). The treatment of cigarette dependence. In *Research advances in alcohol and drug problems,* vol. 4, ed. Y. Israel, F. B. Glaser, H. Kalant, R. E. Popham, W. Schmidt, & R. G. Smart (pp. 441–486). New York: Plenum.

Ray, O., & Ksir, C. (1993). *Drugs, society and human behavior.* St. Louis: Mosby.

Rehm, J., & Sempos, C. T. (1995). Alcohol consumption and all-cause mortality. *Addiction, 90,* 471–480.

Reinisch, J. M., & Sanders, S. A. (1982). Early barbiturate exposure: The brain, sexually dimorphic behavior and learning. *Neuroscience and Biobehavioral Reviews, 6,* 311–319.

Rementiria, J. L., & Bhatt, K. (1977). Withdrawal symptoms in neonates from intrauterine exposure to diazepam. *Journal of Pediatrics, 90,* 123–126.

Restak, R. (1993). Brain by design. *The Sciences,* September/October, 27–33.

Ricciuti, E. R. (1978). *The devil's garden: Facts and folklore of perilous plants.* New York: Walker.

Richards, C. D. (1980). In search of the mechanisms of anesthesia. *Trends in Neuroscience, 3,* 9–13.

Rickels, K. (1983). Benzodiazepines in emotional disorders. *Journal of Psychoactive Drugs, 15*, 49–54.

Rickels, K., Downing, R. W., & Winokur, A. (1978). Antianxiety drugs: Clinical use in psychiatry. In *Handbook of psychopharmacology*, vol. 13, ed. L. L. Iverson, S. D. Iverson, & H. S. Snyder (pp. 395–430). New York: Plenum.

Risner, M. E., & Goldberg, S. R. (1983). A comparison of nicotine and cocaine self-administration in the dog: Fixed ratio and progressive ratio schedules of intravenous drug infusion. *Journal of Pharmacology and Experimental Therapeutics, 224*, 319–326.

Ritchie, M. J. (1975). The xanthines. In *The pharmacological basis of therapeutics,* ed. L. S. Goodman & A. Gillman (pp. 367–378). London: Collier-Macmillan.

Roache, J. D., & Griffiths, R. R. (1987). Lorazepam and meprobamate dose effects in humans: Behavioral effects and abuse liability. *Journal of Pharmacology and Experimental Therapeutics, 243*, 978–988.

Robbins, L. N., Davis, D. H., & Goodwin, D. W. (1974). Drug use by U.S. Army enlisted men in Vietnam: A followup on their return home. *American Journal of Epidemiology, 99*, 235–249.

Robinson, J. H., & Pritchard, W. S. (1992). The role of nicotine in tobacco use. *Psychopharmacology, 108*, 397–407.

Robert, J. C. (1967). *The story of tobacco in America.* Chapel Hill: University of North Carolina Press.

Robertson, D., & Curatolo, P. W. (1984). The cardiovascular effects of caffeine. In *Caffeine: Perspectives from recent research*, ed. P. B. Dews (pp. 77–85). Berlin: Springer-Verlag.

Robinson, D. (1977). Factors influencing alcohol consumption. In *Alcoholism: New knowledge and new responses*, ed. G. Edwards & M. Grant (pp. 60–77). London: Croom Helm.

Robinson, T. E., & Burridge, K. C. (1993). The neural basis of drug craving: An incentive-sensitization theory of addiction. *Brain Research Reviews, 18*, 247–291.

Roffman, M., & Lal, H. (1972). Role of brain amines in learning association with "amphetamine state." *Psychopharmacology, 25*, 196–204.

Romano, C., & Goldstein, A. (1980). Stereospecific nicotine receptors on rat brain membranes. *Science, 210*, 647–649.

Room, R. (1983). Sociological aspects of the disease concept of alcoholism. In R. G. Smart, F. B. Glassier, Y. Israel, H. Kalant, R. E. Popham, and W. Schmidt (Eds.), *Research advances in alcoholism and drug problems*, vol. 7 (pp. 47–91). New York: Plenum Press.

Rorabaugh, W. J. (1979). *The alcoholic republic.* New York: Oxford University Press.

Rosenbaum, G., Cohen, B. D., Luby, D. E., Gottlieb, J. S., & Yellen, D. (1959). Comparison of Sernyl with other drugs—Simulation of schizophrenic performance with Sernyl, LSD-25, and amobarbital (Amytal) sodium: 1. Attention, motor function, and proprioception. *Archives of General Psychiatry, 1*, 651.

Rosett, H. L. (1979). Clinical pharmacology and the fetal alcohol syndrome. In *Biochemistry and pharmacology of ethanol*, vol. 2, ed. E. Majchrowitz & E. P. Noble (pp. 485–510). New York: Plenum.

Rossi, A. M., Babor, T. F., Meyer, R. E., & Mendelson, J. H. (1974). Mood states. In *The use of marijuana: A psychological and physiological inquiry*, ed. J. H. Mendelson, A. M. Rossi, & R. E. Meyer (pp. 115–133). New York: Plenum.

Rossi, A. M., Kuehnle, J. C., & Mendelson, J. H. (1978). Marijuana and mood in human volunteers. *Pharmacology, Biochemistry and Behavior, 8*, 447–453.

Roth, R. H. (1983). Neuroleptics: Functional neurochemistry. In *Neuroleptics: Neurochemical, behavioral, and clinical perspectives*, ed. J. T. Coyle & S. J. Enna (pp. 119–165). New York: Raven Press.

Rothman, K., & Keller, A. (1972). The effects of a joint exposure to alcohol and tobacco on risk of cancer of the mouth and pharynx. *Journal of Chronic Diseases, 25*, 711–716.

Rothschild, A. J., & Locke, C. A. (1991). Reexposure to fluoxetine after serious suicidal attempts by three patients: The role of akathesia. *Journal of Clinical Psychiatry, 52*(12), 491–493.

Rubin, H. B., & Henson, D. B. (1976). Effects of alcohol on male sexual responding. *Psychopharmacologia, 47*, 123–134.

Rudgley, R. (1995). The archaic use of hallucinogens in Europe: An archaeology of altered states. *Addiction, 90*, 63–64.

Rudorfer, M. V., & Potter, W. Z. (1987). Pharmacokinetics of antidepressants. In *Psychopharmacology: A third generation of progress*, ed. H. Y. Meltzer (pp. 1353–1363). New York: Raven Press.

Rumbaugh, C. L., Bergeron, C. L., Fang, H. C., & McCormack, R. (1971). Cerebral anginographic changes in the drug abuse patient. *Radiology, 101*, 335–344.

Rush, C. R., Sullivan, J. T., & Griffiths, R. R. (1995). Intravenous caffeine in stimulant drug abusers: Subjective reports and physiological effects. *Journal of Pharmacology and Experimental Therapeutics, 273,* 351–358.

Russell, C. S., Taylor, R., & Law, C. E. (1968). Smoking in pregnancy: Maternal blood pressure, pregnancy outcome, baby weight and growth, and other related factors. *British Journal of Preventive Social Medicine, 22,* 119.

Russell, M. A. H. (1976). Tobacco smoking and nicotine dependence. In *Research advances in alcohol and drug problems,* vol. 1, ed. R. J. Gibbins, Y. Israel, H. Kalant, R. E. Popham, W. Schmidt, & R. G. Smart (pp. 1–48). New York: Wiley.

Rylander, G. (1969). Clinical and medico-criminological aspects of addiction to central stimulating drugs. In *Abuse of central stimulants,* ed. F. Sjoquist & M. Tottie (pp. 251–274). Stockholm: Almqvist & Wiksell.

Saabag, R. (1994). The cartels would like a second chance. *Rolling Stone,* May 5, 35–37.

Saario, I., & Linnoila, M. (1976). Effects of subacute treatment with hypnotics, alone and combination with alcohol, on psychomotor skills related to driving. *Acta Pharmacologica et Toxicologica, 38,* 382–392.

Safra, M. J., & Oakley, G. P., Jr. (1975). Association between cleft lip with or without cleft palate and perinatal exposure to diazepam. *Lancet, 2,* 478.

Salimenk, C. A. (1976). Pyrolysis of cannabinoids. In *Marijuana: Chemistry, biochemistry and cellular effects,* ed. G. G. Nahas (pp. 31–38). New York: Springer-Verlag.

Saltzman, C., DiMascio, A., Shader, R. I., & Harmatz, J. S. (1969). Chlordiazepoxide, expectation and hostility. *Psychopharmacologia, 14,* 38–45.

Samson, H. H. (1987). Initiation of ethanol-maintained behavior: A comparison of animal models and their implication to human drinking. In *Advances in behavioral pharmacology, vol. 6: Neurobehavioral pharmacology,* ed. T. Thompson, P. B. Dews, & J. E. Barrett (pp. 221–248). Hillsdale, NJ: Erlbaum.

Sanger, D. J., & Blackman, D. E. (1981). Rate dependence and the effects of benzodiazepines. In *Advances in behavioral pharmacology,* vol. 3, ed. T. Thompson, P. B. Dews, & W. A. McKim (pp. 1–20). Orlando, FL: Academic Press.

Sanna, E., & Harris, A. (1993). Neuronal ion channels. In *Recent developments in alcoholism,* vol. 11, ed. M. Galanter (pp. 169–186). New York: Plenum Press.

Schachter, S. (1973). Nesbitt's paradox. In *Smoking behavior: Motives and incentives,* ed. W. L. Dunn (pp. 147–155). Washington, DC: V. H. Winston and Sons.

Schachter, S. (1978). Pharmacological and psychological determinants of smoking. In *Smoking behaviour: Physiological and psychological influences,* ed. R. E. Thornton (pp. 208–228). Edinburgh: Churchill Livingstone.

Schechter, M. D., & Glennon, R. A. (1985). Cathinone, cocaine and methamphetamine: Similarity of behavior effects. *Pharmacology, Biochemistry and Behavior, 22,* 913–916.

Schechter, M. D., & Gordon, T. L. (1993). Comparison of the behavioral effects of ibogaine from three sources: Mediation of discriminative activity. *European Journal of Pharmacology, 249*(1), 79–84.

Schmidt, C. J. (1987). Psychedelic amphetamine, methylendioxymethamphetamine. *Journal of Pharmacology and Experimental Therapeutics, 240,* 1–7.

Schmidt, W. (1977). Cirrhosis and alcohol consumption: An epidemiological perspective. In *Alcoholism: New knowledge and new responses,* ed. G. Edwards & M. Grant (pp. 15–47). London: Croom Helm.

Schmiterlow, C., & Hanson, E. (1965). The distribution of C-14 nicotine. In *Tobacco alkaloids and related compounds,* ed. E. S. Von Euler (pp. 75–86). New York: Macmillan.

Schörring, E., & Hecht, A. (1979). Behavioral effects of low, acute doses of morphine in nontolerant groups of rats in an open-field test. *Psychopharmacology, 64,* 67–71.

Schuckit, M. A. (1985). Genetics and the risk of alcoholism. *JAMA, 254,* 2614–2617.

Schuckit, M. A. (1987). Biology of risk for alcoholism. In *Psychopharmacology: The third generation of progress,* ed. H. Y. Meltzer (pp. 1527–1533). New York: Raven Press.

Schuckit, M. A. (1992). Advances in understanding the vulnerability to alcoholism. In *Addictive states,* ed. C. E. O'Brien & J. H. Jaffe (pp. 93–108). New York: Raven Press.

Schuckit, M. A. (1993). *Drug Abuse and Alcoholism Newsletter, 22*(3), 1–3.

Schuckit, M. A., Smith, T. L., Anthenelli, R., & Irwin, M. (1993). Clinical course of alcoholism in 636 male inpatients. *American Journal of Psychiatry, 150,* 786–792.

Schultes, R. E. (1978). Plants and plant constituents as mind-altering agents throughout history. In *Handbook of psychopharmacology,* vol. 11, ed. L. L. Iverson, S. D. Iverson, & S. H. Snyder (pp. 219–242). New York: Plenum.

Schultes, R. E. (1987). Coca and other psychoactive plants: Magico-religious roles in primitive societies of the world. In *Cocaine: Clinical and behavioral aspects*, ed. S. Fisher, A. Raskin, & E. H. Uhlenhuth (pp. 212–250). New York: Oxford University Press.

Schultes, R. E., & Hoffman, A. (1979). *Plants of the gods: Origins of hallucinogenic use*. New York: McGraw-Hill.

Schultes, R. E., & Hoffman, A. (1980). *The botany and chemistry of hallucinogens*. Springfield, IL: Thomas.

Schuster, C. R. (1970). Psychological approaches to opiate dependence and self-administration by laboratory animals. *Federation Proceedings, 29*, 1–5.

Schuster, C. R. (1975). Drugs as reinforcers in animals and man. *Pharmacological Reviews, 27*, 511–521.

Schuster, C. R., Dockens, W. S., & Woods, J. H. (1966). Behavioral variables affecting the development of amphetamine tolerance. *Psychopharmacologia, 9*, 170–182.

Schuster, C. R., & Pickens, R. (1988). AIDS and intravenous drug abuse. *Problems of drug dependence, 1988*, NIDA Research monograph 90 (pp. 1–13), DHHS Publication No. (ADM)89–1606. Washington, DC: U.S. Government Printing Office.

Schuster, R. M., & Thompson, T. (1969). Self-administration and behavioral dependence on drugs. *Annual Review of Pharmacology, 9*, 483–502.

Schwartz, J. (1994, June 27–July 3). Smoking under siege. *Washington Post, National Weekly Edition*, pp. 6–9.

Schwartz, J.-C., Sokoloff, P., Giros, B., et al. (1990). The dopamine D_3 receptor as a target for antipsychotics. In *Novel antipsychotic drugs*, ed. H. Y. Meltzer (pp. 135–144). New York: Raven Press.

Science News (1992). And you thought you hated mornings. *Science News, 141*, 28.

Scott, C. C., & Chen, K. K. (1944). Comparison of the action of *l*-thyl theobromine and caffeine in animals and man. *Journal of Pharmacology and Experimental Therapeutics, 82*, 89–97.

Scott, J. M. (1969). *The white poppy*. New York: Funk & Wagnalls.

Seallet, A. C. (1991). Neurotoxicity of cannabis and THC: A review of chronic exposure studies in animals. *Pharmacology, Biochemistry and Behavior, 40*(3), 671–676.

Searles, J. S. (1988). The role of genetics in the pathogenesis of alcoholism. *Journal of Abnormal Behavior, 97*, 153–167.

Seeley, J. R. (1960). Death by liver cirrhosis and price of beverage alcohol. *Canadian Medical Association Journal, 83*, 1361–1366.

Seeman, P. (1990). Receptor selectivities of atypical neuroleptics. In *Novel antipsychotic drugs*, ed. H. Y. Meltzer (pp. 145–154). New York: Raven Press.

Seeman, P., Lee, T., Chau-Wing, M., & Wong, K. (1976). Antipsychotic drug dose and neuroleptic/dopamine receptors. *Nature, 261*, 717–718.

Seiden, L. S., & Dykstra, L. A. (1977). *Psychopharmacology: A biochemical and behavioral approach*. New York: Van Nostrand Reinhold.

Sellers, E. M., Ciraulo, D. A., DuPont, R. L., Griffiths, R. R., Kosten, T. R., Romach, M. K., & Woody, G. E. (1993). Alprazolam and benzodiazepine dependence. *Journal of Clinical Psychiatry, 54:*10 (suppl.), 64–75.

Sheppard, S. G. (1994). A preliminary investigation of ibogaine: Case reports and recommendations for further study. *Journal of Substance Abuse Treatment, 11*(4), 379–385.

Sherwood, N., Kerr, J. S., & Hindmarch, I. (1992). Psychomotor performance in smokers following single and repeated doses of nicotine gum. *Psychopharmacology, 108*, 432–436.

Shiffman, S. M. (1989). Tobacco "chippers": Individual differences in tobacco dependence. *Psychopharmacology, 97*, 539–547.

Shiono, P. H., Klebanoff, M. A., Nugent, R. P., et al. (1995). The impact of cocaine and marijuana use and low birthweight and preterm birth: A multicenter study. *American Journal of Obstetrics and Gynecology, 172*, 19–27.

Shopsin, B., Cassano, G. B., & Conti, L. (1981). An overview of new "second generation" antidepressant compounds: Research and treatment implications. In *Antidepressants: Neurochemical, behavioral and clinical perspectives*, ed. S. J. Enna, J. B. Malick, & E. Richelson (pp. 219–252). New York: Raven Press.

Shulgin, A. T. (1978). Psychotomimetic drugs: Structure-activity relationships. In *Handbook of psychopharmacology*, vol. 11, ed. L. L. Iverson, S. D. Iverson, & S. H. Snyder (pp. 243–336). New York: Plenum.

Siegel, R. K. (1977). Hallucinations. *Scientific American, 237*(4), 132–140.

Siegel, R. K. (1981). Inside Castenedas's pharmacy. *Journal of Psychoactive Drugs, 13*, 325–332.

Siegel, R. K. (1982a). Cocaine and sexual dysfunction: The curse of Mama Coca. *Journal of Psychoactive Drugs, 14*, 71–74.

Siegel, R. K. (1982b). Cocaine smoking. *Journal of Psychoactive Drugs, 14*, 271–359.

Siegel, R. K. (1986). MDMA: Medical use and intoxication. *Journal of Psychoactive Drugs, 18*, 349–353.

Siegel, R. K., & Jarvik, M. E. (1975). Drug-induced hallucinations in animals and man. In *Hallucinations: Behavior, experience, and theory*, ed. R. K. Siegel & L. J. West (pp. 81–162). New York: Wiley.

Siegel, S. (1975). Evidence from rats that morphine tolerance is a learned response. *Journal of Comparative and Physiological Psychology, 89*, 489–506.

Siegel, S. (1982). Drug dissociation in the nineteenth century. In *Drug discrimination: Applications in CNS pharmacology*, ed. F. C. Colpaert & J. L. Slangen (pp. 257–262). Amsterdam: Elsevier Biomedical.

Siegel, S. (1983). Classical conditioning, drug tolerance and drug dependence. In *Research advances in alcohol and drug problems*, vol. 7, ed. Y. Israel, F. B. Graser, H. Kalant, W. Popham, W. Schmidt, & R. G. Smart. New York: Plenum.

Siegel, S. (1984). Pavlovian conditioning reports by overdose victims. *Bulletin of the Psychonomic Society, 22*, 428–430.

Siegel, S., Hinson, R. E., Krank, M. D., & McCully, J. (1982). Heroin "overdose" death: Contribution of drug-associated environmental cues. *Science*, 216, 436–437.

Siemens, A. J., Kalant, H., & Nie, J. C. de. (1976). Metabolic interactions between delta-9-tetrahydrocannabinol and other cannabinoids in rats. In *Pharmacology of marijuana*, vol. 1, ed. M. C. Braude & S. Szara (pp. 77–92). Orlando, FL: Academic Press.

Siever, L. J. (1987). Role of noradrenergic mechanisms in the etiology of affective disorders. In *Psychopharmacology: A third generation of progress*, ed. H. Y. Meltzer (pp. 493–504). New York: Raven Press.

Silagy, C., Mant, D., Fowler, G., & Lodge, M. (1994). Meta-analysis of efficacy of nicotine replacement therapies in smoking cessation. *Lancet*, *343*(8890), 139–142.

Silkker, W., Jr., Paule, M. G., Ali, S. F., Scarlett, A. C., & Baily, J. R. (1992). Behavioral, neurochemical and neurophysiological effects of chronic marijuana smoke on the nonhuman primate. In L. Murphy & A. Bartke (Eds.) *Marijuana/cannabinoids neurology and neurophysiology* (pp. 219–274). Boca Raton, FL: CRC Press.

Silverman, K., Kirby, K. C., & Griffiths, R. R. (1994). Modulation of drug reinforcement by behavioral requirements following drug ingestion. *Psychopharmacology*, 114(2), 243–247.

Silverman, K., Mumford, G. K., & Griffiths, R. R. (1994). Enhancing caffeine reinforcement by behavioral requirements following drug ingestion. *Psychopharmacology*, *114*(3), 424–432.

Simon, E. J. (1981). Opiate receptors and endorphins: Possible relevance to narcotic addiction. *Advances in Alcohol and Substance Abuse, 1*(1), 13–31.

Simonson, E., & Brozek, J. (1952). Flicker fusion frequency. *Physiological Review, 32*, 349–378.

Simpson, D. D., Joe, G. W., & Bracy, S. A. (1982). 6-year follow-up of opioid addicts after admission to treatment. *Archives of General Psychiatry, 39*, 1318–1326.

Simpson, G. M., & Singh, H. (1990). Tricyclic antidepressants. In *Pharmacotherapy of depression*, ed. J. D. Amsterdam (pp. 75–91). New York: Marcel Dekker.

Singer, S. J., & Nicholson, G. L. (1972). The fluid mosaic model of the structure of cell membranes. *Science, 175*, 720.

Singh, N. N., & Leung, J. (1988). Smoking cessation through cigarette-fading, self-recording, and contracting: Treatment, maintenance and long-term followup. *Addictive Behaviors, 13*, 101–105.

Single, E. W. (1988). The availability theory of alcohol-related problems. In *Theories on alcoholism*, ed. C. D. Chaudron & D. A. Wilkinson (pp. 325–352). Toronto: Addiction Research Foundation.

Single, E. W. (1995). A harm reduction approach for alcohol: Between the lines of "Alcohol Policy and the Public Good." *Addiction, 90*,195–199.

Small, E. (1979). *The species problem in Cannabis*. Toronto: Corpus.

Smith, C. G. (1964). Effects of *d*-amphetamine upon operant behavior of pigeons: Enhancement of reserpine. *Journal of Pharmacology and Experimental Therapeutics, 146*, 167–174.

Smith, D. E., Buxton, M. E., & Dammann, G. (1979). Amphetamine abuse and sexual dysfunction: Clinical and research considerations. In *Amphetamine use, misuse and abuse*, ed. D. R. Smith (pp. 228–248). Boca Raton, FL: CRC Press.

Smith, D. E., & Wesson, D. R. (1983). Benzodiazepine dependency syndromes. *Journal of Psychoactive Drugs, 15*, 85–96.

Smith, G. M., & Beecher, H. K. (1959). Amphetamine sulfate and athletic performance. *JAMA, 170*, 542.

Smith, G. M., & Beecher, H. K. (1960). Amphetamine, secobarbital and athletic performance: 2. Subjective evaluations of performance, mood states and physical states. *JAMA, 172*, 1502–1514.

Smith, H. W. (1961). *From fish to philosopher*. Garden City, NY: Doubleday.

Sneader, W. (1985). *Drug discovery: The evolution of modern medicines.* Chichester, England: Wiley.

Snyder, S. H. (1977). Opiate receptors and internal opiates. *Scientific American, 236,* 44–56.

Snyder, S. H. (1981). Adenosine receptors and the actions of methylxanthines. *Trends in Neuroscience, 4,* 242–244.

Snyder, S. H. (1984). Adenosine as a mediator of the behavioral effects of caffeine. In *Caffeine: Perspectives from recent research,* ed. P. B. Dews (pp. 129–141). Berlin: Springer-Verlag.

Snyder, S. H. (1986). *Drugs and the brain.* New York: Scientific American Library.

Sofia, R. D. (1978). Cannabis: Structure-activity relationships. In *Handbook of psychopharmacology,* vol. 12, ed. L. L. Iverson, S. D. Iverson, & S. H. Snyder (pp. 319–371). New York: Plenum.

Solomon, D. (1966). *The marijuana papers.* Indianapolis: Bobbs-Merrill.

Spiegel, R., & Aebi, Hans-J. (1981). *Psychopharmacology: An introduction.* Chichester, England: John Wiley & Sons.

Spindel, E. R., & Wurtman, R. J. (1984). The neuroendocrine effects of caffeine in rat and man. In *Caffeine: Perspectives from recent research,* ed. P. B. Dews (pp. 119–128). Berlin: Springer-Verlag.

Spitzer, W. O., Lawrence, V., Dales, R., Gill, G., Archer, M. C., et al. (1990). Links between passive smoking and disease: A best evidence synthesis. *Clinical and Investigative Medicine, 13,* 17–42.

Squires, R. F., & Braestrup, C. (1977). Benzodiazepine receptors in the brain. *Nature, 266,* 732–734.

Sridhar, K. S., Ruab, W. A., Weatherby, N. L., et al. (1994). Possible role of marijuana smoking as a carcinogen in development of lung cancer at a young age. *Journal of Psychoactive Drugs, 26*(3), 285–288.

Stavric, B., & Gilbert, S. G. (1990). Caffeine metabolism: A problem in extrapolating results from animal studies to humans. *Acta Pharmacologica Jugoslavica, 40,* 475–489.

Steinberg, H., Rushton, R., & Tinton, C. (1961). Modification of the effects of an amphetamine-barbiturate mixture by the past experience of rats. *Nature, 192,* 533–535.

Stephenson, F. A. (1987). Benzodiazepines in the brain. *Trends in Neuroscience, 10*(5), 185–186.

Stepney, R. (1982). Human smoking behavior and the development of dependence on tobacco smoking. *Pharmacology and Therapeutics, 15,* 181–206.

Sternback, L. H. (1973). Chemistry of the 1,4-benzodiazepines and some aspects of the structure-activity relationship. In *The benzodiazepines,* ed. S. Garattini, E. Mussini, & L. O. Randall (pp. 1–26). New York: Raven Press.

Stewart, B. S., Lamaire, G. A., Roche, J. D., & Meisch, R. A. (1994). Establishing benzodiazepines as oral reinforcers: Midazolam and diazepam self-administration in rhesus monkeys. *Journal of Pharmacology and Experimental Therapeutics, 271*(1), 200–211.

Stewart, J. (1962). Differential responses based on the physiological consequences of pharmacological agents. *Psychopharmacologia, 3,* 132–138.

Stewart, J., & de Wit, H. (1987). Reinstatement of drug-taking behavior as a method of assessing incentive motivational properties of drugs. In *Methods of assessing the reinforcing properties of abused drugs,* ed. M. A. Bozarth (pp. 211–227). New York: Springer-Verlag.

Stillman, R., Eich, J. E., Weingartner, H., & Wyatt, R. J. (1976). Marijuana-induced state-dependent amnesia and its reversal by cuing. In *Pharmacology of marijuana,* vol. 4, ed. M. C. Braude & S. Szara (pp. 453–456). Orlando, FL: Academic Press.

Stolerman, I. P. (1987). Psychopharmacology of nicotine: Stimulus effects and receptor mechanisms. In *Handbook of psychopharmacology, Vol. 19: New directions in psychopharmacology,* ed. L. L. Iverson, S. D. Iverson, & S. H. Snyder (pp. 241–265). New York: Plenum.

Stolerman, I. P., Fink, R., & Jarvik, M. E. (1973). Acute and chronic tolerance to nicotine as measured by activity in rats. *Psychopharmacologia, 30,* 329–342.

Stolerman, I. P., Pratt, J. A., & Garcha, H. S. (1982). Further analysis of the nicotine cue in rats. In *Drug discrimination: Applications in CNS pharmacology,* ed. F. C. Colpaert & J. L. Slangen (pp. 203–210). Amsterdam: Elsevier Biomedical.

Stoll, W. A. (1949). Ein neues, in sehr kleinen Mengen wirksames Phantasticum. *Schweizerische Archiv von Neurologie, 64,* 483.

Strain, E. C., Mumford, G. K., Silverman, K., & Griffiths, R. R. (1995). Caffeine dependence syndrome, evidence from case histories and experimental evaluations. *JAMA, 272*(13), 1043–1048.

Stripling, J. S., & Ellinwood, E. H., Jr. (1976). Cocaine: Physiological effects of acute and chronic administration. In *Cocaine: Chemical, biological, clinical, social and treatment aspects,* ed. S. J. Mule (pp. 165–186). Boca Raton, FL.: CRC Press.

Sulser, F., Vetulani, J., & Mobley, P. L. (1978). Mode of action of antidepressant drugs. *Biochemical Pharmacology, 27,* 257–261.

Sutherland, G., Stapleton, J. A., Russell, M. A., Jarvis, M. J., Hajek, P., & Belcher, M. (1992). Randomized control trial of nasal nicotine spray. *Lancet, 340*(8815), 324–329.

Syed, I. B. (1976). The effects of caffeine. *Journal of American Pharmaceutical Association, 10,* 568–572.

Tabakoff, B., & Hoffman, P. L. (1987). Biochemical pharmacology of alcohol. In *Psychopharmacology: The third generation of progress*, ed. H. Y. Meltzer (pp. 1521–1526). New York: Raven Press.

Tarriere, C., & Hartemann, F. (1964). Investigation into the effects of tobacco smoke on a visual vigilance task. *Ergonomics: Proceedings of the Second International Congress on Ergonomics*, Dortmund, pp. 5225–5230.

Tart, C. T., & Crawford, H. J. (1970). Marijuana intoxication: Reported effects on sleep. *Psychophysiology, 7,* 348.

Tashkin, D. P., Shapiro, B. D., Ramanna, L., Taplin, G. V., Lee, Y. E., & Harper, C. E. (1976). Chronic effects of heavy marijuana smoking on pulmonary function in healthy young males. In *Pharmacology of marijuana*, vol. 1, ed. M. C. Braude & S. Szara (pp. 291–295). Orlando, FL: Academic Press.

Tatum, A. L., & Seevers, M. H. (1931). Theories of drug addiction. *Physiological Review, 11,* 107–120.

Taylor, J. L., & Tinklenberg, J. R. (1987). Cognitive impairment and benzodiazepines. In *Psychopharmacology: The third generation of progress*, ed. H. Y. Meltzer (pp. 1449–1454). New York: Raven Press.

Teicher, M. H., Glod, C. C., & Cole, J. O. (1990). Emergence of intense suicidal preoccupation during fluoxetine treatment. *American Journal of Psychiatry, 147,* 207–210.

Teschemacher, H. (1978). Endogenous ligands of opiate receptors (endorphins). In *Developments in opiate research*, ed. A. Herz (pp. 67–151). New York: Dekker.

Thompson, T., & Schuster, C. R. (1964). Morphine self-administration, food reinforced and avoidance behaviour in rhesus monkeys. *Psychopharmacologia, 5,* 87–94.

Thompson, T., Trombley, J., Luke, D., & Lott, D. (1970). Effects of morphine on behavior maintained by four simple food reinforcement schedules. *Psychopharmacologia, 17,* 182–192.

Ticku, M. K., & Olsen, R. W. (1978). Interaction of barbiturates with dihydropicrotoxin binding sites related to the GABA receptor-ionophore system. *Life Sciences, 22,* 1643–1652.

Tinklenberg, J. R. (1974). Marijuana and human aggression. In *Marijuana: Effects on human behavior*, ed. L. L. Miller (pp. 339–358). Orlando, FL: Academic Press.

Toit, B. M. du. (1975). Dagga: The history and ethnographic setting of *Cannabis sativa* in southern Africa. In *Cannabis and culture*, ed. V. Rubin (pp. 81–118). The Hague: Mouton.

Tollefson, G. D. (1993). Adverse drug reactions/interactions in maintenance therapy. *Journal of Clinical Psychiatry, 54*(8), 48–58.

Torry, J. M. (1976). A case of suicide with nitrazepam and alcohol. *Practitioner, 217,* 648–649.

Uhlenhuth, E. H., de Wit, H., Balter, M. B., Johanson, C. E., & Mellinger, G. D. (1988). Risks and benefits of long-term benzodiazepine use. *Journal of Clinical Pharmacology, 8*(3), 161–167.

United Nations. (1980). *Bulletin on Narcotics, 32*(3), Special issue devoted to *Catha edulis* (khat).

U.S. DHHS. (1989). *Reducing the health consequences of smoking: 25 years of progress: A report of the surgeon general*. Rockville, MD: U.S. Department of Health and Human Services, Center for Disease Control, Center for Chronic Disease Prevention and Promotion.

U.S. DHHS. (1990a). *The health benefits of smoking cessation: A report of the surgeon general*. Washington, DC: U.S. Department of Health and Human Services, Public Health Service.

U.S. DHHS. (1990b). *Alcohol, tobacco, and other drugs may harm the unborn*. Rockville, MD: U.S. Department of Health and Human Services, Public Health Service, Alcohol, Drug Abuse, and Mental Health Administration, Office for Substance Abuse Prevention.

U.S. DHHS. (1994). *Preliminary estimates from the 1993 national household survey on drug abuse, advance report number 7*, Washington, DC: U.S. Department of Health and Human Services, Substance Abuse and Mental Health Services Administration.

U.S. DHHS. (1995). *Preliminary estimates from the 1994 national household survey on drug abuse, advance report number 10*, Washington, DC: U.S. Department of Health and Human Services, Substance Abuse and Mental Health Services Administration.

U.S. EPA. (1992). *Respiratory health effects of passive smoking: Lung cancer and other disorders*. Washington, DC: Office of Research and Development, Office of Health and Environmental Assessment.

Vaccarino, F. J., Schiff, B. B., & Glickman, S. E. (1989). Biology view of reinforcement. In *Contemporary learning theories*, ed. S. B. Klein & R. R. Mowrer (pp. 111–142). Hillsdale, NJ: Erlbaum.

Vaillant, G. E. (1992). Is there a natural history of addiction? In *Addictive states*, ed. C. E. O'Brien & J. H. Jaffe, (pp. 41–56). New York: Raven Press.

Van Lancker, J. L. (1977). Smoking and disease (NIDA Research Monograph No. 17, DHEW Publ. No. ADM 78–581). In *Research on smoking behavior*, ed. M. E. Jarvik, J. W. Cullen, E. R. Gritz, T. M. Vogt, & L. J. West (pp. 230–280). Washington, DC: U.S. Government Printing Office.

Van Woert, M. H. (1983). Neuroleptics in neurological disorders. In *Neuroleptics: Neurochemical, behavioral, and clinical perspectives*, ed. J. T. Coyle & S. J. Enna (pp. 65–74). New York: Raven Press.

Verebey, K., Alrazi, J., & Jaffe, J. H. (1988). The complications of "ecstasy" (MDMA). [letter], *JAMA, 259*, 1649–1650.

Victor, M., Adams, R. D., & Collins, G. H. (1971). *The Wernicke-Korsakoff syndrome*. Philadelphia: Davis.

Vitiello, M. V., & Woods, S. C. (1975). Caffeine: Preferential consumption by rats. *Pharmacology, Biochemistry and Behavior, 3*, 147–149.

Vogel, J. R. (1979). Objective measurement of human performance changes produced by antianxiety drugs. In *Anxiolytics*, ed. S. Fielding & H. Lal (pp. 343–374). Mt. Kisco, NY: Futura.

Vogel-Sprott, M. (1967). Alcohol effects on human behavior under reward and punishment. *Psychopharmacologia, 11*, 337–344.

Vogel-Sprott, M. (1984). Response measures of social drinking: Research implications and application. *Journal of Studies on Alcohol, 44*, 817–836.

Vree, T. B., & Henderson, P. T. (1980). Pharmacokinetics of amphetamines: In vivo and in vitro studies of factors governing their elimination. In *Amphetamines and related stimulants: Chemical, biological, clinical and sociological aspects*, ed. J. Caldwell (pp. 47–68). Boca Raton, FL: CRC Press.

Vuchinich, R. E., & Tucker, J. A. (1988). Contributions from the behavioral theory of choice to an analysis of alcohol abuse. *Journal of Abnormal Psychology, 97*, 181–195.

Waldorf, D., Murphy, S., Renarman, C., & Joyce, B. (1977). *Doing coke: An ethnography of cocaine users and sellers*. Washington, DC: Drug Abuse Council.

Wallgren, H., & Barry, H., III. (1971). *Actions of alcohol*. Amsterdam: Elsevier.

Wands, J. R. (1979). Ethanol and the immune response. In *Biochemistry and pharmacology of ethanol*, vol. 1, ed. E. Mijchrowitz, & F. P. Noble (pp. 641–658). New York: Plenum.

Warburton, D. M. (1992). Nicotine issues. *Psychopharmacology, 108*, 393–396.

Wasson, R. G. (1972). The divine mushroom of immortality. In *Flesh of the gods*, ed. P. T. Furst (pp. 185–200). New York: Praeger.

Watkins, R. L., and Adler, E. V. (1993). The effect of food on alcohol absorption and elimination patterns. *Journal of Forensic Sciences, JFSCA, 38*(2), 285–291.

Watterson, O., Sells, S. B., & Simpson, D. D. (1976). Death rates and causes of death for opiate addicts in treatment drugs 1972–3. In *Studies in the effectiveness of treatments for drug abuse*, vol. 5, ed. S. B. Sells & D. D. Simpson (pp. 283–318). Cambridge, MA: Ballinger.

Wayner, M. J., Jolicoeur, F. B., Rondeau, D. B., & Baron, F. C. (1976). Effects of acute and chronic administration of caffeine on schedule dependent and schedule induced behavior. *Pharmacology, Biochemistry and Behavior, 5*, 343–348.

Weddington, W. W. (1995). Methadone maintenance for opioid addiction. In *Pharmacological therapies for alcohol and drug addiction*, ed. N. S. Miller & M. S. Gold, (pp. 411–418). New York: Marcel Dekker.

Weil, A., & Rosen, W. (1983). *Chocolate to morphine: Understanding mind-acting drugs*. Boston: Houghton Mifflin.

Weil, A. T. (1979). Nutmeg as a psychoactive drug. In *Ethnopharmacologic search for psychoactive drugs*, ed. D. H. Efron, B. Holmstedt, & N. S. Kline (pp. 188–201). New York: Raven Press.

Weil, A. T., & Zinberg, N. E. (1969). Acute effects of marijuana on speech. *Nature, 222*, 434–437.

Weil, A. T., Zinberg, N. E., & Nelson, J. M. (1968). Clinical and psychological effects of marijuana in man. *Science, 192*, 1234–1242.

Weiss, B. (1969). Enhancement of performance by amphetamine-like drugs. In *Abuse of central stimulants*, ed. F. Sjoquist & M. Tottie (pp. 31–60). Stockholm: Almqvist & Wiksell.

Weiss, B., & Laties, V. G. (1962). Enhancement of human performance by caffeine and the amphetamines. *Pharmacological Review, 14*, 1–36.

Welbert, J. (1972). Tobacco and shamanistic ecstasy among Wararo Indians of Venezuela. In *Flesh of the gods*, ed. P. T. Furst (pp. 55–83). New York: Praeger.

Wenger, J. R., Tiffany, T. M., Bombardier, C., Nicoins, K., & Woods, S. C. (1981). Ethanol tolerance in the rat is learned. *Science, 213*, 575–576.

Wesnes, K., & Warburton, D. M. (1983). Smoking, nicotine and human performance. *Pharmacology and Therapeutics, 21*, 198–208.

Wesson, D. R., & Smith, D. E. (1977). *Barbiturates: Their use, misuse and abuse.* New York: Human Sciences.

Wesson, D. R., & Smith, D. E. (1979). A clinical approach to diagnosis and treatment of amphetamine abuse. In *Amphetamine use, misuse and abuse,* ed. D. R. Smith (pp. 260–274). Boca Raton, FL: CRC Press.

West, G. A. (1970). *Tobacco, pipes and smoking customs of the American Indians.* Westport, CT: Greenwood Press.

West, R. (1993). Beneficial effects of nicotine: Fact or fiction. *Addiction, 88,* 589–590.

White, H. R. (1993). Sociology. In *Recent developments in alcoholism,* vol. 11. New York: Plenum Press.

Whitfield, J. B., & Martin, N. G. (1994). Alcohol consumption and alcohol pharmacokinetics: Interaction within the normal population. *Alcoholism: Clinical and Experimental Research, 18,* 238–243.

Wikler, A. (1980). *Opioid dependence.* New York: Plenum.

Wilder, B. J., & Bruni, J. (1981). *Seizure disorders: A pharmacological approach to treatment.* New York: Raven Press.

Williams, G. D., Clem, D., & Dufour, M. C. (1993). *Surveillance Report #27. Apparent per capita alcohol consumption: National, state, and regional trends, 1977–1991.* Rockville, MD: National Institute on Alcohol Abuse and Alcoholism, Division of Biometry and Epidemiology.

Williams, R., & Davis, M. (1977). Alcoholic liver diseases: Basic pathology and clinical variants. In *Alcoholism: New knowledge and new responses,* ed. G. Edwards & M. Grant (pp. 157–178). London: Croom Helm.

Winger, G., Hoffmann, F. G., & Woods, J. H. (1992). *A handbook on alcohol and drug abuse,* 3rd ed. New York: Oxford University Press.

Winger, G., Stitzer, M. L., & Woods, J. H. (1975). Barbiturate-reinforced responding in rhesus monkeys: Comparisons of compounds with different durations of actions. *Journal of Pharmacology and Experimental Therapeutics, 195,* 505–514.

Winick, C. (1962). Maturing out of narcotic addiction. *Bulletin on Narcotics, 14*(1), 1–8.

Wise, R. (1981). Brain dopamine and reward. In *Theory in psychopharmacology,* vol. 1, ed. S. J. Cooper (pp. 103–121). London: Academic Press.

Wise, R. A. (1995). Brain reward circuits and drug and alcohol addictions. In N. S. Miller, & M. S. Gold, *Pharmacological therapies for drug and alcohol addiction* (pp. 44–52). New York: Marcel Dekker.

Wolfe, S. M., & Victor, M. (1972). The physiological basis of the alcohol withdrawal syndrome. In *Recent advances in the study of alcoholism,* ed. N. K. Mello & J. H. Mendelson (pp. 188–199). Washington, DC: U.S. Government Printing Office.

Wolverton, W., & Johanson, C. (1984). Preference in rhesus monkeys given a choice between cocaine and d,l-cathinone. *Journal of the Experimental Analysis of Behavior, 41,* 35–43.

Wolverton, W., & Johnson, K. M. (1992). Neurobiology of cocaine abuse. *Trends in Pharmacological Sciences, 13,* 193–200.

Woods, N. F. (1984). *Human sexuality in health and illness.* St. Louis, MO: Mosby.

World Health Organization. (1993). *Classification of mental and behavioral disorders (ICD-10): Clinical descriptions and diagnostic guidelines.* Geneva: Word Health Organization.

Worley, C. M., Valdez, A., & Schenk, S. (1994). Reinforcement of extinguished cocaine-taking by cocaine and caffeine. *Pharmacology, Biochemistry and Behavior, 48,* 217–221.

Yablonsky, L., & Dederich, D. E. (1965). Synanon: An analysis of some dimensions of the social structure of an antiaddiction society. In *Narcotics,* ed. D. M. Wilner & G. G. Kassenbaum (pp. 193–216). New York: McGraw-Hill.

Yanagita, T. (1975). Some methodological problems in assessing dependence-producing properties of drugs in animals. *Pharmacological Reviews, 27,* 503–510.

Yanagita, T. (1987). Prediction of drug abuse liability from animal studies. In *Methods for assessing the reinforcing properties of abused drugs,* ed. M. A. Bozarth (p. 189). New York: Springer-Verlag.

Yokel, R. A. (1987). Intravenous self-administration: Response rates, the effects of pharmacological challenges, and drug preferences. In *Methods of assessing the reinforcing properties of abused drugs,* ed. M. A. Bozarth (pp. 1–34). New York: Springer-Verlag.

Zacny, J. P., Stitzer, M. L., Brown, F. J., Yingling, J. E., & Griffiths, R. R. (1987). Human cigarette smoking: Effects of puff and inhalation parameters on smoke exposure. *Journal of Pharmacology and Experimental Therapeutics, 240,* 554–563.

Zuckerman, B., & Frank, D. A. (1994). Prenatal cocaine exposure: Nine years later. *Journal of Pediatrics, 124*(5, part 1), 731–733.

Index

gin, 98, 100
glial cells, 48, 338
glomerulus, 18
glutamate, 56–57, 59, 66
glycine, 56–57
Goldberg, Stephen, 84
grand mal seizure, 338
Grapevine, The, 124
gray matter, 60–61
grayout, 111, 338
green Chinese tea, 193
Griffiths, R.R., 182
Grinspoon, Lester, 307
growth hormone, 56–57
Guarana, 194

H₂-receptor antagonists, 104
habituation, 75
Haight-Ashbury Free Medical Clinic, 232
half-life, 19, 338
  age, 278
  amphetamine, 217
  benzodiazepines, 144
  caffeine, 197
  cathinone, 217
  chlordiazepoxide, 144
  cocaine, 217
  codeine, 240
  delta-9-THC, 291
  fluoxetine, 277–78
  LAAM, 240
  lithium, 278
  LSD, 213
  monoamine oxidase inhibitors (MAOI),
    277
  meperidine, 240
  methadone, 240
  morphine, 240
  nalorphine, 240
  second-generation antidepressant, 277
  SSRI, 277
Hallstrom, Cosmo, 154
hallucinations, 310, 324
  drug state discrimination, 329
  psychotic behavior, 332
  self-administration, 330–31
  serotonin, 311
  stimulus effect, 330
  withdrawal, 330
haloperidol, 80, 113, 258
  performance, 267
Halstead, William Stewart, 245
hand steadiness, 34
hangover, 81, 129
hard liquor, 98
harm reduction, 119
harmaline, 316
harmine, 316
  LSD, 316
  DMT, 316
Harrison Narcotic Act, 235, 238, 249, 338
Harvey, William, 195
hash oil, 288, 338
hashish, 287, 289, 338
heart disease, 132
hemp, 286, 288, 338
  Raleigh, Sir Walter, 289

Washington, George, 289
henbane, Ebers Papyrus, 321
hepatitis, 230
Herodotus, 99
heroin, 45, 80, 93, 236, 238, 246
  AIDS, 239
  antagonist therapies, 254
  distribution, 239
  hepatitis, AIDS, 251
  maturing out, 249
  overdose, 45, 250
  self-administration, 248
  withdrawal, 247, 255
Herrnstein, Richard, 87
Heyman, Gene, 81, 90, 117–19
Hinson, Rily, 45
histamine, 56, 57, 263
hob, 322
Hoffman, Albert, 311
Holmes, Sherlock, 214
hormones, 56
horse tanks, 322
Huxley, Aldous, 327
hyoscyamine, 320
Hyoscyamus niger, 321
hyoskyamos, 321
hyperpolarization, 51, 55, 338
hypogogic states, 324
hypothalamus, 65

iatrogenic self-administration, 158, 338
iboga root, 331
ibogaine, 316–17
  addictions, 316
  alcohol, 317
  heroin, 317
  tobacco, 317
ibogamine, 316
ibotinic acid, 321
  Amanita muscaria, 321
ICD-10, 72
ice, 213
Ilex paraguanyensis, 194
Ilex vomitoria, 194
imipramine, 80, 271, 276
independent variable, 25, 339
indoleamine, 56–57, 212, 339
inebriety, 71
Infanta Catherine, 195
inhalation, 78
inhibition, 53, 54
inhibitory postsynaptic potential (IPSP),
  55–57, 339
inhibitory tone, 146
insulin, 56–57
intemperance, 71
International Life Sciences Institute (ILSI),
  210
interval schedules, 37
intracerebroventricular administration, 78
intracranial administration, 78
intramuscular administration (i.m.), 9,
  22–23, 339
intraperitoneal administration (i.p.), 9, 23,
  339
intravenous administration (i.v.), 9, 23, 78,
  339

introspection, 30, 31, 339
inverse agonist, 146
ion, 13, 50–51, 339
ion channels, 50, 52, 55, 339
  gated, 50–51
  nongated, 50
  voltage gated, 51
ion pump, 17, 50
ion trapping, 15–16, 339
ionophore. See ion channels
iproniazid, 271
IPSP. See inhibitory postsynaptic potential
isoprenaline, 224
isopropyl alcohol, 97
isoproterenol, 224

James, Jack, 209
Jellinek, E.M., 71, 121, 122, 124–25, 127
Johanson, Chris, 85
Johnson, H.J., 173
Joplin, Janis, 250

kappa, 60
Kessler, David, 181
ketamine, 66, 322–23
khat, 213
  reproduction, 231
kicking the habit, 247
kidney, 17–19
King James I, 168
Kluver, Heinrich, 325–24
Koch-Grunberg, 315
Kola tree, 194
Korsakoff's psychosis, 130, 296, 339
Krank, Marvin, 45

l-amphetamine, 212, 218. See also amphetamine
L-dopa, 58, 64, 339
LAAM, 254, 339
  half-life, 240
Laborit, Henri, 261–62
Lader, Malcolm, 154
Lasagana, L., 244
late major syndrome, 115
laudanum, 46, 70, 237, 339
LBJ, 319
LD₅₀, 3, 4
  caffeine, 201
Le Club des Hachichins, Théophile Gautier,
  289
learning, 34
Leary, Timothy, 312, 318
Ledermann, Sully, 115
Lephopora williamsii, 317
letdown, 226
lethal effects, 209
level of arousal, 63
Levontradol, 236, 292
limbic system, 65, 339
Lindesmith, A.R., 76
lipid, 13, 339
lipid bilayer, 13–14
lipid solubility, 16, 143
liqueurs, 98
lithium, 23, 273, 280
  absorption, 277

mixed opiate agonist/antagonist, 241, 324
MMDA, potency, 318
moclobemide, 271, 277
molar theories, 89
molindone, 258
Monardes, 179
monoacetylmorphine, 239
monoamines (MA), 56, 212, 217, 278, 340.
　　See also biogenic amines
　alcohol, 280
　amphetamine, 280
　half-life, 277
　mood, 275
　overdose, 284
　tyramine, 280
monoamine oxidase (MAO), 58, 59, 339
　absorption, 277
　bainsteriopsis, 316
　iproniazid, 275
　MAO-A and MAO-B, 280
　punished behavior, 282
　self-administration, 282–83
monoamine oxidase inhibitors (MAOI), 271, 276, 339
　absorption and excretion, 277
　conditioned behavior, 282
　history, 275–76
　neurophysiology, 278
　self-administration, 282–83
　tyramine, 280
monoamine theory of depression, 275
mood, 33, 275
　5-HT, 279
　amphetamine, 219
　barbiturates, 147
　benzodiazepines, 147
　caffeine, 202
　cocaine, 219–20
　limbic system, 275
　marijuana, 295
　medial forebrain bundle, 275
　mesolimbic system, 275
　morphine, 244
　NE, 275
　nicotine, 174
　opiates, 244
　Raphé system, 275
　ventral tegmentum, 275
mood disorder, 272, 274
Moonstone, The, 46
Moreau de Tors, J.J., 289
morphine, 71, 80–81, 86, 93, 235–36, 246
　distribution, 239
　drug state discrimination, 245
　first pass, 239
　fixed ratio (FR) schedule, withdrawal, 245
　half-life, 240
　Halstead, William Stewart, 244
　intake–abstinence cycles, 249
　mood, 244
　periventricular grey, 242
　physical dependence, 242, 249
　self-administration, 249
　sleep, 242
　SMA, 245
　ventral tegmental area, 242

withdrawal symptoms, 244
morphine-like substances, 57
motoneurons, 62
mu receptor, 60, 246
mucous membrane, 12, 170, 340
muscamole, 322
muscarine, 58, 172
　Amanita muscaria, 322
muscarinic cholinergic receptors, 58, 340
muscatel, 98
muscazone, 322
Musto, David, 103
myelin sheath, 48–49, 340
Myristica fragrans, 320
myristicin, 320

nabilone, 288, 293, 340
nalorphine, 236, 239, 241
　half-life, 240
naloxone, 80, 236, 239, 241, 255, 340
　half-life, 240
naltrexone, 255
narcotic analgesics, 235
narcotic, 235
Narcotic Control Act, 235
　marijuana, 290
narcotics, 235
Native American Church, 327, 340
NE. See norepinephrine
negative reinforcers, 78
negative symptoms, 340
Nembutal, 142
nephron, 17–19, 340
Nero, 99
nerve, 340
Nesbitt's paradox, 174, 340
neuroleptic, 257–58, 267
neuromodulator, 55–56, 292, 340
neuromuscular junction, 60, 173
neuron, 48, 340
neuropharmacology, 108
　cannabinoids, 291
neurophysiology, 240
　amphetamines, 278
　cathinone, 278
　cocaine, 278
　methcathinone, 278
　monoamine oxidase inhibitors, 278
　second-generation antidepressant, 278
　SSRIs, 278
　tricyclics, 278
neurotransmitters, 53, 66
Nicot, Jean, 167
Nicotiana rustica, 166
Nicotiana tabacum, 168
nicotine, 80, 167
　absorption, 170
　ACh, 176
　Addiction Research Center Inventory (ARCI), 175
　Alzheimer's disease, 176
　antidepressants, 174
　arousal, 174, 176
　central nervous system, 173
　cholinergic receptors, 172
　DA, 174
　distribution, 171
　drug state discrimination, 177

EEG, 173
epinephrine, 173, 176
excretion, 171
first pass metabolism, 170
half-life, 172
hallucinogenic use, 179
memory, 176
mesolimbic dopamine system, 174
mood, 174
NE, 174
negatively reinforced behavior, 176
nucleus accumbens, 174
patellar reflex, 173
performance, 175, 178
peripheral nervous system, 173
pKa, 170
positively reinforced behavior, 176
recall, 176
REM, 174
respiration, 173
self-administration, 178
serotonin systems, 174
skin, 173
sleep, 174
spontaneous motor activity (SMA), 176
stomach, 173
substitution therapy, 185
sustained attention, 175
titration, 181
unconditioned behavior, 176
vigilance, 175
vomiting center, 174
weight gain, 177
withdrawal, 171, 174–76
nicotine bolus 171, 184, 340
nicotine bolus theory, 183, 340
nicotine gum, 184, 171, 175
nicotine nasal spray, 171, 175
nicotine patch, 171, 177, 184–85, 340
nicotine-1-N-oxide, 172
nicotinic cholinergic receptors, 58
Niemann, Albert, 214
nigrastriatal system, 265, 340
　stereotyped behavior, 226
nitrazepam (Mogadon), 143, 147
NMDA receptor, 108
No-Dŏz, 192
nod, 227
nomifensine, 271
nondrug substitutes, 92
nonexperimental research, 29
nonproprietary name, 1
norepinephrine (NE), 56, 58, 173, 212, 218, 229, 263, 278, 280
normal saline, 8
norpseudoephedrine, 224
nortriptyline, 271
nuclei, 60
nucleus accumbens (ACC), 65, 94, 109, 264
nutmeg, 320

obsessive–compulsive disorder, 283
obsessive–compulsive personality, 281
Odyssey House, 252
Olds, James, 93
olive oil partition coefficients, 16
ololiuqui, 314
ondansetron, 136